Fifth Edition

Rehabilitation Techniques for Sports Medicine and Athletic Training

William E. Prentice, PhD, PT, ATC, FNATA

Professor, Coordinator of the Sports Medicine Program
Department of Exercise and Sport Science
University of North Carolina at Chapel Hill
Chapel Hill, North Carolina

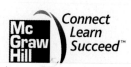

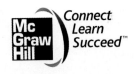

REHABILITATION TECHNIQUES FOR SPORTS AND ATHLETIC TRAINING
FIFTH EDITION
International Edition 2011

10 09 08 07 06 05
20 15 14
CTP   SLP

This text was based on the most up-to-date research and suggestions made by individuals knowledgeable in the field of athletic training. The authors and publisher disclaim any responsibility for any adverse effects or consequences from the misapplications or injudicious use of information contained within this text. It is also accepted as judicious that the coach and/or athletic trainer performing his or her duties is, at all times, working under the guidance of a licensed physician.

When ordering this title, use ISBN 978-007-128953-5 or MHID 007-128953-4

Printed in Singapore

www.mhhe.com

Brief Contents

iii

Contents

PART THREE   The Tools of Rehabilitation

Rehabilitation Techniques for
Specific Injuries

PART FOUR

Preface

This fifth edition of *Rehabilitation Techniques for Sports Medicine and Athletic Training* is for the student of athletic training who is interested in gaining more in-depth exposure to the theory and practical application of rehabilitation techniques used in a sports medicine environment.

The purpose of this text is to provide the athletic trainer with a comprehensive guide to the design, implementation, and supervision of rehabilitation programs for sport-related injuries. It is intended for use in advanced courses in athletic training that deal with practical application of theory in a clinical setting. The contributing authors have collectively attempted to combine their expertise and knowledge to produce a single text that encompasses all aspects of sports medicine rehabilitation.

ORGANIZATION

This fifth edition is divided into four parts. Part One discusses the basics of the rehabilitation process. It begins by discussing the important considerations in designing a rehabilitation program for the injured patient and providing a basic overview of the rehabilitation process (Chapter 1). It is essential for the athletic trainer to understand the importance of the healing process and how it should dictate the course of rehabilitation (Chapter 2). The evaluation process is critical in first determining the exact nature of an existing injury and then designing a rehabilitation program based on the findings of that evaluation (Chapter 3). It is also essential to be aware of the psychological aspects of rehabilitation with which the injured patient must deal (Chapter 4).

Part Two deals with achieving the goals of rehabilitation. The chapters address primary goals of any sports medicine rehabilitation program: establishing core stability (Chapter 5), reestablishing neuromuscular control (Chapter 6), regaining postural stability and balance (Chapter 7), restoring range of motion and improving flexibility (Chapter 8), regaining muscular strength, endurance, and power (Chapter 9), and maintaining cardiorespiratory fitness during rehabilitation (Chapter 10).

Athletic trainers have many rehabilitation "tools" with which they can choose to treat an injured athlete. How they choose to use these tools is often a matter of personal preference. Part Three discusses in detail how these tools can be best incorporated into a rehabilitation program to achieve the goals identified in the first section. The chapters in Part Three focus on primary tools of rehabilitation: plyometric exercise (Chapter 11), open- versus closed-kinetic-chain exercise (Chapter 12), joint mobilization and traction techniques (Chapter 13), proprioceptive neuromuscular facilitation techniques (Chapter 14), aquatic therapy (Chapter 15), and functional progressions and functional testing (Chapter 16).

Part Four of this text goes into great detail on specific rehabilitation techniques that are used in treating a variety of injuries. Specific rehabilitation techniques are included for the shoulder (Chapter 17), the elbow (Chapter 18), the wrist, hand, and fingers (Chapter 19), the groin, hip, and thigh (Chapter 20), the knee (Chapter 21), the lower leg (Chapter 22), the ankle and foot (Chapter 23), and the spine (Chapter 24). Each chapter begins with a discussion of the pertinent functional anatomy and biomechanics of that region. An extensive series of photographs illustrating a wide variety of rehabilitative exercises is presented in each chapter. The last portion of each chapter involves in-depth discussion of the pathomechanics, injury mechanism, rehabilitation concerns, rehabilitation progressions, and finally, criteria for return to activity for specific injuries.

As will become readily apparent, the updated fifth edition of *Rehabilitation Techniques for Sports Medicine and Athletic Training* offers a comprehensive reference and guide emphasizing the most current techniques of sport injury rehabilitation for the athletic trainer overseeing programs of rehabilitation.

COMPREHENSIVE COVERAGE OF RESEARCH-BASED MATERIAL

Compared to some of the other health care specializations, athletic training is still in its infancy. Growth dictates the necessity for expanding our research efforts to identify new and more effective methods and techniques for dealing with sport-related injury. Any athletic trainer charged with the responsibility of supervising a rehabilitation program knows that the most currently accepted and up-to-date rehabilitation protocols tend to change rapidly. A sincere effort has been made by the contributing authors to present the most recent information on the various aspects of injury rehabilitation currently available for the literature.

Additionally, this manuscript has been critically reviewed by selected athletic trainers who are well-respected clinicians, educators, and researchers in this field to further ensure that the material presented is accurate and current.

PERTINENT TO THE ATHLETIC TRAINER

Many texts are currently available on the subject of rehabilitation of injury in various patient populations. However, the fifth edition of this text concentrates exclusively on the application of rehabilitation techniques in a sport-related setting for a unique sports medicine emphasis.

PEDAGOGICAL AIDS

The teaching aids provided in this text to assist the student include the following:

Objectives. These goals are listed at the beginning of each chapter to introduce students to the points that will be emphasized.

Figures and Tables. The number of new photos and tables included throughout the text has been significantly increased in an effort to provide as much visual and graphic demonstration of specific rehabilitation techniques and exercises as possible.

Clinical Decision-Making Exercises. Approximately 150 clinical decision-making exercises are found throughout the text to challenge the student to integrate and apply the information presented in this text to clinical cases that typically occur in an athletic training setting. Solutions for each exercise are presented at the end of each chapter.

Rehabilitation Plans. Rehabilitation Plans can be found in each chapter in Part Four as examples of case studies that help apply the thought process an athletic trainer should use in developing and implementing a rehabilitation program.

Summary. Each chapter has a summary list that reinforces the major points presented.

References. A comprehensive list of up-to-date references is presented at the end of each chapter to guide the reader to additional information about the chapter content.

Glossary. A glossary of terms is provided for quick reference.

ANCILLARIES

Laboratory Manual. A new Laboratory Manual accompanies the fifth edition of *Rehabilitation Techniques for Sports Medicine and Athletic Training.* It has been prepared by Dr. Tom Kaminski of the University of Delaware to provide hands-on directed learning experiences for students using the text. It includes practical laboratory exercises designed to enhance student understanding. The Laboratory Manual is available for download at www.mhhe.com/prenticerehab5e

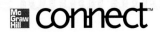

Connect Principles of Athletic Training is a new online learning system composed of interactive exercises and assessments, like those that appear on the NATA's new Board of Certification exam. Videos, animations, and other multimedia features will enable students to visualize complicated concepts ad practice skills. All of the activities are automatically graded and can be submitted to the instructor's grade book. For more information, visit www.mcgrawhillconnect.com

TO THE STUDENT

Connect Principles of Athletic Training is an interactive digital product which can help you study for the NATA's Board of Certification exam. Ask your instructor if this product is available through your bookstore.

ACKNOWLEDGMENTS

The preparation of the manuscript for a textbook is a long-term and extremely demanding effort that requires input and cooperation on the part of many individuals. I would like to personally thank each of the contributing authors. They were asked to contribute to this text because I have tremendous respect for them both personally and professionally. These individuals have distinguished themselves as educators and clinicians dedicated to the field of athletic training. I am exceedingly grateful for their input.

Gary O'Brien, my developmental editor, as always, has been persistent and diligent in the completion of this text. He has patiently encouraged me along, and I certainly have appreciated his support. I have come to rely heavily on Jill Eccher, my project manager. She makes certain that all of the details on a project such as this are taken care of and I greatly appreciate her input and opinions.

The following individuals have invested a significant amount of time and energy as reviewers for this manuscript, and I appreciate their efforts.

Carla Heffner, Texas State University
Joanne Klossner, Indiana University
Henry (Trey) A. Morgan III, Northern Kentucky University
Katherine Newsham, PhD, ATC, University of Indianapolis

Finally, and most importantly, this is for my family—Tena, Brian, and Zach—who make an effort such as this worthwhile.

Bill Prentice

Contributors

Jolene Bennett, MA, PT, OCS, ATC, CertMDT

Clinical Specialist for Orthopedics and Sports Medicine
Spectrum Health Rehabilitation and Sports Medicine
Visser Family YMCA
Grandville, Michigan

Michelle Boling, PhD, LAT, ATC

Assistant Professor
Department of Athletic Training and Physical Therapy
University of North Florida
Jacksonville, Florida

Michael Clark, DPT, MS, PT, PES, CES

President and Chief Executive Officer
National Academy of Sports Medicine
Phoenix, AZ

Bernard DePalma, MEd, PT, ATC

Head Athletic Trainer
Cornell University
Ithaca, New York

Freddie Fu, MD

Chairman and David Silver Professor for the Department
    of Orthopaedic Surgery
University of Pittsburgh School of Medicine and
    University of Pittsburgh Medical Center
Head Team Physician
University of Pittsburgh
Pittsburgh, Pennsylvania

Joe Gieck, EdD, PT, ATC

Professor Emeritus, Sports Medicine
University of Virginia
Charlottesville, Virginia

Kevin Guskiewicz, PhD, ATC, FNATA

Chairman and Professor
Department of Exercise and Sport Science
University of North Carolina
Chapel Hill, North Carolina

Doug Halverson, MA, ATC, CSCS

Staff Athletic Trainer
Campus Health Service
Division of Sports Medicine
University of North Carolina
Chapel Hill, North Carolina

Elizabeth Hedgpeth, EdD

Lecturer, Sport Psychology
Department of Exercise and Sport Science
University of North Carolina
Chapel Hill, North Carolina

Christopher Hirth, MSPT, PT, ATC

Staff Physical Therapist/Athletic Trainer
Campus Health Service
Division of Sports Medicine
University of North Carolina
Chapel Hill, North Carolina

Barbara Hoogenboom, EdD, PT, SCS, ATC

Associate Professor
Physical Therapy Program
Grand Valley State University
Grand Rapids, Michigan

Daniel Hooker, PhD, PT, ATC

Associate Director of Sports Medicine
Coordinator of Physical Therapy and Athletic Training

Essential Considerations in Designing a Rehabilitation Program for the Injured Patient

William E. Prentice

After completing this chapter, the athletic training student should be able to do the following:

- Describe the relationships among the members of the rehabilitation team: the athletic trainers, team physicians, coaches, strength and conditioning specialists, athlete, and athlete's family.

- Express the philosophy of the rehabilitative process in a sports medicine environment.

- Realize the importance of understanding the healing process, the biomechanics, and the psychological aspects of a rehabilitation program.

- Arrange the individual short-term and long-term goals of a rehabilitation program.

- Discuss the components that should be included in a well-designed rehabilitation program.

- Propose the criteria and the decision-making process for determining when the injured patient may return to full activity.

One of the primary goals of every sports medicine professional is to create a playing environment that is as safe as it can possibly be. Regardless of that effort, the nature of participation in sport and physical activity dictates that injuries will eventually occur. Fortunately, few of the injuries that occur in an athletic setting are life-threatening. The majority of the injuries are not serious and lend themselves to rapid rehabilitation. When injuries do occur, the focus of the athletic trainer shifts from injury prevention to injury treatment and rehabilitation. In a sports medicine setting, the athletic trainer generally assumes primary responsibility for the design, implementation, and supervision of the rehabilitation program for the injured athlete.

The athletic trainer responsible for overseeing an exercise rehabilitation program must have as complete an understanding of the injury as possible, including knowledge of how the injury was sustained, the major anatomical structures affected, the degree or grade of trauma, and the stage or phase of the injury's healing.[2,12]

THE REHABILITATION TEAM

Providing a comprehensive rehabilitation program for an injured patient in an athletic environment requires a group effort to be most effective. The rehabilitation process requires communication among a number of individuals, each of whom must perform specific functions relative to caring for the injured athlete. Under ideal conditions, the athletic trainer (and the athletic training students), the athlete, the physician, the coaches, the strength and conditioning specialist, and the injured athlete's family will communicate freely and function as a team. This group is intimately involved with the rehabilitative process, beginning with patient assessment, treatment selection, and implementation, and ending

PART ONE

The Basis of Injury Rehabilitation

C. Buz Swanik, PhD, ATC

Associate Professor
College of Health Sciences
University of Delaware
Newark, Delaware

Michael Voight, PT, DHSc, SCS, OCS, ATC, CSCS

Professor
School of Physical Therapy
Belmont University
Nashville, Tennessee

Steven Zinder, PhD, ATC

Assistant Professor
Department of Exercise and Sport Science
University of North Carolina
Chapel Hill, North Carolina

Pete Zulia, PT, SCS, ATC

Co-founding Partner
Oxford Physical Therapy Centers
Oxford, Ohio

Division of Sports Medicine
University of North Carolina
Chapel Hill, North Carolina

Stuart (Skip) Hunter, PT, ATC

Clemson Sports Medicine
Clemson, South Carolina

Kellie C. Huxel, PhD, ATC

Assistant Professor
Interdisciplinary Health Sciences
A.T. Still University
Arizona School of Health Sciences
Mesa, Arizona

Scott Lephart, PhD, ATC

Chair and Associate Professor
Director, Neuromuscular Research Laboratory
    Department of Sports Medicine and Nutrition
School of Health and Rehabilitation Sciences
Associate Professor of Orthopaedic Surgery
University of Pittsburgh
Pittsburgh, Pennsylvania

Nancy Lomax, PT

Staff Physical Therapist
Spectrum Health Rehabilitation and Sports
    Medicine Services
Visser Family YMCA
Grandville, Michigan

Michael McGee, EdD, LAT, ATC

Chair, School of Health, Exercise and Sport Science
Athletic Training Education Program
    Director and Head Athletic Trainer
Lenoir-Rhyne University
Hickory, North Carolina

Joseph Myers, PhD, ATC

Associate Professor
Department of Exercise and Sport Science
University of North Carolina
Chapel Hill, North Carolina

James Onate, PhD, ATC

Assistant Professor
Director, Sports Medicine Research Laboratory, Old
    Dominion University
Old Dominion University
Norfolk, Virginia

Darin Padua, PhD, ATC

Associate Professor
Department of Exercise and Sport Science
University of North Carolina
Chapel Hill, North Carolina

William Prentice, PhD, PT, ATC, FNATA

Professor, Coordinator of Sports Medicine Specialization
Department of Exercise and Sport Science
University of North Carolina
Chapel Hill, North Carolina

Terri Jo Rucinski, MA, PT, ATC

Staff Physical Therapist/Athletic Trainer
Campus Health Service
Division of Sports Medicine
University of North Carolina
Chapel Hill, North Carolina

Anne Marie Schneider OTR/L, CHT

Certified Hand Therapist/Office Manager
Balanced Physical Therapy
Carrboro/Durham, North Carolina

Rob Schneider PT, MS, LAT, ATC

Co-owner Balanced Physical Therapy
Carrboro/Durham, North Carolina

Steven Tippett, PhD, PT, SCS, ATC

Professor and Department Chair
Department of Physical Therapy and Health Science
Bradley University
Peoria, Illinois

with functional exercises and return to activity. The athletic trainer directs the post-acute phase of the rehabilitation, and it is essential that the patient understand that this part of the recovery is just as crucial as surgical technique to the return of normal joint function and the subsequent return to full activity. All decisions made by the physician, the athletic trainer, and the coaches which dictate the course of rehabilitation ultimately affect the injured patient.

CLINICAL DECISION MAKING   **Exercise 1–1**

A team physician has diagnosed a swimmer with thoracic outlet syndrome. The athletic trainer is developing a rehabilitation plan for this patient. What considerations must be taken into account?

Of all the members of the rehabilitation team charged with providing health care, perhaps none is more intimately involved than the athletic trainer. The athletic trainer is the one individual who deals directly with the patient throughout the entire period of rehabilitation, from the time of the initial injury until the complete, unrestricted return to activity. The athletic trainer is most directly responsible for all phases of health care in an athletic environment, including preventing injuries from occurring, providing initial first aid and injury management, evaluating and diagnosing injuries, and designing and supervising a timely and effective program of rehabilitation that can facilitate the safe and expeditious return to activity.

In 2004 the Board of Certification (BOC) completed the latest role delineation study, which defines the profession of athletic training. This study was designed to examine the primary tasks performed by the entry-level athletic trainer and the knowledge and skills required to perform each task. The panel determined that the roles of the practicing athletic trainer could be divided into six major areas or performance domains: prevention; clinical evaluation and diagnosis; immediate care; organization and administration; professional responsibilities; and treatment, rehabilitation, and reconditioning.

An athletic trainer must work closely with and under the supervision of the team physician with respect to designing rehabilitation and reconditioning protocols that make use of appropriate therapeutic exercise, rehabilitative equipment, manual therapy techniques, or therapeutic modalities. The athletic trainer should then assume the responsibility of overseeing the rehabilitative process, ultimately returning the patient to full activity.

Certainly, the athletic trainer has an obligation to the patient to understand the nature of the injury, the function of the structures damaged, and the different tools available

to safely rehabilitate that patient. Additionally, the athletic trainer must understand the treatment philosophy of the patient's physician and be careful in applying different treatment regimens because what may be a safe but outdated technique in the opinion of one physician may be the treatment of choice to another. The successful athletic trainer must demonstrate flexibility in his or her approach to rehabilitation by incorporating techniques that are evidence-based and effective, but somewhat variable from one patient to another, as well as from one physician to another.

Communication is crucial to prevent misunderstandings and a subsequent loss of rapport with either the patient or the physician. The patient must always be informed and made aware of the why, how, and when factors that collectively dictate the course of an injury rehabilitation program.

Any personal relationship takes some time to grow and develop. The relationship between the coach and the athletic trainer is no different. The athletic trainer must demonstrate to the coach his or her capability to correctly manage an injury and guide the course of a rehabilitation program. It will take some time for the coach to develop trust and confidence in the athletic trainer. The coach must understand that what the athletic trainer wants is exactly the same as what the coach wants—to get an injured patient healthy and back to practice as quickly and safely as possible.

This is not to say, however, that the coaches should not be involved with the decision-making process. For example, when a patient is rehabilitating an injury, there may be drills or technical instruction sessions that the individual can participate in without exacerbating the injury. Thus the coaches, athletic trainer, and team physician should be able to negotiate what that individual can and cannot do safely in the course of a practice.

Athletes are frequently caught in the middle between coaches who tell them to do one thing and medical staff who tell them something else. The athletic trainer must respect the job that the coach has to do and should do whatever can be done to support the coach. Close communication between the coach and the athletic trainer is essential so that everyone is on the same page.

CLINICAL DECISION MAKING   **Exercise 1–2**

A gymnast has just had an anterior cruciate ligament (ACL) reconstruction. The orthopedist has prescribed some active range of motion (AROM) exercises to start the rehabilitation process. The patient is progressing very quickly and wants to increase the intensity of her activity. What should the athletic trainer do to address the patient's request?

When rehabilitating an injured patient, particularly in a high school or junior high school setting, the athletic trainer, the coach, and the physician must take the time to explain and inform the patient's parents about the course of the injury rehabilitation process. With a patient of secondary school age, the parents' decisions regarding health care must be of primary consideration. In certain situations, particularly at the high school and middle school levels, many parents will insist that their child be seen by their family physician rather than by the individual who may be designated as the team physician. This creates a situation in which the athletic trainer must work and communicate with many different "team physicians." The opinion of the family physician must be respected even if that individual has little or no experience with injuries related to sports.

It should be clear that the physician working in cooperation with the athletic trainer assumes the responsibility of making the final decisions relative to the course of rehabilitation for the patient from the time of injury until full return to activity. The coaches must defer to and should support the decisions of the medical staff in any matter regarding the course of the rehabilitative process.

THE PHILOSOPHY OF SPORTS MEDICINE REHABILITATION

The approach to rehabilitation is considerably different in a sports medicine environment than in most other rehabilitation settings.[1] The competitive nature of athletics necessitates an aggressive approach to rehabilitation. Because the competitive season in most sports is relatively short, the patient does not have the luxury of being able to sit around and do nothing until the injury heals. The goal is to return to activity as soon as is safely possible. Consequently, the athletic trainer tends to play games with the healing process, never really allowing enough time for an injury to completely heal. The athletic trainer who is supervising the rehabilitation program usually performs a "balancing act"—walking along a thin line between not pushing the patient hard enough or fast enough and being overly aggressive. In either case, a mistake in judgment on the part of the athletic trainer can hinder return to activity.

Understanding the Healing Process

Decisions as to when and how to alter or progress a rehabilitation program should be based primarily on the process of injury healing. The athletic trainer must possess a sound understanding of both the sequence and the time frames for the various phases of healing, realizing that certain physiological events must occur during each of the phases. Anything that is done during a rehabilitation program that interferes with this healing process will likely increase the length of time required for rehabilitation and slow return to full activity. The healing process must have an opportunity to accomplish what it is supposed to. At best the athletic trainer can only try to create an environment that is conducive to the healing process. Little can be done to speed up the process physiologically, but many things can impede healing (see Chapter 2).

Exercise Intensity.   The **SAID Principle** (an acronym for Specific Adaptation to Imposed Demand) states that when an injured structure is subjected to stresses and overloads of varying intensities, it will gradually adapt over time to whatever demands are placed upon it.[14] During the rehabilitation process, the stresses of reconditioning exercises must not be so great as to exacerbate the injury before the injured structure has had a chance to adapt specifically to the increased demands. Engaging in exercise that is too intense or too prolonged can be detrimental to the progress of rehabilitation. Indications that the intensity of the exercises being incorporated into the rehabilitation program exceed the limits of the healing process include an increase in the amount of swelling, an increase in pain, a loss or a plateau in strength, a loss or a plateau in range of motion, or an increase in the laxity of a healing ligament.[23] If an exercise or activity causes any of these signs, the athletic trainer must back off and become less aggressive in the rehabilitation program.

CLINICAL DECISION MAKING	Exercise 1–3

A baseball player recently underwent surgery to repair a superior labrum anterior and posterior (SLAP) lesion and torn rotator cuff. He wants to know why he can't start throwing right away. What is your reason for why he must progress slowly?

In most injury situations, early exercise rehabilitation involves submaximal exercise performed in short bouts that are repeated several times daily. Exercise intensity must be commensurate with healing. As recovery increases, the intensity of exercise also increases, with the exercise performed less often. Finally, the patient returns to a conditioning mode of exercise, which often includes high-intensity exercise three to four times per week.

Understanding the Psychological Aspects of Rehabilitation

The psychological aspects of how an individual deals with an injury are a critical yet often neglected factor in the rehabilitation process. Injury and illness produce a wide range of emotional reactions; therefore the athletic trainer needs to develop an understanding of the psyche of each patient. Individuals vary in terms of pain threshold, cooperation and compliance, competitiveness, denial of disability, depression, intrinsic and extrinsic motivation, anger, fear, guilt, and the ability to adjust to injury. Besides dealing with the mental aspect of the injury, sports psychology can also be used to improve total athletic performance through the use of visualization, self-hypnosis, and relaxation techniques (see Chapter 4).

Understanding the Pathomechanics of Injury

When a joint or other anatomic structure is damaged by injury, normal biomechanical function is compromised. Adaptive changes occur that alter the manner in which various forces collectively act upon that joint to produce motion. Thus the biomechanics of joint motion are changed as a result of that injury.[11]

It is critical that the athletic trainer supervising a rehabilitation program has a solid foundation in biomechanics and functional human anatomy, to be effective in designing a rehabilitation program. An athletic trainer who does not understand the biomechanics of normal motion will find it very difficult to identify existing adaptive or compensatory changes in motion and then to know what must be done in a rehabilitation program to correct the pathomechanics.

Understanding the Concept of the Kinetic Chain

The athletic trainer must understand the concept of the kinetic chain and must realize that the entire body is a kinetic chain that operates as an integrated functional unit. The kinetic chain is composed of not only the muscular system including muscles, tendons, and fascia, but also the articular system and neural system. Each of these systems functions simultaneously with the others to allow for structural and functional efficiency. The central nervous system sorts the cumulative information from these three systems and allows for *neuromuscular control.* If any system within the kinetic chain is not working efficiently, the other systems are forced to adapt and compensate; this

can lead to tissue overload, decreased performance, and predictable patterns of injury.[3]

The functional integration of the systems allows for optimal neuromuscular efficiency during functional activities. In reality, movements in everyday life require dynamic postural control through multiple planes of motion and at different speeds of motion. Optimal functioning of all contributing components of the kinetic chain results in appropriate length-tension relationships, optimal force-couple relationships, precise arthrokinematics, and optimal neuromuscular control. Efficiency and longevity of the kinetic chain requires optimal integration of each system.[3]

Injury to the kinetic chain rarely involves only one structure. Since the kinetic chain functions as an integrated unit, dysfunction in one system leads to compensations and adaptations in other systems. The myofascial, neuromuscular, and articular systems all play a significant role in the functional pathology of the kinetic chain. Rehabilitation should focus on functional movements that integrate all components necessary to achieve optimal movement performance. Concepts of muscle imbalances, myofascial adhesions, altered arthrokinematics, and abnormal neuromuscular control need to be addressed by the athletic trainer when developing a comprehensive rehabilitation program.[3]

Understanding the Concept of Integrated Functional Movement

To develop a comprehensive rehabilitation program, the athletic trainer must fully understand the concept of the functional kinetic chain and, most importantly, the definition of function. *Function* is integrated, multiplanar movement that requires acceleration, deceleration, and stabilization.[3,21] Functional kinetic chain rehabilitation is a comprehensive approach that strives to improve all components necessary to allow a patient to return to a high level of function. The athletic trainer must understand that the kinetic chain operates as an integrated functional unit. Functional kinetic chain rehabilitation must therefore address each link in the kinetic chain and strive to develop functional strength and neuromuscular efficiency. Functional strength is the ability of the neuromuscular system to reduce force, produce force, and dynamically stabilize the kinetic chain during functional movements in a smooth and coordinated fashion.[3] Neuromuscular efficiency is the ability of the central nervous system (CNS) to allow agonists, antagonists, synergists, stabilizers, and neutralizers to work efficiently and interdependently during dynamic kinetic chain activities.[3]

Traditionally, rehabilitation has focused on isolated absolute strength gains, in isolated muscles, using single planes of motion. However, all functional activities are naturally multiplanar and require a blend of acceleration, deceleration, and dynamic stabilization.[21] Movement may appear to be one plane dominant, but the other planes need to be dynamically stabilized to allow for optimal neuromuscular efficiency.[3] Understanding that functional movements require a highly complex, integrated system allows the athletic trainer to make a paradigm shift. The paradigm shift focuses on training the entire kinetic chain using all planes of movement and establishing high levels of functional strength and neuromuscular efficiency.[3,21] The paradigm shift dictates that we train to allow force reduction, force production, and dynamic stabilization to occur efficiently during all kinetic chain activities.[13,21]

Using the Tools of Rehabilitation

Athletic trainers have many tools at their disposal—such as manual therapy techniques, therapeutic modalities, aquatic therapy, and the use of physician-prescribed medications—that can individually or collectively facilitate the rehabilitative process. How different athletic trainers choose to utilize those tools is often a matter of individual preference and experience.

Additionally, patients differ in their individual responses to various treatment techniques. Thus the athletic trainer should avoid "cookbook" rehabilitation protocols that can be followed like a recipe. In fact, use of rehabilitation "recipes" should be strongly discouraged. Instead the athletic trainer must develop a broad theoretical knowledge base from which specific techniques or tools of rehabilitation can be selected and practically applied to each individual case.

Using Therapeutic Modalities in Rehabilitation. Athletic trainers use a wide variety of therapeutic techniques in the treatment and rehabilitation of sport-related injuries. One of the more important aspects of a thorough treatment regimen is the use of therapeutic modalities. At one time or another, virtually all athletic trainers make use of some type of therapeutic modality. This might involve a relatively simple technique, such as using an ice pack as a first aid treatment for an acute injury, or more complex techniques such as the stimulation of nerve and muscle tissue by electrical currents. There is no question that therapeutic modalities are useful tools in injury rehabilitation. When used appropriately, these modalities can greatly enhance the patient's chances for a safe and rapid return to full activity. The athletic trainer must have knowledge of the scientific basis of the various modalities and their physiological effects on a specific injury. When applied to

practical experience, this theoretical basis can produce an extremely effective clinical method.

A comprehensive rehabilitation program should focus on achieving specific short-term and long-term objectives. Modalities, though important, are by no means the single most critical factor in accomplishing these objectives. Therapeutic exercise that forces the injured anatomic structure to perform its normal function is the key to successful rehabilitation. However, therapeutic modalities certainly play an important role and are extremely useful as adjuncts to therapeutic exercise.

It must be emphasized that the use of therapeutic modalities in any treatment program is an inexact science. There is no way to "cookbook" a treatment plan that involves the use of therapeutic modalities. Athletic trainers should make every effort to understand the basis for using each different type of modality and then make their own decisions as to which will be most effective in a given clinical situation.

Despite the fact that therapeutic modalities are commonly used by athletic trainers as an integral tool in the rehabilitation process, they will not be discussed further in this text. (The reader is referred to W. Prentice, *Therapeutic Modalities for Sports Medicine and Athletic Training*, 6th ed., New York, McGraw-Hill, 2009, for detailed information relative to the use of specific modalities in rehabilitation.)

Using Medications to Facilitate Healing. Prescription and over-the-counter medications can effectively aid the healing process during a rehabilitation program. An athletic trainer supervising a program of rehabilitation must have some knowledge of the potential effects of certain types of drugs on performance during the rehabilitation program. Patients might be expected to respond to medication just as anyone else would, but the patient's situation is not normal. Intense physical activity requires that special consideration be given to the effects of certain types of medication. On occasion, the athletic trainer, working with guidance from the team physician, must make decisions regarding the appropriate use of medications based on knowledge of the indications for use and the possible side effects in patients who are involved in rehabilitation programs.

Those medications commonly used to aid the healing process are discussed in detail in Chapter 2.

Therapeutic Exercise versus Conditioning Exercise

Exercise is an essential factor in fitness conditioning, injury prevention, and injury rehabilitation. To compete successfully at a high level, the patient must be fit. A patient who is not fit is more likely to sustain an injury. Coaches and athletic trainers both recognize that improper conditioning is one of the major causes of sport injuries. It is essential that the patient engage in training and conditioning exercises that minimize the possibility of injury while maximizing performance.[16]

The basic principles of training and conditioning exercises also apply to techniques of therapeutic, rehabilitative, or reconditioning exercises that are specifically concerned with restoring normal body function following injury. The term therapeutic exercise is perhaps most widely used to indicate exercises that are used in a rehabilitation program.[10]

ESTABLISHING SHORT- AND LONG-TERM GOALS IN A REHABILITATION PROGRAM

Designing an effective rehabilitation program is relatively simple if the athletic trainer routinely integrates several basic components. These basic components can also be considered the short-term goals of a rehabilitation program. They should include (1) providing correct immediate first aid and management following injury to limit or control swelling; (2) reducing or minimizing pain; (3) establishing core stability; (4) reestablishing neuromuscular control; (5) improving postural stability and balance; (6) restoring full range of motion; (7) restoring or increasing muscular strength, endurance, and power; (8) maintaining cardiorespiratory fitness; and (9) incorporating appropriate functional progressions. The long-term goal is almost invariably to return the injured patient to practice or competition as quickly and safely as possible.

Establishing reasonable, attainable goals and integrating specific exercises or activities to address these goals is the easy part of overseeing a rehabilitation program. The difficult part comes in knowing exactly when and how to progress, change, or alter the rehabilitation program to most effectively accomplish both long- and short-term goals.

CLINICAL DECISION MAKING   **Exercise 1–4**

A volleyball player has a second-degree ankle sprain. X-rays reveal no fracture. The athletic trainer wants to begin rehabilitation right away so that the patient may be able to play again before the season is over. What are the short- and long-term goals for this patient?

Athletes tend to be goal-oriented individuals. Thus, the athletic trainer should design a goal-oriented rehabilitation program in which the patient can have a series of progressive "successes" in achieving attainable short-term goals throughout the rehabilitation process. Injured athletes are almost always most concerned to know precisely how long they will be out and when exactly they can return to full activity. The athletic trainer should not make the mistake of giving an injured patient an exact time frame or date. Instead, the patient should be given a series of sequenced challenges, involving increasing skill and ability, that must be met before progressing to the next level in his or her rehabilitation program. It is critical that the patient be actively involved in planning the process of rehabilitating his or her injury.[18]

The Importance of Controlling Swelling

The process of rehabilitation begins immediately after injury. Thus, in addition to understanding exactly how the injury occurred, the athletic trainer must be competent in providing correct and appropriate initial care. Initial first aid and management techniques are perhaps the most critical part of any rehabilitation program. The manner in which the injury is initially managed unquestionably has a significant impact on the course of the rehabilitative process.[20]

The one problem all injuries have in common is swelling. Swelling can be caused by any number of factors, including bleeding, production of synovial fluid, an accumulation of inflammatory by-products, edema, or a combination of several factors. No matter which mechanism is involved, swelling produces an increased pressure in the injured area, and increased pressure causes pain.[24] Swelling can also cause neuromuscular inhibition, which results in weak muscle contraction. Swelling is most likely during the first 72 hours after an injury.

Once swelling has occurred, the healing process is significantly retarded. The injured area cannot return to normal until all the swelling is gone. Therefore everything that is done in first aid management of any of these conditions should be directed toward controlling the swelling.[20] If the swelling can be controlled initially in the acute stage of injury, the time required for rehabilitation is likely to be significantly reduced.

To control and significantly limit the amount of swelling, the PRICE principle—Protection, Restricted activity, Ice, Compression, and Elevation—should be applied (Figure 1-1). Each factor plays a critical role in limiting swelling, and all of these elements should be used simultaneously.

Protection.   The injured area should be protected from additional injury by applying appropriate splints, braces, pads, or other immobilization devices. If the injury

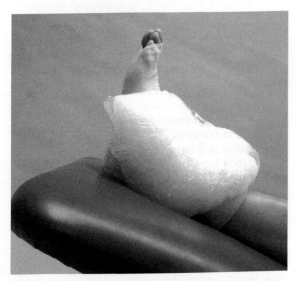

Figure 1-1 The PRICE technique should be used immediately following injury to limit swelling.

involves the lower extremity, it is recommended that the patient go non-weight-bearing on crutches at least until the acute inflammatory response has subsided.

Restricted Activity (Rest). The period of restricted activity following any type of injury is absolutely critical in any treatment program. Once an anatomical structure is injured, it immediately begins the healing process. In an injured structure that is not rested and is subjected to unnecessary external stress and strains, the healing process never really gets a chance to begin. Consequently, the injury does not get well, and the time required for rehabilitation is markedly increased. This is not to minimize the importance of early mobility. Controlled mobility has been shown to be superior to immobilization for scar formation, revascularization, muscle regeneration, and reorientation of muscle fibers and tensile properties.[16] The amount of time necessary for resting varies with the severity of the injury, but most minor injuries should rest for approximately 24 to 48 hours before an active rehabilitation program is begun.

It must be emphasized that rest does not mean that the patient does nothing. The term rest applies only to the injured body part. During this period, the patient should continue to work on cardiovascular fitness and strengthening and flexibility exercises for the other parts of the body not affected by the injury.[25]

Ice. The use of cold is the initial treatment of choice for virtually all conditions involving injuries to the musculoskeletal system.[20] It is most commonly used immediately after injury to decrease pain and promote

local vasoconstriction, thus controlling hemorrhage and edema. Cold applied to an acute injury will lower metabolism in the injured area, and thus the tissue demands for oxygen, thus reducing hypoxia. This benefit extends to uninjured tissue, preventing injury-related tissue death from spreading to adjacent normal cellular structures. It is also used in the acute phase of inflammatory conditions, such as bursitis, tenosynovitis, and tendinitis, in which heat can cause additional pain and swelling. Cold is also used to reduce the reflex muscle guarding and spastic conditions that accompany pain. Its analgesic effect is probably one of its greatest benefits. One explanation of the analgesic effect is that cold decreases the velocity of nerve conduction, although it does not entirely eliminate it. Cold can also bombard cutaneous sensory nerve receptor areas with so many cold impulses that pain impulses are lost. With ice treatments, the patient reports an uncomfortable sensation of cold, followed by burning, an aching sensation, and finally complete numbness.[13,20]

Because of the low thermal conductivity of underlying subcutaneous fat tissues, applications of cold for short periods are ineffective in cooling deeper tissues. For this reason longer treatments of 20 to 30 minutes are recommended. Cold treatments are generally believed to be more effective in reaching deeper tissues than most forms of heat. Cold applied to the skin is capable of significantly lowering the temperature of tissues at a considerable depth. The extent of this lowered tissue temperature depends on the type of cold applied to the skin, the duration of its application, the thickness of the subcutaneous fat, and the region of the body to which it is applied. Ice should be applied to the injured area until the signs and symptoms of inflammation have disappeared and there is little or no chance that swelling will be increased by using some form of heat. Ice should be used for at least 72 hours after an acute injury.[13,20]

Compression. Compression is likely the single most important technique for controlling initial swelling. The purpose of compression is to mechanically reduce the amount of space available for swelling by applying pressure around an injured area. The best way of applying pressure is to use an elastic wrap, such as an Ace bandage, to apply firm but even pressure around the injury.

Because of the pressure buildup in the tissues, having a compression wrap in place for a long time can become painful. However, the wrap must be kept in place despite significant pain because it is so important in the control of swelling. The compression wrap should be left in place continuously for at least 72 hours after an acute injury. In many overuse problems, such as tendinitis, tenosynovitis, and particularly bursitis, which involve ongoing inflammation, the compression wrap should be worn until the swelling is almost entirely gone.

Elevation.   The fifth factor that assists in controlling swelling is elevation. The injured part, particularly an extremity, should be elevated to eliminate the effects of gravity on blood pooling in the extremities. Elevation assists venous and lymphatic drainage of blood and other fluids from the injured area back to the central circulatory system. The greater the degree of elevation, the more effective the reduction in swelling. For example, in an ankle sprain, the leg should be placed in such a position that the ankle is virtually straight up in the air. The injured part should be elevated as much as possible during the first 72 hours.

CLINICAL DECISION MAKING   **Exercise 1–5**

A soccer player has been successfully managing Achilles tendinitis with PRICE, exercises, and anti-inflammatories. The athletic trainer has decided that the patient should begin playing again. What can the athletic trainer do to help the patient prevent further injury?

The appropriate technique for initial management of the acute injuries discussed in this chapter, regardless of where they occur, would be the following:

1. Apply a compression wrap directly over the injury. Wrapping should be from distal to proximal. Tension should be firm and consistent. Wetting the elastic wrap to facilitate the passage of cold from ice packs might be helpful.
2. Surround the injured area entirely with ice bags, and secure them in place. Ice bags should be left on for 45 minutes initially and then 1 hour off and 30 minutes on as much as possible over the next 24 hours. During the following 48-hour period, ice should be applied as often as possible.
3. The injured part should be elevated as much as possible during the initial 72-hour period after injury. Keeping the injured part elevated while sleeping is particularly important.
4. Allow the injured part to rest for approximately 24 hours after the injury.

Controlling Pain

When an injury occurs, the athletic trainer must realize that the patient will experience some degree of pain. The extent of the pain will be determined in part by the severity of the injury, by the patient's individual response to and perception of pain, and by the circumstances in which the injury occurred. The patient's pain is real. The athletic trainer can effectively modulate acute pain by using the PRICE technique immediately after injury.[16] A physician can also make use of various medications to help ease pain.

Persistent pain can make strengthening or flexibility exercises more difficult, thus interfering with the rehabilitation process. The athletic trainer should routinely address pain during each individual treatment session. Making use of appropriate therapeutic modalities—including various techniques of cryotherapy, thermotherapy, and electrical stimulating currents—will help modulate pain throughout the rehabilitation process[20] (Figure 1-2).

To a great extent, pain will dictate the rate of progression. With initial injury, pain is intense and tends to decrease and eventually subside altogether as healing progresses. Any exacerbation of either pain, swelling, or other clinical symptoms during or following a particular exercise or activity indicates that the load is too great for the level of tissue repair or remodeling.

Establishing Core Stability

Core stability is absolutely essential to every aspect of the rehabilitation process (Figure 1-3). The core is considered to be the lumbo-pelvic-hip complex, which functions to dynamically stabilize the entire kinetic chain during functional movements. Without proximal or core stability, the distal movers cannot function optimally to efficiently utilize their strength and power. Chapter 5 will discuss the concept of core stabilization in great detail.[3,9]

Reestablishing Neuromuscular Control

Reestablishing neuromuscular control should be of prime concern to the athletic trainer in all rehabilitation

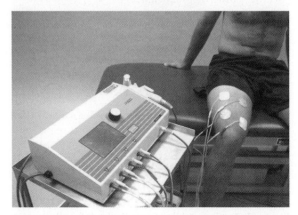

Figure 1-2   Several modalities, including electrical stimulating currents, may be used to modulate pain.

programs[7] (see Chapter 6). The ability to sense the position of a joint in space is mediated by mechanoreceptors found in both muscles and joints, in addition to cutaneous, visual, and vestibular input. Neuromuscular control relies on the central nervous system to interpret and integrate proprioceptive and kinesthetic information and then to control individual muscles and joints to produce coordinated movement.[23]

Following injury and subsequent rest and immobilization, the central nervous system "forgets" how to put together information coming from muscle and joint mechanoreceptors, and from cutaneous, visual, and vestibular input. Regaining neuromuscular control means regaining the ability to follow some previously established sensory pattern.[5] Neuromuscular control is the mind's attempt to teach the body conscious control of a specific movement. Successful repetition of a patterned movement makes its performance progressively less difficult, thus requiring less concentration, until the movement becomes automatic. This requires many repetitions of the same movement, progressing step-by-step from simple to more complex movements. Strengthening exercises, particularly those that tend to be more functional, such as closed kinetic-chain exercises, are essential for reestablishing neuromuscular control.[23] Addressing neuromuscular control is critical throughout the recovery process, but it is perhaps most critical during the early stages of rehabilitation to avoid reinjury.[5]

Restoring Postural Control and Stability (Balance)

Postural stability involves the complex integration of muscular forces, neurological sensory information received from the mechanoreceptors, and biomechanical information.[4,7] The ability to maintain postural stability and balance is essential to acquiring or reacquiring complex motor skills.[23] Patients who show a decreased sense of balance or a lack of postural stability following injury might lack sufficient proprioceptive and kinesthetic information and/or might have muscular weakness, either of which can limit the ability to generate an effective correction response when there is not equilibrium. A rehabilitation program must include functional exercises that incorporate balance and proprioceptive training that prepares the patient for return to activity (Figure 1-4). Failure to address balance problems can predispose the patient to reinjury (see Chapter 7).

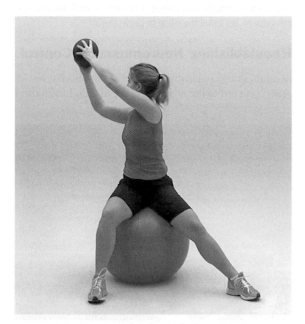

Figure 1-3   Core stability forms the basis for all aspects of a rehabilitation program.

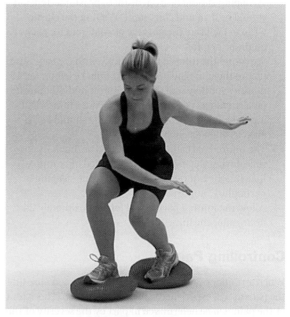

Figure 1-4   Reestablishing neuromuscular control and balance is critical to regaining functional performance capabilities.

Restoring Range of Motion

Following injury to a joint, there will always be some associated loss of motion. That loss of movement can usually be attributed to a number of pathological factors, including resistance of the musculotendinous unit (i.e., muscle, tendon, fascia) to stretch; contracture of connective tissue (i.e., ligaments, joint capsule); or some combination of the two. Muscle imbalances, postural imbalance, neural tension, and joint dysfunction can also lead to a loss in range of motion.

It is critical for the athletic trainer to closely evaluate the injured joint to determine whether motion is limited due to physiological movement constraints involving musculotendinous units or due to limitation in accessory motion (joint arthrokinematics) involving the joint capsule and ligaments. If physiological movement is restricted, the patient should engage in stretching activities designed to improve flexibility (Figure 1-5) (see Chapters 8 and 14). Stretching exercises should be used whenever there is musculotendinous resistance to stretch. If accessory motion is limited due to some restriction of the joint capsule or the ligaments, the athletic trainer should incorporate joint mobilization and traction techniques into the treatment program (Figure 1-6) (see Chapter 14). Mobilization techniques should be used whenever there are tight articular structures.[16] Traditionally, rehabilitation programs tend to concentrate more on passive physiological movements without paying much attention to accessory motions.

Restoring Muscular Strength, Endurance, and Power

Muscular strength, endurance and power are among the most essential factors in restoring the function of a body

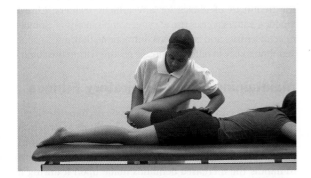

Figure 1-5 Stretching techniques are used with tight musculotendinous structures to improve physiological range of motion.

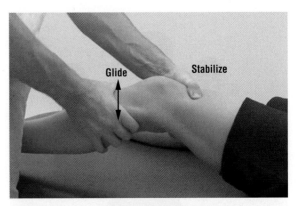

Glide   Stabilize

Figure 1-6 Joint mobilization techniques are used with tight ligamentous or capsular structures to improve accessory motion.

part to preinjury status. Isometric, progressive resistive (isotonic), isokinetic, and plyometric exercises can benefit rehabilitation. A major goal in performing strengthening exercises is to work through a full pain-free range of motion.

Most strength-training programs involve single-plane force production using either free weights or exercise machines. A functional rehabilitative strengthening program should involve exercises in all three planes of motion, concentrating on a combination of concentric, eccentric, and isometric exercises designed both to increase strength through a full multiplanar range of motion and to improve core stabilization and neuromuscular control.[3]

Isometric Exercise. Isometric exercises are commonly performed in the early phase of rehabilitation when a joint is immobilized for a period of time. They are useful when using resistance training through a full range of motion might make the injury worse. Isometrics increase static strength and assist in decreasing the amount of atrophy. Isometrics also can lessen swelling by causing a muscle pumping action to remove fluid and edema (see Chapter 9).

Progressive Resistive Exercise. Progressive resistive exercise (PRE) is the most commonly used strengthening technique in a rehabilitation program. PRE may be done using free weights, exercise machines, or rubber tubing (Figure 1-7). Progressive resistive exercise uses isotonic contractions in which force is generated while the muscle is changing in length. Isotonic contractions may be either concentric or eccentric. In a rehabilitation program the athletic trainer should incorporate both eccentric and concentric strengthening exercises. Traditionally, progressive resistive exercise has concentrated primarily

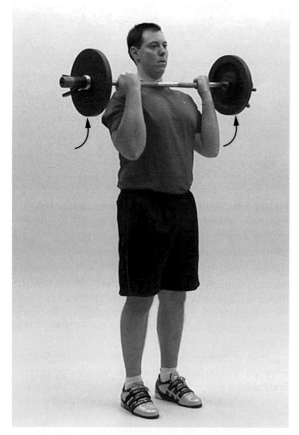

Figure 1-7 Progressive resistive exercise using isotonic contractions is the most widely used rehabilitative strengthening technique.

on the concentric component and has to some extent minimized the importance of the eccentric component (see Chapter 9).

Isokinetic Exercise.   Isokinetic exercise is occasionally used in the rehabilitative process.[17] It is most often incorporated during the later phases of a rehabilitation program. Isokinetics uses a fixed speed with accommodating resistance to provide maximal resistance throughout the range of motion (Figure 1-8). The speed of movement can be altered in isokinetic exercise. Isokinetic measures are commonly used as a criteria for return of the patient to functional activity following injury.

Plyometric Exercise.   Plyometric exercises, also referred to as reactive neuromuscular training, are most often incorporated into the later stages of a rehabilitation program. Plyometrics use a quick eccentric stretch to facilitate a subsequent concentric contraction. Plyometric

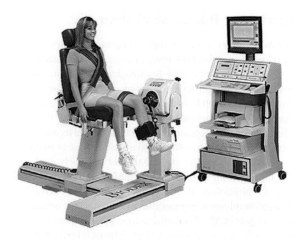

Figure 1-8   Isokinetic exercise is most often used in the later stages of rehabilitation.
(Courtesy Biodex medical systems)

exercises are useful in restoring or developing the patient's ability to produce dynamic movements associated with muscular power (Figure 1-9). The ability to generate force very rapidly is a key to successful performance in many sport activities. It is critical to address the element of muscular power in rehabilitation programs for the injured patient (see Chapter 11).

Open- versus Closed-Kinetic-Chain   Exercise.
The concept of the kinetic chain deals with the anatomical functional relationships that exist in the upper and lower extremities (see Chapter 12). An open kinetic chain exists when the foot or hand is not in contact with the ground or some other surface.[6] In a closed kinetic chain, the foot or hand is weight-bearing (Figure 1-10). In rehabilitation, the use of closed-chain strengthening techniques has become the treatment of choice for any athletic trainers. Closed kinetic-chain exercises use varying combinations of isometric, concentric, and eccentric contractions that must occur simultaneously in different muscle groups within the chain.

Maintaining Cardiorespiratory Fitness

Maintaining cardiorespiratory fitness is perhaps the single most neglected component of a rehabilitation program (see Chapter 10). A patient spends a considerable amount of time preparing the cardiorespiratory system to be able to handle the increased demands made upon it during a competitive season. When injury occurs and the patient is forced to miss training time, cardiorespiratory fitness can decrease rapidly. Thus the athletic trainer must design or

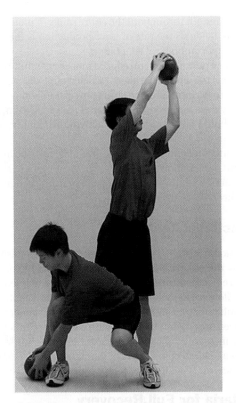

Figure 1-9   Plyometric exercise focuses on improving dynamic, power movements.

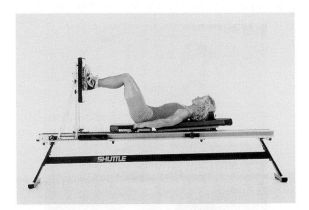

Figure 1-10   Closed-kinetic-chain exercises are widely used in rehabilitation.

substitute alternative activities that allow the patient to maintain existing levels of cardiorespiratory fitness as early as possible in the rehabilitation period[15] (Figure 1-11).

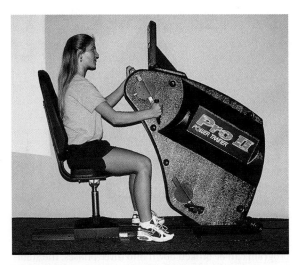

Figure 1-11   Every rehabilitation program must include some exercise designed to maintain cardiorespiratory fitness.

Depending on the nature of the injury, a number of possible activities can help the patient maintain fitness levels. When there is a lower-extremity injury, non-weightbearing activities should be incorporated. Pool activities provide an excellent means for injury rehabilitation. Cycling also can positively stress the cardiorespiratory system.

Functional Progressions

The purpose of any program of rehabilitation is to restore normal function following injury.[8] Functional progressions involve a series of gradually progressive activities designed to prepare the individual for return to a specific activity[22] (see Chapter 16). Those skills necessary for successful participation in a given sport are broken down into component parts, and the patient gradually reacquires those skills within the limitations of his or her own individual progress.[23] Progression through the rehabilitation program may be broken down into three phases: the stabilization phase, the strengthening phase, and the power phase. (Figure 1-12)

The stabilization phase begins with exercises designed to correct the deficits in the structural integrity of the kinetic chain including muscle dysfunction, joint dysfunctions, neuromuscular deficits, and postural control and stability. These deficits must be addressed prior to beginning an aggressive rehabilitation program to correct muscle imbalances, recondition injured structures, prepare tissues for the physical demands of the rehabilitation program,

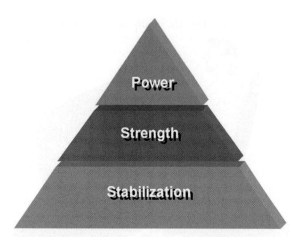

Figure 1-12   Progression through a rehabilitation program can be broken down into three phases: the stabilization phase, the strength phase, and the power phase.

prevent tissue overload through progressive adaptation, improve work capacity, and improve stabilization strength; thus establishing optimal levels of stabilization, strength, and postural control. Exercises should progress from isometric to multiplanar activities designed to recruit joint stabilizers, thus improving neuromuscular efficiency, core stability, functional strength, and functional flexibility.[3]

The strength phase is used to enhance stabilization strength and endurance during functional movement patterns by incorporating high volume resistive exercises that force motor unit recruitment after the prime movers are fatigued. For example, after performing a strength exercise the patient immediately engages in a stabilization exercise that forces neuromuscular stabilization of that movement. During this phase the goal is to achieve several adaptive changes by challenging the neuromuscular system including an increase in the cross sectional diameter of the muscle, increased resistance to fatigue, and increased stabilization strength to control joint translation during functional movements.[3]

The power phase is particularly important for an injured athlete who is attempting to return to high-level physically demanding activity. An athlete who needs high levels of both muscular strength and power should first use exercises that incorporate multiplanar, concentric, eccentric, and isometric contrations to increase strength. Maximal power is then developed by training at 30-45% of maximum strength and by accelerating through the entire range of motion. During this phase the goal is to enhance neuromuscular efficiency and power production by increasing motorneuron excitability thus increasing

speed strength throughout the entire range of motion. For most individuals the rate of force production is the single most important neural adaptation.[3]

Every new activity introduced must be carefully monitored by the athletic trainer to determine the patient's ability to perform and her or his physical tolerance. If an activity does not produce additional pain or swelling, the level should be advanced; new activities should be introduced as quickly as possible.

Functional progressions will gradually help the injured patient achieve normal pain-free range of motion, restore adequate strength levels, and regain neuromuscular control throughout the rehabilitation program.

Functional Testing

Functional testing uses functional progression drills to assess the patient's ability to perform a specific activity (Figure 1-13). Functional testing involves a single maximal effort performed to indicate how close the patient is to a full return to activity. For years athletic trainers have assessed the patients' progress with a variety of functional tests, including agility runs (figure eights, shuttle run, carioca), sidestepping, vertical jump, hopping for time or distance, and co-contraction tests[23] (see Chapter 16).

Criteria for Full Recovery

All exercise rehabilitation plans must determine what is meant by complete recovery from an injury.[21] Often it means that the patient is fully reconditioned and has achieved full

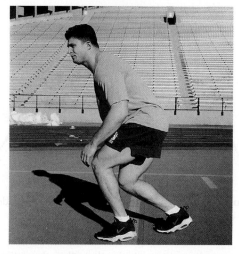

Figure 1-13   Performance on functional tests can determine the athlete's capability to return to full activity.

range of movement, strength, neuromuscular control, cardiovascular fitness, and sport-specific functional skills. Besides physical well-being, the patient must also have regained full confidence to return to his or her activity.

For example, specific criteria for a return to full activity after rehabilitation of the injured knee is largely determined by the nature and severity of the specific injury, but it also depends on the philosophy and judgment of both the physician and the athletic trainer. Traditionally, return to activity has been dictated through both objective and subjective evaluations.

For the patient, criteria for return should be based on functional capabilities as indicated by performance on specific functional tests that are closely related to the demands of a particular activity. Performance on functional tests, such as those described in Chapter 16 (hop test, co-contraction test), should serve as primary determinants of the patient's capability to return to full activity. Data on the majority of these tests are well documented. A number of data-based research studies have objectively quantified performance on various functional tests. These functional tests are extremely useful and valuable tools for determining readiness to return to full activity.

The decision to release a patient recovering from injury to a full return to athletic activity is the final stage of the rehabilitation/recovery process. The decision should be carefully considered by each member of the sports medicine team involved in the rehabilitation process. The team physician should be ultimately responsible for deciding that the patient is ready to return to practice and/or competition. That decision should be based on collective input from the athletic trainer, the coach, and the patient.

In considering the patient's return to activity, the following concerns should be addressed:

- *Physiological healing constraints.* Has rehabilitation progressed to the later stages of the healing process?
- *Pain status.* Has pain disappeared, or is the patient able to play within her or his own levels of pain tolerance?
- *Swelling.* Is there still a chance that swelling could be exacerbated by return to activity?
- *Range of motion.* Is ROM adequate to allow the patient to perform both effectively and with minimized risk of reinjury?
- *Strength.* Is strength, endurance, or power great enough to protect the injured structure from reinjury?
- *Neuromuscular control/proprioception/kinesthesia.* Has the patient "relearned" how to use the injured body part?
- *Cardiorespiratory fitness.* Has the patient been able to maintain cardiorespiratory fitness at or near the level necessary for competition?

- *Sport-specific demands.* Are the demands of the sport or a specific position such that the patient will not be at risk of reinjury?
- *Functional testing.* Does performance on appropriate functional tests indicate that the extent of recovery is sufficient to allow successful performance?
- *Prophylactic strapping, bracing, padding.* Are any additional supports necessary for the injured patient to return to activity?
- *Responsibility of the patient.* Is the patient capable of listening to his or her body and recognizing situations that present a potential for reinjury?
- *Predisposition to injury.* Is this patient prone to reinjury or a new injury when she or he is not 100-percent recovered?
- *Psychological factors.* Is the patient capable of returning to activity and competing at a high level without fear of reinjury?
- *Patient education and preventive maintenance program.* Does the patient understand the importance of continuing to engage in conditioning exercises that can greatly reduce the chances of reinjury?

CLINICAL DECISION MAKING **Exercise 1–6**

After a week of managing a first-degree hamstring strain, a track patient has decided that she is ready to compete. She has no signs of inflammation. She has regained full strength and ROM. What other things should be taken into consideration before she is allowed to compete again?

DOCUMENTATION IN REHABILITATION

Athletic trainers must develop proficiency not only in their ability to constantly evaluate an injury, but also in their ability to generate an accurate report of the findings from that evaluation. Accurate and detailed record keeping that documents initial injury evaluations, treatment records, and notes on progress throughout a rehabilitation program is critical for the athletic trainer. This is particularly true considering the number of malpractice lawsuits in health care. For the athletic trainer working in a clinical setting, clear, concise, accurate record keeping is necessary for third-party reimbursement. Although this may be difficult and time-consuming for the athletic trainer who treats and deals with a large number of patients each day, it is an area that simply cannot be neglected. Documentation and record keeping will be discussed in detail in Chapter 3.

LEGAL CONSIDERATIONS IN SUPERVISING A REHABILITATION PROGRAM

Regarding the treatment and rehabilitation of athletic injuries, currently there is controversy over the specific roles of individuals with various combinations of educational background, certification, and licensure. States vary considerably in their laws governing what an athletic trainer may and may not do in supervising a program of rehabilitation for an injured patient. Many states have specific guidelines in their licensure act that dictate how the athletic trainer may incorporate a variety of treatment tools into the treatment regimen. Each athletic trainer should make sure that any use of a specific tool or technique of rehabilitation is within the limits allowed by the laws of his or her particular state.

Summary

1. The athletic trainer is responsible for the design, implementation, and supervision of the rehabilitation program for the injured patient.
2. The rehabilitation philosophy in sports medicine is aggressive, with the ultimate goal being to return the injured patient to full activity as quickly and safely as possible.
3. To be effective in overseeing a rehabilitation program, the athletic trainer must have a sound understanding of the healing process, the biomechanics of normal movement, and the psychological aspects of the rehabilitative process.
4. The athletic trainer must develop a broad theoretical knowledge base from which specific techniques or tools of rehabilitation can be selected and practically applied to each individual case without relying on "recipe" rehabilitation protocols.
5. Therapeutic exercises are rehabilitative, or reconditioning, exercises that are specifically concerned with restoring normal body function following injury.
6. Short-term goals of a rehabilitation program: (1) providing correct immediate first aid and management following injury to limit or control swelling; (2) reducing or minimizing pain; (3) establishing core stability; (4) reestablishing neuromuscular control; (5) restoring full range of motion; (6) restoring or increasing muscular strength, endurance, and power; (7) improving postural stability and balance; (8) maintaining cardiorespiratory fitness; and (9) incorporating appropriate functional progressions.
7. Controlling swelling immediately following injury is perhaps the single most important aspect of injury rehabilitation in a sports medicine setting. If the swelling can be controlled initially in the acute stage of injury, the time required for rehabilitation is likely to be significantly reduced.

References

1. Buschbacher, R., and R. Braddom. 1994. *Sports medicine and rehabilitation: A sport specific approach.* Philadelphia: Hanley & Belfus.
2. Cahill, J. and C. JeMe. 2006. *Postsurgical Rehabilitation Guidelines for the Orthopedic Clinician.* St. Louis: Mosby.
3. Clark, M. 2001. *Integrated training for the new millennium.* Calabasas, CA: National Academy of Sports Medicine.
4. Guskiewicz, K. and D. Perrin. 1996. Research and clinical applications of assessing balance. *Journal of Sport Rehabilitation* 5(1): 45–63.
5. Hertel, J. and C. Denegar. 1998. A rehabilitation paradigm for restoring neuromuscular control following athletic injury. *Journal of Sport Rehabilitation* 3(5):12.
6. Hillman, S. 1994. Principles and techniques of open kinetic chain rehabilitation. *Journal of Sport Rehabilitation* 3(4): 319–30.
7. Irrgang, J., S. Whitney, and E. Cox. 1994. Balance and proprioceptive training for rehabilitation of the lower extremity. *Journal of Sport Rehabilitation* 3(1): 68–83.
8. Kibler, B. 1998. *Functional rehabilitation of sports and musculoskeletal injuries.* New York: Aspen.
9. King, M. 2000. Core stability: Creating a foundation for functional rehabilitation. *Athletic Therapy Today* 5(2):6.
10. Kisner, C. and A. Colby. 2007. *Therapeutic exercise: Foundations and techniques.* Philadelphia: F. A. Davis.

11. Kirkendall, D. T., W. E. Prentice, and W. E. Garrett. 2001. Rehabilitation of muscle injuries. In *Rehabilitation of sports injuries: Current concepts,* edited by G. Puddu, A. Giombini, and A. Selvanetti. Berlin: Springer.

12. Knight, K. J. 1985. Guidelines for rehabilitation of sports injuries. In *Rehabilitation of the injured patient: Clinics in sports medicine,* vol. 4, no. 3, edited by J. S. Harvey. Philadelphia: W. B. Saunders.

13. Knight, K. L. 1995. *Cryotherapy in sport injury management.* Champaign, IL: Human Kinetics.

14. Logan, G. A., and E. L. Wallis. 1960. *Recent findings in learning and performance.* Paper presented at the Southern Section Meeting, California Association for Health, Physical Education and Recreation, Pasadena, CA.

15. Magnusson, P., and M. McHugh. 1995. Current concepts on rehabilitation in sports medicine. In *The lower extremity and spine in sports medicine,* edited by J. Nicholas and E. Hirschman. St. Louis: Mosby.

16. Malone, T., ed. 1996. *Orthopedic and sports physical therapy.* St Louis: Mosby/Yearbook.

17. Perrin, D. 1993. *Isokinetic exercise and assessment.* Champaign, IL: Human Kinetics.

18. Piccininni, J., and J. Drover. 1999. Patient-patient education in rehabilitation: Developing a self-directed program. *Athletic Therapy Today* 4(6):51.

19. Prentice, W. 2009. *Arnheim's principles of athletic training.* 13th ed. New York: McGraw-Hill.

20. Prentice, W. 2009. *Therapeutic modalities in sports medicine and athletic training.* New York: McGraw-Hill.

21. Sahrmann S. 2001. *Diagnosis and Treatment of Movement Impairment Syndromes.* Philadelphia, PA: Elsevier Publishing.

22. Shamus, E. and J. Shamus. 2001. *Sports injury: Prevention and rehabilitation.* New York: McGraw-Hill.

23. Tippett, S., and M. Voight. 1999. *Functional progressions for sport rehabilitation.* Champaign, IL: Human Kinetics.

24. Voight, M., B. Hoogeboom, and W. Prentice. 2006. *Musculoskeletal interventions: Techniques for therapeutic exercise.* New York: McGraw-Hill.

25. Zachazewski, J., D. Magee, and S. Quillen. 1996. *Athletic injuries and rehabilitation.* Philadelphia: W. B. Saunders.

SOLUTIONS TO CLINICAL DECISION MAKING EXERCISES

1-1 The athletic trainer's decisions about a rehabilitation progression should be based on the following aspects: healing process, pathomechanics of the injury, cardiovascular fitness, and the equipment available. A good understanding of these things will ensure that the athletic trainer is progressing the patient at an appropriate rate.

1-2 Her concerns should be discussed with the orthopedist. The doctor and athletic trainer should maintain open communication throughout a patient's rehabilitation so that a good working relationship is maintained and the doctor's philosophy persists throughout the rehabilitation process.

1-3 He should understand the SAID principle. The muscles and soft tissue will adapt gradually to increasing demands placed on it. If the demands are too great, they can be detrimental to the healing process.

1-4 In general, the short-term goals for rehabilitation of an acute injury are to target inflammation and restore ROM. More specifically, pain and swelling should be controlled using PRICE. Once the patient progresses through the inflammatory phase, the goals become to restore muscular strength, endurance, and power. Neuromuscular control, balance, and cardiorespiratory fitness must also be regained. Long-term goals are to regain functional ability and return to play as soon as possible.

1-5 The patient should be taped and encouraged to keep up with the therapeutic exercise program, while continuing to use ice and anti-inflammatories.

1-6 She should have sufficient neuromuscular control/balance. Her cardiovascular endurance should be at a level that will allow her to be competitive again without reinjury. She should be able to perform a series of functional tests that indicate she will withstand the demands of competition without reinjury. She should also be able to perform with confidence and know when to stop if she is in danger of reinjury.

CHAPTER 2

Understanding and Managing the Healing Process through Rehabilitation

William E. Prentice

After completing this chapter, the athletic trainer should be able to do the following:

- Describe the pathophysiology of the healing process.

- Identify the factors that can impede the healing process.

- Discuss the etiology and pathology of various musculoskeletal injuries associated with various types of tissues.

- Compare healing processes relative to specific musculoskeletal structures.

- Explain the importance of initial first aid and injury management of these injuries and their impact on the rehabilitation process.

- Discuss the use of various analgesics, anti-inflammatories, and antipyretics in facilitating the healing process during a rehabilitation program.

Injury rehabilitation requires sound knowledge and understanding of the etiology and pathology involved in various musculoskeletal injuries that may occur.[24,84,93] When injury occurs, the athletic trainer is charged with designing, implementing, and supervising the rehabilitation program. Rehabilitation protocols and progressions must be based primarily on the physiologic responses of the tissues to injury and on an understanding of how various tissues heal.[39,46] Thus the athletic trainer must understand the healing process to effectively supervise the rehabilitative process. This chapter discusses the healing process relative to the various musculoskeletal injuries that may be encountered by an athletic trainer.

UNDERSTANDING THE HEALING PROCESS

Rehabilitation programs must be based on the cycle of the healing process (Fig. 2-1). The athletic trainer must have a sound understanding of the sequence of the various phases of the healing process. The physiological responses of the tissues to trauma follow a predictable sequence and time frame.[41] Decisions on how and when to alter and progress a rehabilitation program should be primarily based on recognition of signs and symptoms, as well as on an awareness of the time frames associated with the various phases of healing.[57,72]

The healing process consists of the inflammatory-response phase, the fibroblastic-repair phase, and the maturation-remodeling phase. It must be stressed that although the phases of healing are presented as three separate entities, the healing process is a continuum. Phases of the healing process overlap one another and have no definitive beginning or end points.[73]

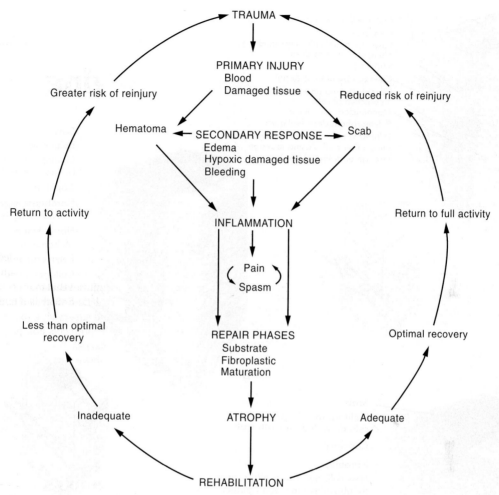

Figure 2-1   A cycle of sport-related injury.
(From Booher and Thibadeau, *Athletic Injury Assessment,* Mosby, 1994.)

Primary Injury

Primary injuries are almost always described as being either chronic or acute in nature, resulting from *macrotraumatic* or *microtraumatic* forces. Injuries classified as macrotraumatic occur as a result of acute trauma and produce immediate pain and disability. Macrotraumatic injuries include fractures, dislocations, subluxations, sprains, strains, and contusions. Microtraumatic injuries are most often called overuse injuries and result from repetitive overloading or incorrect mechanics associated with repeated motion.[59] Microtraumatic injuries include tendinitis, tenosynovitis, bursitis, etc. A *secondary injury* is essentially the inflammatory or hypoxia response that occurs with the primary injury.

Inflammatory-Response Phase

Once a tissue is injured, the process of healing begins immediately[16] (Fig. 2-2A). The destruction of tissue produces direct injury to the cells of the various soft tissues.[35] Cellular injury results in altered metabolism and the liberation of materials that initiate the inflammatory response. It is characterized symptomatically by redness, swelling, tenderness, and increased temperature.[18,54] *This initial inflammatory response is critical to the entire healing process. If this response does not accomplish what it is supposed to or if it does not subside, normal healing cannot take place.*

Inflammation is a process through which *leukocytes* and other *phagocytic cells* and exudates are delivered to the

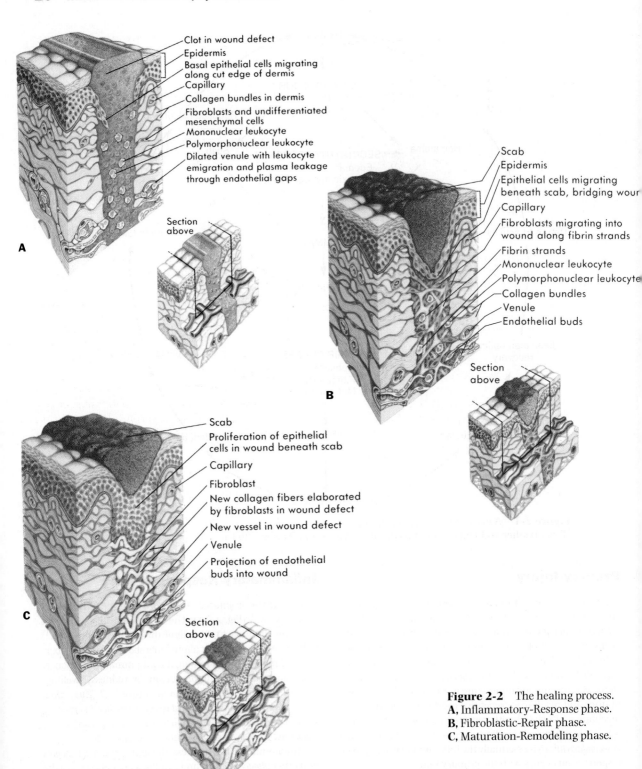

A, Clot in wound defect
Epidermis
Basal epithelial cells migrating along cut edge of dermis
Capillary
Collagen bundles in dermis
Fibroblasts and undifferentiated mesenchymal cells
Mononuclear leukocyte
Polymorphonuclear leukocyte
Dilated venule with leukocyte emigration and plasma leakage through endothelial gaps
Section above

B, Scab
Epidermis
Epithelial cells migrating beneath scab, bridging wound
Capillary
Fibroblasts migrating into wound along fibrin strands
Fibrin strands
Mononuclear leukocyte
Polymorphonuclear leukocyte
Collagen bundles
Venule
Endothelial buds
Section above

C, Scab
Proliferation of epithelial cells in wound beneath scab
Capillary
Fibroblast
New collagen fibers elaborated by fibroblasts in wound defect
New vessel in wound defect
Venule
Projection of endothelial buds into wound
Section above

Figure 2-2   The healing process.
A, Inflammatory-Response phase.
B, Fibroblastic-Repair phase.
C, Maturation-Remodeling phase.

injured tissue. This cellular reaction is generally protective, tending to localize or dispose of injury by-products (e.g., blood and damaged cells) through phagocytosis and thus setting the stage for repair. Local vascular effects, disturbances of fluid exchange, and migration of leukocytes from the blood to the tissues occur.

CLINICAL DECISION MAKING Exercise 2–1

A physical education student fell on his wrist playing flag football. It is very swollen, and he has decreased strength and ROM. The athletic trainer does not suspect a fracture. A decision is made to provide an initial treatment as opposed to sending the student to the emergency room. What should the athletic trainer's goals be at this time?

Vascular Reaction.   The vascular reaction involves vascular spasm, formation of a platelet plug, blood coagulation, and growth of fibrous tissue.[77] The immediate response to tissue damage is a vasoconstriction of the vascular walls in the vessels leading away from the site of injury that lasts for approximately five to ten minutes. This vasoconstriction presses the opposing endothelial wall linings together to produce a local anemia that is rapidly replaced by hyperemia of the area due to vasodilation. This increase in blood flow is transitory and gives way to slowing of the flow in the dilated vessels, thus enabling the leukocytes to slow down and adhere to the vascular endothelium. Eventually there is stagnation and stasis. The initial effusion of blood and plasma lasts for 24 to 36 hours.

Chemical Mediators   The events in the inflammatory response are initiated by a series of interactions involving several chemical mediators. Some of these chemical mediators are derived from the invading organism, some are released by the damaged tissue, others are generated by several plasma enzyme systems, and still others are products of various white blood cells participating in the inflammatory response. Three chemical mediators, *histamine, leukotrienes,* and *cytokines* are important in limiting the amount of exudate, and thus swelling, after injury. Histamine, released from the injured mast cells, causes vasodilation and increased cell permeability, owing to a swelling of endothelial cells and then separation between the cells. Leukotrienes and prostaglandins are responsible for **margination,** in which leukocytes (neutrophils and marcophages) adhere along the cell walls. They also increase cell permeability locally, thus affecting the passage of the fluid and white blood cells through cell walls via diapedesis to form exudate. Therefore vasodilation and active hyperemia are important in exudate (plasma) formation,

in supplying leukocytes to the injured area. Cytokines, in particular chemokines and interleukin, are the major regulators of leukocyte traffic and help to attract leukocytes to the actual site of inflammation. Responding to the presence of chemokines, phagocytes enter the site of inflammation within a few hours. The amount of swelling that occurs is directly related to the extent of vessel damage.

Formation of a Clot   Platelets do not normally adhere to the vascular wall. However, injury to a vessel disrupts the endothelium and exposes the collagen fibers. Platelets adhere to the collagen fibers to create a sticky matrix on the vascular wall, to which additional platelets and leukocytes adhere and eventually form a plug. These plugs obstruct local lymphatic fluid drainage and thus localize the injury response.

The initial event that precipitates clot formation is the conversion of *fibrinogen* to *fibrin.* This transformation occurs because of a cascading effect, beginning with the release of a protein molecule called *thromboplastin* from the damaged cell. Thromboplastin causes *prothrombin* to be changed into *thrombin,* which in turn causes the conversion of fibrinogen into a very sticky fibrin clot that shuts off blood supply to the injured area. Clot formation begins around 12 hours after injury and is completed within 48 hours.

As a result of a combination of these factors, the injured area becomes walled off during the inflammatory stage of healing. The leukocytes phagocytize most of the foreign debris toward the end of the inflammatory phase, setting the stage for the fibroblastic phase. This initial inflammatory response lasts for approximately 2 to 4 days after initial injury.

CLINICAL DECISION MAKING Exercise 2–2

A backstroker suffered a second-degree latissimus dorsi strain. The coach wants to know why he can't be ready to compete the next day. What should the athletic trainer tell the coach about the healing process and how long it may take the strain to heal?

Chronic Inflammation   A distinction must be made between the acute inflammatory response as previously described and chronic inflammation. Chronic inflammation occurs when the acute inflammatory response does not respond sufficiently to eliminate the injuring agent and restore tissue to its normal physiological state. Thus, only low concentrations of the chemical mediators are present. The neutrophils that are normally present during acute inflammation are replaced by macrophages, lymphocytes, fibroblasts, and plasma cells. As this low-grade inflammation persists, damage occurs to connective tissue resulting in tissue necrosis and fibrosis prolonging the healing and repair process. Chronic inflammation involves the production of granulation tissue and fibrous connective tissue. These cells accumulate in a highly vascularized and innervated loose connective tissue matrix in the area of injury. [53] The specific mechanisms that cause an insufficient acute inflammatory response are unknown, but they appear to be related to situations that involve overuse or overload with cumulative microtrauma to a particular structure. [28,53] There is no specific time frame in which the acute inflammation transitions to chronic inflammation. It does appear that chronic inflammation is resistant to both physical and pharmacologic treatments. [44]

Use of Anti-Inflammatory Medications A physician will routinely prescribe nonsteroidal anti-inflammatory drugs (NSAIDs) for a patient who has sustained an injury.[2] These medications are certainly effective in minimizing pain and swelling associated with inflammation and can enhance return to normal activity. However, there are some concerns that the use of NSAIDs acutely following injury might actually interfere with inflammation, thus delaying the healing process.

Fibroblastic-Repair Phase

During the fibroblastic phase of healing, proliferative and regenerative activity leading to scar formation and repair of the injured tissue follows the vascular and exudative phenomena of inflammation[41] (Figure 2-2B). The period of scar formation referred to as *fibroplasia* begins within the first few hours after injury and can last as long as 4 to 6 weeks. During this period, many of the signs and symptoms associated with the inflammatory response subside. The patient might still indicate some tenderness to touch and will usually complain of pain when particular movements stress the injured structure. As scar formation progresses, complaints of tenderness or pain gradually disappear.[39]

During this phase, growth of endothelial capillary buds into the wound is stimulated by a lack of oxygen, after which the wound is capable of healing aerobically.[18] Along with increased oxygen delivery comes an increase in blood flow, which delivers nutrients essential for tissue regeneration in the area.[18]

The formation of a delicate connective tissue called *granulation tissue* occurs with the breakdown of the fibrin clot. Granulation tissue consists of *fibroblasts*, collagen, and capillaries. It appears as a reddish granular mass of connective tissue that fills in the gaps during the healing process.

As the capillaries continue to grow into the area, fibroblasts accumulate at the wound site, arranging themselves parallel to the capillaries. Fibroblastic cells begin to synthesize an extracellular matrix that contains protein fibers of *collagen* and *elastin*, a ground substance that consists of nonfibrous proteins called proteoglycans, glycosaminoglycans, and fluid. On about day 6 or 7, fibroblasts also begin producing collagen fibers that are deposited in a random fashion throughout the forming scar. As the collagen continues to proliferate, the tensile strength of the wound rapidly increases in proportion to the rate of collagen synthesis. As the tensile strength increases, the number of fibroblasts diminishes, signaling the beginning of the maturation phase.

This normal sequence of events in the repair phase leads to the formation of minimal scar tissue. Occasionally, a persistent inflammatory response and continued release of inflammatory products can promote extended fibroplasia and excessive fibrogenesis, which can lead to irreversible tissue damage.[97] Fibrosis can occur in synovial structures, as with adhesive capsulitis in the shoulder, in extra-articular tissues including tendons and ligaments, in bursa, or in muscle.

CLINICAL DECISION MAKING   **Exercise 2–3**

A cross-country runner strained her quadriceps. How will the healing process for this injury differ from the process for a ligamentous injury?

The Importance of Collagen Collagen is a major structural protein that forms strong, flexible, inelastic structures that hold connective tissue together. There are at least 16 types of collagen, but 80—90 percent of the collagen in the body consists of Types I, II, and III. Type I collagen is found in skin, fascia, tendon, bone, ligaments, cartilage, and interstitial tissues; Type II can be found in hyaline cartilage and vertebral disks; and Type III is found in skin, smooth muscle, nerves, and blood vessels. Type III collagen has less tensile strength than does Type I, and tends to be found more in the fibroblastic-repair phase. Collagen enables a tissue to resist mechanical forces and deformation. Elastin, however, produces highly elastic tissues that assist in recovery from deformation. Collagen fibrils are the load-bearing elements of connective tissue. They are arranged to accommodate tensile stress but are not as capable of resisting shear or compressive stress. Consequently the direction of orientation of collagen fibers is along lines of tensile stress.[93]

Collagen has several mechanical and physical properties that allow it to respond to loading and deformation, permitting it to withstand high tensile stress. The mechanical properties of collagen include *elasticity,* which is the capability to recover normal length after elongation; *visco-elasticity*, which allows for a slow return to normal length and shape after deformation; and *plasticity*, which allows for permanent change or deformation. The physical properties include *force relaxation*, which indicates the decrease in the amount of force needed to maintain a tissue at a set amount of displacement or deformation over time; *creep response*, which is the ability of a tissue to deform over time while a constant load is imposed; and *hysteresis*, which is the amount of relaxation a tissue has undergone during deformation and displacement. Injury results when the mechanical and physical limitations of connective tissue are exceeded.[103]

Maturation-Remodeling Phase

The maturation-remodeling phase of healing is a long-term process (Figure 2-2C). This phase features a realignment or remodeling of the collagen fibers that make up scar tissue according to the tensile forces to which that scar is subjected. Ongoing breakdown and synthesis of collagen occur with a steady increase in the tensile strength of the scar matrix. With increased stress and strain, the collagen fibers realign in a position of maximum efficiency parallel to the lines of tension. The tissue gradually assumes normal appearance and function, although a scar is rarely as strong as the normal injured tissue. Usually by the end of approximately 3 weeks, a firm, strong, contracted, nonvascular scar exists. The maturation phase of healing might require several years to be totally complete.

Role of Progressive Controlled Mobility during the Healing Process Wolff's law states that bone and soft tissue will respond to the physical demands placed on them, causing them to remodel or realign along lines of tensile force.[101] Therefore it is critical that injured structures be exposed to progressively increasing loads throughout the rehabilitative process.[73]

In animal models, controlled mobilization is superior to immobilization for scar formation, revascularization, muscle regeneration, and reorientation of muscle fibers and tensile properties.[71] However, a brief period of immobilization of the injured tissue during the inflammatory-response phase is recommended and will likely facilitate the process of healing by controlling inflammation, thus reducing clinical symptoms. As healing progresses to the repair phase, controlled activity directed toward return to normal flexibility and strength should be combined with protective support or bracing.[50] Generally, clinical signs and symptoms disappear at the end of this phase.

As the remodeling phase begins, aggressive active range-of-motion and strengthening exercises should be incorporated to facilitate tissue remodeling and realignment. To a great extent, pain will dictate rate of progression. With initial injury, pain is intense; it tends to decrease and eventually subside altogether as healing progresses. Any exacerbation of pain, swelling, or other clinical symptoms during or after a particular exercise or activity indicate that the load is too great for the level of tissue repair or remodeling. The athletic trainer must be aware of the time required for the healing process and realize that being overly aggressive can interfere with that process.

CLINICAL DECISION MAKING   **Exercise 2–4**

A track athlete is recovering from a grade 1 ankle sprain. Beginning exercises as soon as possible will increase the injured runner's chances of recovering quickly and strongly. Why is this so?

Factors That Impede Healing

Extent of Injury The nature of the inflammatory response is determined by the extent of the tissue injury. *Microtears* or soft tissue involve only minor damage and are most often associated with overuse. *Macrotears* involve significantly greater destruction of soft tissue and result in clinical symptoms and functional alterations. Macrotears are generally caused by acute trauma.[19]

Edema The increased pressure caused by swelling retards the healing process, causes separation of tissues, inhibits neuromuscular control, produces reflexive neurological changes, and impedes nutrition in the injured part. Edema is best controlled and managed during the initial first-aid management period as described previously.[17]

Hemorrhage Bleeding occurs with even the smallest amount of damage to the capillaries. Bleeding produces the same negative effects on healing as does the accumulation of edema, and its presence produces additional tissue damage and thus exacerbation of the injury.[67]

Poor Vascular Supply Injuries to tissues with a poor vascular supply heal poorly and at a slow rate. This response is likely related to a failure in the initial delivery of phagocytic cells and fibroblasts necessary for scar formation.[67]

Separation of Tissue Mechanical separation of tissue can significantly impact the course of healing. A wound that has smooth edges in good apposition will tend to heal by primary intention with minimal scarring. Conversely, a wound that has jagged, separated edges must heal by secondary intention, with granulation tissue filling the defect, and excessive scarring.[76]

Muscle Spasm Muscle spasm causes traction on the torn tissue, separates the two ends, and prevents approximation. Local and generalized ischemia can result from spasm.

Atrophy Wasting away of muscle tissue begins immediately with injury. Strengthening and early mobilization of the injured structure retard atrophy.

Corticosteroids Use of corticosteroids in the treatment of inflammation is controversial. Steroid use in the early stages of healing has been demonstrated to inhibit fibroplasia, capillary proliferation, collagen synthesis, and increases in tensile strength of the healing scar. Their use in the later stages of healing and with chronic inflammation is debatable.

Keloids and Hypertrophic Scars Keloids occur when the rate of collagen production exceeds the rate of collagen breakdown during the maturation phase of healing. This process leads to hypertrophy of scar tissue, particularly around the periphery of the wound.

Infection The presence of bacteria in the wound can delay healing, causes excessive granulation tissue, and frequently causes large, deformed scars.[12]

Humidity, Climate, and Oxygen Tension Humidity significantly influences the process of epithelization. Occlusive dressing stimulates the epithelium to migrate twice as fast without crust or scab formation. The formation of a scab occurs with dehydration of the wound and traps wound drainage, which promotes infection. Keeping the wound moist provides an advantage for the necrotic debris to go to the surface and be shed.

Oxygen tension relates to the neovascularization of the wound, which translates into optimal saturation and maximal tensile strength development. Circulation to the wound can be affected by ischemia, venous stasis, hematomas, and vessel trauma.

Health, Age, and Nutrition The elastic qualities of the skin decrease with age. Degenerative diseases, such as diabetes and arteriosclerosis, also become a concern of the older patient and can affect wound healing. Nutrition is important for wound healing—in particular, vitamins C (for collagen synthesis and immune system), K (for clotting), and A (for the immune system); zinc (for the enzyme systems) and amino acids play critical roles in the healing process.

INJURIES TO ARTICULAR STRUCTURES

Before discussing injuries to the various articular structures, a review of joint structure is in order[66] (Figure 2-3). All *synovial joints* are composed of two or more bones that articulate with one another to allow motion in one or more places. The articulating surfaces of the bone are lined with a very thin, smooth, cartilaginous covering called a hyaline cartilage. All joints are entirely surrounded by a thick, ligamentous joint capsule. The inner surface of this joint capsule is lined by a very thin *synovial membrane* that is highly vascularized and innervated. The synovial membrane produces *synovial fluid*, the functions of which include lubrication, shock absorption, and nutrition of the joint.

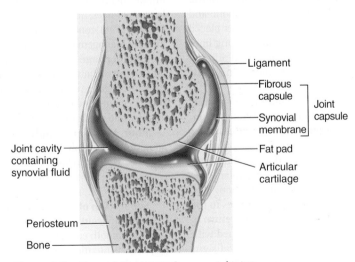

Figure 2-3 General Anatomy of a synovial joint.
From: Saladin, K. S. *Human Anatomy*, 2nd ed, New York: McGraw-Hill, 2008.

Some joints contain a thick fibrocartilage called a *meniscus.* The knee joint, for example, contains two wedge-shaped menisci that deepen the articulation and provide shock absorption in that joint. Finally, the main structural support and joint stability is provided by the ligaments, which may be either thickened portions of a joint capsule or totally separate bands.

Ligament Sprains

Ligaments are composed of dense connective tissue arranged in parallel bundles of collagen composed of rows of fibroblasts. Although bundles are arranged in parallel, not all collagen fibers are arranged in parallel. Ligaments and tendons are very similar in structure. However, ligaments are usually more flattened than tendons, and collagen fibers in ligaments are more compact. The anatomical positioning of the ligaments determines in part what motions a joint can make.

A sprain involves damage to a ligament that provides support to a joint. A ligament is a tough, relatively inelastic band of tissue that connects one bone to another.

A ligament's primary function is threefold: to provide stability to a joint, to provide control of the position of one articulating bone to another during normal joint motion, and to provide proprioceptive input or a sense of joint position through the function of free nerve endings or mechanoreceptors located within the ligament.

If stress is applied to a joint that forces motion beyond its normal limits or planes of movement, injury to the ligament is likely[34] (Figure 2-4). The severity of damage to the ligament is classified in many different ways; however, the most commonly used system involves three grades (degrees) of ligamentous sprain:

Grade 1 sprain: There is some stretching or perhaps tearing of the ligamentous fibers, with little or no joint instability. Mild pain, little swelling, and joint stiffness might be apparent.

Grade 2 sprain: There is some tearing and separation of the ligamentous fibers and moderate instability of the joint. Moderate to severe pain, swelling, and joint stiffness should be expected.

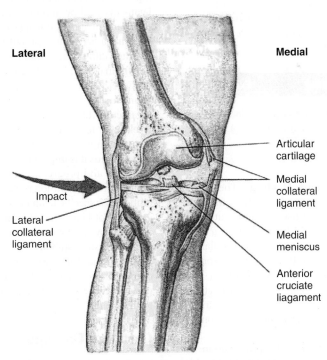

Figure 2-4   Example of a ligament sprain in the knee joint.
From: Voight, M. L., B. J. Hoogenboom, and W.E. Prentice.
Musculoskeletal Interventions, New York: McGraw-Hill, 2006.

CLINICAL DECISION MAKING   **Exercise 2–5**

A basketball player twisted his ankle today in practice. The mechanism and the location of pain suggest an inversion sprain. There is gross laxity with the anterior drawer test and talar tilt test. The swelling is severe and profuse over the lateral side of the ankle. The athlete is incapable of dorsiflexion and has only a few degrees of plantar flexion. He is experiencing very little pain. How would you grade the severity of this injury?

Grade 3 sprain: There is total rupture of the ligament, manifested primarily by gross instability of the joint. Severe pain might be present initially, followed by little or no pain due to total disruption of nerve fibers. Swelling might be profuse, and thus the joint tends to become very stiff some hours after the injury. A third-degree sprain with marked instability usually requires some form of immobilization lasting several weeks. Frequently the force producing the ligament injury is so great that other ligaments or structures surrounding the joint are also injured. With cases in which there is injury to multiple joint structures, surgical repair reconstruction may be necessary to correct an instability.

CLINICAL DECISION MAKING   **Exercise 2–6**

Why is it likely that an athlete with a grade 3 ligament sprain initially will experience little pain, relative to the severity of the injury?

Physiology of Ligament Healing The healing process in the sprained ligament follows the same course of repair as with other vascular tissues. Immediately after injury and for approximately 72 hours there is a loss of blood from damaged vessels and attraction of inflammatory cells into the injured area. If a ligament is sprained outside of a joint capsule (extra-articular ligament), bleeding occurs in a subcutaneous space. If an intra-articular ligament is injured, bleeding occurs inside of the joint capsule until either clotting occurs or the pressure becomes so great that bleeding ceases.

During the next 6 weeks, vascular proliferation with new capillary growth begins to occur along with fibroblastic activity, resulting in the formation of a fibrin clot. It is essential that the torn ends of the ligament be reconnected by bridging of this clot. Synthesis of collagen and ground substance of proteoglycan as constituents of an intracellular matrix contributes to the proliferation of the scar that bridges between the torn ends of the ligament. This scar initially is soft and viscous but eventually becomes more elastic. Collagen fibers are arranged in a random woven pattern with little organization. Gradually there is a decrease in fibroblastic activity, a decrease in vascularity, and an increase to a maximum in collagen density of the scar.[4] Failure to produce enough scar and failure to reconnect the ligament to the appropriate location on a bone are the two reasons why ligaments are likely to fail.

Over the next several months the scar continues to mature, with the realignment of collagen occurring in response to progressive stresses and strains. The maturation of the scar may require as long as 12 months to complete.[4] The exact length of time required for maturation depends on mechanical factors such as apposition of torn ends and length of the period of immobilization.

Factors Affecting Ligament Healing Surgically repaired extra-articular ligaments have healed with decreased scar formation and are generally stronger than unrepaired ligaments initially, although this strength advantage might not be maintained as time progresses. Unrepaired ligaments heal by fibrous scarring effectively lengthening the ligament and producing some degree of joint instability. With intra-articular ligament tears, the presence of synovial fluid dilutes the hematoma, thus preventing formation of a fibrin clot and spontaneous healing.[42]

Several studies have shown that actively exercised ligaments are stronger than those that are immobilized. Ligaments that are immobilized for periods of several weeks after injury tend to decrease in tensile strength and also exhibit weakening of the insertion of the ligament to bone.[72] Thus it is important to minimize periods of immobilization and progressively stress the injured ligaments while exercising caution relative to biomechanical considerations for specific ligaments.[4,68]

It is not likely that the inherent stability of the joint provided by the ligament before injury will be regained. Thus, to restore stability to the joint, the other structures that surround that joint, primarily muscles and their tendons, must be strengthened. The increased muscle tension provided by resistance training can improve stability of the injured joint.[68,88]

Cartilage Damage

Cartilage is a type of rigid connective tissue that provides support and acts as a framework in many structures. It is composed of chondrocyte cells contained in small chambers called lacunae, surrounded completely by an intracellular matrix. The matrix consists of varying ratios of collagen and elastin and a ground substance made of proteoglycans and glycosaminoglycans, which are non-fibrous protein molecules. These proteoglycans act as sponges and trap large quantities of water, which allow cartilage to spring back after being compressed. Cartilage has a poor blood supply, thus healing after injury is very slow. There are three types of cartilage. *Hyaline cartilage* is found on the articulating surfaces of bone and in the soft part of the nose. It contains large quantities of collagen and proteoglycan. *Fibrocartilage* forms the intervertebral disk and menisci located in several joint spaces. It has greater amounts of collagen than proteoglycan and is capable of withstanding a great deal of pressure. *Elastic cartilage* is found in the auricle of the ear and the larynx. It is more flexible than the other types of cartilage and consists of collagen, proteoglycan, and elastin.[79]

Osteoarthrosis is a degenerative condition of bone and cartilage in and about the joint. *Arthritis* should be defined as primarily an inflammatory condition with possible secondary destruction.[6] *Arthrosis* is primarily a degenerative process with destruction of cartilage, remodeling of bone, and possible secondary inflammatory components.

Cartilage fibrillates—that is, releases fibers or groups of fibers and ground substance into the joint.[29] Peripheral cartilage that is not exposed to weightbearing or compression–decompression mechanisms is particularly likely to fibrillate. Fibrillation is typically found in the degenerative process associated with poor nutrition or disuse. This process can then extend even to weightbearing areas, with progressive destruction of cartilage proportional to stresses applied on it. When forces are increased, thus increasing stress, osteochondral or subchondral fractures can occur. Concentration of stress on small areas can produce pressures that overwhelm the tissue's capabilities. Typically, lower-limb joints have to handle greater stresses, but their surface area is usually larger than the surface area of upper limbs. The articular cartilage is protected to some extent by the synovial fluid, which acts as a lubricant. It is also protected by the subchondral bone, which responds to stresses in an elastic fashion. It is more compliant than compact bone, and microfractures can be a means of force absorption. Trabeculae might fracture or might be displaced due to pressures applied on the subchondral bone. In compact bone, fracture can be a means of defense to dissipate force. In the joint, forces might be absorbed by joint movement and eccentric contraction of muscles.[27]

In the majority of joints where the surfaces are not congruent, the applied forces tend to concentrate in certain areas, which increases joint degeneration.

Osteophytosis occurs as a bone attempts to increase its surface area to decrease contact forces. Typically people describe this growth as "bone spurs." *Chondromalacia* is the nonprogressive transformation of cartilage with irregular surfaces and areas of softening. Typically it occurs first in non-weightbearing areas and may progress to areas of excessive stress.[26]

In physically active individuals certain joints maybe more susceptible to a response resembling osteoarthrosis.[70] The proportion of body weight resting on the joint, the pull of the musculotendinous unit, and any significant external force applied to the joint are predisposing factors. Altered joint mechanics caused by laxity or previous trauma are also factors that come into play.[45] The intensity of forces can be great, as in the hip, where the previously mentioned factors can produce pressures or forces four times that of body weight and up to ten times that of body weight on the knee.

Typically, muscle forces generate more stress than body weight itself. Particular injuries are conducive to osteoarthritic changes such as subluxation and dislocation of the patella, osteochondritis dissecans, recurrent synovial effusion, and hemarthrosis. Also, ligamentous injuries can bring about a disruption of proprioceptive mechanisms, loss of adequate joint alignment, and meniscal damage in the knees with removal of the injured meniscus.[40] Other factors that have an impact are loss of full range of motion, poor muscular power and strength, and altered biomechanics of the joint. Spurring and spiking of bone are not synonymous with osteoarthrosis if the joint space is maintained and the cartilage lining is intact. It may simply be an adaptation to the increased stress of physical activity.[29]

Physiology of Cartilage Healing Cartilage has a relatively limited healing capacity. When chondrocytes are destroyed and the matrix is disrupted, the course of healing is variable, depending on whether damage is to cartilage alone or also to subchondral bone. Injuries to the articular cartilage alone fail to elicit clot formation or a cellular response. For the most part the chondrocytes adjacent to the injury are the only cells that show any signs of proliferation and synthesis of matrix. Thus the defect fails to heal, although the extent of the damage tends to remain the same.[33,58]

If subchondral bone is also affected, inflammatory cells enter the damaged area and formulate granulation tissue. In this case, the healing process proceeds normally, with differentiation of granulation tissue cells into chondrocytes occurring in about 2 weeks. At approximately 2 months, normal collagen has been formed.

Injuries to the knee articular cartilage are extremely common, and until recently, methods for treatment did not produce good long-term results. A better understanding of how articular cartilage responds to injury has produced various techniques that hold promise for long-term success.[91] One such technique is autologous chondrocyte implantation, in which a patient's own cartilage cells are harvested, grown ex vivo, and reimplanted in a full-thickness articular surface defect. Results are available with up to 10 years of follow-up, and more than 80 percent of patients have shown improvement with relatively few complications.

INJURIES TO BONE

Bone is a type of connective tissue consisting of both living cells and minerals deposited in a matrix (Figure 2-5). Each bone consists of three major components. The *epiphysis* is an expanded portion at each end of the bone that articulates with another bone. Each articulating surface is covered by an articular, or hyaline, cartilage. The *diaphysis* is the shaft of the bone. The *epiphyseal* or *growth plate* is the major site of bone growth and elongation. Once bone growth ceases, the plate ossifies and forms the epiphyseal

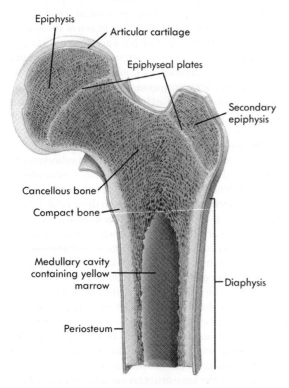

Figure 2–5 Structure of bone shown in cross section.

line. With the exception of the articulating surfaces, the bone is completely enclosed by the *periosteum*, a tough, highly vascularized and innervated fibrous tissue.[55]

The two types of bone material are *cancellous*, or spongy, bone and *cortical*, or compact, bone. Cancellous bone contains a series of air spaces referred to as trabeculae, whereas cortical bone is relatively solid. Cortical bone in the diaphysis forms a hollow medullary canal in long bone, which is lined with *endosteum* and filled with bone *marrow*. Bone has rich blood supply that certainly facilitates the healing process after injury. Bone has the functions of support, movement, and protection. Furthermore, bone stores and releases calcium into the bloodstream and manufactures red blood cells.[93]

Fractures

Fractures are extremely common injuries among the athletic population. They can be generally classified as being either open or closed. A closed fracture involves little or no displacement of bones and thus little or no soft-tissue disruption. An open fracture involves enough displacement of the fractured ends that the bone actually disrupts the cutaneous layers and breaks through the skin. Both fractures can be relatively serious if not managed properly, but an increased possibility of infection exists in an open fracture. Fractures may also be considered complete, in which the bone is broken into at least two fragments, or incomplete, where the fracture does not extend completely across the bone.

The varieties of fractures that can occur include greenstick, transverse, oblique, spiral, comminuted, avulsion, and stress. A *greenstick fracture* (Figure 2-6A) occurs most often in children whose bones are still growing and have not yet had a chance to calcify and harden. It is called a greenstick fracture because of the resemblance to the splintering that occurs to a tree twig that is bent to the point of breaking. Because the twig is green, it splinters but can be bent without causing an actual break.

CLINICAL DECISION MAKING   **Exercise 2–7**

A Little League player collided with the catcher when sliding home. Radiographs did not show a fracture, but a bone scan shows a hot spot. What type of fracture would you suspect this young athlete has?

A *transverse fracture* (Figure 2-6B) involves a crack perpendicular to the longitudinal axis of the bone that goes all the way through the bone. Displacement might occur;

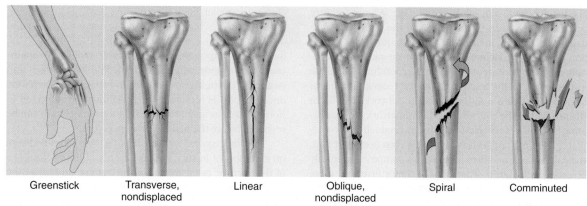

| Greenstick | Transverse, nondisplaced | Linear | Oblique, nondisplaced | Spiral | Comminuted |

Figure 2–6 Fractures of bone. **A,** Greenstick. **B,** Transverse. **C,** Linear. **D,** Oblique. **E,** Spiral. **F,** Comminuted. From McKinley, M and O Loughlin, V: *Human Anatomy,* New York: McGraw-Hill, 2006.

however, because of the shape of the fractured ends, the surrounding soft tissue (for example, muscles, tendons, and fat) sustains relatively little damage.

A *linear fracture* runs parallel to the long axis of a bone and is similar in severity to a transverse fracture (Figure 2-6C).

An *oblique fracture* (Figure 2-6D). results in a diagonal crack across the bone and two very jagged, pointed ends that, if displaced, can potentially cause a good bit of soft-tissue damage. Oblique and spiral fractures are the two types most likely to result in compound fractures.

A *spiral fracture* (Figure 2-6E) is similar to an oblique fracture in that the angle of the fracture is diagonal across the bone. In addition, an element of twisting or rotation causes the fracture to spiral along the longitudinal axis of the bone. Spiral fractures used to be fairly common in ski injuries occurring just above the top of the boot when the bindings on the ski failed to release when the foot was rotated. These injuries are now less common due to improvements in equipment design.

A *comminuted fracture* (Figure 2-6F) is a serious problem that can require an extremely long time for rehabilitation. In the comminuted fracture, multiple fragments of bone must be surgically repaired and fixed with screws and wires. If a fracture of this type occurs to a weightbearing bone in the leg, a permanent discrepancy in leg length can develop.

An *avulsion fracture* occurs when a fragment of bone is pulled away at the bony attachment of a muscle, tendon, or ligament. Avulsion fractures are common in the fingers and some of the smaller bones but can also occur in larger bones where tendinous or ligamentous attachments are subjected to a large amount of force.

Perhaps the most common fracture resulting from physical activity is the *stress fracture.* Unlike the other types of fractures that have been discussed, the stress fracture results from overuse or fatigue rather than acute trauma.[49] Common sites for stress fractures include the weightbearing bones of the leg and foot. In either case, repetitive forces transmitted through the bones produce irritations and microfractures at a specific area in the bone. The pain usually begins as a dull ache that becomes progressively more painful day after day. Initially, pain is most severe during activity. However, when a stress fracture actually develops, pain tends to become worse after the activity is stopped.[80]

The biggest problem with a stress fracture is that often it does not show up on an X-ray film until the osteoblasts begin laying down subperiosteal callus or bone, at which point a small white line, or a callus, appears. However, a bone scan might reveal a potential stress fracture in as little as 2 days after onset of symptoms. If a stress fracture is suspected, the patient should stop any activity that produces added stress or fatigue to the area for a minimum of 14 days. Stress fractures do not usually require casting but might become normal fractures that must be immobilized if handled incorrectly.[92] If a fracture occurs, it should be managed and rehabilitated by a qualified orthopedist and physical athletic trainer.

Physiology of Bone Healing Healing of injured bone tissue is similar to soft-tissue healing in that all phases of the healing process can be identified, although bone regeneration capabilities are somewhat limited. However, the functional elements of healing differ significantly from those of soft tissue. Tensile strength of the scar is the single most critical factor in soft-tissue healing, whereas bone has to contend with a number of additional forces, including torsion, bending, and compression.[46] Trauma to bone can vary from contusions of the periosteum to closed, nondisplaced fractures to severely displaced open fractures that also involve significant soft-tissue damage. When a fracture occurs, blood vessels in the bone and the periosteum are damaged, resulting in bleeding and subsequent clot formation (Figure 2-7). Hemorrhaging from the marrow is contained by the periosteum and the surrounding soft tissue in the region of the fracture. In about 1 week, fibroblasts begin laying down a fibrous collagen network. The fibrin strands within the clot serve as the framework for proliferating vessels. *Chondroblast* cells begin producing fibrocartilage, creating a *callus* between the broken bones. At first, the callus is soft and firm because it is composed primarily of collagenous fibrin. The callus becomes firm and more rubbery as cartilage beings to predominate. Bone-producing cells called *osteoblasts* begin to proliferate and enter the callus, forming cancellous bone trabeculae, which eventually replace the cartilage. Finally the callus crystallizes into bone, at which point remodeling of the bone begins. The callus can be divided into two portions, the external callus located around the periosteum on the outside of the fracture and the internal callus found between the bone fragments. The size of the callus is proportional both to the damage and to the amount of irritation to the fracture site during the healing process. Also during this time *osteoclasts* begin to appear in the area to resorb bone fragments and clean up debris.[42,46,83]

The remodeling process is similar to the growth process of bone in that the fibrous cartilage is gradually replaced by fibrous bone and then by more structurally efficient lamellar bone. Remodeling involves an ongoing process during which osteoblasts lay down new bone and osteoclasts remove and break down bone according to the forces placed upon the healing bone.[62] Wolff's law maintains that a bone will adapt to mechanical stresses and strains by changing size, shape, and structure. Therefore, once the cast is removed, the bone must be subjected to normal stresses and strains so that tensile strength can be regained before the healing process is complete.[36,90]

The time required for bone healing is variable and based on a number of factors, such as severity of the fracture, site of the fracture, extensiveness of the trauma, and age of the patient. Normal periods of immobilization range from as short as 3 weeks for the small bones in the hands and feet to as long as 8 weeks for the long bones of the upper and lower extremities. In some instances, such as fractures in the four small toes, immobilization might not be required for healing. The healing process is certainly not complete when the splint or cast is removed. Osteoblastic and osteoclastic activity might continue for 2 to 3 years after severe fractures.[49,62]

INJURIES TO MUSCULOTENDINOUS STRUCTURES

Muscle is often considered to be a type of connective tissue, but here it is treated as the third of the fundamental tissues. The three types of muscles are smooth (involuntary),

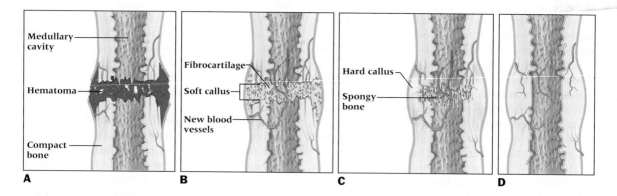

Figure 2-7 The healing of a fracture. **A,** Blood vessels are broken at the fracture line; the blood clots and forms a fracture hematoma. **B,** Blood vessels grow into the fracture and a fibrocartilage soft callus forms. **C,** The fibrocartilage becomes ossified and forms a bony callus made of spongy bone. **D,** Osteoclasts remove excess tissue from the bony callus and the bone eventually resembles its original appearance.
From: Prentice, W. *Principles of Athletic Training*, 13th Edition, New York: McGraw-Hill, 2009.

cardiac, and skeletal (voluntary) muscles. *Smooth muscle* is found with the viscera, where it forms the walls of the internal organs, and within many hollow chambers. *Cardiac muscle* is found only in the heart and is responsible for its contraction. A significant characteristic of the cardiac muscle is that it contracts as a single fiber, unlike smooth and skeletal muscles, which contract as separate units. This characteristic forces the heart to work as a single unit continuously; therefore, if one portion of the muscle should die (as in myocardial infarction), contraction of the heart does not cease.[79]

Skeletal muscle is the striated muscle within the body, responsible for the movement of bony levers (Figure 2-8). Skeletal muscle consists of two portions: (1) the muscle belly, and (2) its tendons, which are collectively referred to as a musculotendinous unit. The muscle belly is composed of separate, parallel elastic fibers called myofibrils. Myofibrils are composed of thousands of small sarcomeres, which are the functional units of the muscle. Sarcomeres contain the contractile elements of the muscle, as well as a substantial amount of connective tissue that holds the fibers together. Myofilaments are small contractile elements of protein within the sarcomere. There are two distinct types of myofilaments: thin actin myofilaments and thicker myosin myofilaments. Fingerlike projections, or crossbridges, connect the actin and myosin myofilaments.[83] When a muscle is stimulated to contract, the crossbridges pull the myofilaments closer together, thus shortening the muscle and producing movement at the joint that the muscle crosses.[25]

The *muscle tendon* attaches the muscle directly to the bone. The muscle tendon is composed primarily of collagen fibers and a matrix of proteoglycan, which is produced by the tenocyte cell. The collagen fibers are grouped together into *primary bundles*. Groups of primary bundles join together to form hexagonal-shaped *secondary bundles*. Secondary bundles are held together by intertwined loose connective tissue containing elastin, called the *endotenon*. The entire tendon is surrounded by a connective tissue layer, called the *epitenon*. The outermost layer of the tendon is the *paratenon*, which is a double-layer connective tissue sheath lined on the inside with synovial membrane[56] (Figure 2-9).

All skeletal muscles exhibit four characteristics: (1) elasticity, the ability to change in length or stretch; (2) extensibility, the ability to shorten and return to normal length; (3) excitability, the ability to respond to stimulation from the nervous system; and (4) contractility, the ability to shorten and contract in response to some neural command.[55]

Skeletal muscles show considerable variation in size and shape. Large muscles generally produce gross motor movements at large joints, such as knee flexion produced by contraction of the large, bulky hamstring muscles. Smaller skeletal muscles, such as the long flexors of the fingers, produce fine motor movements. Muscles producing movements that are powerful in nature are usually thicker and longer, whereas those producing finer movements requiring coordination are thin and relatively shorter.[42,83] Other muscles may be flat, round, or fan-shaped.[42,83] Muscles may be connected to a bone by a single tendon or by two or three separate tendons at either end. Muscles that have two separate muscle and tendon attachments are called *biceps,* and muscles with three separate muscle and tendon attachments are called *triceps.*

Muscles contract in response to stimulation by the central nervous system. An electrical impulse transmitted from the central nervous system through a single motor nerve to a group of muscle fibers causes a depolarization of those fibers. The motor nerve and the group of muscle fibers that it innervates are collectively referred to as a *motor unit.* An impulse coming from the central nervous system and traveling to a group of fibers through a particular motor nerve causes all the muscle fibers in that motor unit to depolarize and contract. This is referred to as the *all-or-none response* and applies to all skeletal muscles in the body.[42]

Muscle Strains

If a musculotendinous unit is overstretched or forced to contract against too much resistance, exceeding the extensibility limits or the tensile capabilities of the weakest component within the unit, damage can occur to the muscle fibers, at the musculotendinous juncture, in the tendon, or at the tendinous attachment to the bone.[34] Any of these injuries may be referred to as a *strain* (Figure 2-10). Muscle strains, like ligament sprains, are subject to various classification systems. The following is a simple system of classification of muscle strains:

Grade 1 strain: Some muscle or tendon fibers have been stretched or actually torn. Active motion produces some tenderness and pain. Movement is painful, but full range of motion is usually possible.

Grade 2 strain: Some muscle or tendon fibers have been torn and active contraction of the muscle is extremely painful. Usually a palpable depression or divot exists somewhere in the muscle belly at the spot where the muscle fibers have been torn. Some swelling might occur because of capillary bleeding.

Grade 3 strain: There is a complete rupture of muscle fibers in the muscle belly, in the area where the

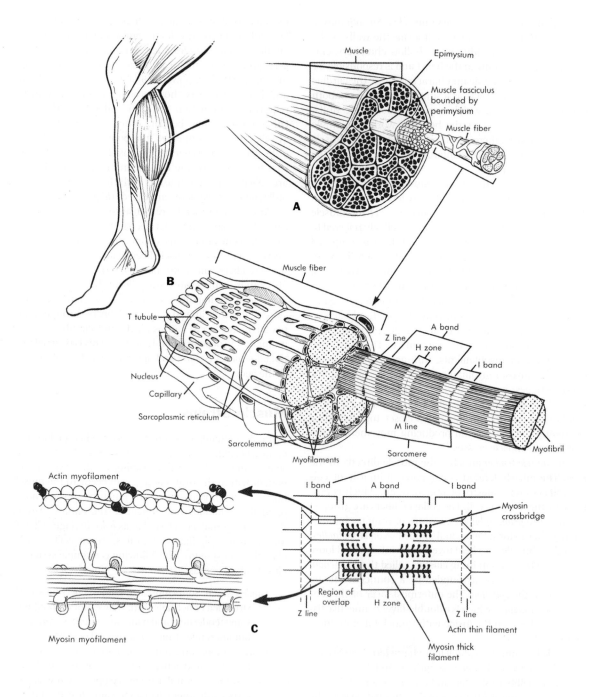

Figure 2-8 Parts of a muscle. **A,** Muscle is composed of muscle fasciculi, which can be seen by the unaided eye as striations in the muscle. The fasciculi are composed of bundles of individual muscle fibers (muscle cells). **B,** Each muscle fiber contains myofibrils in which the banding patterns of the sarcomeres are seen. **C,** The myofibrils are composed of actin myofilament and myosin myofilaments, which are formed from thousands of individual actin and myosin molecules.

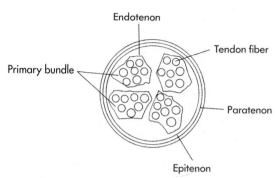

Figure 2-9   Structure of a tendon.

muscle becomes tendon, or at the tendinous attachment to the bone. The patient has significant impairment to, or perhaps total loss of, movement. Pain is intense initially but diminishes quickly because of complete separation of the nerve fibers. Musculotendinous ruptures are most common in the biceps tendon of the upper arm or in the Achilles heelcord in the back of the calf. When either of these tendons rupture, the muscle tends to bunch toward its proximal attachment. With the exception of an Achilles rupture, which

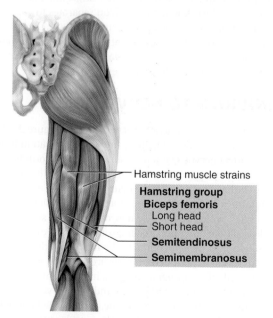

── Hamstring muscle strains

Hamstring group
Biceps femoris
Long head
Short head
Semitendinosus
Semimembranosus

Figure 2-10   A muscle strain results in tearing or separation of fibers.
From: Saladin, K. S. *Anatomy and physiology*, 2nd ed. Dubuque, IA: McGraw-Hill, 2001.

is frequently surgically repaired, the majority of third-degree strains are treated conservatively with some period of immobilization.

Physiology of Muscle Healing   Injuries to muscle tissue involve similar processes of healing and repair as discussed for other tissues. Initially there will be hemorrhage and edema followed almost immediately by phagocytosis to clear debris. Within a few days there is a proliferation of ground substance, and fibroblasts begin producing a gel-type matrix that surrounds the connective tissue, leading to fibrosis and scarring. At the same time, myoblastic cells form in the area of injury, which will eventually lead to regeneration or new myofibrils. Thus regeneration of both connective tissue and muscle tissue begins.[13]

Collagen fibers undergo maturation and orient themselves along lines of tensile force according to Wolff's law. Active contraction of the muscle is critical in regaining normal tensile strength.[6,60]

Regardless of the severity of the strain, the time required for rehabilitation is fairly lengthy. In many instances, rehabilitation time for a muscle strain is longer than that for a ligament sprain. These incapacitating muscle strains occur most frequently in the large, force-producing hamstring and quadriceps muscles of the lower extremity. The treatment of hamstring strains requires a healing period of at least 6 to 8 weeks and a considerable amount of patience. Attempts to return to activity too soon frequently cause reinjury to the area of the musculotendinous unit that has been strained, and the healing process must begin again.

Tendinitis

Of all the overuse problems associated with physical activity, tendinitis is among the most common.[48] *Tendinitis* is a catchall term that can describe many different pathological conditions for a tendon. It essentially describes any inflammatory response within the tendon without inflammation of the paratenon.[87] *Paratenonitis* involves inflammation of the outer layer of the tendon only and usually occurs when the tendon rubs over a bony prominence. *Tendinosis* describes a tendon that has significant degenerative changes with no clinical or histological signs of an inflammatory response.[20]

In cases of what is most often called *chronic tendinitis*, there is evidence of significant tendon degeneration, loss of normal collagen structure, loss of cellularity in the area, but absolutely no inflammatory cellular response in the tendon.[81] The inflammatory process is an essential part of healing. Inflammation is supposed to be a brief process with an end point after its function in the healing process has been fulfilled. The point or the cause in the pathological process where the acute inflammatory cellular response terminates and the chronic degeneration begins is difficult to determine. As mentioned previously, with chronic tendinitis the cellular response involves a replacement of leukocytes with macrophages and plasma cells.[99]

During muscle activity a tendon must move or slide on other structures around it whenever the muscle contracts. If a particular movement is performed repeatedly, the tendon becomes irritated and inflamed. This inflammation is manifested by pain on movement, swelling, possibly some warmth, and usually crepitus. Crepitus is a crackling sound similar to the sound produced by rolling hair between the fingers by the ear. Crepitus is usually caused by the adherence of the paratenon to the surrounding structures while it slides back and forth. This adhesion is caused primarily by the chemical products of inflammation that accumulate on the irritated tendon.[20]

The key to treating tendinitis is rest. If the repetitive motion causing irritation to the tendon is eliminated, chances are that the inflammatory process will allow the tendon to heal.[65] Unfortunately a patient who is seriously involved with some physical activity might have difficulty in resting for 2 weeks or more while the tendinitis subsides. Anti-inflammatory medications and therapeutic modalities are also helpful in reducing the inflammatory responses. An alternative activity, such as bicycling or swimming, is necessary to maintain fitness levels to a certain degree, while allowing the tendon a chance to heal.[30]

Tendinitis most commonly occurs in the Achilles tendon in the back of the lower leg in runners or in the rotator cuff tendons of the shoulder joint in swimmers or throwers, although it can certainly flare up in any tendon in which overuse and repetitive movements occur.

Tenosynovitis

Tenosynovitis is very similar to tendinitis in that the muscle tendons are involved in inflammation. However, many tendons are subject to an increased amount of friction due to the tightness of the space through which they must move. In these areas of high friction, tendons are usually surrounded by synovial sheaths that reduce friction on movement. If the tendon sliding through a synovial sheath is subjected to overuse, inflammation is likely to occur. The inflammatory process produces by-products that are "sticky" and tend to cause the sliding tendon to adhere to the synovial sheath surrounding it.[51]

Symptomatically, tenosynovitis is very similar to tendinitis, with pain on movement, tenderness, swelling, and crepitus. Movement may be more limited with tenosynovitis

because the space provided for the tendon and its synovial covering is more limited. Tenosynovitis occurs most commonly in the long flexor tendons of the fingers as they cross over the wrist joint and in the biceps tendon around the shoulder joint. Treatment for tenosynovitis is the same as that for tendinitis. Because both conditions involve inflammation, mild anti-inflammatory drugs, such as aspirin, might be helpful in chronic cases.[51]

Physiology of Tendon Healing Unlike most soft-tissue healing, tendon injuries pose a particular problem in rehabilitation.[40] The injured tendon requires dense fibrous union of the separated ends and both extensibility and flexibility at the site of attachment. Thus an abundance of collagen is required to achieve good tensile strength. Unfortunately, collagen synthesis can become excessive, resulting in fibrosis, in which adhesions form in surrounding tissues and interfere with the gliding that is essential for smooth motion. Fortunately, over a period of time the scar tissue of the surrounding tissues becomes elongated in its structure because of a breakdown in the cross-links between fibrin units and thus allows the necessary gliding motion. A tendon injury that occurs where the tendon is surrounded by a synovial sheath can be potentially devastating.

A typical time frame for tendon healing would be that during the second week when the healing tendon adheres to the surrounding tissue to form a single mass and during the third week when the tendon separates to varying degrees from the surrounding tissues. However, the tensile strength is not sufficient to permit a strong pull on the tendon for at least 4 to 5 weeks, the danger being that a strong contraction can pull the tendon ends apart.[85]

INJURIES TO NERVE TISSUE

The final fundamental tissue is nerve tissue (Figure 2-11). This tissue provides sensitivity and communication from the central nervous system (brain and spinal cord) to the muscles, sensory organs, various systems, and the periphery. The basic nerve cell is the neuron. The neuron cell body contains a large *nucleus* and branched extensions called *dendrites*, which respond to neurotransmitter substances released from other nerve cells. From each nerve cell arises a single *axon*, which conducts the nerve impulses. Large axons found in peripheral nerves are enclosed in sheaths composed of *Schwann cells*, which are tightly wound around the axon. A nerve is a bundle of nerve cells held together by some connective tissue, usually a lipid-protein layer called the *myelin sheath*, on the outside of the axon.[93] Neurology is an extremely complex science, and only a brief presentation of its relevance to musculoskeletal injuries is covered here.[16]

and neuromuscular control of movement as an integral part of a rehabilitation program. This will be discussed in great detail in Chapter 6.

Physiology of Nerve Healing

Nerve cell tissue is specialized and cannot regenerate once the nerve cell dies. In an injured peripheral nerve, however, the nerve fiber can regenerate significantly if the injury does not affect the cell body (Figure 2-12). The proximity of the axonal injury to the cell body can significantly affect the time required for healing. The closer an injury is to the cell body, the more difficult is the regenerative process. In the case of severed nerve, surgical intervention can markedly enhance regeneration.[79]

For regeneration to occur, an optimal environment for healing must exist. When a nerve is cut, several degenerative changes occur that interfere with the neural pathways (Figure 2-12). Within the first 3 to 5 days the portion of the axon distal to the cut begins to degenerate and breaks into irregular segments. There is also a concomitant increase in metabolism and protein production by the nerve cell body to facilitate the regenerative process. The neuron in the cell body contains the genetic material and produces chemicals necessary for maintenance of the axon. These substances cannot be transmitted to the distal part of the axon, and eventually there will be complete degeneration.[83]

In addition, the myelin portion of the Schwann cells around the degenerating axon also degenerates, and the myelin is phagocytized. The Schwann cells divide, forming a column of cells in place of the axon. If the cut ends of the axon contact this column of Schwann cells, the chances are good that an axon may eventually reinnervate distal structures. If the proximal end of the axon does not make contact with the column of Schwann cells, reinnervation will not occur.

The axon proximal to the cut has minimal degeneration initially and then begins the regenerative process with growth from the proximal axon. Bulbous enlargements and several axon sprouts form at the end of the proximal axon. Within about 2 weeks, these sprouts grow across the scar that has developed in the area of the cut and enter the column of Schwann cells. Only one of these sprouts will form the new axon, while the others will degenerate. Once the axon grows through the Schwann cell columns, remaining Schwann cells proliferate along the length of the degenerating fiber and form new myelin around the growing axon, which will eventually reinnervate distal structures.[42]

Regeneration is slow, at a rate of only 3 to 4 mm/day. Axon regeneration can be obstructed by scar formation

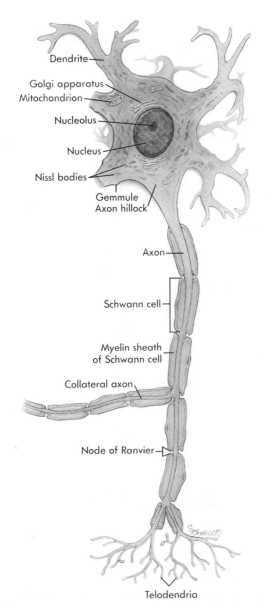

Figure 2-11   Structural features of a nerve cell.

Dendrite
Golgi apparatus
Mitochondrion
Nucleolus
Nucleus
Nissl bodies
Gemmule
Axon hillock
Axon
Schwann cell
Myelin sheath of Schwann cell
Collateral axon
Node of Ranvier
Telodendria

Nerve injuries usually involve either contusions or inflammations. More serious injuries involve the crushing of a nerve or complete division (severing). This type of injury can produce lifelong physical disability, such as paraplegia or quadriplegia, and should therefore not be overlooked in any circumstance.

Of critical concern to the athletic trainer is the importance of the nervous system in proprioception

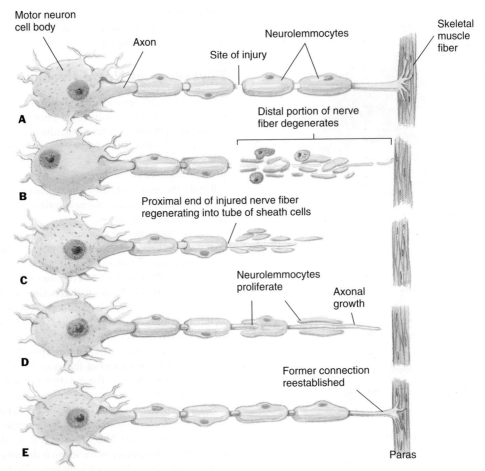

Figure 2-12   Neuron regeneration. **A,** If a neuron is severed through a myelinated axon, the proximal portion may survive but **B,** the distal portion will degenerate through phagocytosis. **C–D,** The myelin layer provides a pathway for regeneration of the axon, and **E,** innervation is restored.
From: Van De Graaff, K. *Human anatomy,* 6th ed, Dubuque, IA: McGraw-Hill, 2002.

due to excessive fibroplasia. Damaged nerves within the central nervous system regenerate very poorly compared to nerves in the peripheral nervous system. Central nervous system axons lack connective tissue sheaths, and the myelin-producing Schwann cells fail to proliferate.[42,83]

ADDITIONAL MUSCULOSKELETAL INJURIES

Dislocations and Subluxations

A dislocation occurs when at least one bone in an articulation is forced out of its normal and proper alignment and stays out until it is either manually or surgically put back into place or reduced.[10] Dislocations most commonly occur in the shoulder joint, elbow, and fingers, but they can occur wherever two bones articulate.[15,64,82]

A subluxation is like a dislocation except that in this situation a bone pops out of its normal articulation but then goes right back into place. Subluxations most commonly occur in the shoulder joint, as well as in the kneecap in females.

Dislocations should never be reduced immediately, regardless of where they occur. The patient should have an X-ray to rule out fractures or other problems before reduction. Inappropriate techniques of reduction might only exacerbate the problem. Return to activity after dislocation or subluxation is largely dependent on the degree of soft-tissue damage.[15]

Bursitis

In many areas, particularly around joints, friction occurs between tendons and bones, skin and bone, or two muscles. Without some mechanism of protection in these high-friction areas, chronic irritation would be likely.[93]

Bursae are essentially pieces of synovial membrane that contain small amounts of synovial fluid. This presence of synovium permits motion of surrounding structures without friction. If excessive movement or perhaps some acute trauma occurs around these bursae, they become irritated and inflamed and begin producing large amounts of synovial fluid. The longer the irritation continues or the more severe the acute trauma, the more fluid is produced. As the fluid continues to accumulate in a limited space, pressure tends to increase and causes irritation of the pain receptors in the area.

Bursitis can be extremely painful and can severely restrict movement, especially if it occurs around a joint. Synovial fluid continues to be produced until the movement or trauma producing the irritation is eliminated.

A bursa that occasionally completely surrounds a tendon to allow more freedom of movement in a tight area is referred to as a *synovial sheath.* Irritation of this synovial sheath may restrict tendon motion.

All joints have many bursae surrounding them. Perhaps the three bursae most commonly irritated as a result of various types of physical activity are the subacromial bursa in the shoulder joint, the olecranon bursa on the tip of the elbow, and the prepatellar bursa on the front surface of the patella. All three of these bursae have produced large amounts of synovial fluid, affecting motion at their respective joints.

Muscle Soreness

Overexertion in strenuous muscular exercise often results in muscular pain. At one time or another almost everyone has experienced muscle soreness, usually resulting from some physical activity to which we are unaccustomed.

There are two types of muscle soreness. The first type of muscle pain is acute and accompanies fatigue. It is transient and occurs during and immediately after exercise. The second type of soreness involves delayed muscle pain that appears approximately 12 hours after injury. It becomes most intense after 24 to 48 hours and then gradually subsides so that the muscle becomes symptom-free

after 3 or 4 days. This second type of pain may best be described as a syndrome of delayed muscle pain, leading to increased muscle tension, edema formation, increased stiffness, and resistance to stretching.[61]

The cause of *delayed-onset muscle soreness* (DOMS) has been debated. Initially it was hypothesized that soreness was due to an excessive buildup of lactic acid in exercised muscles. However, recent evidence has essentially ruled out this theory.[1]

It has also been hypothesized that DOMS is caused by the tonic, localized spasm of motor units, varying in number with the severity of pain. This theory maintains that exercise causes varying degrees of ischemia in the working muscles. This ischemia causes pain, which results in reflex tonic muscle contraction that increases and prolongs the ischemia. Consequently a cycle of increasing severity is begun.[25] As with the lactic acid theory, the spasm theory has also been discounted.

Currently there are two schools of thought relative to the cause of DOMS. DOMS seems to occur from very small tears in the muscle tissue, which seem to be more likely with eccentric or isometric contractions.[1] It is generally believed that the initial damage caused by eccentric exercise is mechanical damage to either the muscular or the connective tissue. Edema accumulation and delays in the rate of glycogen repletion are secondary reactions to mechanical damage.[69]

DOMS might be caused by structural damage to the elastic components of connective tissue at the musculotendinous junction. This damage results in the presence of hydroxyproline, a protein by-product of collagen breakdown, in blood and urine.[19] It has also been documented that structural damage to the muscle fibers results in an increase in blood serum levels of various protein/enzymes, including creatine kinase. This increase indicates that there is likely some damage to the muscle fiber as a result of strenuous exercise.[1]

Muscle soreness can best be prevented by beginning at a moderate level of activity and gradually progressing the intensity of the exercise over time. Treatment of muscle soreness usually also involves some type of stretching activity.[39] As for other conditions discussed in this chapter, ice is important as a treatment for muscle soreness, particularly within the first 48 to 72 hours.

Contusions

Contusion is synonymous with *bruise.* The mechanism that produces a contusion is a blow from some external object that causes soft tissues (e.g., skin, fat, muscle, ligaments, joint capsule) to be compressed against the hard bone underneath.[100]

If the blow is hard enough, capillaries rupture and allow bleeding into the tissues. The bleeding, if superficial enough, causes a bluish-purple discoloration of the skin that persists for several days. The contusion may be very sore to the touch. If damage has occurred to muscle, pain may be elicited on active movement. In most cases the pain ceases within a few days, and discoloration disappears in usually 2 to 3 weeks.

The major problem with contusions occurs where an area is subjected to repeated blows. If the same area, or more specifically the same muscle, is bruised over and over again, small calcium deposits might begin to accumulate in the injured area. These pieces of calcium might be found between several fibers in the muscle belly, or calcium might form a spur that projects from the underlying bone. These calcium formations, which can significantly impair movement, are referred to as *myositis ossificans.* In some cases myositis ossificans develops from a single trauma.[8]

The key to preventing myositis ossificans from occurring from repeated contusions is protection of the injured area by padding.[8] If the area is properly protected after the first contusion, myositis ossificans might never develop. Protection, along with rest, might allow the calcium to be reabsorbed and eliminate any need for surgical intervention. The two areas that seem to be the most vulnerable to repeated contusions during physical activity are the quadriceps muscle group on the front of the thigh and the biceps muscle on the front of the upper arm.[100] The formation of myositis ossificans in either of these or any other areas can be detected on X-ray films.

CLINICAL DECISION MAKING   **Exercise 2–8**

A field hockey player suffered a contusion from a ball on the elbow just superior to the medial epicondyle. She sustained some ulnar nerve damage. In general, what is the likelihood that the nerve will repair itself ?

INCORPORATING THERAPEUTIC EXERCISE TO AFFECT THE HEALING PROCESS

Rehabilitation exercise progressions can generally be subdivided into three phases, based primarily on the three stages of the healing process: phase 1, the acute phase; phase 2, the repair phase; and phase 3, the remodeling phase. Depending on the type and extent of injury and the individual response to healing, phases will usually overlap. Each phase must include carefully considered goals and criteria for progressing from one phase to another.[72]

Presurgical Exercise Phase

This phase would apply only to those patients who sustain injuries that require surgery. If surgery can be postponed, exercise may be used as a means to improve its outcome. By allowing the initial inflammatory-response phase to resolve, by maintaining or, in some cases, increasing muscle strength and flexibility, levels of cardiorespiratory fitness, and improving neuromuscular control, the patient may be better prepared to continue the exercise rehabilitative program after surgery.

Phase 1, the Acute Injury Phase

Phase 1 begins immediately when injury occurs and can last as long as day 4 following injury. During this phase, the inflammatory stage of the healing process is attempting to "clean up the mess," thus creating an environment that is conducive to the fibroblastic stage. As indicated in Chapter 1, the primary focus of rehabilitation during this stage is to control swelling and to modulate pain by using the PRICE (Protection, Restricted activity, Ice, Compression, and Elevation) technique immediately following injury. Ice, compression, and elevation should be used as much as possible during this phase[73] (Figure 2-13).

Rest of the injured part is critical during this phase. It is widely accepted that early mobility during rehabilitation is essential. However, if the athletic trainer becomes overly aggressive during the first 48 hours following injury, and does not allow the injured part to be rested during the inflammatory stage of healing, the inflammatory process never really gets a chance to accomplish what it is supposed

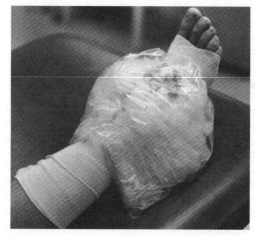

Figure 2-13   Musculoskeletal injuries should be treated initially with protection, restricted activity, ice, compression, and elevation.

to. Consequently, the length of time required for inflammation might be extended. Therefore, immobility during the first 24 to 48 hours following injury is necessary to control inflammation. If the injury involves the lower extremity, the patient should be encouraged to be non-weightbearing for the first 24 hours and progressively bear more weight as pain permits.

By day 2 or 3, swelling begins to subside and eventually stops altogether. The injured area may feel warm to the touch, and some discoloration is usually apparent. The injury is still painful to the touch, and some pain is elicited on movement of the injured part.[98] Following injury there will almost always be some loss in range of motion. Acutely that loss can be attributed primarily to pain and thus modalities (i.e., ice, electrical stimulation) which modulate pain should be routinely incorporated into each treatment session. At this point the patient should begin active mobility exercises, working through a pain-free range of motion. In this phase strengthening is less important than regaining range of motion but should not be entirely ignored.

A physician may choose to have the patient take NSAIDs to help control swelling and inflammation. It is usually helpful to continue this medication throughout the rehabilitative process.[2]

Phase 2, the Repair Phase

Once the inflammatory response has subsided, the repair phase begins. During this stage of the healing process, fibroblastic cells are laying down a matrix of collagen fibers and forming scar tissue. This stage might begin as early as 2 days after the injury and can last for several weeks. At this point, swelling has stopped completely. The injury is still tender to the touch but is not as painful as it was during the previous stage. There is less pain on active and passive motion.[73]

As soon as inflammation is controlled, the athletic trainer should immediately begin to incorporate into the rehabilitation program activities that can maintain levels of cardiorespiratory fitness, restore full range of motion, restore or increase strength, and reestablish neuromuscular control. The athletic trainer should design exercises that simultaneously challenge the neural, muscular, and articular systems to help the patient regain neuromuscular control. As neuromuscular control improves strength will also improve. The patient very quickly "forgets" how to correctly execute even simple motor patterns such as walking, and the central nervous system must relearn how to integrate visual, proprioceptive, and kinematic information that collectively produces coordinated movement.

As in the acute phase, modalities should be used to control pain and swelling. Cryotherapy should still be used

during the early portion of this phase to reduce the likelihood of swelling. Electrical stimulating currents can help with controlling pain and improving strength and range of motion.[73]

Phase 3, the Remodeling Phase

The remodeling phase is the longest of the three phases and can last for several years, depending on the severity of the injury. The ultimate goal during this maturation stage of the healing process is return to activity. The injury is no longer painful to the touch, although some progressively decreasing pain might still be felt on motion. The collagen fibers must be realigned according to tensile stresses and strains placed upon them during functional exercises.

The focus during this phase should be on regaining functional skills. Functional training involves the repeated performance of movement or skill for the purpose of perfecting that skill. Strengthening exercises should progressively place on the injured structures stresses and strains that would normally be encountered during activity. Plyometric strengthening exercises can be used to improve muscle power and explosiveness.[40] Functional testing should be done to determine specific skill weaknesses that need to be addressed prior to normal activity return.

At this point some type of heating modality is beneficial to the healing process. The deep-heating modalities, ultrasound, or the diathermies should be used to increase circulation to the deeper tissues. Massage and gentle mobilization may also be used to reduce guarding, increase circulation, and reduce pain. Increased blood flow delivers the essential nutrients to the injured area to promote healing, and increased lymphatic flow assists in breakdown and removal of waste products.[73]

USING MEDICATIONS TO AFFECT THE HEALING PROCESS

Medications are most commonly used in rehabilitation for pain relief. A patient may be continuously in pain that can be associated with even minor injury.

The over-the-counter nonnarcotic analgesics often used include aspirin (salicylate), acetaminophen, naproxen sodium ketoprofen, and ibuprofen. These belong to the group of drugs called nonsteroidal anti-inflammatory drugs (NSAIDs). Aspirin is one of the most commonly used drugs in the world.[78] Because of its easy availability, it is also likely the most misused drug. Aspirin is a derivative of salicylic acid and is used for its analgesic, anti-inflammatory, and antipyretic capabilities.

Analgesia can result from several mechanisms. Aspirin can interfere with the transmission of painful impulses in the thalamus.[78] Soft-tissue injury leads to tissue necrosis. This tissue injury causes the release of arachidonic acid from phospholipid cell walls. Oxygenation of arachidonic acid by cyclooxygenase produces a variety of prostaglandins, thromboxane, and prostacyclin that mediate the subsequent inflammatory reaction.[2] The predominant mechanism of action of aspirin and other NSAIDs is the inhibition of prostaglandin synthesis by blocking the cyclooxygenase pathway.[95] Pain and inflammation are reduced by the blockage of accumulation of proinflammatory prostaglandins in the synovium or cartilage.

Stabilization of the lysosomal membrane also occurs, preventing the efflux of destructive lysosomal enzymes into the joints.[47] Aspirin is the only NSAID that irreversibly inhibits cyclooxygenase; the other NSAIDs provide reversible inhibition. Aspirin can also reduce fever by altering sympathetic outflow from the hypothalamus, which produces increased vasodilation and heat loss through sweating.[22,47] Among the side effects of aspirin usage are gastric distress, heartburn, some nausea, tinnitus, headache, and diarrhea. More serious consequences can develop with prolonged use or high dosages.[3]

A patient should be very cautious about selecting aspirin as a pain reliever, for a number of reasons. Aspirin inhibits aggregation of platelets and thus impairs the clotting mechanism should injury occur.[3] Aspirin's irreversible inhibition of cyclooxygenase, which leads to reduced production of clotting factors, creates a bleeding risk not present with the other NSAIDs.[94] Prolonged bleeding at an injured site will increase the amount of swelling, which has a direct effect on the time required for rehabilitation.

Use of aspirin as an anti-inflammatory medication should be recommended with caution. Other antiinflammatory medications do not produce as many undesirable side effects as aspirin. Generally prescription antiinflammatories are considered to be equally effective.

Aspirin sometimes produces gastric discomfort. Buffered aspirin is no less irritating to the stomach than regular aspirin, but enteric-coated tablets resist aspirin breakdown in the stomach and might minimize gastric discomfort. Regardless of the form of aspirin ingested, it should be taken with meals or with large quantities of water (8–10 oz/tablet) to reduce the likelihood of gastric irritation.

Ibuprofen is classified as an NSAID; however, it also has analgesic and antipyretic effects, including the potential for gastric irritation. It does not affect platelet aggregation as aspirin does. Ibuprofen administered at a dose of 200 mg does not require a prescription and at that dosage may be used for analgesia. At a dose of 400 mg, the effects are both analgesic and anti-inflammatory.[9] Dosage forms greater than 200 mg require a prescription. For names and recommended doses of prescription NSAIDs, refer to Table 2–1.

Acetaminophen, like aspirin, has both analgesic and antipyretic effects, but it does not have significant anti-inflammatory capabilities. Acetaminophen is indicated for relief of mild somatic pain and fever reduction through mechanisms similar to those of aspirin.[3]

The primary advantage of acetaminophen is that it does not produce gastritis, irritation, or gastrointestinal bleeding. Likewise, it does not affect platelet aggregation and thus does not increase clotting time after an injury.[75]

For the patient who is not in need of an anti-inflammatory medication but who requires some pain-relieving medication or an antipyretic, acetaminophen should be the drug of choice. If inflammation is a consideration, physician may elect to use a type of NSAID. Most NSAIDs are prescription medications that, like aspirin, have not only anti-inflammatory but also analgesic and antipyretic effects.[47] They are effective for patients who cannot tolerate aspirin because of associated gastrointestinal distress. Patients who have the aspirin allergy triad of (1) nasal polyps, (2) associated bronchospams/asthma, and (3) history of anaphylaxis should not receive any NSAID. Caution is advised when using NSAIDs in persons who might be subject to dehydration. NSAIDs inhibit prostaglandin synthesis and therefore can compromise the elaboration of prostaglandins within the kidney during salt and/or water deficits. This can lead to ischemia within the kidney.[47,63] Adequate hydration is essential to reduce the risk of renal toxicity in patients taking NSAIDs.

NSAID anti-inflammatory capabilities are thought to be equal to those of aspirin, their advantages being that NSAIDs have fewer side effects and relatively longer duration of action. NSAIDs have analgesic and antipyretic capabilities; the short-acting over-the-counter NSAIDs may be used in cases of mild headache or increased body temperature in place of aspirin or acetaminophen. They can be used to relieve many other mildly to moderately painful somatic conditions like menstrual cramps and soft-tissue injury.[9]

It has been recommended that patients receiving long-acting NSAIDs have monitoring of liver function enzymes during the course of therapy because of case reports of hepatic failure associated with the use of long-acting NSAIDs.[74]

The NSAIDs are used primarily for reducing the pain, stiffness, swelling, redness, and fever associated with localized inflammation, most likely by inhibiting the synthesis of prostaglandins.[9] The athletic trainer must be aware

■ **TABLE   2-1**   **NSAIDs Frequently Used: Prescription Required**

Drug	Dosage Range (mg) And Frequency	Maximum Daily Dose (mg)
Aspirin	325–650, every 4 hours	4,000
Voltaren	50–75, twice a day	200
Cataflam	50–75, twice a day	200
Dolobid	500–1,000, followed by 250–500 mg 2–3 times a day	1,500
Nalfon	300–600, 3–4 times a day	3,200
Motrin	400–800, 3–4 times a day	3,200
Indocin	5–150, a day in 3–4 divided doses	200
Orudis	75, 3 times a day or 50 mg 4 times a day	300
Ponstel	500, followed by 250 mg every 6 hours	1,000
Naprosyn	250–500, twice a day	1,250
Anaprox	550, followed by 275 mg every 6–8 hours	1,375
Feldene	20, per day	20
Clinoril	200, twice a day	400
Tolectin	400, 3–4 times a day	1,800
Ansaid	50–100, 2–3 times a day	300
Toradol	10, every 4–6 hours for pain: Not to be used for more than 5 days	40
Lodine	200–400, every 6–8 hours for pain	1,200
Relafin	1,000, once or twice a day	2,000
Myobic	7.5, once per day	15
Daypro	1,200, once per day	1,800

that inflammation is simply a response to some underlying trauma or condition and that the source of irritation must be corrected or eliminated for these anti-inflammatory medications to be effective. Both naproxen and ketoprofen (now available without a prescription) have been shown to provide additional benefit when administered concomitantly with physical therapy.[63]

Muscle spasm and guarding accompany many musculoskeletal injuries. Elimination of this spasm and guarding should facilitate programs of rehabilitation. In many situations, centrally acting oral muscle relaxants are used to reduce spasm and guarding. However, to date the efficacy of using muscle relaxants has not been substantiated, and they do not appear to be superior to analgesics or sedatives in either acute or chronic conditions.[7]

Many analgesics and anti-inflammatory products are available over the counter in combination products (i.e., those containing two or more nonnarcotic analgesics with or without caffeine). Chronic use of analgesics containing aspirin and phenacetin or acetaminophen contributes to the development of papillary necrosis and analgesic-associated nephropathy. The presence of caffeine plays a role in dependency on these products leading to chronic use.

REHABILITATION PHILOSOPHY

The rehabilitation philosophy relative to inflammation and healing after injury is to assist the natural process of the body while doing no harm.[53] The course of rehabilitation chosen by athletic trainers must focus on their knowledge of the healing process and its therapeutic modifiers to guide, direct, and stimulate the structural function and integrity of the injured part. The primary goal should be to have a positive influence on the inflammation and repair process to expedite recovery of function in terms of range of motion, muscular strength and endurance, neuromuscular control, and cardiorespiratory endurance.[29] The athletic trainer must try to minimize the early effects of excessive inflammatory processes including pain modulation, edema control, and reduction of associated muscle spasm, which can produce loss of joint motion and contracture. Finally, the athletic trainer should concentrate on preventing the recurrence of injury by influencing the structural ability of the injured tissue to resist future overloads by incorporating various therapeutic exercises.[53] The subsequent chapters of this book can serve as a guide for the athletic trainer in using the many different rehabilitation tools available.

Summary

....

1. The three phases of the healing process are the inflammatory-response phase, the fibroblastic-repair phase, and the maturation-remodeling phase. These occur in sequence but overlap one another in a continuum.
2. Factors that can impede the healing process include edema, hemorrhage, lack of vascular supply, separation of tissue, muscle spasm, atrophy, corticosteroids, hypertrophic scars, infection, climate and humidity, age, health, and nutrition.
3. Ligament sprains involve stretching or tearing the fibers that provide stability at the joint.
4. Fractures can be classified as greenstick, transverse, oblique, spiral, comminuted, impacted, avulsive, or stress.
5. Osteoarthritis involves degeneration of the articular cartilage or subchondral bone.
6. Muscle strains involve a stretching or tearing of muscle fibers and their tendons and cause impairment to active movement.
7. Tendinitis, an inflammation of a muscle tendon that causes pain on movement, usually occurs because of overuse.
8. Tenosynovitis is an inflammation of the synovial sheath through which a tendon must slide during motion.
9. Dislocations and subluxations involve disruption of the joint capsule and ligamentous structures surrounding the joint.
10. Bursitis is an inflammation of the synovial membranes located in areas where friction occurs between various anatomic structures.
11. Muscle soreness can be caused by spasm, connective tissue damage, muscle tissue damage, or some combination of these.
12. Repeated contusions can lead to the development of myositis ossificans.
13. All injuries should be initially managed with protection, rest, ice, compression, and elevation to control swelling and thus reduce the time required for rehabilitation.
14. A patient who requires an analgesic for pain relief should be given acetaminophen because aspirin may produce gastric upset and slow clotting time.
15. For treating inflammation, NSAIDs are recommended because they do not produce many of the side effects associated with aspirin use.

....

References

1. Allen, T. 2004. Exercise-induced muscle damage: Mechanisms, prevention, and treatment. *Physiother Can* 56(2):67–79.
2. Almekinders, L. C. 1999. Anti-inflammatory treatment of muscular injuries in sport: An update of recent studies. *Sports Med* 28(6):383–388.
3. Alper, B. 2004. Evidence-based medicine. Update: Acetaminophen effective in osteoarthritis (NSAIDs more effective). *Clin Adv Nurse Pract* 7(12):98–99.
4. Arnoczky, S. P. 1991. Physiologic principles of ligament injuries and healing. In *Ligament and Extensor Mechanism Injuries of the Knee*, Scott W. N. ed. St. Louis, MO: Mosby.
5. Athanasiou, K. A., A. R. Shah, R. J. Hernandez, and R. G. LeBaron 2001. Basic science of articular cartilage repair. *Clin Sports Med* 20(2):223–247.
6. Bandy, W., and K. Dunleavy 1996. Adaptability of skeletal muscle: Response to increased and decreased use. In *Athletic Injuries and Rehabilitation*, Zachazewski, J., D. Magee and W. Quillen, eds. Philadelphia: WB Saunders.
7. Beebe, F. 2005. A clinical and pharmacologic review of skeletal muscle relaxants for musculoskeletal conditions. *Amer J Ther* 12(2):151–171.
8. Beiner, J. 2002. Muscle contusion injury and myositis ossificans traumatica. *Clin Orthop Relat Res* 403S(Suppl): S110–119.
9. Biederman, R. 2005. Pharmacology in rehabilitation: Nonsteroidal anti-inflammatory agents. *J Orthop Sports Phys Ther* 35(6):356–367.
10. Bottoni, C., and L. Hart. 2003. Recurrent shoulder dislocations after arthroscopic stabilization or nonoperative treatment. *Clin J Sport Med* 13(2):128–129.
11. Briggs, J. 2001. Soft and bony tissues–injury, repair and treatment implications. In *Sports Therapy: Theoretical and Practical Thoughts and Considerations*, Briggs, J. ed. Chichester, UK: Corpus.
12. Booher, J. M., and G. A. Thibodeau 2000. *Athletic Injury Assessment*, 4th ed. St. Louis, MO: McGraw-Hill.
13. Brothers, A. 2003. Basic clinical management of muscle strains and tears: Following appropriate treatment, most patients can return to sports activity. *J Musculoskelet Med* 20(6):303–307.
14. Bryant, M. W. 1997. Wound healing. *CIBA Clin Symp* 29(3):2–36.

15. Burra, G. 2002. Acute shoulder and elbow dislocations in the patient. *Orthop Clin N Am* 33(3):479–495.
16. Butler, D. Nerve structure, function, and physiology. 1996. In *Athletic Injuries and Rehabilitation.* Zachazewski, J., D. Magee and W. Quillen eds. Philadelphia: WB Saunders.
17. Cailliet, R. 1996 *Soft Tissue Pain and Disability,* 3rd ed. Philadelphia: F. A. Davis.
18. Carrico, T. J., A. I. Mehrhof and I. K., Cohen 1984. Biology and wound healing. *Surg Clin N Am* 64(4):721–734.
19. Clancy, W. 1990. Tendon trauma and overuse injuries. In *Sports-Induced Inflammation,* Leadbetter, W., J. Buckwalter, and S. Gordon, eds. Park Ridge, IL: American Academy of Orthopaedic Surgeons.
20. Clarkson, P. M., and I. Tremblay. 1988. Exercise-induced muscle damage, repair and adaptation in humans. *J Appl Physiol* 65:1–6.
21. Cox, D. 1993. Growth factors in wound healing. *J Wound Care* 2(6):339–342.
22. Curtis, J. 2005. A group randomized trial to improve safe use of nonsteroidal anti-inflammatory drugs. *Amer J Manag Care* 11(9):537–543.
23. Curwin, S. 1996. Tendon injuries, pathophysiology and treatment. In *Athletic Injuries and Rehabilitation,* Zachazewski J, D. Magee, and W. Quillen. eds. Philadelphia: WB Saunders.
24. Damjanov, I. 1996. *Anderson's Pathology,* 10th ed. St. Louis, MO: Mosby.
25. deVries, H. A. 1996. Quantitative EMG investigation of spasm theory of muscle pain. *Amer J Phys Med* 45:119–134.
26. Di Domenica, F. 2005. Physical and rehabilitative approaches in osteoarthritis. *Semin Arthritis Rheum* 34(6; Suppl 2):62–69.
27. Dieppe, P. 2005. Pathogenesis and management of pain in osteoarthritis. *Lancet* 365(9463):965–973.
28. Fantone, J. 1990. Basic concepts in inflammation. In *Sports-Induced Inflammation* Leadbetter W., J. Buckwalter, and S. Gordon, eds. Park Ridge, IL: American Academy of Orthopaedic Surgeons.
29. Felson, D. 2005. Osteoarthritis. *Curr Opin Rheumatol* 17(5): 624–656, 684–697.
30. Fitzgerald, G. K. 2000. Considerations for evaluation and treatment of overuse tendon injuries. *Athlet Ther Today* 5(4): 14–19.
31. Frank, C. 1996. Ligament injuries: Pathophysiology and healing. In *Athletic Injuries and, Rehabilitation* Zachazewski, J., D. Magee and W. Quillen. eds. Philadelphia: WB Saunders.
32. Frank, C., N. Shrive, H. Hiraoka, N. Nakamura, Y. Kaneda, and D. Hart 1990. Optimization of the biology of soft tissue repair. *J Sci Med Sport* 2(3):190–210.
33. Gelberman, R., V. Goldberg, and K-N An, et al. 1988. Soft tissue healing. In *Injury and Repair of Musculoskeletal Soft Tissues,* Woo, SL-Y, and J. Buckwalter, eds. Park Ridge, IL: American Academy of Orthopaedic Surgeons.
34. Glick, J. M. 1980. Muscle strains: Prevention and treatment. *Physician Sports Med* 8(11):73–77.
35. Goldenberg, M. 1996. Wound care management: Proper protocol differs from athletic trainers' perceptions. *J Athlet Train* 31(1):12–16.
36. Gradisar, I. A. 1985. Fracture stabilization and healing. In *Orthopaedic and Sports Physical Medicine,* Gould, J. A, and G. J. Davies, eds. St. Louis, MO: Mosby.
37. Gross, A., D. Cutright, and S. Bhaskar, et al. 1972 Effectiveness of pulsating water jet lavage in treatment of contaminated crush wounds. *Amer J Surg* 124:73–75.
38. Guyton, A. C., and J. Hell 2006. *Pocket Companion to Textbook of Medical Physiology.* Philadelphia: WB Saunders.
39. Hart, L. 2003. Effects of stretching on muscle soreness and risk of injury: A meta-analysis. *Clin J Sport Med* 13(5):321–322.
40. Henning, C. E. 1988. Semilunar cartilage of the knee: Function and pathology. In *Exercise and Sport Science Review,* Pandolf, K. B., ed. New York: Macmillan.
41. Hettinga, D. L. 1985. Inflammatory response of synovial joint structures. In *Orthopaedic and Sports Physical Therapy,* Gould, J. A., and G. J. Davies, eds. St. Louis, MO: Mosby.
42. Hole, J. 2007. *Human Anatomy and Physiology.* St. Louis, MO: McGraw-Hill.
43. Houglum, P. 1992. Soft tissue healing and its impact on rehabilitation. *J Sport Rehabil* 1(1):19–39.
44. Hubbel, S., and R. Buschbacher 1994. Tissue injury and healing: Using medications, modalities, and exercise to maximize recovery. In *Sports Medicine and Rehabilitation: A Sport Specific Approach,* Bushbacher, R. and R. Branddom, eds. Philadelphia: Hanley & Belfus.
45. James, C. B., and T. L. Uhl 2001. A review of articular cartilage pathology and the use of glucosamine sulfate. *J Athlet Train* 39(4): 413–419.
46. Junge, T. 2002. Bone healing. *Surg Technol* 34(5):26–29.
47. Kaplan, R. 2005. Current status of nonsteroidal anti-inflammatory drugs in physiatry: Balancing risks and benefits in pain management. *Amer J Phys Med Rehabil* 84(11): 885–894.
48. Khan, K. M., J. L. Cook, J. E. Taunton, and F. Bonar 2000. Overuse tendinosis, not tendinitis. Part 1: a new paradigm for a difficult clinical problem. *Physician Sports Med* 28(5): 38–43, 47–48.
49. Kelly, A. 2005. Managing stress fractures in patients. *J Musculoskelet Med* 22(9):463–465, 468–470, 472.
50. Kibler, W. B. 1990. Concepts in exercise rehabilitation of athletic injury. In *Sports-Induced Inflammation,* Leadbetter, W., J. Buckwalter, S. Gordon, eds. Park Ridge, IL: American Academy of Orthopaedic Surgeons.
51. Kibler, W. 2003. Current concepts in tendinopathy. *Clin Sports Med* 22(4):xi, xiii, 675–684.
52. Knight, K. L. 1995. *Cryotherapy in Sport Injury Management.* Champaign, IL: Human Kinetics.
53. Leadbetter, W. 1990. Introduction to sports-induced soft-tissue inflammation. In *Sports-Induced Inflammation,* Leadbetter, W., J. Buckwalter, and S. Gordon, eds. Park Ridge, IL: American Academy of Orthopaedic Surgeons.

54. Leadbetter, W., J. Buckwalter, and S. Gordon. 1990. *Sports-Induced Inflammation*. Park Ridge, IL: American Academy of Orthopaedic Surgeons.

55. Loitz-Ramage, B., and R. Zernicke 1996. Bone biology and mechanics. In *Athletic Injuries and Rehabilitation*, Zachazewski, J., D. Magee, and W. Quillen, eds. Philadelphia: WB Saunders.

56. Maffulli, N., and F. Benazzo 2000. Basic science of tendons. *Sports Med Arthrosc Rev* 8(1):1–5.

57. Marchesi, V. T. 1996. Inflammation and healing. In *Andersons' Pathology*, 9th ed., Kissane, J. M., ed. St. Louis, MO: Mosby.

58. Martinez-Hernanadez, A., and P. Amenta 1990. Basic concepts in wound healing. In *Sports-Induced Inflammation*, Leadbetter, W., J. Buckwalter, and S. Gordon, eds. Park Ridge, IL: American Academy of Orthopaedic Surgeons.

59. Matheson, G., J. MacIntyre, and J. Taunton 1989. Musculoskeletal injuries associated with physical activity in older adults. *Med Sci Sports Exerc* 21:379–385.

60. Malone, T., W. Garrett, and J. Zachewski. Muscle: Deformation, injury and repair. In *Athletic Injuries and Rehabilitation*, Zachazewski, J., D. Magee, and W. Quillen, eds. Philadelphia: WB Saunders.

61. Malone, T., and T. McPhoil, eds. 1997. *Orthopaedic and Sports Physical Therapy*. St. Louis, MO: Mosby.

62. Mayo Clinic 2002. Fracture healing: What it takes to heal a break. *Mayo Clin Health Lett* 20(2):1–3.

63. McCormack, K., and K. Brune 1993. Toward defining the analgesic role of non-steroidal anti-inflammatory drugs in the management of acute and soft tissue injuries. *Sports Med* 3:106–117.

64. Mehta, J. 2004. Elbow dislocations in adults and children. *Clin Sports Med* 23(4):609–627.

65. Murrell, G. A. C., D. Jang, E. Lily, and T. Best 1999. The effects of immobilization and exercise on tendon healing–abstract. *J Sci Med Sport* 2(1 Suppl):40.

66. Levangie, P., and C. Norkin 2005. *Joint Structure and Function: A Comprehensive Analysis*. Philadelphia: FA Davis.

67. Norris, S., B. Provo, and N. Stotts 1990. Physiology of wound healing and risk factors that impede the healing process. *AACN Clin Issues Crit Care Nurs* 1(3):545–552.

68. Ng, G. 2002. Ligament injury and repair: Current concepts. *Hong Kong Physiother J* 20:22–29.

69. O'Reilly, K., M. Warhol, and R. Fielding, et al. 1987. Eccentric exercise induced muscle damage impairs muscle glycogen depletion. *J Appl Physiol* 63:252–256.

70. Panush, R. S., and D. G. Brown 1987. Exercise and arthritis. *Sports Med* 4:54–64.

71. Peterson, L., and P. Renstrom 2001. Injuries in musculoskeletal tissues. In *Sports Injuries: Their Prevention and Treatment*, 3rd ed. Peterson, L., ed., Champaign, IL: Human Kinetics.

72. Prentice, W. 2009. *Arnheim's Principles of Athletic Training*, 13th ed. New York: McGraw-Hill.

73. Prentice, W.E., ed. 2009. *Therapeutic Modalities in Sports Medicine and Athletic Training*. New York: McGraw-Hill.

74. Purdum, P., S. Shelden, and J. Boyd 1994. Oxaprozinin-duced hepatitis. *Ann Pharmacother* 28:1159–1161.

75. Rahusen, F. 2004. Nonsteroidal anti-inflammatory drugs and acetaminophen in the treatment of an acute muscle injury. *Amer J Sports Med* 32(8):1856–1859.

76. Robbins, S. L., R. S. Cotran, and V. Kumar 2004. *Pathologic Basis of Disease*, 3rd ed. New York: Elsevier Science.

77. Rywlin, A. M. 1996. Hemopoietic system. In *Anderson's Pathology*, 8th ed. Kissane, J. M., ed. St. Louis, MO: Mosby.

78. Sachs, C. 2005. Oral analgesics for acute nonspecific pain. *Amer Fam Physician* 71(5):913–918, 847–849.

79. Saladin, K. 2006. *Anatomy and Physiology*. New York: McGraw-Hill.

80. Sanderlin, B. 2003. Common stress fractures. *Amer Fam Physician* 68(8):1527–1532, 1478–1479.

81. Sandrey, M. A. 2000. Effects of acute and chronic pathomechanics on the normal histology and biomechanics of tendons: A review. *J Sport Rehabil* 9(4):339–352.

82. Schenck, R. 2003. Classification of knee dislocations. *Oper Tech Sports Med* 11(3):193–198.

83. Seeley, R., T. Stephens, and P. Tate 2005. *Anatomy and Physiology*. St. Louis, MO: McGraw-Hill.

84. Seller, R. H. 2007. *Differential Diagnosis of Common Complaints*. Philadelphia: Elsevier Health Sciences.

85. Sharma, P. 2005. Tendon injury and tendinopathy: Healing and repair. *J Bone Joint Surg* 87A(1):187–202.

86. Shrier, I., and S. Stovitz 2005. Best of the literature: Do anti-inflammatory agents promote muscle healing? *Physician Sports Med* 33(6):12.

87. Stanish W. D., S. Curwin, and S. Mandell 2000. *Tendinitis: Its Etiology and Treatment*. Oxford: Oxford University Press.

88. Soto-Quijano, D. 2005. Work-related musculoskeletal disorders of the upper extremity. *Crit Rev Phys Rehabil Med* 17(1):65–82.

89. Stewart, J. 2001. *Clinical Anatomy and Physiology*. Miami, FL: MedMaster.

90. Stone, M. H. 1988. Implications for connective tissue and bone alterations resulting from rest and exercise training. *Med Sci Sports Exerc* 20(5):S162–168.

91. Terry, M., and A. L. Fincher 2000. Postoperative management of articular cartilage repair. *Athlet Ther Today* 5(2):57–58.

92. Tuan, K. 2004. Stress fractures in patients: Risk factors, diagnosis, and management. *Orthopedics* 27(6):583–593.

93. Van de Graaff, K. 2006. *Human Anatomy*. New York: McGraw-Hill.

94. Vane, J. 1971. Inhibition of prostaglandin synthesis as a mechanism of action for aspirin-like drugs. *Nature (New Biol)* 231:232–235.

95. Vane, J. 1987. The evolution of nonsteroidal anti-inflammatory drugs and their mechanism of action. *Drugs* 33(1):18–27.

96. Walker, J. 1996. Cartilage of human joints and related structures. In *Athletic Injuries and Rehabilitation*, Zachazewski J., D, Magee, and W. Quillen, eds. Philadelphia: WB Saunders.

97. Wahl, S., and P. Renstrom. 1990. Fibrosis in soft-tissue injuries. In *Sports-Induced Inflammation*, Leadbetter, W., J. Buckwalter, and S. Gordon, eds. Park Ridge, IL: American Academy of Orthopaedic Surgeons.

98. Wells, P. E., V. Frampton, and D. Bowsher. 1988. *Pain Management in Physical Therapy*. Norwalk, CT: Appleton & Lange.

99. Wilder, R. 2004. Overuse injuries: Tendinopathies, stress fractures, compartment syndrome, and shin splints. *Clin Sports Med* 23(1):55–81.

100. Wissen, W. T. 2000. An aggressive approach to managing quadriceps contusions. *Athlet Ther Today* 5(1):36–37.

101. Woo, SL-Y, and J. Buckwalter, eds. 1988. *Injury and Repair of Musculoskeletal Soft Tissues*. Park Ridge, IL: American Academy of Orthopaedic Surgeons.

102. Wroble, R. R. 2000. Articular cartilage injury and autologous chondrocyte implantation: Which patients might benefit? *Phys Sports Med* 28(11):43–49.

103. Zachezewski, J. 1990. Flexibility for sports. In *Sports Physical Therapy*, Sanders, B., ed. Norwalk, CT: Appleton & Lange.

SOLUTIONS TO CLINICAL DECISION MAKING EXERCISES

2-1   Immediate action to control swelling can expedite the healing process. The athletic trainer should first provide compression and elevation. Applying ice, which decreases the metabolic demands of the uninjured cells, can prevent secondary hypoxic injury. Ice also slows nerve conduction velocity, which will decrease pain and thus limit muscle guarding.

2-2   The athletic trainer should explain to the coach that it can take up to 3 or 4 days for the inflammatory response to subside. During this time, the muscle is initializing repair by containing the injury by clot formation. Too much stress during this time could increase the time it takes the muscle to heal. After that, it may take a couple of weeks before fibroblastic and myoblastic activity has restored tissue strength to a point where the tissue can withstand the stresses of training.

2-3   Muscle healing generally takes longer. While fibroblasts are laying down new collagen for connective tissue repair, myoblasts are working to replace the contractile tissue.

2-4   Once the injured structure has progressed through the inflammatory phase and repair has begun, sufficient tensile stress should be provided to ensure optimal repair and positioning of the new fibers (according to Wolff 's law). Efforts should be made right away to avoid the strength loss that comes with immobility due to pain.

2-5   The presence of gross laxity would suggest a grade 3 sprain. The athlete should be referred to the team physician for further evaluation.

2-6   In a complete ligament tear, it is likely that the nerves in that structure will also be completely disrupted. Therefore, no pain signals can be transmitted.

2-7   It is likely that this young boy has a greenstick fracture. Such fractures are common in athletes of this age.

2-8   Peripheral nerves are likely to regenerate if the cell body has not been damaged. The closer the injury is to the cell body, the more difficult the healing process is. If a nerve is severed, surgical intervention can significantly improve chances of regeneration.

CHAPTER 3

The Evaluation Process in Rehabilitation

Darin A. Padua

After completion of this chapter, the athletic training student should be able to do the following:

- Identify the components of the systematic differential evaluation process.

- Explain the role of the systematic injury evaluation process in establishing a rehabilitation plan and treatment goals.

- Describe various ways to differentiate between normal and pathological tissue.

- Discuss special tests that should be incorporated into an evaluation scheme.

- Review ways to perform injury risk screenings and describe how the findings can be incorporated into injury prevention training programs.

- Recognize how to establish short-term and long-term rehabilitation goals based on the findings of the injury evaluation.

Injury evaluation is the foundation of the rehabilitation process. To effectively coordinate the rehabilitation process, the athletic trainer must be able to perform a systematic differential evaluation and identify the pathological tissue. According to Cyriax,[5] the injury evaluation process involves applying one's knowledge of anatomy to differentiate between provoked and normal tissue:

Provoked tissue − Normal tissue = Pathological tissue

Once the pathological tissue is identified, the athletic trainer must then consider the contraindications and determine the appropriate course of treatment:

Pathological tissue − Contraindications = Treatment (rehabilitation plan)

The athletic trainer determines the appropriate rehabilitation goals and plan based on the information gathered from the evaluation. In designing the rehabilitation plan, the athletic trainer must consider the severity, irritability, nature, and stage of the injury.[21] Throughout the rehabilitation process, the athletic trainer must continuously reevaluate the status of the pathological tissue in order to make appropriate adjustments to the rehabilitation goals and plan.

The athletic trainer might conduct multiple injury evaluations of the following kinds for varying purposes during the course of athletic injury management:

1. On-site evaluation at the time of injury (on-field)
2. On-site evaluation just following injury (sideline)
3. Off-site evaluation that involves the injury assessment and rehabilitation plan
4. Follow-up evaluation during the rehabilitation process to determine the patient's progress
5. Preparticipation physical evaluation (preseason screening)

All forms of injury evaluation will involve similar steps and procedures. However, it is important to note the difference between the on-site injury evaluation processes and the off-site evaluation performed when designing a rehabilitation program. The goal of an on-site injury evaluation is to quickly, but thoroughly, evaluate the patient and determine the injury severity, whether immobilization is needed, whether medical referral is needed, and the manner of transportation from the field. The off-site injury evaluation is more detailed and used to gain information to effectively design the rehabilitation program. This chapter will focus on the steps and procedures involved during the off-site injury evaluation and incorporating this information into the rehabilitation plan.

THE SYSTEMATIC DIFFERENTIAL EVALUATION PROCESS

The key to a successful injury evaluation is to establish a sequential and systematic approach that is followed in every case. A systematic approach allows the athletic trainer to be confident that a thorough evaluation has been performed. However, the athletic trainer must keep in mind that each injury may be unique in some manner. Thus, the athletic trainer must maintain a systematic approach but not be inflexible during the evaluation process. The Injury Evaluation Checklist in Figure 3-1 is provided as an example of the steps and procedures that may be included in a sequential and systematic evaluation scheme.

The systematic differential evaluation process is composed of subjective and objective elements. During the **subjective evaluation** the athletic trainer gathers information on the injury history and the symptoms experienced by the patient. This is performed through an initial interview with the patient. The athletic trainer attempts to relate information gathered during the subjective evaluation to observable signs and other quantitative findings obtained during the objective evaluation. The **objective evaluation** involves observation and inspection, acute injury palpation, range of motion assessment (active and passive), muscle strength testing, special tests, neurological assessment, subacute or chronic injury palpation, and functional testing. After completing the subjective and objective evaluation, the athletic trainer will arrive at an assessment of the injury based on the information gathered.

Subjective Evaluation

The subjective evaluation is the foundation for the rest of the evaluation process. Perhaps the single most revealing component of the injury evaluation is the information gathered during the subjective evaluation. Essentially, during the subjective evaluation the athletic trainer engages in an orderly, sequential process of questions and dialogue with the patient. In addition to gathering information about the injury, the subjective evaluation serves to establish a level of comfort and trust between the patient and the athletic trainer.

The injury history and the symptoms are the key elements of the subjective evaluation. A detailed injury history is the most important portion of the evaluation. The remainder of the evaluation will focus on confirming the information taken from the patient's history.

History of Injury.   In gathering a detailed history, the athletic trainer should focus on gathering information relative to the patient's impression of the injury, site of injury, mechanism of injury, previous injuries, and general medical health. The history should be taken in an orderly sequence. This information will then be used to determine the appropriate components to incorporate during the objective evaluation.

When taking the patient's history, the athletic trainer should initially use nonleading, open-ended questions. As the subjective evaluation progresses, the athletic trainer may move to more close-ended questions once a clear picture of the injury has been presented. Open-ended questions involve narrative information about the injury; close-ended questions ask for specific information.[13]

The history relies on the athletic trainer's ability to clearly communicate with the injured patient. Thus, the athletic trainer should avoid the use of scientific and medical jargon and use simple terminology that is easy to understand. The use of simple terminology ensures that the patient will understand any close-ended questions the athletic trainer may ask.

Patient's impression.   Allow the patient to describe in his or her own words how the injury occurred, where the injury is located, and how they feel. While listening to the patient, the athletic trainer should be generating close-ended questions. Once the patient has given his or her impression of the injury the athletic trainer should ask more specific questions that fill in specific details.

Site of injury.   Have the patient describe the general area where the injury occurred or pain is located. Further isolate the site of injury by having the patient point with one finger to the exact location of injury or pain. If the patient is able to locate a specific area of injury or pain, the athletic trainer should make note of the anatomic structures in the general area and consider this tissue as provoked tissue. A major purpose of the remaining evaluation phases is to further differentiate the identified provoked tissue from the normal tissue.[5] Differentiating between

SUBJECTIVE PHASE

History
____ Patient's impression
____ Site of injury
____ Mechanism of injury
____ Previous injury
____ Behavior of symptoms (PQRST)
 ____ Provocation of symptoms
 ____ Quality of symptoms
 ____ Region of symptoms
 ____ Severity of symptoms
 ____ Timing of symptoms

OBJECTIVE PHASE

Observation and Inspection
____ Postural alignment (see postural alignment checklist)
____ Gait (lower-extremity injury) or upper-extremity functional motion (upper-extremity injury)
____ Signs of trauma
 ____ Deformity
 ____ Bleeding
 ____ Swelling
 ____ Atrophy
 ____ Skin color

Palpation
____ Temperature
____ Dermatome assessment
____ Bone palpation
____ Soft tissue palpation
 ____ Muscle
 ____ Tendon
 ____ Ligament and joint capsule
 ____ Superficial nerves
*Palpate all structures accessible in a specific position before repositioning patient.
*Palpate areas above and below the injured region.

Range of Motion
____ Active range of motion
____ Passive range of motion
____ Resistive range of motion
*Perform range-of-motion testing in all cardinal planes of motion.
*Assess end-feels by applying overpressure.
*Assess arthrokinematic motions if normal range of motion altered.
*Be aware of capsular patterns for specific joint tested

Resistive Strength Testing
____ Mid-range of motion muscle tests
____ Specific muscle tests
*Specific muscle tests should be based on results of mid-range of motion muscle tests
*Rate or grade strength assessment

Figure 3-1 Injury evaluation checklist.

Muscle Imbalances
____ Review range of motion and resistive strength testing findings

*Determine whether muscle imbalances appear to exist

Special Tests
____ Joint stability tests
____ Joint compression tests
____ Passive tendon stretch tests
____ Diagnostic tests

Neurologic Testing
____ Dermatomes
____ Myotomes
____ Reflexes
 ____ Deep tendon reflexes
 ____ Superficial reflexes
 ____ Pathologic reflexes

Functional Testing
____ Movement patterns that facilitate similar stresses as encountered during normal activity (i.e., activity specific)

Figure 3-1 (continued)

provoked tissue and **normal tissue** allows the athletic trainer to identify the **pathological tissue.**[5] The athletic trainer must be able to identify the pathological tissue in order to develop an appropriate rehabilitation plan.

 Mechanism of injury. Musculoskeletal injury results from forces acting on the anatomic structures and ultimately results in tissue failure. Thus, it is imperative to identify the nature of the forces acting on the body and relate these to the anatomic function of the underlying anatomic structures. The athletic trainer should determine whether the injury was caused by a single traumatic force (macrotrauma) or resulted from the accumulation of repeated forces (microtrauma). In dealing with an acute injury, it is important to identify the body position at time of injury, the direction of applied force, the magnitude of applied force, and the point of application of the applied force. The athletic trainer must then apply knowledge of anatomy, biomechanics, and tissue mechanics to determine which tissues may have been injured. When dealing with recurrent or chronic injuries, it is important to establish what factors influence the patient's symptoms, such as changes in training, routine, equipment use, and posture. The accumulation of this information should be used to further identify the pathological tissue.

 Any sound or sensation noted at the moment of or immediately after injury is also important information to gather. The athletic trainer may be able to relate certain sounds and sensations with possible injuries, hence identifying pathological tissue:

- Pop = joint subluxation, ligament tear
- Clicking = cartilage or meniscal tear
- Locking = cartilage or meniscal tear (loose body)
- Giving way = reflex inhibition of muscles in an attempt to minimize muscle or joint loading

 Previous injury. Tissue reinjury or injury of tissue surrounding previously injured tissue is common. The athletic trainer should determine whether the current injury is similar to previous injuries. If so, what anatomic structures were previously injured? How often has the injury recurred? How was the previous injury managed, from a rehabilitation standpoint? Have there been any residual effects since the original injury? Was surgery or medication given for the previous injury? Who evaluated the previous injury?

 Previous injuries may influence the evaluation process of the current injury as well as the rehabilitation plan. Secondary pathology may be present in cases of recurrent injury, such as excessive scar tissue development, reduced soft-tissue elasticity, muscle contracture, inhibition or weakness of surrounding musculature, altered postural alignment, increased joint laxity, or diminished joint play/accessory motions. The athletic trainer must consider these possibilities and investigate them during the objective evaluation.

Behavior of Symptoms.   During the second phase of the subjective evaluation, the athletic trainer explores specific details of the symptoms discovered during the history. Again, this should be performed in a systematic and sequential process. Moore[14] describes the PQRST mnemonic to guide this phase of the subjective evaluation (P = provocation or cause of symptoms; Q = quality or description of symptoms; R = region of symptoms; S = severity of symptoms; T = time symptoms occur or recur).

Provocation of symptoms.   This information is primarily gathered through a detailed mechanism-of-injury description by the patient. Additional information may be gathered by asking the patient if they are able to recreate their symptoms by performing certain movements. However, the athletic trainer should not have the patient recreate these movements at this phase of the evaluation. This will be performed during range-of-motion assessment in the objective evaluation.

Typically, musculoskeletal pain is worse with movement and better with rest. Symptoms caused by excessive inflammation may be constant and not alleviated with rest. Symptoms associated with prolonged postures may be indicative of prolonged stress being placed on the surrounding soft-tissue structures, which ultimately causes breakdown.

Quality of symptoms.   The patient should be asked to describe the quality of their symptoms. The patient might describe their pain as being sharp, dull, aching, burning, or tingling. The athletic trainer should attempt to relate the patient description of the quality of symptoms to possible pathological tissue. Magee[13] describes different descriptions of the quality of symptoms as being associated with different anatomic structures:

- Nerve pain: sharp, bright, shooting (tingling), along line of nerve distribution
- Bone pain: deep, nagging, dull, localized
- Vascular pain: diffuse, aching, throbbing, poorly localized, may be referred
- Muscular pain: hard to localize, dull, aching, may be referred

Region of symptoms.   The majority of this information is given during the patient's description of the site of injury. The region of symptoms might correlate with underlying injured or pathological tissue. However, the athletic trainer must be aware of possible referred pain patterns and not assume that the pathological tissue is located directly within the region of symptoms. Once the region of symptoms has been identified, there are several other items that should be noted. Do the symptoms stay localized, or do they spread to peripheral areas? Do the symptoms feel deep or superficial? Do the symptoms seem to be located within the joint or in the surrounding area?

Pain that radiates to other areas may be due to pressure on the nerve or from active trigger points in the myofascial tissue. Symptoms that are well localized in a small area might indicate minor injury or chronic injury. Symptoms that are diffuse in nature may be indicative of more severe injury.

Severity of symptoms.   The severity of symptoms may give insight into the severity of injury. However, the athletic trainer should be cautions in equating the patient's description of severity with actual injury severity. Individuals' perceptions of severity are highly subjective and likely vary to a large extent from one person to the next. Hence, information relative to perceived severity of symptoms is an unreliable indicator of injury severity. More appropriately, reports of symptom severity may be used during the rehabilitation process to track the patient's progress. Improvement of symptoms indicates that the rehabilitation plan is succeeding. Worsening of symptoms may indicate that the injury is getting worse or that the rehabilitation plan is not appropriate at this time.

The patient should quantify their pain in order to most efficiently track the patient's progress during the rehabilitation process. The athletic trainer should instruct the patient to rate their pain on a scale of 0 to 10, where 0 is no pain (normal) and 10 is the worst pain imaginable. Having the patient rate their pain does not provide an objective assessment. Rather, this information will be used to make relative comparisons of the patient's progress during rehabilitation.[10]

Timing of symptoms.   The onset of symptoms may help determine the nature of the injury. Symptoms with a slow and insidious onset that tend to progressively worsen over time are often associated with repetitive microtrauma. In contrast, macrotrauma injuries typically result in a sudden, identifiable onset of symptoms. Injuries resulting from repetitive microtrauma may include stress fractures, trigger point formation, tendinitis, or other chronic inflammatory conditions. Macrotraumatic injuries may result in ligament sprains, muscle strains, acute bone fractures, or other acute soft-tissue injuries.

Duration and frequency of symptoms may be used to determine whether the injury is progressing or worsening. An improvement in symptoms is demonstrated by reductions in their duration and frequency. The opposite may be reported in the situation of a worsening injury.

Response of symptoms to activity or rest may also be used to identify the nature of the injury. Magee[13] describes several injury classifications that may be related to the response of symptoms to activity or rest:

- Joint adhesion = pain during activity that decreases with rest
- Chronic inflammation and edema = initial morning pain and stiffness that is reduced with activity

- Joint congestion = pain or aching that progressively worsens throughout the day with activity
- Acute inflammation = pain at rest and pain that is worse at the beginning of activity in comparison to the end of activity
- Bone pain or organic/systemic disorders = pain that is not influenced by either rest or activity
- Peripheral nerve entrapment = pain that tends to worsen at night
- Intervertebral disc involvement = pain that increases with forward or lateral trunk bending

Objective Evaluation

At the completion of the subjective evaluation the athletic trainer should have developed a list of potential provoked tissues. In some cases, the experienced athletic trainer may be able to identify the specific injury and pathological tissue at this point of the evaluation. During the objective evaluation, the athletic trainer will perform several procedures as a process of eliminating normal tissue from being considered as provoked tissue. These procedures will serve to differentiate between provoked and normal tissues, allowing the pathological tissue to be identified.

The athletic trainer should plan the objective evaluation.[14] After completing the subjective evaluation, the athletic trainer should create a mental list of specific procedures and tests to perform during the objective evaluation. At this point the athletic trainer may expect to get specific findings during the objective evaluation. However, the athletic trainer is reminded to stay open-minded and not become too focused during this stage of the evaluation.

Observation and Inspection.   The beginning of the objective evaluation consists of a visual inspection of the injured patient as they enter the medical facility. The athletic trainer focuses on the patient's overall appearance and specific body regions that were identified during the subjective evaluation as being a potential site of provoked tissue. For example, if the lower extremity is identified as a potential area of injury, the athletic trainer will pay close attention to the patient's gait patterns. If an upper-extremity injury is suspected, the carrying position of the injured extremity and movement patterns when removing an item of clothing would be noted. In observing the patient's movement patterns, the athletic trainer should be looking for compensatory patterns, muscle guarding, antalgic movements, and facial expressions. All observations should be made with a bilateral comparison of the uninvolved side.

Postural alignment.   Overall postural alignment should be assessed during the observation, especially in patients suffering from chronic or overuse-type injuries.[12,13,22] Many chronic and overuse injuries are due to postural malalignments that create repeated stress on a specific tissue. Over time the repeatedly loaded tissue may become pathological or lead to additional postural alignment alterations as compensatory mechanisms to reduce tissue stress. In addition, postural alignment can influence muscle function.

If postural malalignments are present, the athletic trainer should consider the patterns of muscle tightness and weakness that would correspond to such a postural malalignment. Altered postural alignment can be caused by muscle imbalances, not just bony deformity.[2,3] It is important that the athletic trainer determine whether postural malalignments are due to muscle imbalances or bony deformity, as this might influence the rehabilitation options. Postural malalignments that are due to muscle imbalances may be addressed through physical rehabilitation using appropriate muscle flexibility and strengthening techniques to restore muscle balance, hence improving normal postural alignment.

There are many elements involved with a detailed postural alignment assessment. The athletic trainer may consider using a checklist approach to ensure that all elements are covered. It is important that the patient be viewed in a weightbearing position (standing) from multiple vantage points (anterior, posterior, medial, lateral). In general, the athletic trainer should be checking for neutral alignment, symmetry, balanced muscle tone, and specific postural deformities (genu valgum, genu varum, etc.). A detailed checklist for postural alignment is provided as an example in Figure 3-2.

Signs of trauma.   During the postural alignment assessment, the athletic trainer should also be checking

---

CLINICAL DECISION MAKING   **Exercise 3–1**

While taking a patient's history, the athletic trainer records the following information:

- Site of pain: Knee joint
- Mechanism of injury: Direct blow to knee causing knee to be forced into excessive valgus and rotation
- Behavior of symptoms: Pain is described as "deep, nagging, dull, and localized," pain increases with weight bearing, reports a clicking and locking sensation in knee joint

Based on the findings from the history, what types of special tests should the athletic trainer consider performing?

Frontal View (Anterior): Arms relaxed, palms facing lateral thighs

Line bisecting: (plumb line)
____ Nose
____ Mouth
____ Sternum
____ Umbilicus
____ Pubic bones

Level:
____ Earlobes
____ Acromion process
____ Nipples
____ Fingertip ends
____ Anterior superior iliac spine
____ Greater trochanter
____ Patella
____ Medial malleoli

Neutral Rotational Alignment
____ Shoulder (direction of olecranon process)
____ Patella
____ Feet (direction of toes)

Balanced Muscle Tone
____ Deltoids
____ Trapezius
____ Pectoralis major
____ Quadriceps

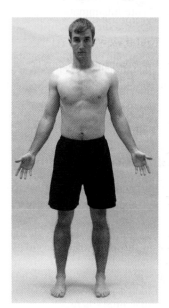

Is there evidence of:

Cubitus valgus	L	R	B
Cubitus varus	L	R	B
Internal shoulder rotation	L	R	B
External shoulder rotation	L	R	B
Pes planus	L	R	B
Pes cavus	L	R	B
Forefoot valgus	L	R	B
Forefoot varus	L	R	B
Hallux valgus	L	R	B
Genu valgus	L	R	B
Genu varus	L	R	B
Internal tibial rotation	L	R	B
External tibial rotation	L	R	B
Femoral anteversion	L	R	B
Femoral retroversion	L	R	B
Unequal weight bearing	L	R	

Line bisecting: (plumb line)
____ External auditory meatus
____ Cervical vertebral bodies
____ Acromion process

Figure 3-2   Postural alignment checklist.

_____ Deltoid
_____ Mid-thoracic region

Asymmetric stance width   L   R

Frontal view (posterior)

Line bisecting: (plumb line)
_____   Head
_____   Cervical through lumbar spinous processes
_____   Sacrum

Level:
_____   Earlobes
_____   Acromion process
_____   Inferior angle of scapula
_____   Gluteal fold
_____   Posterior superior Iliacs spine
_____   Greater trochanter
_____   Popliteal crease
_____   Medial malleoli

Normal Scapular Alignment:
_____   Vertebral borders rest against thorax
_____   Superior and inferior angles are equal distance from vertebrae
_____   Superior and inferior angles sit at ribs 2 and 7, respectively

Perpendicular to Floor
_____   Line bisecting calcaneus
_____   Line bisecting Achilles tendon

Balanced Muscle Tone
_____   Trapezius
_____   Deltoids
_____   Rhomboids
_____   Latissimus dorsi
_____   Erector spinae group
_____   Gluteus maximus
_____   Hamstrings
_____   Triceps surae

Is there evidence of?

Winging scapula	L	R	B
Rearfoot valgus	L	R	B
Rearfoot varus	L	R	B
Scoliosis	L	R	S
Lateral shift		L	R

Saggital View (bilateral)

Line bisecting: (plumb line)
_____   External auditory meatus
_____   Cervical vertebral bodies
_____   Acromion process

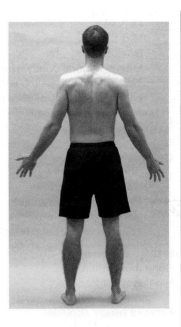

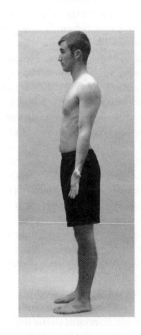

Figure 3-2(continued)

_____ Deltoid
_____ Mid-thoracic region
_____ Greater trochanter
_____ Lateral femoral condyle (slightly anterior)
_____ Tibia (parallel to plumb line)
_____ Lateral malleolus (slightly posterior)

Level:
_____ ASIS and PSIS

General (normal)
_____ Chin tucked slightly
_____ Mild cervical curvature
_____ Mild thoracic curvature
_____ Mild lumbar curve
_____ Knees straight, but not locked

Is there evidence of?

Genu recurvatum	L	R	B
Hip flexor contracture (anterior pelvic tilt)	L	R	B
Forward head / shoulder	L	R	B

Figure 3-2 (continued)

for signs of trauma. In acute injuries, observing for signs of trauma might be the primary purpose of the observation. Gross deformity along the bone's long axis or joint line may be present in cases of fractures of joint dislocations. Visible swelling, bleeding, or signs of infection at the injury site should also be noted, as should the nature of its onset. Swelling that is rapid and immediate could be indicative of acute trauma; gradual and slow-onset swelling may be more indicative of chronic overuse injury. The athletic trainer should attempt to quantify the amount of swelling by taking girth or volumetric measurements. Quantification of swelling can help establish rehabilitation goals and aid in tracking rehabilitation progress. Atrophy of the surrounding muscles may be present in the case of chronic injury. Skin color and texture should also be assessed. The patient's skin might have red (inflammation), blue (cyanosis, indicating vascular compromise), or black-blue (contusion), coloration. If the skin appears to be shiny, to have lost elasticity, or to have lost overlying hair, or if there is skin breakdown, there might be a peripheral nerve lesion.

The information collected during the observation should be related to the findings of the subjective evaluation. This will allow the athletic trainer to further confirm or differentiate possible pathological tissue.

CLINICAL DECISION MAKING   **Exercise 3–2**

As you assess a patient's postural alignment, you observe excessive anterior pelvic tilting and increased lumbar lordosis. How would these observations guide your evaluation during the range-of-motion and resistive strength-testing phases?

Palpation

The question of when palpation should be performed during the objective evaluation is debatable. Some feel that palpation should be performed immediately following the observation; others feel that palpation should be performed later during the objective evaluation. If an acute injury is being evaluated, palpation may be appropriate immediately following observation in order to detect any obvious, but not visible, soft-tissue or bony deformities.[14] Such findings may warrant termination of the evaluation and immediate referral to a physician. However, if the injury is subacute or chronic in nature, palpation may be performed later in the objective evaluation. The disadvantage of performing palpation early in the objective evaluation is that such manual probing can elicit a pain response that will distract from findings during the later subphases of the objective evaluation (range-of-motion, strength, and special tests).[15]

Regardless of when palpation is performed, the primary purpose of palpation is to localize as closely as possible the potential pathological tissues involved. To gain the patient's confidence, palpation should start with a gentle and assuring touch and the trainer should frequently communicate with the patient. Palpation should be performed in a sequential manner and include the anatomic and joint structures that are above and below the site of the injury. Palpation should begin on the uninjured side so that the patient knows what to expect and the examiner knows what is "normal" and has an objective comparison when palpating the injured side. Palpation of the injured side begins with the anatomic structures distal to the site of pain and then progressively works toward the potential pathological tissues. To systematically palpate all possible tissues, it may be helpful to develop a specific sequencing of tissues to palpate.[22] For example, the athletic trainer might first palpate all bones, then ligaments and tendons, and then the muscles and corresponding tendons. Consideration should be given to positioning of the patient as one develops the sequencing of tissues to palpate. Minimizing patient movement is important, as excessive motion can cause the patient's symptoms to worsen. Thus, the athletic trainer should palpate all possible anatomic structures in a given position prior to repositioning the patient.

During palpation, the athletic trainer should take note of point tenderness, trigger points, tissue quality, crepitus, temperature, and symmetry.[9,10,13 - 16,21,22] Point tenderness is noted by indications of pain over the area being palpated. If point tenderness is noted, the patient should be asked to rate their point tenderness on a scale of 0 to 10, where 0 is no pain (normal) and 10 is the worst pain imaginable. Similar to rating one's symptoms, this does not provide an objective assessment. Rather, this information will be used to make relative comparisons of the patient's progress during rehabilitation. Trigger points may be located in the muscle and feel like a small nodule or muscle spasm. The trigger point may be identified as an area that upon palpation refers pain to another body area. Increased tissue temperature may be present if infection or inflammation is present. Calcification or change in tissue density may be present in a poorly managed hematoma formation, or might indicate effusion or hemarthrosis of the joint. Crepitus is a crunching or crackling sensation along the tendon, bone, or joint. Crepitus along the length of a tendon can indicate tenosynovitis or tendinitis. The presence of crepitus along the bone or joint may indicate damage to the bone (fracture), cartilage, bursa, or joint

capsule. Rupture of a muscle or tendon may present as a gap at the point of separation.

All information gathered during palpation should be used to further confirm the findings of the initial evaluation steps. At this point the athletic trainer should be further able to differentiate between the normal and provoked tissue. Before beginning the next subphase of the objective evaluation, the athletic trainer should review the findings and further organize the remainder of the objective evaluation.

Special Tests

Range of Motion. Range-of-motion assessment involves determining the patient's ability to move a limb through a specific pattern of motion. There are several general principles that should be applied during range-of-motion testing. Motions will be performed passively, actively, and against resistance to fully quantify the patient's status.[14,22] Testing should first be performed on the patient's uninjured limb through each of the joint's cardinal planes of motion and the quantity of motion available should be recorded. Then range-of-motion testing is repeated on the injured limb. The athletic trainer can then compare the range of motion of the injured limb to that of the uninjured limb and/or against established normative data.[22] In addition, range-of-motion records will serve an important role in tracking the patient's progress during rehabilitation. Active range-of-motion testing should be performed first, followed by passive, then resistive, range-of-motion assessment.[14,22] If possible, the athletic trainer should perform movement patterns that facilitate pain at the end to prevent a carryover effect to following movement patterns. This should be evident based on the previous steps performed during the evaluation process. Range-of-motion assessment should also be performed at the joints proximal and distal to the involved area for a comprehensive evaluation.[22] These general guidelines allow the athletic trainer to efficiently assess range of motion.

One of the primary goals of range-of-motion testing is to assess the integrity of the inert and contractile tissue components of the joint complex. Inert tissues are sometimes referred to as anatomic joint structures and include bone, ligament, capsule, bursae, periosteum, cartilage, and fascia.[5] The contractile tissues, also referred to as physiological joint structures, include muscle, tendon, and nerve structures.[5] Cyriax developed a method to differentiate between inert and contractile pathological tissues as part of the range-of-motion assessment.[5] Differentiating between inert or contractile tissue pathology is performed by selectively applying passive and active tension to joint structures and making note of where pain is located.[5] The ability to differentiate between inert and contractile tissue pathology is an important step in setting up the rehabilitation plan and identifying the appropriate tissue to treat.

Inert tissue pathology is indicated when the patient reports pain occurring during both active and passive range of motion in the same direction of movement.[5] Typically, pain due to inert tissue pathology will occur near the end of the range of motion as the tissue becomes compressed between the bony segments. Example: The patient reports pain in the anterior shoulder region when actively and passively moving the humerus into the end range of shoulder flexion. Because pain was present in the same direction of motion (direction of shoulder flexion = anterior shoulder) during active and passive movements, pathology of an inert tissue structure of the shoulder would be indicated.

Contractile tissue pathology is indicated when the patient reports pain in the same direction of motion during active range of motion, then reports pain in the opposite direction of motion during passive range of motion.[5] Contractile tissue pain occurs due to increased tension placed on the tissue. However, the cause of contractile tissue tension differs between active and passive range-of-motion testing. During active range of motion, contractile tissue tension increases due to the voluntary agonist muscle contraction generated to move the limb. In contrast, passive range of motion increases contractile tissue tension as the muscle is stretched by the athletic trainer. Example: The patient reports anterior shoulder pain when actively bringing the humerus into shoulder flexion (pain in same direction as motion) and when passively bringing the humerus into shoulder extension as it is stretched by the athletic trainer (pain in opposite direction as motion). It is not possible to determine the specific location of either inert or contractile tissue pathology through range-of-motion assessment. This is accomplished by incorporating manual muscle and special tests to locate the exact location of pathology.

Active range of motion. Having the patient "actively" contract their muscles as they take their limb through the desired cardinal plane of motion assesses active range of motion, location of pain, and painful arcs.[15] A painful arc is pain that occurs at some point during the range of motion but later disappears as the limb moves past this point in either direction.[15,22] Typically, a painful arc is present due to impingement of tissue between bony surfaces. Painful arcs may be present during either active or passive range-of-motion testing.

Overpressure may be applied at the end range of motion to assess end-point feels, if active range of motion is full and pain-free.[14] Pain or limited range of motion prohibits applying overpressure during active range-of-motion

assessment and may indicate waiting until the passive range-of-motion testing. If range of motion is limited or elicits pain, the athletic trainer should consider the cause of these findings, as this will have direct implications on the rehabilitation plan. Limited range of motion can be caused by several factors, including swelling, joint capsule tightness, agonist muscle weakness/inhibition, or antagonist muscle tightness/contracture.[10]

Passive range of motion. When passive range of motion is assessed, the patient should be positioned so that the contractile tissues are relaxed and do not influence the findings due to active muscle contraction. The athletic trainer then takes the limb through the desired passive movement pattern until the point of pain or end range of motion. Upon reaching the end range of motion, gentle overpressure should be applied and particular attention should be directed toward the sensation of the end-point feel.

The end-point feel encountered at the end range of motion has been given several normal and abnormal classification schemes.[5] End-point feel assessment may be useful in helping determine the type of pathological tissue[5] (Table 3-1).

The athletic trainer should determine whether differences exist between the ranges of motion available during active and passive testing. Reduced range of motion during active compared to passive testing may indicate deficiency in the contractile tissue. Contractile tissue deficiencies may be caused by muscle spasm or contracture, muscle weakness, neurological deficit, or muscle pain.[22] Such deficiencies should be addressed during the rehabilitation plan to restore normal range of motion.

The presence of crepitus or clicking is also of significance during passive range of motion testing.[15] Crepitus or clicking along the joint line or between two bones may indicate damage to the articular cartilage or a possible loose body in the joint. Similar sensations along the muscle or tendon may indicate adhesion formation or tendon subluxation.

CLINICAL DECISION MAKING   **Exercise 3–3**

During knee flexion range-of-motion testing, a patient complains of pain in the same direction of motion during active range of motion, but no pain during passive range of motion. Upon testing knee extension range of motion, the patient indicates that pain occurs in the opposite direction of motion during passive range of motion. What type of tissue may be suspected to have been injured, based on these findings?

■ **TABLE   3-1**   End-Feel Categorization Scheme.

Normal End-Feels

Soft-tissue approximation	Soft and spongy, a gradual painless stop (e.g., elbow flexion)
Capsular	An abrupt, hard, firm end point with only a little give (e.g., shoulder rotation)
Bone-to-bone	A distinct and abrupt end point where two hard surfaces come in contact with one another (e.g., elbow extension)

Abnormal End-Feels

Empty	Movement definitely beyond the anatomical limit, or pain prevents the body part from moving through the available range of motion (e.g., ligament rupture)
Spasm	Involuntary muscle contraction that prevents normal range of motion due to pain (guarding) (e.g., muscle spasm)
Loose	Extreme hypermobility (e.g., chronic ankle sprain, chronic shoulder subluxation/dislocation)
Springy block	A rebound at the end point of motion (e.g., meniscal tear, loose body formation)

Capsular patterns of motion.   Irritation to the joint capsule may cause a progressive loss of available motion in different cardinal planes of motion. When identifying a capsular pattern, movement restrictions are listed in order, with the first being the motion pattern that is most affected.[15] Each joint has a specific pattern of progressive motion loss in different planes of motion. For example, the capsular pattern of the glenohumeral joint involves significant limitation to external rotation, followed by abduction and internal rotation. Presence of a capsular pattern indicates a total joint reaction that may involve muscle spasm, joint capsule tightening (most common), and possible osteophyte formation.[13] The athletic trainer must determine which joint structures may be involved with the capsular pattern in order to adequately plan the patient's rehabilitation. This will be performed through assessment of joint end-feels, muscle strength, and various special tests.

Noncapsular patterns of motion.   Noncapsular patterns of motion result from irritation to structures located outside of the joint capsule and do not follow the progressive loss of motion patterns as observed with a capsular pattern. Cyriax has classified the following lesions as producing noncapsular patterns of motion.[5]
- Ligamentous adhesion occurs after injury and may result in a movement restriction in one plane, with a full pain-free range in other planes.
- Internal derangement involves a sudden onset of localized pain resulting from the displacement of a loose body within the joint. The mechanical block restricts motion in one plane while allowing normal, pain-free

motion in the opposite direction. Movement restrictions can change as the loose body shifts its position in the joint space.
- Extra-articular lesion results from adhesions occurring outside the joint. Movement in a plane that stretches that adhesion results in pain, whereas motion in the opposite direction is pain-free and nonrestricted.

Accessory motion and joint play (arthrokinematic motion).   Accessory or joint play motions occur between joint surfaces as the joint undergoes passive and active motions.[13] The motion occurring between the joint surfaces is also referred to as arthrokinematic motion. Arthrokinematic motions are not actively produced by the patient. However, arthrokinematic motion is necessary for full active and passive joint range of motion to be achieved. As such, accessory motion/joint play assessment should be evaluated during a comprehensive assessment of joint range of motion.[17]

Three types of arthrokinematic motions can occur: roll, glide, and spin. A detailed description of the arthrokinematic motions is provided in Chapter 13. In brief, for normal joint motion to occur there must be normal arthrokinematic motion available. An example of arthrokinematic motion can be easily demonstrated at the knee in the open-kinetic-chain position as the knee moves from a flexed position into full extension (femur is stationery, tibia is moving). During this motion the tibia rolls and glides anteriorly and spins externally (external rotation) relative to the femur. Because arthrokinematic motions are involuntary, assessment requires specific manual techniques. Techniques used for assessment of accessory motion are the same as those used in joint mobilization treatment and are discussed in detail in Chapter 13.

During arthrokinematic motion assessment, the examiner is looking for alterations in either hypomobility (restricted arthrokinematic motion) or hypermobility (excessive arthrokinematic motion). In addition to assessing the amplitude of arthrokinematic motion, the examiner should also note signs of joint stiffness, quality of motion, end-feel, and pain.[10]

It is particularly important to evaluate arthrokinematic motion in patients that have reduced passive or active range of motion. It is possible that limited passive and active range of motion arises from altered arthrokinematic motions. Reduced arthrokinematic motions may be due to joint capsule or ligamentous adhesions and tightness. To restore normal passive and active range of motion in the patient demonstrating reduced arthrokinematic motion, it will be important to incorporate joint mobilization techniques during the rehabilitation process.

CLINICAL DECISION MAKING   **Exercise 3–4**

You determine that a patient's active and passive range of motion is limited. Based on this information you assess the patient's arthrokinematic motion and find that it is hypomobile. What types of exercises would you consider incorporating into the patient's rehabilitation plan to address these findings?

Resistive Strength Testing   Resistive strength testing is used to assess the state of contractile tissue (muscle, tendon, and nerve).[13,14] Typically, resistive strength testing is performed as the patient performs an isometric contraction while the athletic trainer performs a "break test." The break test assesses the amount of isometric force the patient can generate prior to allowing joint motion (i.e., "breaking" the isometric contraction). In general, two types of resistive strength testing are used during the injury evaluation process: midrange-of-motion muscle testing and specific muscle testing.[14]

Midrange-of-motion muscle testing.   The athletic trainer should perform midrange-of-motion muscle testing before performing specific muscle testing. It is important to perform midrange motion to allow for isolation of contractile tissue. Muscle testing performed near the end range of motion may involve the inert tissue structures. When pain or weakness is noted during muscle testing at the end range of motion, it will be difficult to determine whether pain

arises from contractile or inert tissues.[14] The athletic trainer should be aware of any type of compensatory motions the patient may perform as an attempt to compensate for weak or limited motion.

Midrange-of-motion muscle testing is performed by placing the joint in its approximate midrange of motion for a specific movement pattern. The athletic trainer tells the patient "Don't let me move you," and then applies a manual force to initiate the break test. Midrange-of-motion muscle testing should be performed in each of the cardinal planes of motion and compared bilaterally to the uninjured limb. Midrange-of-motion muscle testing focuses on muscle groups, not specific muscles. Thus, performing specific muscle testing of the agonist and synergistic muscles acting in that cardinal plane of motion should be included as a follow-up for noted weakness or pain during midrange-of-motion muscle testing.[14] Essentially, the results of the midrange-of-motion muscle testing will guide the examiner through specific muscle testing.

During the midrange-of-motion muscle testing the athletic trainer does not "grade" strength, but instead assesses the motion as strong, weak, painful, or painless.[14] According to Cyriax,[5] the athletic trainer can identify the type of lesion through muscle testing (Table 3-2).

CLINICAL DECISION MAKING   **Exercise 3–5**

During midrange-of-motion muscle testing, you note that the patient has pain and weakness when performing hip extension. Based on this finding, what muscles should be tested during specific muscle testing?

Specific muscle testing.   Specific muscle testing is used to assess the strength and integrity of specific muscles, not simply muscle groups. Muscles tested during specific muscle testing should be based upon information obtained from midrange-of-motion muscle testing, range-of-motion assessment, and the patient's history. Similar to midrange-of-motion muscle testing, the athletic trainer will apply a break test to assess muscle function. However, the joint is placed in various positions in an attempt to isolate stress on the muscle of interest. Detailed positioning of the joint to isolate specific muscles is described in detail in Daniels and Worthingham[7] as well as Kendall.[12]

During specific muscle testing the athletic trainer will note any pain and grade the patient's muscle strength. This information will be compared to the injured side and be used during rehabilitation to track the patient's progress in regaining muscle strength. Several grading scales

■ **TABLE   3-2**   Midrange-of-Motion Muscle Testing Scheme.

Cyriax System for Differentiating Muscular Lesions

Strong and painless = normal muscle

Strong and painful = minor lesion in some part of muscle or tendon (first- or second-degree strain)

Weak and painless = complete rupture of muscle or tendon or some nervous system disorder

Weak and painful = gross lesion of contractile tissue (muscle or tendon rupture, peripheral nerve or nerve root involvement; if movement is weak and pain-free, neurological involvement or a tendon rupture should be first suspected)

■ **TABLE   3-3**   Specific Muscle Testing Grading Scheme.

Grade 5	Normal	Complete AROM against gravity, with maximum resistance
Grade 4	Good	Complete AROM against gravity, with some resistance
Grade 3	Fair	Complete AROM against gravity, with no resistance
Grade 2	Poor	Complete AROM, with gravity eliminated
Grade 1	Trace	Evidence of slight muscle contraction, with no joint motion
Grade 0	Zero	No evidence of muscle contraction

have been reported; numerical systems are the most common[7] (Table 3-3). Weakness or pain elicited during resistive strength testing may be caused by several factors, including muscle strain, pain/reflex inhibition, peripheral nerve injury, nerve root lesion (myotome), tendon strain, avulsion, or psychological overlay.[13] The athletic trainer should always consider the source of muscular deficiency and not simply focus on assigning a muscle strength grade. Through appropriate use of neurological tests and various special tests, the athletic trainer should be able to accurately identify the source of muscular deficiency. This is imperative in order to efficiently manage the injury throughout the rehabilitation process.

Muscle Imbalances. After evaluating both range-of-motion and resistive strength testing, the athletic trainer should review the findings to determine whether muscle imbalances can be identified. Muscle imbalances arise between an agonist muscle and its functional antagonist muscle, disrupting the normal force-couple relationship between the agonist and antagonist muscle.[2,3,18] Muscle tightness or hyperactivity of one muscle or muscle group is often the initial cause of muscle imbalances and initiates a predictable pattern of kinetic dysfunction.[2,3,18] Tightness or hyperactivity in the agonist muscle can cause inhibition of the antagonist muscle. This is explained by Sherrington's law of reciprocal inhibition. Reciprocal inhibition causes decreased neural drive to the antagonist muscle, which ultimately facilitates a functional weakness of the antagonist muscles. Agonist muscle tightness and hyperactivity combined with inhibition and weakness of the antagonist muscles results in disruption of the normal force-couple relationship between these muscles, hence a muscle imbalance.[2,3]

Initial disruption of the normal force-couple relationship between agonist and antagonist muscles stimulates a series of events that further perpetuates the altered force couple relationship. Due to the force imbalance between agonist and antagonist muscles, the joint tends to position itself in the direction of the tight agonist muscle and normal postural alignment can be adversely affected.[2,3] Alterations to postural alignment allow the agonist muscle to move into a more shortened position. Conversely, the antagonist muscle is lengthened from its normal position. Increasing the resting length of the antagonist muscle is believed to alter the normal length-tension relationship of the muscle, which further reduces the antagonist muscle's ability to generate force. Reduced antagonist muscle force generation due to lengthening is explained by the length–tension relationship. As the antagonist muscle is lengthened, there are fewer crossbridges that can be aligned, hence reduced muscle force capacity. Reduced antagonist muscle force output further disrupts the normal force-couple relationship and may bring about additional postural alignment alterations.[2,3]

To compensate for weakness of the antagonist muscle group, the patient might compensate by placing greater reliance on muscles that act as synergists to the weakened muscles. This is referred to as synergistic dominance.[2,3] The synergist muscles are now forced to perform greater work to accelerate and decelerate the bony segments. This places greater demands on the synergist muscles, which increases the risk of injury to these muscles.[2,3] This series of events is summarized in Figure 3-3.

Janda has identified several common muscle imbalances that may be observed by the athletic trainer.[11] The basic concept is to separate muscles into two basic groups

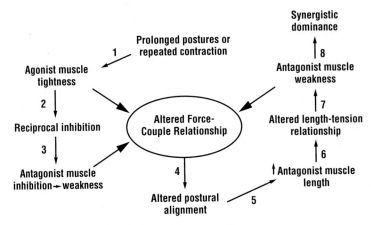

Figure 3-3   Muscle imbalance injury paradigm.

based on their function: movement and stabilization. **Movement group muscles** are characterized as being:

- Prone to developing tightness (hyperactive)
- More active during functional movements (hyperactive)
- More active when the individual becomes fatigued or when performing new movement patterns (hyperactive)

Stabilization group muscles are characterized as being:

- Prone to developing inhibition and weakness (reduced force capacity)
- Less active during functional movements (reduced force capacity)
- Easily fatigued during dynamic movements (reduced force capacity)

According to Janda, several specific muscles in the movement and stabilization groups are extremely prone to developing tightness and weakness, respectively.[11] These muscles are indicated in Table 3-4.

It is important for the examiner to address muscle imbalances during the rehabilitation process in order to restore normal postural alignment and force-couple relationships. The athletic trainer must pay special attention to whether limited range of motion in one muscle is accompanied by weakness in its functional antagonist. If a muscle imbalance is revealed, the athletic trainer must work to restore the normal force-couple relationship during rehabilitation in order to reestablish postural alignment. In general, restoring normal balance between muscles is accomplished by first stretching the tight muscle to restore normal range of motion before attempting to strengthen the weak antagonist muscle. Failure to address muscle imbalances can result in a failed rehabilitation program where the examiner is constantly treating the symptoms, but never the cause.

Additional Special Tests

At this point in the evaluation, the athletic trainer should have considerably narrowed the list of possible pathological tissues involved and be judicious in choosing the special tests to perform. Suspicion of a fracture or joint dislocation may contraindicate performance of various special tests that could exacerbate the current injury. Also, if the patient is in a considerable amount of pain, performance of special tests may yield findings of questionable validity. In cases where the patient is in a considerable amount of pain it is best to wait until the patient's symptoms have subsided to perform the special tests.

The special tests performed at this phase should be used to further differentiate between pathological and normal tissue.[14] The athletic trainer should perform special tests only on those tissues that they suspect to be pathological based on the findings from the previous evaluation phases.[14] The experienced athletic trainer performs only those special tests that confirm their previous findings and eliminate other tissues from being involved. To isolate pathological tissue, special tests are designed to asses the integrity of specific body tissues, such as muscle, ligament, tendon, joint surface, and nerve.

There are several types of special tests. **Joint stability tests** assess the integrity of the inert joint tissues, specifically the joint capsule and ligaments. Joint stability testing is performed by applying to the joint a manual force that places strain on specific capsular or ligamentous structures. The manual force is applied until reaching the end point of the specific joint motion. The athletic trainer then grades the amount of joint laxity (displacement) and end-feel and notes the presence of pain. For example, the

■ **TABLE 3-4** Janda Classification of Functional Muscle Groupings.

Muscles Prone to Tightness (Movement Group)

Gastrocnemius
Soleus
Short hip adductors
Hamstrings
Rectus femoris
Iliopsoas
Tensor fascia latae
Piriformis
Erector spinae (especially lumbar, thoracolumbar,
   and cervical portions)
Quadratus lumborum
Pectoralis major
Upper trapezius
Levator scapulae
Sternocleidomastoid
Scalenes
Flexors of the upper limb

Muscles Prone to Weakness (Stabilization Group)

Peroneals
Anterior tibialis
Posterior tibialis
Gluteus maximus
Gluteus medius
Abdominals
Serratus anterior
Rhomboids
Lower trapezius
Short cervical flexors
Extensors of the upper limb

Anterior Drawer Test at the knee assesses the integrity of the anterior cruciate ligament. Based on these findings the athletic trainer may estimate the extent of injury to the specific capsular or ligamentous structures tested. Table 3-3 indicates the grading system commonly used to assess joint stability. **Joint compression tests** assess the integrity of inert joint tissues that line the joint surface, such as the articular cartilage and meniscus. Joint compression testing is performed as the athletic trainer manually applies a compressive load across the joint, typically combined with some form of rotary stress. This type of combined motion places significant stress across the joint surface and may elicit a painful or crepitus/clicking sensation at the joint

level. The McMurray's Test at the knee is an example of a joint compression test. Passive tendon stretch tests are used to determine the presence of tendinitis or tenosynovitis. The athletic trainer applies a passive stretch along the tendon that when positive elicits a painful or crepitus like sensation along the tendon.

Another form of special tests that may be useful are **anthropometric assessments** of the patient of injured area.[14] Anthropometric assessments range from being as simple as qualitatively assessing the patient's somatotype (general body structure) to as detailed as performing body composition assessment (e.g., underwater weighing). Such information may be useful in situations where the patient will be required to miss a significant amount of physical activity for a prolonged period of time. The athletic trainer may be able to compare the patient's body composition pre- or immediately postinjury to their body composition during rehabilitation or before returning to activity. Anthropometric assessments might also be performed on the limb and might include measurements of limb girth and volume. Limb anthropometric measurements can be useful in tracking rehabilitation progress to assess swelling or muscle atrophy/hypertrophy.[14,22]

Neurological Testing. There is some debate as to how often neurological testing should be performed. Some believe that neurological testing should be performed any time the patient reports of symptoms that affect their distal extremities, such as below the acromion process or gluteal folds,[4,10] especially if the mechanism of injury was not directly witnessed. However, other professionals do not feel that neurological testing is warranted for orthopedic evaluations, unless the results from the previous evaluation phases suggest nervous system involvement.[8,14] Neurological testing may be indicated from the history if the patient describes unexplained loss of strength, paresthesia, or numbness, or has sustained an injury to the vertebral region that may have involved the spine.[22]

Neurological testing typically involves three components: sensory (dermatomes), motor (myotomes), and reflex (deep tendon, superficial, and pathological reflexes) testing.[8] Neurological testing of these three components assesses the integrity of the spinal nerve roots and peripheral nerves. The evaluator's challenge is to determine whether the nerve root or peripheral nerve is the source of the symptoms. Nerve root damage typically involves abnormal motor and sensory function over a large area. In contrast, peripheral nerve damage will be confined to a more localized area innervated by the nerve.[14] Other possible neurological testing components include cranial nerve assessment, neuropsychological assessment (cognitive ability), and cerebellar function (coordinated movements: finger to nose).[13,22]

Dermatome testing. Dermatomes are areas of the skin whose sensory distribution is innervated by a specific nerve root. Assessment of dermatomes involves a bilateral comparison of light touch discrimination. During dermatome testing the examiner should alter or remove the pressure applied to one side in order to determine whether the patient can distinguish changes in pressure. Sensory testing may also include sharp and dull discrimination, hot and cold discrimination, and two-point discrimination to assess peripheral nerve injury.[22] Dermatomes for the body are illustrated in Figure 3-4.

Myotome testing. Myotomes represent a group of muscles that are innervated from a specific nerve root. Essentially, myotomes are the motor equivalent to dermatomes.[14] Myotomes may be assessed for various muscle groups of the upper and lower extremities. Myotome testing is performed through sustained isometric contraction of a specific muscle. Common muscles tested during myotome assessment are listed in Table 3-5.

Reflex testing. Reflex testing may involve the assessment of deep tendon reflexes, superficial reflexes, and pathological reflexes. Testing for deep tendon reflexes assesses the integrity of the stretch reflex arc for a specific nerve root and provides further information on the

■ TABLE 3-5   Myotome Assessment.

C5 = Middle deltoid
C6 = Biceps brachii
C7 = Triceps brachii
C8 = Finger flexors
T1 = Finger interossei (DAB & PAD)
T12 – L3 = Hip flexion
L2 – L4 = Quadriceps
L5 – S1 = Hamstrings
L4 – L5 = Ankle dorsiflexion
S1 – S2 = Ankle plantar flexion

integrity of the specific nerve root.[8] Testing of deep tendon reflexes typically involves the use of a reflex hammer. The athletic trainer strikes over the tendon in order to place a slight quick-stretch on the tendon. If done properly, the slight stretching of the tendon will elicit a reflex response (i.e., a muscle jerk response). Applying a quick stretch to almost any tendon can facilitate the reflex response, if done properly. There are several upper- and lower-extremity deep tendon reflexes that may be tested (Table 3-6). However, not all nerve roots have a specific deep tendon reflex. The common deep tendon reflexes assessed in the upper and lower extremities include the biceps, brachioradialis, triceps, patella, hamstrings medial, hamstrings lateral, tibialis posterior, and the Achilles tendon. Grading of deep tendon reflexes uses a 5-point scale to characterize the stretch reflex response and compare it bilaterally to the uninjured limb (Table 3-7).

Superficial reflexes are assessed as the athletic trainer provides a superficial stoking of the patient's skin, usually using a sharp object.[8,13] During this time the examiner notes the movement of the patient's skin or distal extremities. Commonly, several superficial reflexes are described.[8,13] These include the upper-abdominal, lower-abdominal, cremasteric, plantar, gluteal, and anal reflexes.

Pathological reflexes normally are not present. The presence of a pathological reflex is a sign that there might be a lesion in either the upper or the lower motor neuron.[8,13] An upper motor neuron lesion may be present if the pathological reflex is present bilaterally.[13] A lesion of the lower motor neuron may be indicated by the unilateral presence of the pathological reflex.[13] Assessment of pathological reflexes can involve stoking, squeezing, tapping, or pinching of various anatomical structures to elicit a response. Perhaps the best-known pathological reflex is the Babinski reflex.

The athletic trainer must consider the source of any altered neurological test findings. Neurological test

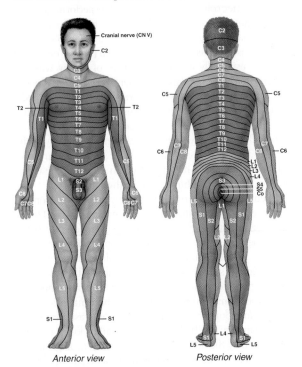

Anterior view   *Posterior view*

Figure 3-4 Dermatome assessment.
From: McKinley, M & O' Loughlin, V. *Human Anatomy,* 1st ed., NY: McGraw-Hill, 2006.

■ **TABLE   3-6**   Deep Tendon Reflex Assessment.

C6 = Biceps brachii
C7 = Triceps brachii
C8 = Brachiradialis
L4 = Patella tendon
S1 = Achilles tendon

■ **TABLE   3-7**   Deep Tendon Reflex Grading Scheme.

Grade 0	Absent: no reflex elicited
Grade 1	Diminished: reflex elicited with reinforcement (precontracting muscle)
Grade 2	Normal
Grade 3	Exaggerated: hyperresponsive reflex
Grade 4	Clonus: spasmlike response followed by relaxation

findings can be altered due to nerve root compression, nerve root stretch, or motor neuron lesion. The examiner should utilize the neurological test findings to further differentiate the source of the patient's symptoms. In addition, the information gained from the neurological assessment might dictate the need for further medical evaluation or diagnostic testing.

Functional Testing. Functional testing is an important component of the evaluation process, especially during the follow-up evaluations to track the patient's progress and their potential to return to previous activities. In sports medicine, functional testing typically involves observing the patient perform various functional movement patterns. It is important that the functional assessment reflect the type of stresses that the patient will experience during normal activities (i.e., the assessment should be sport-specific). Examples of sport-specific movement factors the athletic trainer should consider in designing a functional testing protocol include explosive movement, multi-joint coordination, neuromuscular control, fatigue, and repeated motions. Functional testing performed on an offensive lineman who has sustained a knee injury, for instance, may include observing the patient rapidly get in and out of a three-point stance, perform blocking drills and side-shuffle maneuvers, and perform plant and pivot maneuvers on the injured limb.

The athletic trainer should make note of any pain or discomfort experienced by the patient. In addition, the athletic trainer must be looking for compensatory movement patterns the patient uses to achieve the goals of the functional test. Should compensatory movement patterns be observed, the athletic trainer should address these deficiencies during the rehabilitation process.

Optimally, functional tests performed may be quantified or graded according to the patient's performance. For example, the athletic trainer might use a timed test to determine how quickly the patient can perform the functional task. The athletic trainer might also consider creating a grading system that focuses on body positioning and errors committed during assessment. The Balance Error Scoring System (BESS) is an example of a grading system where the examiner counts the number of errors the patient commits during an assessment of balance.[19,20] Errors are predefined and include such variables as taking hands off of hips, opening eyes, excessive hip abduction, taking a step to regain balance, or committing a stumble or fall. The greater the number of errors committed during testing, the worse the performance of the patient.

Functional testing should not only be performed after injury has occurred. The athletic trainer might perform a battery of functional tests on the uninjured patient during preparticipation examinations in order to establish baselines for comparison during the rehabilitation process should injury occur. Comparison of postinjury scores to preinjury baseline measures can help the athletic trainer determine whether the patient is ready to return to activity. An objective criterion might be set—for example, that the patient be able to perform at 90 to 95 percent of their preinjury levels before they will be allowed to perform functional activities or return to play.

INJURY PREVENTION SCREENING

Injury prevention screening may be performed as part of the preparticipation physical examination in order to identify individuals that may be at risk for injury. There is little scientific research on what the athletic trainer should focus on during injury risk screening. However, knowledge of basic biomechanics and anatomy can help the athletic trainer identify movement patterns that put stress and strain on tissue, hence increasing risk of injury.

When the athletic trainer has identified movement patterns that place the athlete at greater risk of injury, he or she can devise an injury prevention training program to address the cause of the inefficient movements. By incorporating training in injury prevention, the athletic trainer may be able to reduce the incidence of injury; this has been demonstrated in several research studies looking at the incidence of lower-extremity injury, specifically ACL injury.[1,6]

Several clinicians have developed injury risk screening protocols.[3] In general, these protocols involve the individual performing a dynamic movement pattern in a slow and controlled manner. The athletic trainer then observes the individual's movement pattern at each of the involved joints. By noting inefficient movement patterns, the athletic trainer may be able to identify preexisting muscle imbalances that alter the normal force-couple relationships, postural alignment, joint kinematics, and neuromuscular control.

Essentially, the athletic trainer observes whether the individual can maintain a neutral alignment of limb segments while performing the dynamic movement patterns. If the individual's limb segment moves out of neutral alignment, this may be due to muscle tightness or weakness. Muscle tightness may be present in the muscles in the direction of limb motion. Excessively tight muscles are believed to pull the limb into the direction of tightness, away from neutral alignment. Muscle inhibition or weakness might also be present in the muscles acting in the opposite direction of limb motion. Weak and inhibited muscles are believed to be unable to generate the magnitude of force necessary to maintain neutral alignment. Both situations cause altered joint kinematics that can place greater stress on the surrounding tissues and push these tissues closer to their point of failure during repeated movements. On pages 65 and 66, we provide two examples of injury risk screenings that may be incorporated for the lower extremity during preparticipation physical examinations (Figures 3-5 and 3-6).

DOCUMENTING FINDINGS

Often overlooked in the rehabilitation process is the fact that good record keeping is essential to the rehabilitation program's success. The examiner must be able to refer back to previous evaluation records to determine the patient's progress and make the appropriate adjustments to the rehabilitation plan.

SOAP Notes

The records of the evaluation process should be recorded in SOAP (Subjective, Objective, Assessment, Plan) note format (Figure 3-7).
- S (*Subjective*). This component of the SOAP note includes relevant information gathered during the subjective phase of the evaluation when taking the patient's history. This information might include the patient's general impression, site of injury, mechanism of injury, previous injuries, and symptoms.[16]

- O (*Objective*). The objective component of the SOAP note includes relevant information gathered during the objective phase of the evaluation. The athletic trainer should record only the significant signs and symptoms revealed during the objective evaluation. An asterisk may be placed by information of particular importance. This often helps the athletic trainer readily find such information during subsequent reevaluations to assess patient progress.[16]
- A (*Assessment*). Assessment of the injury is the athletic trainer's professional judgment with regard to the impression and nature of injury. Although the athletic trainer may be unable to determine the exact nature of the injury, information pertaining to the suspected site and pathological tissues involved is appropriate. In addition, a judgment of injury severity may be included.[16]
- P (*Plan*). The treatment plan should include the initial first aid performed and the athletic trainer's intentions relative to disposition.[16] Disposition may include referral for more definitive evaluation or simply application of splint, wrap, or crutches and a request to report for reevaluation the following day. Formulating the treatment plan is the final step of the SOAP note. The plan for treatment should include short-term and long-term goals for the patient.[10,14] Short- and long-term goals should be objective and include timelines. This will allow the athletic trainer to judge the success of the rehabilitation program and make any needed adjustments after determining whether the patient was able to meet the goals.

The athletic trainer should attempt to make all information recorded as quantitative as possible.[14] This will allow the athletic trainer to better monitor the patient's progress during rehabilitation and make the adjustments and progressions to treatment accordingly, as indicated by reevaluation and comparison with previous evaluation notes.

Setting Rehabilitation Goals

Great attention should be made when developing the short- and long-term goals as these will be key factors in developing the actual rehabilitation program, as the exercises and modalities utilized during rehabilitation selected should be based on these goals. Rehabilitation goals should be included as part of the treatment plan in the SOAP note. The rehabilitation goals should be based upon the information gathered during the evaluation and should address signs and symptoms recorded in the SOAP note.[14] For every significant sign and symptom listed in the SOAP note, the examiner

Performance:
A-Start Position   B-Stop Position   C-Side View

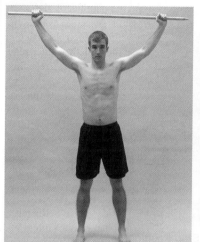 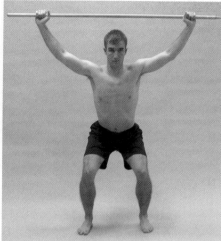 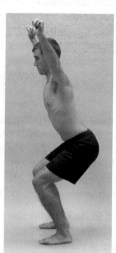

What to look for:
Foot & Ankle
- Foot pronation: Y / N
- Externally rotation: Y / N

Knees
- Valgus collapse: Y / N
- Varus: Y / N

Lumbo-Pelvic-Hip Complex
- Asymmetrical weight shift: Y / N
- Lumbar lordosis: Y / N
- Hip adduction: Y / N
- Hip internal rotation: Y / N

What to do with findings:
Foot pronation & external rotation
- Tightness: Soleus, lateral gastrocnemius, biceps femoris, peroneals, piriformis

Knee Valgus & Internal Rotation
- Tightness: Gastrocnemius / soleus, adductors, IT band
- Weakness: Gluteus medius

Lumbar Lordosis
- Tightness: Erector Spinae & psoas
- Weakness: Transverse abdominis, internal obliques

Hip Adduction
- Tightness: Hip adductors
- Weakness: Gluteus medius

Hip Internal Rotation
- Weakness: Gluteus maximus, hip external rotators

Figure 3-5   Overhead squat test (Clark, 2001).

Repeat procedures for Overhead Squat Test while performing a forward lunge.

What to look for:
Foot & Ankle
- Foot pronation: Y / N
- Externally rotation: Y / N

Knees
- Valgus collapse: Y / N
- Varus: Y / N

Lumbo-Pelvic-Hip Complex
- Lumbar lordosis: Y / N
- Lateral trunk flexion: Y / N
- Trunk rotation: Y / N
- Hip adduction: Y / N
- Hip internal rotation: Y / N

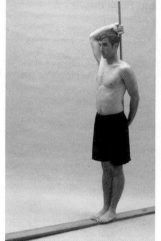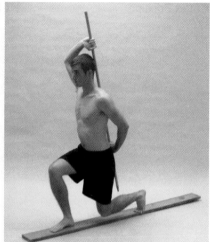

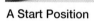
A Start Position   B Stop Position

What to do with findings:
Foot pronation &
external rotation
- Tightness: Soleus, lateral gastrocnemius, biceps femoris, peroneals, piriformis

Knee Valgus & Internal Rotation
- Tightness: Gastrocnemius / soleus, adductors, IT band
- Weakness: Gluteus medius

Lumbar Lordosis
- Tightness: Erector spinae & psoas
- Weakness: Transverse abdominis, internal obliques

Lateral Trunk Flexion
- Weakness: Core musculature

Trunk Rotation
- Weakness: Core musculature

Hip Adduction
- Tightness: Hip adductors
- Weakness: Gluteus medius

Hip Internal Rotation
- Weakness: Gluteus maximus, hip external rotators

Figure 3-6   Lunge test (Clark, 2001).

should develop a corresponding goal. Typically, the duration of short-term goals is 2 weeks.[10,14] Following the evaluation or reevaluation the examiner should consider what goals could reasonably be achieved within this time frame. Long-term goals are the final goals the patient should achieve in order to be ready to return to normal activities.[14] A different set of short- and long-term goals will be developed for each injured patient depending upon the findings from the injury

evaluation. For example, a soccer player presenting with a knee injury may have restricted knee flexion and extension range of motion, decreased knee extension strength, and significant knee joint swelling. The short-term goals for this case may be to increase range of motion by a specific amount (e.g., increase by 10 degrees), improve knee extension strength by a specific amount (e.g., increase by 10 lbs), and reduce swelling by a specific amount

---

Patient Name _____   **Date of Injury** _____

Injury Site   R   L _____   **Today's Date** _____

Subjective Findings (history):

Objective Findings (observation/inspection, palpation, range of motion, strength, & special tests):

Assessment (clinical impression):

Plan (treatment administered, disposition, rehabilitation goals, treatment plan):

Figure 3-7   SOAP note.

(e.g., decrease by 1 inch during girth measurement) within a specified time period (typically 1—2 weeks for short-term goals). Thus, short-term goals should provide an immediate, achievable target that the athletic trainer can use to evaluate the success of their rehabilitation program. The long-term goal for this patient may be to play soccer without limitations after 8 weeks. Long-term goals help the patient understand what they can expect to achieve over the course of the rehabilitation process. The patient should be encouraged to achieve each short-term goal, and the athletic trainer should closely monitor the patient's progress. Understand that the goals may change over time depending upon how the patient progresses with the rehabilitation program. The following are examples of short- and long-term goals that may be included for a grade-2 inversion ankle sprain.

Short-Term Goals
- Decrease swelling by 30 percent within 4 days
- Increase active range of motion by 50 percent within 1 week
- Progress to full weight bearing during walking gait within 1 week
- Reduce acute pain by 50 percent within 4 days
- Increase eversion ankle strength by 50 percent in 4 days
- Increase plantarflexion ankle strength by 50 percent in 4 days

Long-Term Goals
- Return to limited practice using protective tape support within 2 weeks

- Return to full practice using protective tape support within 2.5 weeks
- Return to full competition using protective taping within 3 weeks

---

CLINICAL DECISION MAKING   **Exercise 3–6**

You perform an injury evaluation on a soccer patient. After completing the injury evaluation, you determine the following information from the objective phase:
- Active range of motion for knee extension limited by 10 degrees
- Passive range of motion for knee flexion limited by 20 degrees
- Presence of swelling and discoloration over anterior thigh
- Decreased quadriceps strength compared to uninjured side

Based on these findings, how would you write up the treatment goals for this injured patient?

Progress Evaluations

The athletic trainer who is overseeing a rehabilitation program must constantly monitor the progress of the patient toward full recovery throughout the rehabilitative process. In many instances the athletic trainer will be able to treat the injured patient on a daily basis. This close supervision gives the athletic trainer the luxury of being able to continuously adjust or adapt the treatment program based on the progress made by the patient on a day-to-day basis.

The progress evaluation should be based on the athletic trainer's knowledge of exactly what is occurring in the healing process at any given time. The timelines of injury healing dictate how the athletic trainer should progress the rehabilitation program. The athletic trainer must understand that little can be done in rehabilitation to speed up the healing process and that progression will be limited by the constraints of that process.

Progress evaluations will be more limited in scope than the detailed evaluation sequence previously described. The off-field evaluation should be thorough and comprehensive, taking time to systematically rule out information that is not pertinent to the present injury. Once the extraneous information has been eliminated, the subsequent progress evaluations can focus specifically on how the injury appears today compared with yesterday. Is the patient better or worse as a result of the treatment program rendered on the previous day?

To ensure that the progress evaluation will be complete, it is still necessary to go through certain aspects of history, observation, palpation, and special testing.

History
• How is the pain today, compared to yesterday?
• Are you able to move better and with less pain?
• Do you think that the treatment done yesterday helped or made you more sore?

Observation
• How is the swelling today? More or less than yesterday?
• Is the patient able to move better today?

• Is the patient still guarding and protecting the injury?
• How is the patient's attitude—upbeat and optimistic, or depressed and negative?

Palpation
• Does the swelling have a different consistency today, and has the swelling pattern changed?
• Is the injured structure still as tender to touch?
• Is there any deformity present today that was not as obvious yesterday?

Special Tests
• Does ligamentous stress testing cause as much pain, or has assessment of the grade of instability changed?
• How does a manual muscle test compare with yesterday?
• Has either active or passive range of motion changed?
• Does accessory movement appear to be limited?
• Can the patient perform a specific functional test better today than yesterday?

Progress Notes. Progress notes should be routinely written following progress evaluations done throughout the course of the rehabilitation program. Progress notes can follow the SOAP format outlined earlier in this chapter. They can be generated in the form of an expanded treatment note, or may be done as a weekly summary. Information in the progress note should concentrate on the types of treatment received and the patient's response to that treatment, progress made toward the short-term goals established in the SOAP note, changes in the previous treatment plan and goals, and the course of treatment over the next several days.[1]

Summary

1. The components of the systematic differential evaluation process are split into subjective and objective phases. The subjective phase involves a detailed patient history. The objective phase includes observation/inspection of the injured patient, range-of-motion testing, resistive strength testing, assessment of muscle imbalances, performance of special tests based on previous findings, neurological testing, and functional testing.

2. The systematic injury evaluation process establishes the foundation for designing an effective rehabilitation program. All significant findings from the systematic differential evaluation will be used to identify the pathological tissues as well as any related deficiencies in the surrounding tissues. The rehabilitation plan and treatment goals will then focus on reestablishing normal function to the tissues and structures revealed to be pathological or deficient.

3. By applying knowledge of anatomy and the systematic differential evaluation process, the athletic trainer should be able to determine what tissue is pathological. This is accomplished by differentiating between normal tissue asymptomatic) and provoked tissue (symptomatic).

4. Injury risk screenings may be performed to determine whether the individual uses movement patterns during functional activities that may place greater stress on the surrounding tissues. By identifying such movement patterns in the early stages, the athletic trainer may be able to incorporate preventative training exercises to reduce the risk of injury at a later time.

5. Short-term and long-term goals should be based on the significant findings from the systematic differential evaluation. All significant findings should have a corresponding rehabilitation goal. All goals should be quantifiable and have a given time period in which they should be achieved. Typically, short-term goals are those that can be achieved within a 2-week time period. Long-terms goals are the final goals that the patient should achieve in order to be ready to return to normal activities.

References

1. Caraffa, A., G. Cerulli, M. Projett, G. Aisa, and A. Rizzo. 1996. Prevention of anterior cruciate ligament injuries in soccer: A prospective controlled study of proprioceptive training. *Knee Surgery Sports Traumatology Arthroscopy* 4: 19–21.

2. Clark, M. 2001. Muscle energy techniques in rehabilitation. In *Techniques in musculoskeletal rehabilitation*, edited by Prentice, W. and M. Voight. NY: McGraw-Hill.

3. Clark, M., and A. Russell. 2001. *Optimum performance training for the performance enhancement specialist.* Calabasas, CA: National Academy of Sports Medicine.

4. Corrigan, B., and G. Maitland. 1989. *Practical orthopedic medicine.* London: Butterworth.

5. Cyriax, J. 1982. *Textbook of orthopedic medicine.* 8th ed. London: Bailliere Tindal.

6. Hewett, T., T. Lindenfeld, J. Riccobene, and F. Noyes. 1999. The effect of neuromuscular training on the incidence of knee injury in female athletes: A prospective study. *American Journal of Sports Medicine* 27(6):699–706.

7. Hislop, H. 2007. *Montgomery J. Daniels and Worthingham's Muscle Testing.* 7th ed. Philadelphia: W. B. Saunders.

8. Hoppenfeld, S. 1977. *Orthopaedic neurology: A diagnostic guide to neurologic levels.* Philadelphia: Lippincott.

9. Hoppenfeld, S. 1976. *Physical examination of the spine and extremities.* Norwalk, CT: Appleton & Lange.

10. Houglum, P. 2005. *Therapeutic exercise for athletic injuries.* Champaign, IL: Human Kinetics.

11. Janda, V. 1983. *Muscle function testing.* London: Butterworth.

12. Kendall, F., E. McCreary, and P. Provance. 2005. *Muscles, testing and function.* 5th ed. Baltimore: Lippincott, Williams & Wilkins.

13. Magee, D. 2007. *Orthopedic physical assessment.* 5th ed. Philadelphia: W. B. Saunders.

14. Moore, R., B. Mandelbaum, and D. Wantabe. 2005. Evaluation of neuromusculoskeletal injuries. In *Athletic training and sports medicine,* edited by Starkey, C. 4th ed. Rosemont, IL: American Academy of Orthopaedic Surgeons.

15. Perrin, D. 1999. The evaluation process in rehabilitation. In *Rehabilitation techniques in sports medicine,* edited by Prentice, W. 3rd ed. NY: McGraw-Hill.

16. Prentice, W. 2009. *Arnheim's principles of athletic training.* 13th ed. NY: McGraw-Hill.

17. Prentice, W. 2010. Mobilization and traction techniques in rehabilitation. In *Rehabilitation techniques in sports medicine and athletic training,* edited by Prentice, W. 5th ed. NY: McGraw-Hill.

18. Richardson, C., G. Jull, P. Hodges, and J. Hides. 1999. *Therapeutic exercise for spinal segmental stabilization in low back pain.* Edinburgh: Churchill Livingstone.

19. Riemann, B., K. Guskiewicz, and E. Shields. 1999. Relationship between clinical and forceplate measures of postural stability. *Journal of Sport Rehabilitation* 8(2): 1–7.

20. Riemann, B., and K. Guskiewicz. 2000. Effects of mild head injury on postural stability as measured through clinical balance testing. *Journal of Athletic Training* 35(1): 19–25.

21. Shultz, S., D. Perrin, and P. Houglum. 2000. *Assessment of athletic injuries.* Champaign, IL: Human Kinetics.

22. Starkey, C., and J. Ryan. 2002. *Evaluation of orthopedic and athletic injuries.* 2nd ed. Philadelphia: F. A. Davis.

SOLUTIONS TO CLINICAL DECISION MAKING EXERCISE

3-1 The athletic trainer should perform special tests on only those tissues they suspect to be pathological based on the findings from the previous evaluation phases. The special tests should be used to confirm previous findings and eliminate other tissues from being involved. Given the patient's history, the athletic trainer might suspect meniscal or articular cartilage damage and perform special tests that focus on these structures.

3-2 It is important to understand that altered postural alignment can be caused by muscle force imbalances. Muscles crossing the body segment may be excessively tight or weak, causing an altered postural alignment. The athletic trainer should pay special attention to those muscles that may alter postural alignment due to tightness or weakness during range-of-motion and resistive strength testing. For example, the patient might demonstrate tight/overactive hip flexor and erector spinae muscles or weak/inhibited abdominal and gluteus maximus muscles.

3-3 Cyriax states that pain in the same direction of motion during active range of motion, combined with pain in the opposite direction of motion during passive range of motion, is indicative of contractile tissue injury. Based on these findings, the athletic trainer may suspect injury to the hamstring muscle group.

3-4 Always consider the potential causes for reduced range of motion based upon your findings. Because normal arthrokinematic motion was altered, the athletic trainer will need to address this during rehabilitation. Joint mobilization techniques may be performed in addition to traditional stretching exercises to regain normal range of motion. Failure to address all possible causes (altered arthrokinematics) will result in an ineffective rehabilitation plan.

Long-term goals may include:
- Return to soccer practice in 2 weeks
- Return to full soccer participation in 2 1/2 weeks

3-5 The findings from midrange-of-motion muscle testing should be used to help determine which muscles to test during specific muscle testing. The athletic trainer should perform specific muscle testing for all muscles that assist with the symptomatic movement pattern tested. Given that the patient demonstrated pain and weakness during hip extension, the athletic trainer should perform specific muscle tests on the gluteus maximus and hamstring muscles.

3-6 Rehabilitation goals should be based upon the evaluation findings. Each significant finding should have a corresponding rehabilitation goal. The athletic trainer should include both short-term and long-term goals.

Short-term goals may include:
- Decrease swelling by 25 percent in 3 days
- Increase knee extension active range of motion by 50 percent in 1 week
- Increase knee flexion passive range of motion by 50 percent in 1 week
- Increase quadriceps strength by 30 percent in 1 week

CHAPTER 4

Psychological Considerations for Rehabilitation of the Injured Athlete

Elizabeth G. Hedgpeth
Joe Gieck

After completion of this chapter, the athletic training student should be able to do the following:

- Identify various predictors of injury and interventions.

- Recognize stressors in the athlete's life.

- Understand the concept of using buffers for stress management.

- Explain the progressive reactions to injury, dependent on length of rehabilitation.

- Integrate interventions for the four time periods of rehabilitation.

- Recognize irrational thinking and its resolution.

- Explain the importance of athletes taking responsibility for their actions in regard to injury.

- Compare and contrast compliance and adherence.

- Analyze the importance of rehabilitation compliance and its deviations.

- Identify signs and symptoms of clinical depression and suicide intention.

- Discuss goal setting and rehabilitation compliance.

- Review the coping skills necessary for successful rehabilitation.

- Recognize the importance of the relationship between the athletic trainer and the athlete.

Athletic injuries are considered to be one of the major health hazards of sport.[55] The fear of injury might cause a negative view of participation in an activity that has a positive impact on the health and well-being of millions of participants.[45] Sports medicine and athletic training are still inexact sciences. Nowhere is this more evident than in the psychological process of responding to injury in a rational and productive manner and completing the rehabilitation process to the best of the athlete's ability. Early writings often mention that one should never attempt to cure the body without curing the soul.

ACCULTURATION

An overlooked stressor for injured athletes is *acculturation*, which refers to the moving of the injured athletes from the familiar sport culture to the unfamiliar rehabilitation culture (Figure 4-1). In the culture of sport, they know

Uninjured athlete	Injured athlete in rehab
Familiar activity	Unfamiliar activity
Familiar rules	Unfamiliar rules
Familiar field	Unfamiliar area
Veteran player	Rookie player
Familiar pain	Unfamiliar pain
Coach in charge	ATC's in charge
Instant feedback	Feedback deferred
Control	Loss of control
Measure success	Different measure
Vigorous	Loss of vigor

Figure 4-1   Acculturation: Injured athletes moving from the culture of sport to the culture of injury rehabilitation (Hedgpeth, 1997).

how the game is played, what the rules are, and who is in charge. Once injured, they move out of their comfort zone of sport and into the world of rehabilitation where the rules are changed and they are in foreign territory. Without even dealing with the injury, the athletes are stressed. They are veteran players of their sport and now they are in a new game. The coach has always had the power and now the athletic trainer and the sports medicine team have the power. Pain is a factor and that pain is different from the normal pain of working out and playing.

The athletic trainer now tells them "Listen to your body" where coaches have often said "Suck it up and play tough." Coaches give instant feedback on the play; athletic trainers say wait and see how your body reacts.

Loss of control is also a major factor. Athletes know that if they work out and practice hard, they have a chance to play—unlike rehabilitation, where they may or may not get well even if they do all the treatments and exercises as ordered. They can do all that is asked in rehabilitation and still not make progress due to factors out of their control. The bone might not heal properly, or infection might set in, or any number of other things could go wrong. Uninjured athletes measure success by amount of playing time, number of runs scored, or whatever accomplishments are specific to their sport. In the athletic training clinic, the score is measured in terms of how it feels, how strong it is, how many reps can be done, and so on.

Loss of vigor is easily seen in athletes who feel that they are not progressing fast enough or that the exercises are boring. Vigor is regained when the athletes return to practice and play. Loss of vigor might be masked as depression, but over time it clears on its own. Therefore, though

it might appear that injured athletes are stressed for no reason, the acculturation from sport to rehabilitation is a stressor in and of itself.

Most athletes have the self-confidence to adapt to a mild or moderate injury, and most have the support, understanding, and proper encouragement to adapt to more severe injury, but even the most self-confident athletes have their doubts. One athlete put it this way, expressing the positive aspects of returning to competition but also some of the doubts involved: "The best competitors like to compete, and to me this is just a game—an inner game. It's an inner soul game. Can I beat my knee back?" But he also expressed doubts about the real test when a tackler "takes a whack at the knee": "I haven't thought about it, but I've had nightmares about it. My buddy told me he broke his ankle. He said once you get that real good hit and you pop up and it pops up with you, then everything is going to fall into place and you're going to be rolling. You're going to go out there like it's never been hurt and just play."

With the emergence of sport psychology, more attention is being paid to getting the mind ready to return to competition to match the adjustment of the body. Athletes have begun to describe the nightmares, fears, and anxiety of returning to competition. Also, in the current trend of professional athletes receiving extremely high salaries, some athletes describe their injuries and surgery as the most important things in their lives because the ability to play will either make or break them. Surgery and subsequent rehabilitation can determine whether athletes make either millions of dollars in an athletic career or only thousands in a regular job if the injury ends their career.

Athletes don't all deal with injury in the same manner. Rotella[57] describes how one might view the injury as disastrous, another might view it as an opportunity to show courage, whereas another athlete might relish the injury as a means to avoid embarrassment over poor performance, to escape from a losing team, or to discourage a domineering parent. When injuries are career-threatening, athletes whose lives have revolved around a sport may have to make major adjustments in how they perceive themselves as well as how they are perceived within their society. Olympic and other top-caliber athletes are often emotionally and socially years behind their chronological peers because they have spent so much time in their sport that their social interactions have suffered. Therefore many top or single-minded athletes have difficulty with emotional control when they sustain a serious injury. Figure 4-2 demonstrates the physical and emotional aspects of return to performance. The return to performance is either enhanced or negated by the physiological results of both elements.

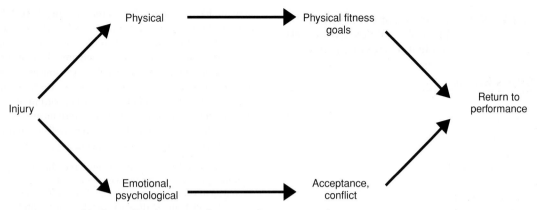

Figure 4-2   The physical and emotional aspects of return to performance.

PREDICTORS OF INJURY

The Injury-Prone Athlete

Some athletes seem to have a pattern of injury, whereas others in exactly the same position with the same physical makeup are injury-free. Certain researchers suggest that some psychological traits might predispose the athlete to a repeated injury cycle.[50,53,65,71,] No one particular personality type has been recognized as injury-prone. However, the individual who likes to take risks seems to represent the injury-prone athlete.[29] Other factors that are seen as predisposing an athlete to risk of injury are being reserved, detached, tender-minded,[36] apprehensive, overprotective, or easily distracted.[56] These individuals usually also lack the ability to cope with the stress associated with the risks and their consequences. Sanderson[58] suggests some other factors leading to a propensity for injury, such as attempts to reduce anxiety by being more aggressive, fear of failure, or guilt over unobtainable or unrealistic goals.

Stress and Risk of Injury

Much has been written about life stress events and the likelihood of illness.[2,14,34,73] Stressors are both positive (e.g., making All-American) and negative (e.g., not making the starting lineup or failing a drug test). Stressors that seem to predispose an athlete to injury are the negative stressors.[73]

Andersen and Williams[2] suggest that negative stressors lead to a lack of attentional focus and to muscle tension, which in turn lead to the stress-injury connection. Loss of attentional focus can cause the athlete to miss cues during a play, setting the stage for a possible injury. Muscle tension

(bracing or guarding) leads to reduced flexibility, reduced motor coordination, and reduced muscle efficiency, which set the athlete up for a variety of injuries (e.g., getting hit by a golf ball or missing an obstacle during a run).

Attentional focusing is perceived on two planes (width and directional). A major component is the ability to change focus when the situation demands it. Width of focus ranges from broad (attending to a number of cues) to narrow (attending to one cue), and direction of focus is internal (attending to feelings or thoughts) or external (attending to events outside of the body). The trick is not only to be able to change focus, but to know the optimal time to make the change in order to minimize the possibility of injury or reinjury. For instance, a football player can be blindsided and take an unanticipated hit, or the gymnast can be distracted and miss a landing.

Life stress is a more global assessment, taking into account events that cause stress over the past year to 18 months. The Life Events Survey for Collegiate Athletes (LESCA) asks collegiate-athlete-specific questions, eliciting a negative or positive response on a Likert-type 8-point scale.[53] Typical events asked about are "major change in playing status" and "pressure to gain or lose weight for sport participation." Another life events assessment is the Social and Athletic Readjustment Rating Scale[7] (SARRS). The events most likely to elicit a negative stress response are listed in Table 4-1.

Profiles of Mood States[46] (POMS) is a more immediate response inventory assessing moods within the last few days or at the most the last few weeks. The POMS identifies six mood states. Five are negative, and one (vigor) is positive. The six mood states are (1) tension-anxiety; (2) depression-dejection; (3) anger-hostility; (4) vigor-activity; (5) fatigue-inertia; and (6) confusion-bewilderment. When

■ **TABLE 4-1** Examples of Events in the Lives of Athletes Most Likely to Elicit a Stress Response.

....

Life Stress Events

Death of family member
Detention or jail
Injury
Death of close friend
Playing for a new coach
Playing on a new team
Personal achievements
Change in living habits
Social readjustments
Change to new school
Change in social activities

....

the POMS results were compared using elite athletes and the general population, a visual "iceberg profile" was noted for the elite athletes by Morgan.[49] The elite athletes' scores on the five negative scales fall below the 50th percentile, and their scores on the sixth, positive scale (vigor) peak considerably above the 50th percentile, indeed resembling the silhouette of an "iceberg."

The POMS has been used to measure the mood states of athletes at the time of injury as well as at 2-week intervals during the rehabilitation process.[64] When the POMS was used within 2 days of injury, the injured athletes showed significant elevations in depression and anger, no change in tension and vigor, but less fatigue and confusion as compared to the college norms. When the athletes were divided into groups according to severity of injury based on length of rehabilitation, the data is more explicit concerning reactions to injury and rehabilitation. Group 1 consists of athletes with less than 1 week of rehabilitation; they had less tension, depression, fatigue, and confusion. Group 2 consists of athletes in rehabilitation for more than 2 weeks but less than 4 weeks; they had more anger but less fatigue and confusion. Group 3 consists of athletes in rehabilitation more than 4 weeks; they had more tension, depression, and anger, and less vigor. This finding is important in that it sends a wake-up call to the sports medicine team to be aware of the ramifications of severe injury that entails a long rehabilitation period.

Interventions for Stress Reduction

Not all athletes need or want counseling, and the close relationship between the athlete and the athletic trainer

is invaluable in making this decision (Figure 4-3). Athletic trainers are now taking a more active role in the psychological aspects of injury and rehabilitation. They are the closest to the athlete and often spend as much time as the athletes at practice and games. Athletic trainers are now aware of the psychological impact of injury and have a working knowledge of counseling techniques for various situations.[12,26,51] Few athletes react to stress events by verbalizing their feelings of stress, yet most handle them very well by themselves. James Michener[48] makes the following point:

> For many athletes physical activity, rather than talking things out, appears to offer a means of expressing feelings and aggressions. Perhaps this substitution of actions for words contributes to the seeming reluctance of athletes to come to a service that requires that they articulate their feelings.

Unfortunately, many coaches do not have the interest or ability to work with athletes who need help. Some sort of screening device should be used to identify athletes who are experiencing life situations that they are unprepared to handle. Obviously the staff of a smaller team is more familiar with the athletes and their problems and can more effectively deal with them,[31] but larger teams' staffs should attempt to deal with the athlete through the position coach or other available support personnel (e.g., counseling centers, sport psychologists, grief support groups).

Using Buffers. In many instances athletes feel that their sport is the one positive thing in life that helps them get through times of extreme stress. Areas outside of sports are often stressful, and athletes tend to respond to interventions that are within their framework of emotional comfort. The use of buffers might be all the athlete

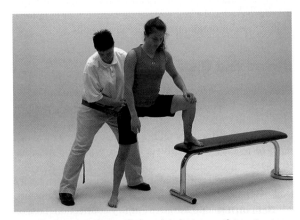

Figure 4-3 A close relationship between the patient and the athletic trainer is invaluable.

needs to handle the stress of injury and rehabilitation. Buffers are techniques that allay the symptom of stress but do not address the problem that originally caused the stressors. Several buffers that can be beneficial in reducing the stress of injury and rehabilitation are progressive relaxation with or without imagery, aerobic exercise, diet modifications (e.g., reduction of caffeine), treatment of sleep disorders, and time management programs.

CLINICAL DECISION MAKING　　　　　**Exercise 4–1**

Julie is a women's lacrosse player at a Division I school playing in the starting lineup as a sophomore. She had played her entire high school years without injury, so having a severe ankle sprain at the end of this season was a shock. Julie is not accustomed to having the normal activities of daily living take so much time, and she feels she never has time to go to the athletic training room for her rehabilitation. What can the athletic trainer do to help Julie alter her schedule to include time for rehabilitation?

Abdominal Breathing.　Deep abdominal breathing for relaxation is a product of yoga and has been practiced for more than 5,000 years.[69] The practice was brought to the West in the 1960s. Deep abdominal breathing is simple to learn and is effective as a tool for relaxation and relief from stress and pain.[61] It is used in the Lamaze childbirth method to relieve pain and stress during the birthing process.[69] Deep abdominal breathing[41] is simple and can be mastered in a few days. Following is a simple way to teach it to an athlete:

> Lie on your back in a quiet place with one hand on chest and one hand on your stomach. Inhale through your nose and have the air fill up your belly without your chest moving. Now breathe out through your mouth and feel your belly go down. Breathe slowly and pay attention to the air moving in and out of your lungs. This can be used for pain and tension relief by paying attention to the sore and tense muscle groups in the body during the inhale phase. During the exhale phase feel your pain and tension being 'blown out' of the body with the exhaled breath.

Once the athlete has mastered the lying-down position, move on to sitting and then standing positions. The beauty of this practice is that it can be performed anywhere and anytime and enables athletes in rehabilitation to control their pain and stress.[61]

Relaxation Techniques.　Progressive relaxation techniques[37] are most effective for athletes who tend to be stressed regarding an injury and who have problems

sleeping, tension headaches, or general muscle bracing or tightness. Relaxation training, with or without imagery, allows athletes to control their feelings of stress and anxiety with a series of deep breathing, voluntary muscular contraction, and relaxation exercise.[4] Relaxation and imagery are used by athletes to reduce the symptoms of anxiety associated with the reaction to injury and rehabilitation. Athletes who are coping well on their own should not be forced to spend extra time on relaxation training.

Jacobsen's[38] progressive relaxation technique is thought to be effective because of the assumption that it is impossible to be nervous or tense when the muscles are relaxed. The tenseness of the involuntary muscles and organs can be reduced when the contiguous skeletal muscles are relaxed. The muscles are tensed and relaxed in order for the athlete to become familiar with how the muscle feels in a relaxed state and in a tense state. The relaxation method involves the tensing and relaxing of muscles in a predetermined order. The arm and hand are done first because the difference in tense and relaxed muscles is more apparent in these muscle groups. The repetitions should last approximately 10 to 15 seconds for the tension segment and 15 to 20 seconds for the relaxation segment, with about three repetitions for each muscle group. After the athlete is comfortable with the relaxation training, then imagery can be introduced.

CLINICAL DECISION MAKING　　　　　**Exercise 4–2**

Tim is a 17-year-old tennis player at a prep school known for turning out exceptional tennis players ready to play at the Division I level. He developed elbow tendinitis at the end of last season and has spent the summer doing rehabilitation. The medical staff cleared him to play, but Tim is unable to keep from tensing up when he knows he is being observed by recruiters. His whole body is stiff and tight, and his usual warm-up stretching is not sufficient to keep his muscles relaxed. How can the athletic trainer help Tim manage this problem?

Imagery.　Imagery is the use of one's senses to create or recreate an experience in the mind.[6] Visual images used in the rehabilitation process include visual rehearsal, emotive imagery rehearsal, and body rehearsal.[15,66] Visual rehearsal uses both coping and mastery rehearsal. Coping rehearsal has athletes visually rehearsing problems they feel might stand in the way of a return to competition. They then rehearse how they will overcome these problems. Mastery rehearsal aids in gaining confidence and motivational skills. Athletes visualize their successful return to competition, beginning with early practice drills and continuing on to the game situation.

In emotive rehearsal, the athlete gains confidence and security by visualizing scenes relating to positive feelings of enthusiasm, confidence, and pride—in other words, the emotional rewards of praise and success from participating well in competition. Body rehearsal empirically helps athletes in the healing process. It is suggested that athletes visualize their bodies healing internally both during the rehabilitation procedures and throughout their daily activities.[28] To do this, the athletes have to have a good understanding of the injury and of the type of healing occurring during the rehabilitation process. Ievleva and Orlick[35] had athletes use imagery during physiotherapy by imagining that the ultrasound was increasing blood flow and thus promoting recovery.

Care should be taken to explain the healing and rehabilitative process clearly but not to overwhelm athletes with so much information that they become intimidated and fearful. This mistake is often made by the inexperienced athletic trainer who wants to impress the athletes. Educate athletes only to the amount of knowledge required. By the same token, don't hold back information athletes require for this imagery.

PROGRESSIVE REACTIONS DEPEND ON LENGTH OF REHABILITATION

The literature on reactions to injury has dispelled the stage theory of reaction to injury, according to an extensive literature review by Wortman and Silver.[79] However, there are factors that are commonly seen among athletes going through adjustment to injury and rehabilitation in the athletic training room. Severity of injury usually determines length of rehabilitation. Regardless of length of rehabilitation, the injured patient has to deal with three reactive phases of the injury and rehabilitation process (Figure 4-4). These phases are reaction to injury, reaction to rehabilitation, and reaction to return to competition or career termination. These reactions can be cumulative in nature depending on the length of rehabilitation. Other factors that influence reactions to injury and rehabilitation are the patient's coping skills, past history of injury, social support, and personality traits. These reactions fall into four time frames: short-term (less than 4 weeks), long-term (more than 4 weeks), chronic (recurring), and termination (career-ending). Reactions are primary and secondary, but patients do not all have all reactions, nor do all reactions fall into the suggested sequence.

Length of rehabilitation	Reaction to injury	Reaction to rehabilitation	Reaction to return
Short (< 4 weeks)	Shock Relief	Impatience Optimism	Eagerness Anticipation
Long (> 4 weeks)	Fear Anger	Loss of vigor Irrational thoughts Alienation	Acknowledgment
Chronic (recurring)	Anger Frustration	Dependence or independence Apprehension	Confident or skeptical
Termination (career-ending)	Isolation Grief process	Loss of athletic identify	Closure and renewal

Figure 4-4   Progressive reactions of injured athletes based on severity of injury and length of rehabilitation.

DEALING WITH SHORT-TERM INJURY

Short-term injuries are usually less than 4 weeks but may be a few days over depending on how the length is measured in terms of the end of rehabilitation. For practical purposes the rehabilitation is complete when the patient and the sports medicine team feel it is safe for the patient to return, when an appropriate level of competitive fitness has been reached, and the athlete feels ready physically and psychologically to return to competition. Short-term injuries can include, but are not limited to, first- or second-degree sprains/strains, bruises, and simple dislocations. These are the types of injuries that are fairly common and are part of playing the game.

Reactions to Short-Term Injury

The primary reaction to these injuries is the **shock** of surprise—the shock that the injury cannot be just "walked off" or "shaken off." At the time of the injury, the athlete tries to walk it off or shake it off on the court or playing field. Athletes have probably experienced this type of injury before with no residual complaint and need time to accept that, this time, it is not immediately going away. Rehabilitation compliance is often compromised when athletes envision themselves returning in a couple of days without treatment. The athletic trainer assesses the patient's injury and explains the process of rehabilitation to the patient.

The secondary reaction is **relief**—relief that it is not something really major, given that it couldn't be discounted as just a "nick" or "ding." The sense of relief is contingent on the patient's trust in the athletic trainer. At this point, the relationship between the athletic trainer and the patient is forged and trust is established. This sets the tone for the success or failure of the rehabilitation process.

Reactions to Rehabilitation of Short-Term Injury

Once short-term injury rehabilitation begins, the primary reaction the patient displays is **impatience**—an impatience to get started, to do something, to get on with the program as quickly as possible. During this time the patient is often experiencing peaks and valleys in the recovery process. The athlete is accustomed to two speeds: no speed and full speed. Athletes often express the belief that they should heal faster because they are in better shape, and they are not happy to spend time in the sequential phases of reha-

bilitation. If it is a sprained ankle, the athlete does not react with exhilaration to the crutch phase, then the walking phase, then the walk-jog phase, then the jog-run phase, then the run phase, and then finally the full-speed activity phase. The athletic trainer can reassure the patient that the phases are necessary and that to push it could set back the rehabilitation time.

The secondary reaction is one of **optimism.** This optimism is due to the confidence and trust established between the athletic trainer and the patient. The patient is able to believe the athletic trainer's assessment that because the injury turned out to be less serious than originally thought, it stands to reason that the rehabilitation will work out as well. It is important that compliance be consistent with the athletic trainer's treatment plan and that the injured patient does not try to return to practice or play too soon. This level of injury has a good track record for excellent recovery.

Intervention for Short-Term Injury

Intervention should include allowing the patient to vent frustrations and reiterating that there is a light at the end of the tunnel. At the collegiate level, athletes have frequently had this type of injury and consider it to be part and parcel of playing the game. The injured athlete should be encouraged to remain involved with the team, attending practices while performing rehabilitation, attending team meetings, and interacting with teammates after hours. At this stage the athletic trainer and the patient will have to conduct some reality checks to ascertain that the concerns that come up are in the realm of the patient's control. Losing their spot on the team, losing their speed, or losing their best shot is not within the athletes' control. Doing effective rehabilitation on a consistent basis is within their control. Staying current with the team will keep them current with plays and coaching changes. Effective rehabilitation is the only way to return to their sport. Compliance is not usually a factor for short-term injuries.

Reactions to Return to Competition after Short-Term Injury

The primary reaction to returning to competition is **eagerness** and the secondary reaction is **anticipation.** At the time of return to competition, the patients with short-term injuries are usually eager to begin to practice and play. They anticipate that they will return to their preinjury competence the first day back. By the time the athletic trainer feels the patient is ready to return, it is assumed that a level of trust has been established. The patient and the athletic trainer must agree on a realistic plan for return to activity so that the transition will be safe and satisfactory for all concerned.

DEALING WITH LONG-TERM INJURY

Long-term injuries are considered to have a rehabilitation time of more than 4 weeks and can be anywhere from 4 weeks to 6 months to a year. These injuries are the most severe and tend to be the most difficult for the patient to handle because of the length of inactivity and the lack of rapid progress during rehabilitation. Long-term injuries include, but are not limited to, fractures, orthopedic surgery, general surgery, second- and third-degree sprains/strains, and debilitating illness.

Reaction to Long-Term Injury

The primary reaction to long-term injury is **fear**—fear that they will never get better, fear that they can never play again, fear that they cannot handle a long rehabilitation period, fear of pain, and fear of the unknown (Figure 4-5). Most athletes have heard the horror stories of the individual who had this same injury and never came back for a multitude of reasons. They hear stories of individuals who came back but were never again as fast or as talented or as fearless . . . the list goes on. At this point the athletic trainer must allay the fear with pertinent information in terms that are easy to understand. It is not helpful to overload the patient with all the latest information on that particular

injury. The rule of thumb is to present the truth in appropriate doses that the patient can handle. Again, establishing a trusting relationship with the athletic trainer is a vital component of this long-term process.

The secondary reaction to a long-term injury is **anger**—anger that the injury happened, that it happened to them, that it happened at the time it did, and so on. Anger cannot be reasoned with, and the sports medicine team must understand and not react to the patient's anger. An angry, hostile, or surly attitude toward the personnel or program should not offend the athletic trainer. Whoever happens to be around the patient often bears the brunt of the anger. This response is merely an emotional release. With anger the patient is usually reacting to the situation and not necessarily to the individual.

Reaction to Long-Term Rehabilitation

The primary reaction to **long-term rehabilitation** is twofold: loss of vigor and irrational thoughts. At this point the athletic trainer needs to be aware that a loss of vigor can be masked as depression, although depression can also be a possible reaction. The patient appears to be lacking the usual vim, vigor, and vitality but does not have the common signs and symptoms of a true depression (Figure 4-6). Understanding this phenomenon will enable the athletic trainer to understand the patient's change in temperament and disposition. The patient should understand that it is reasonable to feel somewhat discouraged concerning the injury, as long as there are no other presenting symptoms of clinical depression.

In one study, it was found that clinical depression occurs in only 4.8 percent of the injured athletic population.[8] The

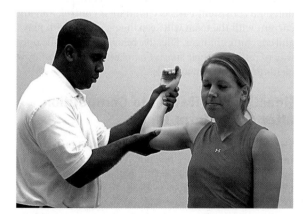

Figure 4-5   The athletic trainer assists the patient to quell the fear associated with long-term injuries.

1. Change in eating and/or sleeping habits either more or less than usual
2. Difficulty in concentration
3. Lack of interest in activities previously enjoyed
4. Inappropriate reaction to stressful situations: aggression, extreme agitation, rage or no re-action: "I don't care," "Doesn't bother me," "Whatever"
5. Flat affect—a void of the normal fluctuation of facial expressions
6. Decreased involvement with normal social support such as teammates, friends, and family
7. History of depression in the past or family history of depression

Figure 4-6   Common signs and symptoms of clinical depression.

possibility of attempted suicide by the clinically depressed patient warrants the vigilance of the sports medicine team. If signs of clinical depression (loss of appetite, sleep disruption, withdrawal, change in mood state, thoughts of or plans for attempting suicide, etc.) are present, then the possibility of attempted suicide must be addressed (Figure 4-7). According to Smith and Milliner,[63] the incidence of attempted suicide is high among the age group of 15 to 24 years. In Smith and Milliner's study of five athletes who had attempted suicide, the common factors were a serious injury that required surgical intervention, rehabilitation of 6 weeks to a year while not participating in sport, diminished athletic skill upon return after successful rehabilitation, and being replaced in their position on the team. Adaptation to the physical, mental, and emotional frustration is hard work during the rehabilitative process. The work the athlete is doing is not producing the same rewards as participation in the sport; plus the athlete is becoming anxious about falling farther behind in the sport. At this point it is prudent to ask the athlete if psychological intervention is needed or desired, since not all athletes require or desire psychological intervention.

The other primary reaction to long-term rehabilitation is **irrational thoughts** (Figure 4-8). If irrational thoughts are persistent, interfere with the normal routine of daily life, and disrupt the rehabilitation process, then

1. Has signs and symptoms of being clinically depressed
2. Has feelings of helplessness and hopelessness such as seeing no way out of stressful situation except suicide
3. Has thoughts of suicide or a previous attempt, or has a close friend, family member, or acquaintance who committed suicide
4. Has an irreversible plan to commit suicide (taking pills as opposed to jumping from the top of a building)
5. Making plans to not be around, such as giving away possessions, writing letters, getting affairs in order, saying good-bye to friends
6. Expresses intention to commit suicide (taking demographics into account—women make more attempts but men are more successful)

Figure 4-7   Common signs of possible suicidal intentions.

psychological intervention is recommended and is frequently effective. Irrational thoughts can be negative perceptions of pain, fear of reinjury, lack of social support, poor performance, and so on. These patients might harbor thoughts of not returning to play or not being able

Irrational Thinking toward Injury and Rehabilitation

Exaggeration: Severity or mildness and significance or insignificance of injury— "I'm in great shape, so my broken leg will heal faster than it would for someone who is out of shape." "How bad can a sprain be?"

Disregard: Neglecting or overdoing rehabilitation treatment— "I'll wait a few weeks and see if it gets better on its own." "If one repetition of five sets is good, then two of ten will be twice as good."

Oversimplification: Thinking of rehabilitation as good or bad, right or wrong, necessary or unnecessary— "No one ever came back from ACL surgery." "I don't see any reason to do rehab exercises if I am going to have surgery in two weeks."

Generalization: Generalizing the outcome of one athlete's injury to all injuries, or one athlete's outcome of rehabilitation to all rehabilitation— "All sprains heal in two weeks." "Rehab is necessary only if you plan to compete again."

Unwarranted Conclusions: Conclusions based on unsound thinking or false information— "I know an athlete who did everything they told him to do and his arm never got better." "They say that once you break a bone you never can run as fast."

Figure 4-8   Examples of thought patterns athletes might have concerning injury and rehabilitation.

to return to their previous level of play. Previously rational and positive perceptions of situations now become negative and irrational as self-destructive emotions color the thought process. Emotional reaction is exacerbated when the patient fails to heal or return faster than the nonathlete. Frequently, athletes feel that because they are in better shape at the time of injury, they should heal faster than nonathletes who are out of shape at the time of injury. The athlete has often put in years of training and imposes pressures to heal faster and return quicker. The athlete's common sense and judgment become altered. This mood change might occur daily or weekly, so continual interaction between the athletic trainer and the patient is necessary to restore rationality and change negative thoughts.

The secondary reaction to long-term rehabilitation is a feeling of **alienation.** With an injury that requires weeks or months of rehabilitation before the athlete's return to competition, the athlete often feels that the coaches have ceased to care, teammates have no time to spend with them, friends are no longer around, and their social life consists of time put into rehabilitation. The injured athletes may have had little support from coaches and teammates, since the coaches are concerned with the results of the team. Injured athletes feel neglected if their daily activities have revolved around the sport and they are no longer part of the sport.

The injured athlete must understand that the coach cares but has no expertise in injury management and must be concerned with getting the rest of the team ready. The athletic trainer has no expertise in coaching but is primarily interested in getting the injured athlete back to optimal fitness. Coaches work with players on playing their sport, athletic trainers work with patients on rehabilitating injuries: two different fields, two different abilities, two different areas of expertise. Some coaches, unfortunately, might also want the injured athlete kept away from other players to remove the reminder that injury is a possibility.[20]

The injured athlete may feel unable to maintain or regain normal relationships with teammates. The injured athlete is a reminder that injury can happen, and teammates might pull away from that constant reminder. Friendships based on athletic identification are now compromised because the athletic identification is gone, and they can be related to in athletic terms only by what they did yesterday or as injured teammates and not as individuals. Injured athletes no longer have the camaraderie of the dressing room, the practice bashing, the travel to away events, and the other interactions mired in tradition that give athletes a sense of belonging, a sense of being important. When injured athletes can remain involved

with the team, however, they feel less isolated and less guilty for not putting it on the line to help the team.

Intervention for Long-Term Rehabilitation

Whenever possible, anger should not be challenged, because no one can reason with anger. Instead, the athletic trainer should wait until the individual is in control of the anger and then discuss the inappropriate behavior that cannot be tolerated in the rehabilitation setting. Then the athletic trainer and the patient can work out the cause of the anger and together arrive at a solution. The athletic trainer must act as an emotional blotter and, if possible, not further aggravate the situation by attempting to exert power to calm down the patient. It is as important to listen to what the patient is feeling in addition to what the patient is saying. At this point the patient has a need to vent the anger, and the athletic trainer must simply listen to the patient's reaction.

At this time active listening by the athletic trainer is a move toward developing a supportive and trusting relationship with the patient. Having a trusting relationship between the patient and the athletic trainer can make all the difference in getting the patient into the proper frame of mind for successful completion of the rehabilitation process.

One of the more difficult aspects of adjusting to injury is stopping negative thoughts, which are devastating to a successful rehabilitation process. These thoughts have to be recognized by the patient and then controlled.[60] Controlling inner thoughts determines future behavior. This process is one of awareness, education, and encouragement for ultimate positive change.

Negative thoughts have a detrimental effect on both mental and physical performance.[57] It is helpful to keep a daily record of when these thoughts take place, as well as the correlated physical progress and the time and circumstances in which they occur. Then patients are helped to stop these negative thoughts and instill a positive regimen. This step is followed by an evaluation of the whole negative thought-stopping program on a regular basis. In this manner, injured athletes have the practice and feedback to begin their own positive outlook in terms of constructive thoughts, concentration, cues, images, and calming responses to change inappropriate attitudes. This positive outlook, plus seeing physical progress, can help patients return more quickly to competition with better abilities to perform. The reinforcement of sayings such as "You will get better" and "This too will pass" aid in the blockage of the negative thoughts. Negative thoughts block the athlete's road to recovery by increasing pain, anxiety, and anger. Patients should be encouraged to put their efforts into recovery rather than into the downward spiral of self-pity. Thoughts create emotions, therefore these negative thoughts have to be recognized and dealt with for a more rapid recovery. The patient should never be allowed to say "I can't" but rather should substitute "I'll try."

The technique of restructuring perceptions helps the patient become aware of these destructive, self-defeating behaviors. The patient, however, might fall into the mode of "I can't do it, I'll never get well." This irrational thinking produces anxiety, fear, and possibly depression, which are detrimental to progress in rehabilitation. The patient might be illogical, distort perceptions of events, or reach unrealistic decisions and conclusions. The patient has replaced the old set of worries about simply playing well and helping the team win with the set of "Woe is me," with its resultant anxiety. Obviously, these thought patterns are detrimental to the positive attitude necessary in the rehabilitation process.

The athletic trainer must recognize and challenge irrational thinking. Examination of these thoughts with patients reassures them that it is normal to feel unhappy, frustrated, angry, or insecure, but that the injury is not hopeless, they do not lack courage, and all is not lost and life is not over. The patient should be challenged to replace irrational thoughts with positive and rational ones. In short, the injury is aggravating and unfortunate, but it can be handled and overcome. The injury is placed in perspective and viewed in the same way as the athlete would consider preparation for the next athletic contest. The patient must identify faulty thinking, gain understanding of it, and actively work for its change. Research[5,76] indicates that the self-thoughts, images, and attitudes during the recovery period impact the length and quality of the rehabilitation.

Lost social support can be replaced by organizing support groups or similar injury groups or mentoring by athletes who have completed rehabilitation successfully.[23] A supporting relationship between the patient and the athletic trainer can be the mainstay in attainment of successful rehabilitation (Figure 4-9). Establishing this relationship may be difficult for athletes who have been catered to when healthy and are now in a reversed role. At this time patients question many aspects of the rehabilitation procedure. They question the doctor's diagnosis, the athletic trainer for working them possibly too much, and the coach for not paying attention to them. They question whether they are thought of as malingerers. They question whether the rehabilitation personnel know how important competition is to them.

Toward the end of rehabilitation, the patient should begin sport-specific drills during practice time with the team. The patient then begins to re-enter the team culture and is not isolated from the team environment. Thus more effort is put into functional sport-specific situations that are generally less boring to the athlete. In so doing, the athlete gains a more realistic appreciation of the skills needed to attain preinjury performance levels. The rehabilitation routine is more easily tolerated by patients if they can see some carryover to their particular sport.

After injury, patients need the support of teammates. To prevent possible feelings of negative self-worth and problems of loss of identity for athletes, their support groups need to stress that they are interested in the patient as a person as well as a team member. If the athletic trainer and sports medicine team have established prior personal contact with the patient as a worthwhile person, this transition can be easier.

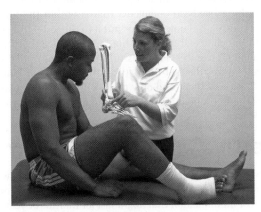

Figure 4-9   The patient and the athletic trainer develop a relationship of respect and trust.

Reaction to Return to Competition for Long-Term Injury

The primary reaction to return to competition from a long-term injury is an **acknowledgment** that the rehabilitation process is completed. This is a feeling of "I have done my best and all that I can do in the area of rehabilitation." The patient might go down a checklist of performance abilities. The team physician who has the final vote on medically clearing an athlete to return to competition has given the OK to return. The athletic trainer has set functional criteria to be followed before returning to play. The athletic trainer and the patient have discussed the use of additional padding, the wearing of a brace, or other equipment adjustments to minimize reinjury. The physician, the athletic trainer, the sport psychologist, and the coach have determined that the athlete is ready to play at 100 percent, the athlete fits back into the chemistry of the current lineup, the athlete is knowledgeable about recent changes in coaching strategy, and the athlete feels psychologically ready. The athlete and the sports medicine team have discussed feelings of confidence about returning, willingness to play with pain or soreness, and willingness to risk reinjury or permanent damage. The athlete has gained the emotional self-control to think rationally about the injury and cope successfully with the return to competition. It is now up to the athlete to make the decision to return to play.

After going through the checklist of concerns that the athlete feels are important, the secondary reaction is **trust**—trust that everything has been done to be as prepared as possible to return to play. Trust at this time is trust that everything has been done, not that the injury is healed—this won't come until it has been tested and proven. When the athlete has been cleared to return, everything has been completed that is within the athlete's control. It is now time to "put it to the test—to step up to the plate and give it a shot." Acceptance that the rehabilitation process is successful will not come until the athlete makes the first move, takes the first hit, or runs the first race. Then, and only then, will the athlete play with the freedom and confidence she or he had prior to the injury.

DEALING WITH CHRONIC INJURY

Chronic injury can be defined as an injury having a slow, insidious onset, most often starting with pain and/or signs of inflammation that might last for months or years and giving the impression of recurring over time.[1] These injuries are usually overuse injuries and can include tendinitis, stress fractures (shin splints), compartment syndrome, and other second- or third-degree injuries.

Reaction to Chronic Injury

The primary reaction to a chronic injury is **anger.** Often the patient has done everything the athletic trainer suggested as far as rehabilitation and even maintenance rehabilitation, and still the injury recurred. The patient desperately wants to return to previous form and remembers that rehabilitation is going to be another long, drawn-out process. The athletic trainer often has to explain over and over that setbacks occur even without provocation. Such repetition is necessary because an angry patient has selective hearing and a short attention span. It might take several meetings for the athlete to cool down enough to hear what is being said. Because many chronic injuries are overuse injuries, rest and inactivity are frequently the treatment of choice. Athletes often describe this inactivity during injury as being harder than playing. When they are playing, all their energy is directed toward the goal of running, throwing, jumping, or whatever other activity is part of their sport. When they are doing rehabilitation for a chronic injury, most physical activity screeches to a halt.

Inactivity leads to **frustration,** the secondary reaction to chronic injury. The fact that many of these injuries are overuse injuries increases the frustration brought on by a sense of somehow having caused the recurrence or at least done something to increase the chance of it. "If I hadn't run the extra mile." "If I hadn't played the second set." If the athlete has used sport as a buffer to control stress, that outlet is gone for the time being. Stress then accelerates. Often these athletes are used to being very active and the forced inactivity is frustrating. These athletes are well acquainted with the rehabilitation process to come, the emotional ups and downs, the time commitment, the expense, and the hard work that goes into successful rehabilitation. The thoughts of going through the process again with no real expectation of a permanent solution is indeed frustrating.

Reaction to Rehabilitation of Chronic Injury

The primary reactions to rehabilitation of a chronic injury are **dependence** and **independence.** These reactions are manifested by athletes reacting to the rehabilitation process as if they have no control or as if they have complete control. The stance is either reactive or proactive and is seen in the patient's either not taking control or responsibility for getting better or assuming total control over the rehabilitation process.

There is very little middle ground for these patients in the treatment protocol: they either try everything new or they are unwilling to try anything new. They either question every treatment the athletic trainer recommends or accept every treatment the athletic trainer recommends. Patients might swing from one end of the spectrum to the other, depending on factors such as how well the last rehabilitation worked, how fast the last rehabilitation moved, how well they liked the last athletic trainer, where they are in their season, and any other situation they perceive as warranting a change.

Dependent patients don't take part in the decisions of rehabilitation, they don't give their input concerning what did, or didn't, work before and they often leave all decisions up to the athletic trainer or team physician. Often these patients become dependent on the athletic trainer and relinquish all power regarding rehabilitation decisions. These patients want someone else to be responsible for their welfare and to meet their every need at their whim and command. They demand that more time be spent on them. Failure of one athletic trainer to meet their demands results in their selecting an athletic trainer who will meet their demands. Athletic trainers with the greatest need to help others will be easily taken advantage of, at the sacrifice of time needed for other patients.

The independent reaction is just the opposite. These patients want to call all the shots and are up-to-date on the latest fads. They are likely to change the treatment plan—or the athletic trainer—if progress is not as fast or as productive as they expect or want. They have a strong urge to find the perfect treatment by trying new techniques, changing physicians and athletic trainers, or shopping around for any solution that might work better and faster. The athletic trainer must not take this personally. It is important to accept that shopping around is not a rejection of the athletic trainer but a reaction to the chronic injury rehabilitation.

The secondary reaction to chronic injury rehabilitation is **apprehension.** Patients with chronic injuries know that although they might get through this flare-up, there is a strong possibility that the injury will return, for in fact it never completely heals. They approach rehabilitation with trepidation, not knowing what will work this time and what will last. They tend to feel stress over every sign and symptom that the rehabilitation is not going as well or as rapidly as expected. Dependent patients react to this apprehension by being overcompliant, thinking that

they just need to work harder at what the athletic trainer suggests. Independent patients, reacting to apprehension, tend to make more changes if rehabilitation is not going well—trying new and different things, looking for the perfect treatment.

CLINICAL DECISION MAKING   Exercise 4–4

Christine is a 15-year-old Junior Level diver who has been competing since she was 9 years old. She has had chronic back pain and muscle spasms for 3 months. For several weeks she has been making irrational complaints: "No divers I know have ever been able to dive once back pain starts." "Rehabilitation never works for back pain." How can the athletic trainer help Christine change her opinion?

Interventions for Chronic Injury

If patients become dependent and they no longer receive the special attention they feel they deserve, they often lash out in anger or frustration. The athletic trainer needs to head off this response by firmly explaining the restrictions on time and what is required of the patient in terms of rehabilitation. This response should be pointed out to the patient as inappropriate, and it should be examined by the athletic trainer and the patient if it becomes a continual problem, because it is only a detriment to recovery. At this time the patient is encouraged to transfer the time and energy formerly given to the sport into the rehabilitation process. The patient has to become an active, not a passive, participant. The injury is now the competitor, rather than next week's opponent. Care should be taken to prevent the patient from becoming a dependent patient.

In order to be more proactive rather than reactive, the dependent patient is encouraged to take part in the rehabilitation. This does not mean that the patient assumes the role of the athletic trainer, but it does mean that they work as a team. This is where the trust and respect between the athletic trainer and the patient is of paramount importance. It is a two-way street where the athletic trainer provides the expertise concerning the injury and the patient has the expertise concerning his or her body.

The independent patient is encouraged to develop a relationship with the athletic trainer that is one of respect and trust. At this point the athletic trainer can facilitate this trust by being current with the latest literature on the patient's particular injury. Knowledge of the injury, its healing mechanism, and the rehabilitation progression

gives patients an orderly timetable within which to pro-
ceed. It will help if the athletic trainer and the patient have
a plan that is mutually acceptable. The athletic trainer can
make an effort to be particularly flexible when working
with these patients; this will go a long way in strengthening the relationship of trust and respect so necessary to a
smooth rehabilitation.

All patients are participants in the rehabilitation process, but they must be active participants and become
engaged in the process. Patients have to be encouraged and
believe in future success. All efforts should point toward
a positive result, with the patients working with what is
available and not with wishful thinking.

Reaction to Chronic Injury Recovery

Recovery from chronic injury is in some ways a misnomer,
because the very nature of the injury assumes it will recur
if the athlete continues to play. The single level reaction is
twofold—either skeptical or confident.

The **skeptical reaction** is not necessarily a negative
reaction but one born of multiple experiences with rehabilitation. Skeptical patients are realistic in their options
and have usually made peace with the nature of a chronic
injury. This is not to say defeat is accepted, but that reality is acknowledged. They have not given up hope, but the
hope is tempered with acceptance of factors that they have
no power to control. These patients rehabilitate to the best
of their ability but accept that some things are not within
their control.

The **confident reaction** to recovery from chronic
injury is not necessarily an unrealistic or unenlightened
reaction regarding the course of this injury. These patients
have an unyielding faith that is untarnished by repeated
experiences with recurrence of a chronic injury. Often
confidence is more global for these patients and is not
necessarily an injury-specific reaction. This may be a personality trait and is not tied into the injury or lack of participation in their sport. Identity for these patients is not
contingent upon sport. This does not mean these patients
do not care, but just that they do not allow the injury to
design and mandate their disposition or to define and out-
line their life.

It is unclear whether one reaction comes before the
other. It can be assumed that patients are not relegated to
one or the other reaction but can move between the two.
The mitigating factors for moving between the two could
be maturity, experience with rehabilitation, length of time
playing a sport, the particular time in the season, or the
meaning of the sport to the patient.

DEALING WITH A CAREER-ENDING INJURY

One of the hardest adjustments an athlete has to make
is when to end participation in a sport. It does appear to
matter if this is an abrupt ending (injury, illness, cut from
team) or one with some advance warning (retirement, age,
ability).[20] For the athlete whose career ends unexpectedly,
there is a feeling of not being able to complete goals due
to unexpected termination.[75] The athletes who ended
careers voluntarily, who chose the time to leave, and who
had played the sport longer had a smoother transition.

Injuries that fall into this category include spinal cord
injuries, extensive hardware implants (screws, plates, etc.),
multiple surgeries with declining benefits, and persistent
debilitating or incapacitating illness.

Reaction to a Career-Ending Injury

Isolation is the primary reaction to termination of sport
and is dependent upon the athlete's perception of the
importance of participation. Many athletes have spent
years as part of a team that has offered a well-defined
and meaningful activity. The very nature of sport is one
of exact boundaries (rules of play, precise beginnings
and endings, codes of conduct, etc.), and the athletes in
turn have defined roles within these boundaries (position
played, rankings, roles within the team structure, etc.).
At the time of termination, the disruption of a significant
attachment affiliation, coupled with a large time commitment and expansion of injury, all set these athletes up for
the debilitating effects of depression.[20]

The secondary reaction is that these athletes must go
through a process of **grief**—grieving for a loss of not only
a career, but an identity, an extended family, a place in society where they know the rules and can play the game. Sport
for the athlete is a community, where they are productive
members, where they excel, where they feel accepted, and
where they feel they belong. These athletes grieve for what
they no longer have: their place in the group, their place in
society, their identity as an athlete, their job or career, their
place of comfort, their sense of belonging.

The grief process is an adjustment period, and the form
it takes and how long it lasts depend on the individual's
personality and the importance the sport had in forming
that personality. There are many theories of the process
of grief. A good review can be found in Baillie and Danish[3] or Evans and Hardy.[21] The grief process is a sequential progression: the grief process must take place before
acceptance, the acceptance process must take place before

career change, and the career change attempts to fill the void created after the end of the dream of competition.

Reaction to Rehabilitation for a Career-Ending Injury

Loss of athletic identity is the primary reaction to rehabilitation of an injury that terminates participation in a sport. It is a feeling of "Who am I? Where do I belong? What is my purpose, my reason for being?" The rehabilitation involves the psychological adjustment to the loss of self. Baillie and Danish[3] suggest that athletes have taken anywhere from 2 to 10 years to adjust to termination from sport.

The injured athlete enters physical rehabilitation half-heartedly, if at all. The patient often says, "Who cares?" "What does it matter?" "Who will know?" in response to setting a rehabilitation plan. These patients might go through the motions of rehabilitation, but the inner spark to get back to competition is missing. At this point the athletic trainer must decide whether the patient needs to be referred to a counselor or sport psychologist. The criterion for referral is usually an established protocol and consists of determining whether the patient is able to maintain a sense of control and engaging in activities while emotionally working through the grief process.

Intervention in a Career-Ending Injury

Interventions for career-ending injuries are decided on an individual basis. Intervention can have the nature of psychological counseling (stress management, alcohol or drug counseling, etc.), career counseling (school enrollment, job placement, etc.), financial planning (investments, tax shelters, etc.), or whatever the patient needs. Adjustment to termination is better for athletes who had participated longer, were aware of chronic injuries, knew of the possibility of being cut, or had planned on retiring from the team. Poor adjustment is associated with sudden unexpected injury that occurs in the prime of the career and results in a forced retirement.[3]

Reaction to Recovery from a Career-Ending Injury

The primary reaction to recovery from a terminating injury is to see it as both an ending and beginning. **Closure** and **renewal** are intertwined, with closure being necessary to give full energy to renewal. Once they reach the acceptance stage, these athletes can put closure on a career that has

ended and focus their other talents, long overshadowed by athletic prowess, toward a new career. This might be either in the field of athletics (coaching, announcer, sponsor, etc.) or in a totally unrelated field. Baillie and Danish[3] found that Olympic athletes and college athletes were better prepared and made a better adjustment to new careers than did older professional athletes. The reason for this might be better education, more choices of careers, more assistance in career planning—in other words, more options. Many athletes make a satisfactory adjustment to termination from sport when it is in their time frame and of their choosing, but termination forced by an unexpected event such as injury is received with less than enthusiasm.

CLINICAL DECISION MAKING	Exercise 4–5

Joe is a 20-year-old junior at a Division I school where he played football for 3 years. He had dreamed of playing in the NFL until a severe concussion put an end to those dreams. How can the athletic trainer help Joe deal with this realization?

COMPLIANCE AND ADHERENCE TO REHABILITATION

Compliance to athletic injury rehabilitation programs is abysmal, considering the purpose of rehabilitation.[22,30,59] The goal of athletic rehabilitation is to return the patient to the level of performance present prior to injury. The primary treatment is exercise to retrain the muscles that have been damaged due to injury. The psychological ramification of unsuccessful rehabilitation is that the patient tends to focus on the injury, resulting in guarding or muscle tension and/or lack of attentional focus, setting up the scenario for reinjury. Following we discuss, first, definitions of compliance and adherence; second, incidents of compliance in other fields; third, measures of compliance; fourth, deterrents to compliance; and fifth, incentives to increase compliance.

Compliance and Adherence Defined

According to Meichenbaum and Turk,[47] *compliance* is a term from the medical profession and means obedience of the patient to the physician's or health caregiver's instruction. The concept of compliance is more passive than active, and carries the connotation that if patients are noncompliant, they are at fault. This assigns an authoritative position to the caregiver. The implication is: "I tell you what to do, and you do it." The concept of compliance mainly applies to immediate short-term treatment that has been prescribed for a patient. Adherence is a term from the exercise discipline and carries the meaning of active voluntary choice, a mutuality in treatment planning. Adherence involves long-term change on a more voluntary basis and suggests a behavioral change sought by the participant. Usually when adherence is the term used, it carries the implication that the service was sought out as opposed to being prescribed—for instance, when people seek an exercise program or a weight-loss program, instead of being ordered by the physician to enroll in one. These are usually long-term commitments.

For the purpose of this discussion about rehabilitation, the term compliance will be used, but either is acceptable. The term compliance has been chosen because there are certain guidelines for treatments that produce the desired result of rehabilitation of an injury. The patient needs to comply with a certain regimen for the short term to facilitate healing, then adhere to a program of exercise to decrease the risk of reinjury. In rehabilitation, a *comply now—adhere later* approach is the best descriptor for successful return to the previous level of fitness.

Incidences of Compliance in Other Disciplines

In the field of athletic injury, compliance is the biggest deterrent to successful rehabilitation.[59] The fields of medicine and exercise fare no better. In medicine, compliance is roughly 50 percent, with the rule of thumb being that one-third always comply, one-third sometimes comply, and one-third never comply.[47] In a study of glaucoma (high intraocular fluid pressure), patients were told that if they didn't use drops 3 times a day, they would go blind. Only 42 percent complied with treatment recommended by the physician. Several weeks later at revisit, they were told they were in danger of losing sight in one eye if they did not comply with treatment. Compliance only increased by 16 percent, according to Vincent.[72] In other words, only 58 percent were compliant when the likely result of being noncompliant was to go blind in one eye!

The exercise literature[18] shows similar findings: There is a 30 to 70 percent dropout rate in the first 3 months of exercise programs. Sixty-six percent of Americans do not exercise on a regular basis; 44 percent do not exercise at all.[18] Self-improvement programs do not fare any better. The dropout rate for obesity, smoking, and stress management programs is 20 to 80 percent. Only 16 to 59 percent of people wear seat belts. There is limited literature on the compliance rate for athletes. Before all hope is lost, it should be understood that maybe 100 percent compliance is not necessary to achieve total rehabilitation. In medicine it was found that less than 100 percent compliance was adequate to bring about desired results.[47] It is important to keep in mind that we are looking at a range, not an absolute. Is the athlete who gets back to preinjury standards without doing 100 percent of treatments noncompliant? They are only if 100 percent compliance is considered to be the gold standard.

Measurements of Compliance

How compliance is measured might be an indicator of the problem. In medicine and exercise, compliance is usually measured in one of three ways: self-report, attendance, and therapeutic outcome.[47] Self-report consists of just asking whether the person has been compliant, through either a structured questionnaire, self-monitoring with record keeping, or corroboration (someone else keeps track). These methods can be inaccurate due to poor memory, trying to please the investigator, or channeling the behavior to please the investigator. Keeping track of attendance is the most common and most direct method. The problem with attendance is that it doesn't say what was done, it just indicates that the patients showed up. The patients could be doing exercises somewhere else, or forget to sign in, or sign in and then leave without exercising, or do only a portion of the prescribed rehabilitation exercises. Therapeutic outcome is not completely reliable, as it can be confounded by other factors. In a weight-loss program the athlete could be gaining muscle weight but losing fat weight, could lose weight due to exercising but not due to recommended changes in eating habits, or could lose weight because of illness without exercising or change in eating habits.

In order to start at the beginning of measuring compliance, the Hedgpeth/Gansneder Athletic Rehabilitation Indicators[32] were designed to determine what treatments were used, and what percentage of the time they were used, in a Division I university. The basic areas assessed are aerobic conditioning, strength conditioning, balance, modalities, and long-term strategies (bracing, taping, protective equipment). Athletes are asked what percentage of the time the treatment was done. A range of compliance is measured, with 0–10 percent being the lowest compliance, and 91–100 percent being the highest compliance. A category of N/A was included to indicate that the athletic trainer had not suggested the treatment. At the same time, athletic trainers were asked to complete the indicator. Preliminary reports suggest an 87-percent reliability rate for the indicator. Until such a time as what is being done in the athletic training room setting is determined, it is premature to discuss why it is or is not being done.

Factors Influencing Compliance

Shank[62] found that patients who are committed to the rehabilitation program work harder and thus return to competition more quickly with better results than those who are nonadherents. Their pain tolerance is greater and of less concern, and they are more self-motivated, as opposed to the apathy of the nonadherents.

Also, support from peers, coaches, and rehabilitation staff is important in influencing compliance.[5] Patients with support show a greater effort to fit the rehabilitation effort into their schedules. They are more likely to keep commitments to those who support them. Patients who are nonadherents respond better to support and motivation from their support group than do the adherents. Thus extra encouragement from this support group for the nonadherent patients can really pay dividends in getting them motivated to successfully complete their rehabilitation.

Attitude is another important consideration when dealing with injured patients. If the athletic trainer expects the patient to be nonadherent, this can create the self-fulfilling prophecy.[74] If the athletic trainer feels the patient is going to be nonadherent, then it is less likely that the athletic trainer will work to motivate the patient to comply with the treatment program. Webborn et al.[74] suggest that if instructions are written down—even in the face of the patient's denial of the need for written instruction—the more likely it is that the patient will follow through with the treatment plan. Athletic trainers have an impact on compliance through enhancing the patient's belief in the efficacy of the treatment as well as providing a supportive environment[19] (Figure 4-10).

Injured athletes are expected to report for rehabilitation, but the coach is the disciplinarian, not the athletic trainer, and the coach institutes punishment for lack of participation in the rehabilitation process. The coach must support the rehabilitation concept. Patients soon know if rehabilitation is not a priority with the coach and begin to lose interest if they are not highly motivated to return to competition.

The real challenge of rehabilitation is how to motivate patients to do their best in the rehabilitation process. Patients who are not reporting for rehabilitation have a reason. Everything is done for some need. The rehabilitation program must be established within these needs. If patients are not reporting for rehabilitation, either something is more important to them than a hastened recovery, or they have not had the importance of the process adequately explained

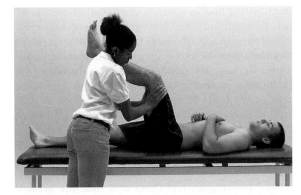

Figure 4-10   A supportive environment and a belief in the effectiveness of the treatment improves compliance.

to them. Reexamine the program and the patient's goals. If the program has not been well explained and the patient is not committed to the program, the program either is doomed to failure or will be less than successful. Motivation must come from within, but the athletic trainer can provide the encouragement and positive reinforcement necessary for the patient to make a commitment.

Lack of commitment might indicate frustration, boredom, or feelings of a lack of progress. In this case, further explanations or changes in routine are necessary. The patient might need the opportunity to comment on the program and make a commitment to the rehabilitation before being structured into a strict regimen of rehabilitative procedures. The athletic trainer should keep in mind that patients may have many activities in their daily schedules, and fitting the rehabilitation to their schedules rather than the reverse can also encourage compliance. The more the patient is allowed input and flexibility, the more successful the compliance will be.

Another aspect of compliance has to do with patients' perception of their ability. Patients who perceive themselves as continuing on to a more advanced level of competition tend to shirk rehabilitation. They usually are the better athletes. They do not have to work as hard as, but perform better than, their peers, so they assume the same attitude about rehabilitation. With this attitude, these good athletes never become truly great athletes because of their lack of commitment to their sport. Once they have risen to the top level where most athletes have the same skills, the work habit is not there to put them in the top of the elite athletic group.

Other factors of compliance for athletes are the length of time at a particular school, semester grade-point average, perception of class load, career goals, amount of participation time in contests, perception of time available for treatments, and previous experience with rehabilitation programs. The more formal education a person has, the higher the level of compliance to treatments; the higher the semester grade-point average, the higher the treatment compliance. Interestingly enough, an inverse relationship exists between athletes' perception of difficulty of their class load and compliance. Often athletes do better academically during the season than at other times, possibly because they budget their time with better discipline during the season, and this approach carries over into the rehabilitation setting. Athletes who have better-defined career goals and those who have the greatest amount of participation time have higher levels of compliance, as do those who perceive they have a greater amount of time available for treatments and those who have previous experience with rehabilitation programs.

PAIN AS A DETERRENT TO COMPLIANCE

Almost all rehabilitation should be pain-free, and what is not is usually detrimental to the return to competition. Painful exercise, therefore, is not only harmful but also reduces compliance, especially in the nonadherent athlete.[22] Rehabilitation programs should be examined to determine the aspects that may be painful.

Pain is subjective, and the caregivers must assume that the pain is as severe or persistent as the athlete says it is. Although the symptoms of pain must be treated to ensure compliance, the cause needs to be addressed.[68] In general, it is more productive in the long run for the athletic trainer to determine the cause of pain than to treat the symptoms and disregard the cause. For instance, if swelling is the cause of the pain, then treatment to reduce the swelling is of a more lasting benefit than treating the pain and disregarding or masking the underlying cause of the pain. Pain that persists and does not respond to adjustments in the rehabilitation process (e.g., decreases in the amount of weights, number of sets, or number of repetitions) should be reevaluated by the athletic trainer or team physician.

Athletes often say "You can play hurt, you can't play injured." But the difference is in what pain means to the athlete. There is the pain of performance, the pain of training, the pain of rehabilitation, the pain of acute injury, and the chronic pain of overuse. Pain can be assessed across intensity (0 = none to 10 = worst) and quality (burning, aching, stabbing, stinging, etc.), but pain is subjective. Factors affecting pain can be culture,[78] type (contact versus noncontact) of sport,[39] and individual versus team sport.[44]

One technique for pain management that is frequently used and easy to apply is dissociation.[11,70] Dissociation involves thinking about something other than the pain, such as a favorite location, a mountain cabin with the smell of fresh crisp air and the magnificent view of mountains, or a beach cottage with the feel and smell of the salty breeze and the calming rhythmic sound of the surf. Another tactic is one Norman Cousins[11] used to distract his thoughts from intractable pain from cancer as well as to prolong the action of pain medication. He watched funny, vintage, slapstick movies such as Laurel and Hardy, the Three Stooges, and Abbott and Costello. Any activity that engages the mind can be used.[25] The athlete could visualize playing a round of golf from tee to green, playing a football game from kickoff to the final whistle, or playing a final NCAA basketball game from tip-off until the buzzer.

Goal Setting as a Motivator to Compliance

Goal setting in and of itself has been shown to be an effective motivator for compliance to rehabilitation of an athletic injury[16,27] as well as reaching goals in a general sport setting.[10,43] Athletes have been setting goals since they started competing, usually from an early age. They set goals to run faster, jump higher, shoot straighter, throw longer, hit harder, and so on. These goals have all had one thing in common, and that is that they were not achieved with one burst of effort but came as the result of many short-term goals having been met prior to the achievement of the long-term goal. For a comprehensive explanation on goal setting in general, see Locke,[42] or for goal setting specifically in sport, see Locke and Lathan.[43] Heil[33] suggests nine guides for goal setting: it should be specific and measurable; use positive rather than negative language; be challenging but realistic; have a timetable; integrate short-, medium-, and long-term goals; and link outcome to process; involve internalized goals; and involve monitoring and evaluating goals and sport goals linked to life goals.

In athletic rehabilitation, patients need to know exactly what the goal is and have a sense that it can be met. This could be accomplished by, for instance, telling a patient that by a certain day the patient should be partial weight bearing with crutches. However, this is neither specific or measurable. It is more effective to say that by achieving a certain range of motion and strength level, the foot can be placed on the ground with weight bearing. The measurement of success is that the partial weight bearing is to be without pain. The goal must be a challenge, but one that the patient can reach with reasonable rehabilitation effort. Goals that are easily reached have no reward in success. Goals must be personal and internally satisfying, not imposed on the athlete by the coach or athletic trainer. The setting of goals needs to be a joint venture between the athlete and the athletic trainer to be successful.[17] The patient has to take responsibility for the progress of the injury and be responsible for doing the necessary rehabilitation.

Goal setting incorporates a multitude of other motivating factors that intuitively appear to increase the odds of compliance by reducing the stress associated with injury rehabilitation. These buffers incorporated within the goal setting paradigm include: positive reinforcement when goals are met, time management for incorporating goals into a lifestyle, a feeling of social support when goals are set with the athletic trainer, the feelings of increased self-efficacy when goals are achieved, etc. Goals should be easily understood by the patient, be concrete, be active events, and be a natural part of their sport that requires no additional time commitment.[9] Goals can be daily for a sense of accomplishment, weekly for a sense of progress, and monthly or yearly for long-term achievement (Figure 4-11).

CLINICAL DECISION MAKING	Exercise 4–6

George is a second-year Division I goalie on the soccer team. He tore his ACL in the first game of the season, had surgery, and is now starting rehabilitation. He is frustrated with the projected length of rehabilitation and is overwhelmed with thoughts of not being able to return to his previous level of play. What should the athlete trainer do to help George establish attainable goals for his rehabilitation program?

RETURN TO COMPETITION

The saying "You have to play with pain" has been interpreted more literally to mean that the athlete has to play through an injury. The difference is that some injuries may be mild and only somewhat painful, resulting in no reinjury in competition, whereas a more severe injury is made worse by continuing to compete. The competitive athlete might be more "body aware" than the general public and therefore more apt to respond to injury with the use of protection, rest, ice, compression, and elevation (PRICE) in order to promote healing. The general public, on the other hand, is more likely to respond to the pain of injury rather than the healing process.[52] Therefore the athlete might want to return to competition in spite of pain, whereas the nonathlete wants the pain to be treated before engaging in any activity. The importance of an athletic trainer for making the decision of when it is safe to compete and when reinjury is a possibility is obvious.

Unfortunately, untrained personnel, such as fellow teammates, parents, and coaches, assume this responsibility when no athletic trainer is present or when the athletic trainer is easily intimidated by the coach and not backed up by the athletic director and sports medicine physician. Either situation results in poor medical care and leaves the management vulnerable to legal action as a result of negligence. Courts expect competent medical care to be provided to the athletes. That care can be provided only by a qualified athletic trainer or a sports medicine physician.

Flint and Weiss[24] found that coaches returned players on the basis of status and game situation, whereas athletic trainers' decisions were determined by the player's injury. Players who feel that a missed practice or a game will relegate them to the bench for the year, or those who have

Weeks 1–3	Set a goal to use relaxation techniques or abdominal breathing before and after treatments. This will lessen the fear that can make pain more intense or more evident when going from knee extension to weight bearing to balance exercises.
Weeks 4–7	This block of time can be monotonous and frustrating. Athletes should set goals to use imagery to see themselves using these movements in their sport. The imagery will be an effective motivator to continue rehabilitation.
Weeks 8–11	The goal for this block of time is to use dissociation to handle the pain that accompanies the increased use of muscles when jogging, rope jumping, and stair running.
Weeks 12–15	Goals at this level should be more reality checks, such as "I am closer to returning to play" or "I can see the light at the end of the tunnel."
Week 15 to return to play	Goals here are to remain positive and to use positive affirmations, such as "I am almost there—each day I am getting stronger and more ready to play."

Figure 4-11 Process goals for rehabilitation.

been encouraged to play no matter what, are candidates for injury and reinjury. Usually what happens, however, is that they are performing poorly because they are not at full strength, thus they only reinforce the coach's decision to play someone else. The role of the athletic trainer is to determine when the player is functioning at optimal physical fitness without risk of injury or reinjury and to keep the coach abreast of the player's status. It is important that the athlete have a clear perception of the injury and its limitations.[13] An important role of the athletic trainer is to inform the athlete of the difference between pain and injury.

The athlete who continues to play with an unhealed or poorly rehabilitated injury is constantly reducing her or his chances for a healthy life of physical activity. The athlete has to live past the few years of competition. Most athletes, however, have difficulty seeing past the present season, or at best have the goal of participating in their sport until they can no longer compete, regardless of the consequences. The rewards of competition and the admiration of others take sports out of perspective and retard a healthy attitude toward sports. The athlete's attitude is "Give it up for the sport" and "I'm invincible." Lack of this attitude is viewed by some as weakness or not being a team player. Athletes with this attitude have difficulty adjusting to injury, especially a career-ending one.

Neglecting injured athletes or giving them the perception that they are "outcasts" also can contribute to injury and reinjury. Coaches who foster this attitude are saying to the players that they have no worth if they are injured. Some coaches go so far as to prevent team contact with injured players until they are ready to return, or to belittle them in front of their peers, believing that this will make the athlete want to get back to competition quicker. This tactic might work with some players with minor injuries, but it only causes major adjustment difficulties for athletes who suffer severe injury.

Some coaches refuse to talk to the injured athlete, or tell others that the athlete really doesn't want to play or isn't tough enough. The coach and athlete are experiencing frustration with the injury. Counseling the coach in this situation to point out the effects of such attitudes may be helpful. Unfortunately, these coaches are not in the minority. During this period, either the sports medicine team shows its concern for the athlete and in return wins the athlete's loyalty and dedication down the road, or they undermine the athlete's trust and set up a future situation to be let down when the athlete gets in the position of controlling the outcome of a contest—the athlete might underperform out of spite. Commitment is a two-way street. The athletic trainer has to show their commitment to the athlete to receive commitment from the athlete. By the same token the athletic trainer must not become the power broker and in essence say "He can't play because I say so." Showing the coach that the athlete who usually has 4.5 speed can presently run only a 5.0 illustrates to the coach that the athlete is not ready for competition. It will also illustrate to the athlete that more time and effort are necessary to get ready to return.

INTERPERSONAL RELATIONSHIP BETWEEN ATHLETE AND ATHLETIC TRAINER

The athletic trainer is often the first person athletes interact with after injury and the one who will direct the recovery. As a result, the athletic trainer has to deal with the athlete as a person and not as just an injury. When an injured athlete enters the treatment setting, they should get the perception that the athletic trainer cares for him or her as a person and not just as part of the job. Their perception of the athletic trainer makes a difference in terms of recovery time and effort. First they have to respect the athletic trainer as a person before they can trust the athletic trainer in the rehabilitative setting. Successful communication between the athletic trainer and the patient is essential for effective rehabilitation. Taking an interest in athletes before injuries have occurred enables the athletic trainer to know the athletes' personalities and be able to work with them in helping to build their confidence.

Active listening is one of the athletic trainer's most important skills. One must learn to listen to the patient beyond the complaining. The athletic trainer should listen for fear, anger, depression, or anxiety in the patient and in his or her voice. With fear, the patient might be wondering what the pain means in terms of function and whether she or he will be accepted by peers. Anger is often a feeling of being victimized by the injury and the unfairness of it. A depressed patient will have an overwhelming feeling of hopelessness or loneliness. Patients who feel anxiety wonder how they can survive the injury and what will happen if they cannot return to full competition.[54]

Body language is important as well. The athletic trainer who continues to work on paperwork while talking to the patient is sending a message of noncaring. The athletic trainer needs to be concerned, and look the patient in the eye with a genuine interest in their problems. This will go a long way toward gaining confidence and respect. It is important for the athletic trainer to consider the patient as an individual instead of the "sprained ankle." If the injury is the only consideration, the patient becomes just an injury and not a person. As a result the attitude projected to the patient is just that, thus the athletic trainer is perceived as caring for the patient only superficially (Figure 4-12).

The relationship between the athletic trainer and the patient should be one of person to person and not of a coach to a player or one of a judgmental nature. When the patient is treated as an equal, the relationship is improved, and it helps the patient accept responsibility for his or her own rehabilitation. With injury, athletes lose control over their physical efforts. They have gone from 4 or 5 hours a day of practice or competition to no activity. They are in a temporary lifestyle change. Their feelings are going to affect the success or failure of the rehabilitation process. The athletic trainer must establish rapport and a sense of genuine concern and caring for the patient, who is not fooled by superficiality.

During an injury evaluation, the athletic trainer should allow the patient to provide as much input about her or his injury as possible. Paraphrasing or restating the information to the patient will be invaluable to the athletic trainer who is unsure of the mechanism of injury or its results. Statements such as "I see" or "Go ahead" or simple silence to allow athletes to fully express themselves are of value. One of the most important bits of information can be the question posed at the end of gathering subjective information: "What else have I not asked you or do I need to know about this injury?" Then give the patient input into the decision of where to go from here.

The athletic trainer is often the person who effectively explains the injury to the patient. Care should be taken to explain the situation to the patient in understandable terms. In most cases the simplest explanation acceptable to the patient is the best. With mild and moderate injuries, the use of the term *sprain, strain,* or *bruise* suffices. The example of a sprained knee and torn ligaments of the knee can be descriptions of the same grade II injury, but the patient

might interpret the two terms altogether differently and react in a totally different way to the explanation.

Patients must have injuries explained to them to their satisfaction. Disseminating injury information appropriate to the patient's emotional and intellectual level can be a real challenge. The rate and degree of acceptance is not the same with all patients. Severity of injury is certainly important, but the patient's perception of that severity is what matters in the rehabilitation process.[13] Thus the physiological must be interrelated with the psychological. In working with patients, the athletic trainer should be not only empathetic but also nonjudgmental.

The addition of a sport psychologist to the rehabilitation team can facilitate the athlete's transition from the sport culture into the rehabilitation culture. Each culture has specific rules as well as defined roles that the members of that culture must follow. An understanding of the different rules and roles can assist the athlete's transition after the injury from the sport culture to the rehabilitation culture. The role of the sport psychologist is to understand the impact this transition has on the athlete who is injured and has to assimilate into a totally new environment, follow new rules, and assume a new role. For example, the concept of pain in the football culture is entirely different from the concept of pain in the rehabilitation culture. In the football culture, "Suck it up" and "Play through the pain" are the norm. In the rehabilitation culture, pain can be an indication that needs to be evaluated. The athlete and athletic trainer need to reevaluate the rehabilitation exercises or activity level, decrease the amount of repetitions, change the type of exercise, or consult with the team physician. If the pain is something the athlete must assimilate into his or her lifestyle, then the sport psychologist can teach the athlete how to deal with it. This can be done through pain management (dissociation) or pain perceptions (pain versus soreness).

Type of athletic trainer	Knowledgeable	Convincing	Sincerely concerned
Great athletic trainer	X	X	X
Good athletic trainer	X	X	O
Fair athletic trainer	X	O	O
Quack	O	X	O
Bad athletic trainer	O	O	O

Figure 4-12 The effectiveness of an athletic trainer is based on three factors.

The amount of stress associated with playing a sport, and the meaning the sport has to the patient, can impact the patient's compliance with rehabilitation.[2] The patient has a more successful rehabilitation when engaged fully in the activity of rehabilitation, much as the athlete will have a more successful sport career when more interested and involved in the sport. Stress can be a deterrent to engaging in rehabilitation. Several techniques the sport psychologist can use (relaxation, imagery, cognitive restructuring, thought stopping) can lessen the stressful reaction to injury. Often a change in the patient's perception of the injury and rehabilitation can affect outcome. Systematic rationalization[67] can facilitate changing the patient's reaction to injury and rehabilitation through changing how the athlete perceives events.

Returning to competition is another area where the sport psychologist can help the injured athlete. Often individuals perceive themselves as ready to return but not being allowed to, or as being forced to return before ready. The sport psychologist can assist the patient to make a decision based on the facts and not clouded by emotions.

The addition of a sport psychologist to the sports medicine team can be an effective link when athletes are unable or unwilling to continue to participate in their sport. Frequently an athlete's identity is intertwined with the sport played. The transition into a completely different culture can be a traumatic experience. It is stressful to enter a culture and not know one's place or identity in that culture. To not know what the game is and what the rules are is frustrating for the injured athlete.

The treatment of athletic injury and rehabilitation involves more than the physical, emotional, and psychological aspects of the individual. The impact of the environment, the support of the athletic community, and the culture in which the athlete resides at the time of injury combine to influence the course the athlete takes from injury, through rehabilitation, to return to competition. Treating the athlete's physical injury and attending to the extraneous factors influencing the injured athlete are the challenges facing the sports medicine team.

Summary

1. There are no absolutes when it comes to how an athlete will react to an injury. However, there are some guidelines for progressive reactions to injury based on length of rehabilitation. These guidelines allow the athletic trainer to conceptualize individual stress reactions to injury and to implement psychological interventions to facilitate successful rehabilitation.

2. The athlete must take responsibility for rehabilitating his or her injury, but the interpersonal relationship between the athlete and the sports medicine team can promote a positive adjustment to the rehabilitation process.

3. The use of psychological techniques such as dissociation for pain management, the use of buffers for stress reduction, and goal setting for motivation can assist the athlete in taking control of and managing her or his successful rehabilitation.

4. The key to successful rehabilitation is compliance. Advances in the field of medicine have allowed injuries that 10 years ago would have ended an athlete's career to now be successfully repaired. Without compliance to the rehabilitation process, these medical advances are moot.

References

1. American Academy of Orthopaedic Surgeons. 1991. *Athletic training and sports medicine.* 2nd ed. Park Ridge, IL: American Academy of Orthopaedic Surgeons.

2. Andersen, M. B., and J. M. Williams. 1988. A model of stress and athletic injury: Predictions and prevention. *Journal of Sport and Exercise Psychology* 10:294–306.

3. Baillie, P. H. F., and S. J. Danish. 1992. Understanding the career transition of athletes. *Sport Psychologist* 6:77–98.

4. Benson, H. 1976. *The relaxation response.* New York: Morrow.

5. Bianco, T. 2001. Social support and recovery from sport injury: Elite skiers share their experiences. *Research Quarterly for Exercise and Sport* 72(4): 376–88.

6. Block, N. 1981. *Imagery.* Boston: MIT Press.

7. Bramwell, S. T., M. Masuda, N. N. Wagnor, and T. H. Holmes. 1975. Psychosocial factors in athletic injuries: Development

and application of the social and athletic readjustment rating scale. *Journal of Human Stress* 1:6–20.

8. Brewer, B. W. 1994. Review and critique of models of psychological adjustment to athletic injury. *Journal of Applied Sport Psychology* 6:87–100.

9. Brewer, B. W., K. E. Jeffers, A. J. Petitpas, and J. L. Van Raalte. 1994. Perceptions of psychological interventions in the context of sport injury rehabilitation. *Sport Psychologist* 8:176–88.

10. Carron, A. V. 1984. *Motivation: Implications for coaching and teaching.* London, Ontario: Pear Creative.

11. Cousins, N. 1981. *Anatomy of an illness as perceived by the patient: Reflections on healing and regeneration.* New York: Bantam.

12. Cramer Roh, J., and F. Perna. 2000. Psychology/counseling: A universal competency in athletic training. *Journal of Athletic Training* 35(4): 458–65.

13. Crossman, J., and J. Jamieson. 1985. Differences in perceptions of seriousness and disrupting effects of athletic injury as viewed by athletes and their trainer. *Perceptual and Motor Skills* 61:1131–34.

14. Cryan, P. D., and W. F. Alles. 1983. The relationship between stress and college football injuries. *Journal of Sports Medicine* 23:52–58.

15. Cupal, D., and B. Brewer. 2001. Effects of relaxation and guided imagery on knee strength, reinjury anxiety and pain following anterior cruciate ligament reconstruction. *Rehabilitation Psychology* 46:28–43.

16. Danish, S. 1986. Psychological aspects in the care and treatment of athletic injuries. In *Sports injuries: The unthwarted epidemic,* 2nd ed., edited by P. E. Vineger and E. F. Hoerner. Boston: PSG.

17. DePalma, M. T., and B. DePalma. 1989. The use of instruction and the behavioral approach to facilitate injury rehabilitation. *Athletic Training* 24:217–19.

18. Dishman, R. K. 1982. Compliance/adherence in health related exercise. *Health Psychology* 3:237–67.

19. Duda, J. L., A. E. Smart, and M. K. Tappe. 1989. Predicators of adherence in the rehabilitation of athletic injuries: An application of personal investment theory. *Journal of Sport and Exercise Psychology* 11:367–81.

20. Ermler, K. L., and C. E. Thomas. 1990. Interventions for the alienating effects of injury. *Athletic Training* 25:269–71.

21. Evans, L., and L. Hardy. 1995. Sport injury and grief response: A review. *Journal of Sport and Exercise Psychology* 17:227–45.

22. Fisher, A. C. 1990. Adherence to sport injury rehabilitation programs. *Sports Medicine* 9:151–58.

23. Flint, F. A. 1993. Seeing helps believing: Modeling in injury rehabilitation. In *Psychological bases of sport injuries,* edited by D. Pargman. Morgantown, WV: Fitness Information Technology.

24. Flint, F. A., and M. R. Weiss. 1992. Returning injured athletes to competition: A role and ethical dilemma. *Canadian Journal of Sport Science* 17:34–40.

25. Fordyce, W. E. 1988. Pain and suffering: A reappraisal. *American Psychologist* 43:276–83.

26. Francis, S., M. Andersen., and P. Maley. 2000. Physiotherapists' and male professional athletes' views on psychological skills for rehabilitation. *Journal of Medicine and Science in Sport* 3(1):17–29.

27. Gilbourn, D., and A. Taylor. From theory to practice: The integration of goal perspective theory and life development approaches within an injury-specific goal-setting program. *Journal of Applied Sport Psychology* 10(1):124–39.

28. Green, L. B. 1992. Imagery in the rehabilitation of injured athletes. *Sport Psychologist* 6:416–28.

29. Grove, D. 1987. Why do some athletes choose high risk sports? *Physician and Sports Medicine* 15:190–93.

30. Grove, J. R., R. M. L. Stewart, and S. Gordon. 1990. Emotional reactions of athletes to knee rehabilitation. Paper presented at the annual meeting of Australian Sports Medicine Federation (abstract).

31. Hedgpeth, E., and C. Sowa. 1998. Incorporating stress management into athletic injury rehabilitation. *Journal of Athletic Training* 33(4):372–74.

32. Hedgpeth, E. G. Hedgpeth/Gansneder Athletic Rehabilitation Indicator (unpublished).

33. Heil, J. 1993. *Psychology of sport injury.* Champaign, IL: Human Kinetics.

34. Holmes, T. H., and R. H. Rahe. 1976. The social readjustment rating scale. *Journal of Psychosomatic Research* 11:213.

35. Ievleva, L., and T. Orlick. 1991. Mental links to enhanced healing: An exploratory study. *Sport Psychologist* 5:25–40.

36. Jackson, D. W., H. Jarrett, D. Bailey, J. Kausek, J. Swanson, and J. Powell. 1978. Injury prediction in the young athlete: A primary report. *American Journal of Sports Medicine* 6:6–14.

37. Jacobsen, E. 1929. *Progressive relaxation.* Chicago: University of Chicago Press.

38. Jacobsen, E. 1931. Variation of specific muscles contracting during muscle imagination. *American Journal of Physiology* 96:101–2.

38a. Jacobsen, F. 1957. *You must relax.* 4th ed. New York: McGraw-Hill.

39. Jaremko, M. E., L. Silbert, and T. Mann. 1981. The differential ability of athletes and non-athletes to cope with two types of pain: A radical behavioral model. *Psychological Record* 31:265–75.

40. Kerr, G., and H. Minden. 1988. Psychological factors related to the occurrence of athletic injuries. *Journal of Sport and Exercise Psychology* 10:167–73.

41. Krucoff, C. 2000. Right under your nose. *Washington Post,* May 2.

42. Locke, E. A. 1968. Toward a theory of task motivation and incentives. *Organizational Behavior and Human Performance* 3:157–58.

43. Locke, E. A., and G. P. Latham. 1985. The application of goal setting to sport. *Journal of Sport Psychology* 7:205–22.

44. Martens, R., and D. M. Landers. 1969. Coaction effects on a muscular endurance task. *Research Quarterly* 40:733–36.

45. McGinnis, J. 1992. The public health burden of a sedentary lifestyle. *Medicine and Science in Sports and Exercise* 24(suppl.):S196–S200.

46. McNair, D. M., M. Lorr, and L. F. Droppleman. 1971. *Profiles of mood states.* San Diego: Educational and Industrial Testing Service.

47. Meichenbaum, D., and D. C. Turk. 1987. *Facilitating treatment adherence: A practitioner's guidebook.* New York: Plenum Press.

48. Michener, J. 1976. *Sports in America.* New York: Random House.

49. Morgan, W. P. 1980. Test of champions: The iceberg profile. *Psychology Today,* pp. 92, 93, 99, 102, 108.

50. Morgan, W. P., and M. L. Pollock. 1977. Psychological characterizations of the elite distance runner. *Annals of the New York Academy of Science* 301:382–403.

51. Ninedek, A., and G. Kolt. 2000. Sport physiotherapists' perceptions of psychological strategies in sport injury rehabilitation. *Journal of Sport Rehabilitation* 9(3):191–206.

52. Norris, C. 1993. *Psychological aspects of sports injury: Diagnosis and management for physiotherapists.* London: Butterworth Heinemann.

53. Petrie, T. A. 1992. Psychosocial antecedents of athletic injury: The effects of life stress and social support on women collegiate gymnasts. *Behavioral Medicine* 18:127–38.

54. Pitt, R. 1992. *Physical Therapy Forum,* 16, September.

55. Requa, R. K., L. N. DeAvilla, and J. G. Garrick. 1993. Injuries in recreational adult fitness activities. *American Journal of Sports Medicine* 21:461–67.

56. Reilly, T. 1975. An ergonomic evaluation of occupational stress in professional football. Unpublished doctoral thesis. Polytechnic University, Liverpool, England.

57. Rotella, R. J. 1985. Psychological care of the injured athlete. In *The injured athlete,* 2nd ed., edited by D. Kuland. Philadelphia: Lippincott.

58. Sanderson, F. H. 1992. Psychology and injury prone athletes. *British Journal of Sports Medicine* 11:56–57.

59. Saterfield, M. J., D. Dowden, and K. Yasumura. 1990. Patient compliance for successful stress fracture rehabilitation. *Journal of Orthopaedic and Sports Physical Therapy* 11:321–24.

60. Scherzer, C. B., B. W. Brewer, A. E. Cornellis, J. L. Van Raalte, A. J. Petitpas, et al. 2001. Psychological skills and adherence to rehabilitation after reconstruction of the anterior cruciate ligament. *Journal of Sport Rehabilitation* 10(3):165–72.

61. Seward, B. L. 1994. *Managing stress.* Boston: Jones & Bartlett.

62. Shank, R. H. 1989. Academic and athletic factors related to predicting compliance by athletes for treatment. *Athletic Training* 24:123.

63. Smith, A. M., and E. K. Milliner. 1994. Injured athletes and the risk of suicide. *Journal of Athletic Training* 29:337.

64. Smith, A. M., S. G. Scott, W. M. O'Fallon, and M. L. Young. 1990. Emotional responses of athletes to injury. *Mayo Clinic Proceedings* 65:38–40.

65. Smith, A. M., M. J. Stuart, D. M. Wiese-Bjornstal, E. K. Milliner, W. M. O'Fallon, and C. S. Crowson. 1993. Competitive athletes: Preinjury and postinjury mood states and self-esteem. *Mayo Clinic Proceedings* 68:939–47.

66. Sordoni, C., C. Hall, and L. Forwell. 2000. The use of imagery by athletes during injury rehabilitation. *Journal of Sport Rehabilitation* 9:329–38.

67. Sowa, C. J. 1992. Understanding clients' perceptions of stress. *Journal of Counseling Development* 71:179–83.

68. Taylor, J., and S. Taylor. 1998. Pain education and management in the rehabilitation from sports injury. *Sport Psychologist* 12(1):68–88.

69. Tomlinson, C. 2000. *Simple yoga.* Edison, NJ: Castle.

70. Turk, D. C., D. Meichenbaum, and M. Genest. 1983. *Pain and behavioral medicine: A cognitive behavioral perspective.* New York: Guilford Press.

71. Valiant, P. M. 1981. Personality and injury in competitive runners. *Perceptual and Motor Skills* 53:251–53.

72. Vincent, P. 1971. Factors influencing patient compliance: A theoretical approach. *Nursing Research* 20:509–16.

73. Vinokur, A., and M. L. Selzer. 1975. Desirable versus undesirable life events: Their relationship to stress and distress. *Journal of Personality and Social Psychology* 32:329–37.

74. Webborn, A. D. J., R. J. Carbon, and B. P. Miller. 1997. Injury rehabilitation programs: "What are we talking about?" *Journal of Sport Rehabilitation* 6:54–61.

75. Werthner, P., and T. Orlick. 1986. Retirement experiences of successful athletes. *International Journal of Sport Psychology* 17:337–63.

76. Wiese, D. M., and M. R. Weiss. 1987. Psychological rehabilitation and physical injury: Implications for the sports medicine team. *Sport Psychologist* 1:318–30.

77. Williams, J. M., T. D. Hogan, and M. B. Andersen. 1993. Positive states of mind and injury risk. *Psychosomatic Medicine* 55:468–72.

78. Wolff, B. B. 1985. Ethnocultural factors influencing pain and illness behavior. *Clinical Journal of Pain* 1:23–30.

79. Wortman, C. B., and R. C. Silver. 1989. The myth of coping with loss. *Journal of Consulting and Clinical Psychology* 57:349–57.

SOLUTIONS TO CLINICAL DECISION MAKING EXERCISES

4-1 Julie and the athletic trainer sat down and mapped out a plan to fit what she needed to get accomplished into a reasonable amount of time. Julie first made a list of her priorities. She decided just what activities she needed to get done and which ones she could delete or postpone. After she had the list of necessary activities, she blocked out several 30-minute stretches of time for "catch-up" or "thinking time."

These 30-minute periods allow Julie to not be rushed throughout the entire day. Julie and the athletic trainer were able to combine activities to save time and to come to the athletic training room during off-hours when it was less crowded. Julie came to realize that, with a bit of creativity and some organizational skills, she could use time management as a buffer for stress.

4-2   The athletic trainer helped Tim realize that his whole body and mind need to be relaxed by using the progressive relaxation technique. By tightening and relaxing all his muscle groups in progression, Tim was able to have a low-intensity workout for the high intensity motions to be performed during the match. Tim also did some yoga abdominal breathing, which cleared his mind and allowed him to become more centered. This amounts to a mind and body dress rehearsal for the performance match. Tim was then able to go out and play in a more relaxed state with less pain and a more fluid motion.

4-3   The athletic trainer and Dana will work on changing the negatives to positive in two ways. The first is by changing the words such as *can't* to *can, won't* to positive terms like *will*. For example: "I can swing my club freely" or "My turn is smooth." The second change can be in the mental picture she has of herself hitting the shot. This works best if Dana can replay the video in her mind of the correct result, much as one retapes over an existing video. She can see herself swinging the club without pain in a very fluid and effortless manner. In her mind she can project that image on her mind-tape. Dana will become very imaginative at creating the tapes she chooses to have in her mind's recorder.

4-4   The athletic trainer will need to continually remind Christine that rehabilitation will help her back. Offer examples of athletes who have returned from back problems. Allow Christine to vent her irrational thoughts, but counter them with reality checks such as "Just last year one of your teammates came back from back problems and is diving now." The athletic trainer can work with Christine to keep her assessment of her condition based on the medical facts, not her irrational fears.

4-5   Joe and the athletic trainer need to discuss what Joe's options are for the future. Joe must first decide if he wants to stay in sports, or rethink his career goals. He can use imagery to daydream what it would look like and feel like to be in another field. Joe can "see" himself as a color commentator for the NFL and get some idea of what that experience would involve. A different field entirely may suit his personality and he can explore his options. It is important that he see the career change as a challenge to be overcome, not a defeat. This will be long and rocky process, and one he has been forced to take. What he does have control over is choosing how he sees himself in a new role. Imaging allows him time to get used to his new identity.

4-6   The athletic trainer and George start with short-term goals to make the process more manageable and allow George to achieve satisfaction with short-term accomplishments. George and the athletic trainer set goals that are realistic, positive, and measurable. These process goals can be monitored and measured. George is now able to see that the plan is in place and the end is in sight. Process goals act as stepping stones to the end result. George understands that he is moving forward toward the long-term goal of returning to play.

PART TWO

Achieving the Goals of Rehabilitation

CHAPTER 5

Establishing Core Stability in Rehabilitation

Mike Clark
Barbara J. Hoogenboom
Jolene L. Bennett

After completing this chapter, the athletic training student should be able to do the following:

- Describe the functional approach to kinetic chain rehabilitation.

- Define the concept of the core.

- Discuss the anatomic relationships between the muscular components of the core.

- Explain how the core functions to maintain postural alignment and dynamic postural equilibrium during functional activities.

- Describe procedures for assessing the core.

- Discuss the rationale for core stabilization training and relate to efficient functional performance of activities.

- Identify appropriate exercises for core stabilization training and their progressions.

- Discuss the guidelines for core stabilization training.

A dynamic, core stabilization training program should be a hallmark component of all comprehensive functional rehabilitation programs.[10,13,22,23,28,31,55] A core stabilization program will improve dynamic postural control, ensure appropriate muscular balance, and affect joint arthrokinematics around the lumbo-pelvic-hip complex. A carefully crafted core stabilization program will allow for the expression of dynamic functional strength and improve neuromuscular efficiency throughout the entire kinetic chain.[1,11,16,28,29,31,51,61,64–66,88,89]

WHAT IS THE CORE?

The *core* is defined as the lumbo-pelvic-hip complex.[1,28] The core is where our center of gravity is located and where all movement begins.[33,34,78,79] There are 29 muscles that have an attachment to the lumbo-pelvic-hip complex.[7,8,28,80] An efficient core allows for maintenance of the normal length-tension relationship of functional agonists and antagonists, which allows for the maintenance of the normal force-couple relationships in the lumbo-pelvic-hip complex. Maintaining the normal length-tension relationships and force-couple relationships allows for the maintenance of optimal arthrokinematics in the lumbo-pelvic-hip complex during functional kinetic-chain movements.[88,89,96] This provides optimal neuromuscular efficiency in the entire kinetic chain, allowing for optimal acceleration, deceleration, and dynamic stabilization of the entire kinetic chain during functional movements. It also provides proximal stability for efficient lower-extremity and upper-extremity movements.[1,28,33,34,43,55,78,79,88,89]

The core operates as an integrated functional unit, whereby the entire kinetic chain works synergistically to produce force, reduce force, and dynamically stabilize against abnormal force.[1] In an efficient state, each structural component distributes weight, absorbs force, and transfers ground reaction forces.[1] This integrated, interdependent system needs to be trained appropriately to allow it to function efficiently during dynamic kinetic-chain activities.

Core stabilization exercise programs have been labeled many different terms, some of which include dynamic lumbar stabilization, neutral spine control, muscular fusion, and lumbopelvic stabilization. The authors of this chapter use the terms "butt and gut" to educate their patients, colleagues, and health care students. This catchy phrase illustrates the importance of the entire abdominal and pelvic region working together to provide functional stability and efficient movement.

CORE STABILIZATION TRAINING CONCEPTS

Many individuals develop the functional strength, power, neuromuscular control, and muscular endurance in specific muscles that enable them to perform functional activities.[1,28,46,55] However, few people develop the muscles required for spinal stabilization.[43,46,47] The body's stabilization system has to be functioning optimally to effectively use the strength, power, neuromuscular control, and muscular endurance developed in the prime movers. If the extremity muscles are strong and the core is weak, then there will not be enough trunk stabilization created to produce efficient upper extremity movements. A weak core is a fundamental problem of many inefficient movements that leads to injury.[43,46,47,55]

The core musculature is an integral component of the protective mechanism that relieves the spine of deleterious forces inherent during functional activities.[14] A core stabilization training program is designed to help an individual gain strength, neuromuscular control, power, and muscle endurance of the lumbo-pelvic-hip complex. This approach facilitates a balanced muscular functioning of the entire kinetic chain.[1] Greater neuromuscular control and stabilization strength will offer a more biomechanically efficient position for the entire kinetic chain therefore allowing optimal neuromuscular efficiency throughout the kinetic chain.

Neuromuscular efficiency is established by the appropriate combination of postural alignment (static/dynamic) and stability strength, which allows the body to decelerate gravity, ground reaction forces, and momentum at the right joint, in the right plane, and at the right time.[12,31,54] If the neuromuscular system is not efficient, it will be unable to respond to the demands placed on it during functional activities.[1] As the efficiency of the neuromuscular system decreases, the ability of the kinetic chain to maintain appropriate forces and dynamic stabilization decreases significantly. This decreased neuromuscular efficiency leads to compensation and substitution patterns, as well as poor posture during functional activities.[29,88,89] Such poor posture leads to increased mechanical stress on the contractile and non-contractile tissue, leading to repetitive microtrauma, abnormal biomechanics, and injury.[16,29,62,63]

CLINICAL DECISION MAKING   **Exercise 5–1**

A gymnast has been having low back pain. She is otherwise a very fit and healthy athlete. You suspect that her pain might be disc related. How might core weakness be contributing to her problem, and how can core strengthening benefit her?

REVIEW OF FUNCTIONAL ANATOMY

To fully understand functional core stabilization training and rehabilitation, the athletic trainer must fully understand functional anatomy, lumbo-pelvic-hip complex stabilization mechanisms, and normal force-couple relationships.[4,7,8,80]

A review of the key lumbo-pelvic-hip complex musculature will allow the athletic trainer to understand functional anatomy and therefore develop a comprehensive kinetic-chain rehabilitation program. The key lumbar spine muscles include the transversospinalis group, erector spinae, quadratus lumborum, and latissimus dorsi (Figure 5-1). The key abdominal muscles include the rectus abdominus, external oblique, internal oblique, and transversus abdominus (TA) (Figure 5-2). The key hip musculature includes the gluteus maximus, gluteus medius, and psoas (Figure 5-3).

The transversospinalis group includes the rotatores, inter-spinales, intertransversarii, semispinalis, and multifidus. These muscles are small and have a poor mechanical advantage for contributing to motion.[27,80] They contain primarily type I muscle fibers and are therefore designed mainly for stabilization.[27,80] Researchers[80] have found that the transversospinalis muscle group contains two to six times the number of muscle spindles found in larger muscles. Therefore, it has been established that this group is primarily responsible for providing the CNS with proprioceptive information.[80] This group is also responsible for inter- or intrasegmental stabilization and segmental

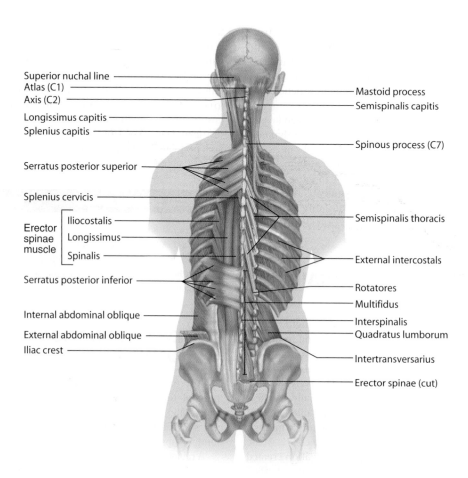

Superior nuchal line
Atlas (C1)
Axis (C2)
Longissimus capitis
Splenius capitis

Mastoid process
Semispinalis capitis

Spinous process (C7)

Serratus posterior superior

Splenius cervicis

Erector spinae muscle
— Iliocostalis
— Longissimus
— Spinalis

Semispinalis thoracis

External intercostals

Serratus posterior inferior

Rotatores
Multifidus
Internal abdominal oblique
Interspinalis
External abdominal oblique
Quadratus lumborum
Iliac crest
Intertransversarius
Erector spinae (cut)

Figure 5-1   Spinal muscles.

eccentric deceleration of flexion and rotation of the spinal unit during functional movements.[4,80] The transversospinalis group is constantly put under a variety of compressive and tensile forces during functional movements and therefore needs to be trained adequately to allow dynamic postural stabilization and optimal neuromuscular efficiency of the entire kinetic chain.[80] The multifidus is the most important of the transversospinalis muscles. It has the ability to provide intrasegmental stabilization to the lumbar spine in all positions.[27,97] Wilke et al.[97] found increased segmental stiffness at L4-L5 with activation of the multifidus.

Additional key back muscles include the erector spinae, quadratus lumborum, and the latissimus dorsi. The erector spinae muscle group functions to provide dynamic intersegmental stabilization and eccentric deceleration of trunk flexion and rotation during kinetic-chain activities.[80] The quadratus lumborum muscle functions primarily as a frontal plane stabilizer that works synergistically with the gluteus medius and tensor fascia lata. The latissimus dorsi has the largest moment arm of all back muscles and therefore has the greatest effect on the lumbo-pelvic-hip complex. The latissimus dorsi is the bridge between the upper extremity and the lumbo-pelvic-hip complex. Any functional upper-extremity kinetic-chain rehabilitation must pay particular attention to the latissimus and its function on the lumbo-pelvic-hip complex.[80]

The abdominals are made up of four muscles: rectus abdominus, external oblique, internal oblique, and most importantly, the transversus abdominus (TA).[80] The abdominals operate as an integrated functional unit, which helps maintain optimal spinal kinematics.[4,7,8,80] When working efficiently, the abdominals offer sagittal, frontal, and transversus plane stabilization by controlling forces that reach the lumbo-pelvic-hip complex.[80] The rectus abdominus eccentrically decelerates trunk extension

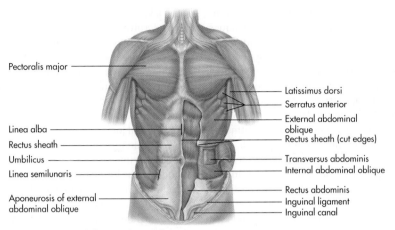

Figure 5-2   Abdominal muscles.

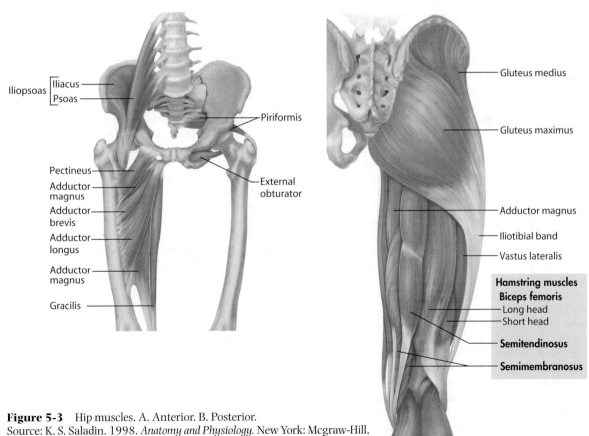

Figure 5-3   Hip muscles. A. Anterior. B. Posterior.
Source: K. S. Saladin. 1998. *Anatomy and Physiology.* New York: Mcgraw-Hill,
pp. 363 and 367.

and lateral flexion, as well as providing dynamic stabilization during functional movements. The external obliques work concentrically to produce contralateral rotation and ipsilateral lateral flexion, and work eccentrically to decelerate trunk extension, rotation, and lateral flexion during functional movements.[80] The internal oblique works concentrically to produce ipsilateral rotation and lateral flexion and works eccentrically to decelerate extension, rotation, and lateral flexion. The internal oblique attaches to the posterior layer of the thoracolumbar fascia. Contraction of the internal oblique creates a lateral tension force on the thoracolumbar fascia, which creates intrinsic translational and rotational stabilization of the spinal unit.[34,43] The transversus abdominus is probably the most important of the abdominal muscles. The TA functions to increase intra-abdominal pressure (IAP), provide dynamic stabilization against rotational and translational stress in the lumbar spine, and provide optimal neuromuscular efficiency to the entire lumbo-pelvic-hip complex.[43,46–48,58] Research has demonstrated that the TA works in a feedforward mechanism.[43] Researchers have demonstrated that contraction of the TA precedes the initiation of limb movement and all other abdominal muscles, regardless of the direction of reactive forces.[26,43] Cresswell et al.[25,26] demonstrated that like the multifidus, the TA is active during all trunk movements, suggesting that this muscle has an important role in dynamic stabilization.[46]

Key hip muscles include the psoas, gluteus medius, gluteus maximus, and hamstrings.[7,8,80] The psoas produces hip flexion and external rotation in the open chain position, and produces hip flexion, lumbar extension, lateral flexion, and rotation in the closed-chain position. The psoas eccentrically decelerates hip extension and internal rotation, as well as trunk extension, lateral flexion, and rotation. The psoas works synergistically with the superficial erector spinae and creates an anterior shear force at L4-L5.[80] The deep erector spinae, multifidus, and deep abdominal wall (transversus, internal oblique, and external oblique)[80] counteract this force. It is extremely common for clients to develop tightness in their psoas. A tight psoas increases the anterior shear force and compressive force at the L4-L5 junction.[80] A tight psoas also causes reciprocal inhibition of the gluteus maximus, multifidus, deep erector spinae, internal oblique, and TA. This leads to extensor mechanism dysfunction during functional movement patterns.[51,61,63,65,66,80,89] Lack of lumbo-pelvic-hip complex stabilization prevents appropriate movement sequencing and leads to synergistic dominance by the hamstrings and superficial erector spinae during hip extension. This complex movement dysfunction also decreases the ability of the gluteus maximus to decelerate femoral internal rotation during heel strike, which predisposes an individual

with a knee ligament injury to abnormal forces and repetitive microtrauma.[14,19,51,65,66]

The gluteus medius functions as the primary frontal plane stabilizer of the pelvis and lower extremity during functional movements.[80] During closed-chain movements, the gluteus medius decelerates femoral adduction and internal rotation.[80] A weak gluteus medius increases frontal and transversus plane stress at the patellofemoral joint and the tibiofemoral joint.[80] A weak gluteus medius leads to synergistic dominance of the tensor fascia latae and the quadratus lumborum.[19,51,53] This leads to tightness in the iliotibial band and the lumbar spine. This will affect the normal biomechanics of the lumbo-pelvic-hip complex and the tibiofemoral joint as well as the patellofemoral joint. Research by Beckman and Buchanan[9] has demonstrated decreased electromyogram (EMG) activity of the gluteus medius following an ankle sprain. Athletic trainers must address the altered hip muscle recruitment patterns or accept this recruitment pattern as an injury-adaptive strategy and thus accept the unknown long-term consequences of premature muscle activation and synergistic dominance.[9,29]

The gluteus maximus functions concentrically in the open chain to accelerate hip extension and external rotation. It functions eccentrically to decelerate hip flexion and femoral internal rotation.[80] It also functions through the iliotibial band to decelerate tibial internal rotation.[80] The gluteus maximus is a major dynamic stabilizer of the sacroiliac (SI) joint. It has the greatest capacity to provide increased compressive forces at the SI joint secondary to its anatomic attachment at the sacrotuberous ligament.[80] It has been demonstrated by Bullock-Saxton[15,16] that the EMG activity of the gluteus maximus is decreased following an ankle sprain. Lack of proper gluteus maximus activity during functional activities leads to pelvic instability and decreased neuromuscular control. This can eventually lead to the development of muscle imbalances, poor movement patterns, and injury.

The hamstrings work concentrically to flex the knee, extend the hip, and rotate the tibia. They work eccentrically to decelerate knee extension, hip flexion, and tibial rotation. The hamstrings work synergistically with the anterior cruciate ligament.[80] All of the muscles mentioned play an integral role in the kinetic chain by providing dynamic stabilization and optimal neuromuscular control of the entire lumbo-pelvic-hip complex. These muscles have been reviewed so the athletic trainer realizes that muscles not only produce force (concentric contractions) in one plane of motion, but also reduce force (eccentric contractions) and provide dynamic stabilization in all planes of movement during functional activities. When isolated, these muscles do not effectively achieve stabilization of the lumbo-pelvic-hip complex. It is the synergistic, interdependent functioning of the entire lumbo-pelvic-hip complex that enhances stability and neuromuscular control throughout the entire kinetic chain.

TRANSVERSUS ABDOMINUS AND MULTIFIDUS ROLE IN CORE STABILIZATION

The transversus abdominus muscle is the deepest of the abdominal muscles and plays a primary role in trunk stability. The horizontal orientation of its fibers has a limited ability to produce torque to the spine necessary for flexion or extension movement although it has been shown to be an active trunk rotator.[81] The TA is a primary trunk stabilizer via modulation of IAP, tension through the thoracolumbar fascia, and compression of the SI joints.[25,91] For many decades, IAP was believed to be an important contributor to spinal control by the pressure within the abdominal cavity putting force on the diaphragm superiorly and pelvic floor inferiorly to extend the trunk.[6,35,73] It was hypothesized that IAP would provide an extensor moment and thus reduce the muscular force required by the trunk extensors and decrease the compressive load on the lumbar spine.[95] Recent research by Hodges et al.[42] utilized electrical stimulation applied to the phrenic nerve in humans to produce an involuntary increase in IAP without abdominal or extensor muscle activity. IAP was increased by the contraction of the diaphragm, pelvic floor muscles, and the TA with no flexor moment noted. It has been demonstrated through research that IAP may directly increase spinal stiffness.[45] Hodges et al.[42] used a tetanic contraction of the diaphragm to produce IAP which resulted in increased stiffness in the spine. Bilateral contraction of the TA assists in IAP and thus enhances spinal stiffness.

The role of the thoracolumbar fascia in trunk stability has also been discussed in the literature, and it has been theorized that the contraction of the TA could produce an extensor torque via the horizontal pull of the TA via its extensive attachment into the thoracolumbar fascia.[34] Recently, this theory was tested by Tesh et al.[93] by placing tension on the thoracolumbar fascia of cadavers. No approximation of the spinous processes or trunk extension movement was noted although a small amount of compression on the spine was noted. This small amount of compression may play a role in the control of intervertebral shear forces. Hodges et al.[42] electrically stimulated contraction of the TA in pigs and demonstrated that when tension was developed in the thoracolumbar fascia, without an associated increase in IAP, there was no significant effect on the intervertebral stiffness. In the next step of that same research study, the thoracolumbar fascial attachments were cut and an increase

in IAP decreased the spinal stiffness. This demonstrates that the thoracolumbar fascia and IAP work in concert to enhance trunk stability.[42] Trunk stability is also dependent on the joints caudal to the lumbar spine. The SI joint is the connection between the lumbar spine and the pelvic region, which ultimately connects the trunk to the lower extremities. The SI joint is dependent on the compressive force between the sacrum and ilia. The horizontal direction and anterior attachment on the ilium of the TA produces the compressive force necessary for spinal stability. Richardson et al.[84] utilized ultrasound to detect movement of the sacrum and ilium while having subjects voluntarily contract their transverse abdominals. They demonstrated that a voluntary contraction of the TA reduced the laxity of the SI joint. This study also pointed out that this reduction in joint laxity of the SI joint was greater than that during a bracing contraction. The researchers did note that they were unable to exclude changes in activity in other muscles such as the pelvic floor, which may have reduced the laxity via counternutation of the sacrum.[84] The aforementioned research findings illustrate that the TA plays an important role in maintaining trunk stability by interacting with IAP, thoracolumbar fascia tension, and compressing the SI joints via muscular attachments.

The multifidi are the most medial of the posterior trunk muscles, and they cover the lumbar zygapophyseal joints except for the ventral surfaces.[81] The multifidi are primary stabilizers when the trunk is moving from flexion to extension. The multifidi contribute only 20 percent of the total lumbar extensor moment, while the lumbar erector spinae contribute 30 percent, and the thoracic erector spinae function as the predominant torque generator at 50 percent of the extension moment arm.[56] The multifidus, lumbar, and thoracic erector spinae muscles have a high percentage of type I fibers and are postural control muscles similar to the TA.[56] The multifidus has been shown to be active during all antigravity activities including static tasks, such as standing, and dynamic tasks, such as walking.[97]

Clinical observation and experimental evidence confirm that when the TA contracts, the multifidi are also activated.[81] A girdlelike cylinder of muscular support is produced due to the coactivation of the TA, multifidus, and the thick thoracolumbar fascial system. EMG evidence suggests that the TA and internal obliques contract in anticipation of movement of the upper and lower extremities, often referred to as the feed forward mechanism. This feed forward mechanism gives the TA and multifidus muscular girdle a unique ability to stabilize the spine regardless of the direction of limb movements.[44,45] As noted previously, the pelvic floor muscles play an important role in the development of IAP and thus enhance trunk stability. It has also been demonstrated that the pelvic floor is active during repetitive arm movement tasks independent of the direction of movement.[49] Sapsford et al.[90] discovered that maximal contraction of the pelvic floor was associated with activity of all abdominal muscles and submaximal contraction of the pelvic floor muscles was associated with a more isolated contraction of the TA. In this same study it was also determined that the specificity of the response was better when the lumbar spine and pelvis were in a neutral position.[90] Clinically this information is helpful in guiding the patient in the process of TA contraction by instructing them to perform a submaximal pelvic floor isometric hold. Another interesting fact to note is that men and women with incontinence have almost double the incidence of low back pain than people without incontinence issues.[30] In summary, the lumbopelvic region may be visualized as a cylinder with the inferior wall being the pelvic floor, the superior wall being the diaphragm, the posterior wall being the multifidus, and the transversus abdominal muscles forming the anterior and lateral walls. All walls of the cylinder must be activated and taut for optimal trunk stabilization to occur with all static and dynamic activities.

CLINICAL DECISION MAKING   **Exercise 5–2**

Last year a tennis player suffered a knee injury. She tore her ACL, MCL, and meniscus. She is competing now but complains of recurrent back pain. She has rather poor posture and significant postural sway. Could she benefit from core training, and how would you go about selecting exercises for her?

POSTURAL CONSIDERATIONS

The core functions to maintain postural alignment and dynamic postural equilibrium during functional activities. Optimal alignment of each body part is a cornerstone to a functional training and rehabilitation program. Optimal posture and alignment will allow for maximal neuromuscular efficiency because the normal length-tension relationship, force-couple relationship, and arthrokinematics will be maintained during functional movement patterns.[14,28,29,50,51,53,55,58,62,64,88,89] If one segment in the kinetic chain is out of alignment, it will create predictable patterns of dysfunction throughout the entire kinetic chain. These predictable patterns of dysfunction are referred to as *serial distortion patterns*.[28] Serial distortion patterns represent the state in which the body's structural integrity is compromised because segments in the kinetic chain are out of alignment. This leads to abnormal distorting forces being placed on the segments in the kinetic chain that are above and below the dysfunctional segment.[14,28,29,55]

To avoid serial distortion patterns and the chain reaction that one misaligned segment creates, we must emphasize stable positions to maintain the structural integrity of the entire kinetic chain.[16,28,55,65,66] A comprehensive core stabilization program will prevent the development of serial distortion patterns and provide optimal dynamic postural control during functional movements.

MUSCULAR IMBALANCES

An optimally functioning core helps to prevent the development of muscle imbalances and synergistic dominance. The human movement system is a well-orchestrated system of interrelated and interdependent components.[16,61] The functional interaction of each component in the human movement system allows for optimal neuromuscular efficiency. Alterations in joint arthrokinematics, muscular balance, and neuromuscular control affect the optimal functioning of the entire kinetic chain.[16,88,89] Dysfunction of the kinetic chain is rarely an isolated event. Typically a pathology of the kinetic chain is part of a chain reaction involving some key links in the kinetic chain and numerous compensations and adaptations that develop.[61] The interplay of many muscles about a joint is responsible for the coordinated control of movement. If the core is weak, normal arthrokinematics are altered. Changes in normal length-tension and force-couple relationships in turn affect neuromuscular control. If one muscle becomes weak, tight, or changes its degree of activation, then synergists, stabilizers, and neutralizers have to compensate.[16,29,61,64–66,88,89] Muscle tightness has a significant impact on the kinetic chain. Muscle tightness affects the normal length-tension relationship.[89] This impacts the normal force-couple relationship. When one muscle in a force couple becomes tight, it changes the normal arthrokinematics of two articular partners.[14,61,89] Altered arthrokinematics affect the synergistic function of the kinetic chain.[14,29,61,89] This leads to abnormal pressure distribution over articular surfaces and soft tissues. Muscle tightness also leads to reciprocal inhibition.[14,29,50–53,61,92,96] Therefore, if one develops muscle imbalances throughout the lumbo-pelvic-hip complex, it can affect the entire kinetic chain. For example, a tight psoas causes reciprocal inhibition of the gluteus maximus, TA, internal oblique, and multifidus.[47,51,53,77,80] This muscle imbalance pattern may decrease normal lumbo-pelvic-hip stability. Specific substitution patterns develop to compensate for the lack of stabilization, including tightness in the iliotibial band.[29] This muscle imbalance pattern will lead to increased frontal and transverse plane stress at the knee. Dr. Vladamir Janda has proposed a syndrome named the "crossed pelvis syndrome" in which a weak abdominal wall and weak gluteals are counterbalanced with tight hamstrings and hip flexors.[51] A strong core with optimal neuromuscular efficiency can help to prevent the development of muscle imbalances. Therefore, a comprehensive core stabilization training program should be an integral component of all rehabilitation programs. A strong, efficient core provides the stable base upon which the extremities can function with maximal precision and effectiveness. It is important to remember that the spine, pelvis, and hips must be positioned in proper alignment with proper activation of all muscles during any core strengthening exercise. No one muscle works in isolation, thus attention should be paid to the position and activity of all muscles during open- and closed-chain exercises.

NEUROMUSCULAR CONSIDERATIONS

A strong and stable core can improve optimal neuromuscular efficiency throughout the entire kinetic chain by helping to improve dynamic postural control.[37,43,47,57,83,88,89] A number of authors have demonstrated kinetic-chain imbalances in individuals with altered neuromuscular control.[9,14–16,43,46–48,50–54,61–66,76,77,83,88] Research has demonstrated that people with low back pain have an abnormal neuromotor response of the trunk stabilizers accompanying limb movement, significantly greater postural sway, and decreased limits of stability.[46,47,77] Research has also demonstrated that approximately 70 percent of patients suffer from recurrent episodes of back pain. Furthermore, it has been demonstrated that individuals have decreased dynamic postural stability in the proximal stabilizers of the lumbo-pelvic-hip complex following lower-extremity ligamentous injuries,[9,14–16] and that joint and ligamentous injury can lead to decreased muscle activity.[29,92,96] Joint and ligament injury can lead to joint effusion, which in turn leads to muscle inhibition. This leads to altered neuromuscular control in other segments of the kinetic chain secondary to altered proprioception and kinesthesia.[9,16] Therefore, when an individual with a knee ligament injury has joint effusion, all of the muscles that cross the knee can be inhibited. Several muscles that cross the knee joint are attached to the lumbo-pelvic-hip complex.[80] Therefore, a comprehensive rehabilitation approach should focus on reestablishing optimal core function in order to positively affect peripheral joints.

Research has also demonstrated that muscles can be inhibited from an arthrokinetic reflex.[14,61,92,96] This is referred to as athrogenic muscle inhibition. Arthrokinetic reflexes are mediated by joint receptor activity. If an individual has abnormal arthrokinematics, the muscles that move the joint will be inhibited. For example, if an individual has a sacral torsion, the multifidus and the gluteus medius can be inhibited.[41] This will lead to abnormal movement in the kinetic chain. The tensor fascia latae will become synergistically dominant and the primary frontal plane stabilizer.[80] This can lead to tightness in the iliotibial band. This can also decrease the frontal and transverse plane control at the knee. Furthermore, if the multifidus is inhibited,[41] the erector spinae and the psoas become facilitated. This will further inhibit the lower abdominals (internal oblique and TA) and the gluteus maximus.[43,46] This also decreases frontal and transverse plane stability at the knee. As previously mentioned, an efficient core will improve neuromuscular efficiency of the entire kinetic chain by providing dynamic stabilization of the lumbo-pelvic-hip complex and therefore improve pelvofemoral biomechanics. This is yet another reason that all rehabilitation programs should include a comprehensive core stabilization training program.

CLINICAL DECISION MAKING	**Exercise 5–3**

As part of a preparticipation screening you want to look for athletes who may be prone to low back pain. What evaluative test can you use to do this?

SCIENTIFIC RATIONALE FOR CORE STABILIZATION TRAINING

Most individuals train their core stabilizers inadequately compared to other muscle groups.[1] Although adequate strength, power, muscle endurance, and neuromuscular control are important for lumbo-pelvic-hip stabilization, performing exercises incorrectly or that are too advanced is detrimental. Several authors have found decreased firing of the TA, internal oblique, multifidus, and deep erector spinae in individuals with chronic low back pain.[43,46–48,77,82] Performing core training with inhibition of these key stabilizers leads to the development of muscle imbalances and inefficient neuromuscular control in the kinetic chain. It has been demonstrated that abdominal training without proper pelvic stabilization increases intradiscal pressure and compressive forces in the lumbar spine.[3,10,43,46–48,74,75] Furthermore, hyperextension training without proper pelvic stabilization can increase intradiscal pressure to dangerous levels, cause buckling of the ligamentum flavum, and lead to narrowing of the intervertebral foramen.[3,10,75]

Research has also shown decreased stabilization endurance in individuals with chronic low back pain.[10,18,33,34] The core stabilizers are primarily type I slow-twitch muscle fibers.[33,34,78,79] These muscles respond best to time under tension. Time under tension is a method of contraction that lasts for 6–20 seconds and emphasizes hypercontractions at end ranges of motion. This method improves intramuscular coordination, which improves static and dynamic stabilization. To get the appropriate training stimulus, you must prescribe the appropriate speed of movement for all aspects of exercises.[22,23] Core strength endurance must be trained appropriately to allow an individual to maintain dynamic postural control for prolonged periods of time.[3]

Research has demonstrated decreased cross-sectional area of the multifidus in subjects with low back pain and that there was not spontaneous recovery of the multifidus following resolution of symptoms.[41] It has also been demonstrated that the traditional curl up increases intradiscal pressure and increases compressive forces at L2-L3.[3,10,74,75]

Additional research has demonstrated increased EMG activity and pelvic stabilization when an abdominal drawing-in maneuver was performed prior to initiating core training.[3,10,13,22,36,37,48,72,76,83] Also, maintaining the cervical spine in a neutral position during core training will improve posture, muscle balance, and stabilization. If the head protracts during movement, then the sternocleidomastoid is preferentially recruited. This increases the compressive forces at the C0-C1 vertebral junction. This can also lead to pelvic instability and muscle imbalances secondary to the pelvo-occular reflex. This reflex is important to keep the eyes' level.[62,63] If the sternocleidomastoid muscle is hyperactive and extends the upper cervical spine, then the pelvis will rotate anteriorly to realign the eyes. This can lead to muscle imbalances and decreased pelvic stabilization.[62,63]

CLINICAL DECISION MAKING Exercise 5–4

You have had a track athlete on a core stabilization program for several weeks. She has been progressing well but needs a different challenge. What can you do to change up her program?

ASSESSMENT OF THE CORE

Before a comprehensive core stabilization program is implemented, an individual must undergo a comprehensive assessment to determine muscle imbalances, arthrokinematic deficits, core strength, core muscle endurance, core neuromuscular control, core power, and overall function of the lower-extremity kinetic chain. Assessment tools include activity-based tests that are performed in the clinical setting, EMG with surface or indwelling electrodes, and technologically advanced testing and training techniques using real-time ultrasound. Real-time ultrasound has been used extensively in research settings and has been proven to be a reliable tool in evaluating the activation patterns of various abdominal muscles.[38,94] Real-time ultrasound, although not currently readily available in clinical settings, is a great asset in the laboratory setting. Perhaps the future will allow for more use of real-time ultrasound in clinical practice.

It has been previously stated that muscle imbalances and arthrokinematic deficits can cause abnormal movement patterns to develop throughout the entire kinetic chain. It is therefore extremely important to thoroughly assess each individual with a kinetic-chain dysfunction for muscle imbalances and arthrokinematic deficits. It is recommended that the interested reader use the reference list to explain a comprehensive muscle imbalance assessment procedure thoroughly.[1,14,19,22,23,28,48,52,54,55,64,88,89,96]

Core strength can be assessed by using the straight leg-lowering test.[3,48,58,76,88,89] The individual is placed supine. A pressure biofeedback device called the Stabilizer.® (Figure 5-4) is placed under the lumbar spine at approximately L4-L5. The cuff pressure is raised to 40 mm Hg. The individual's legs are maintained in full extension while flexing the hips to 90 degrees (Figure 5-5). The individual is instructed to perform a drawing-in maneuver (pull belly button to spine) and then flatten the back maximally into the table and pressure cuff. The individual is instructed to lower the legs toward the table while maintaining the back flat. The test is over when the pressure in the cuff decreases. The hip angle is then measured with a goniometer to determine the angle using a rating scale developed by Kendall[59] (Figure 5-6). This test provides a basic idea of how strong the lower abdominal muscle groups (rectus abdominus and external obliques) are. Using the pressure feedback device ensures that there is no compensation

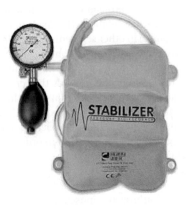

Figure 5-4 Stabilizer pressure feedback unit.
(Courtesy, Chattanooga Group)

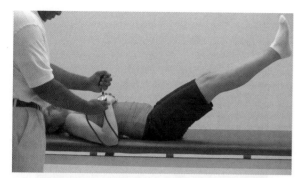

Figure 5-5 Core strength can be assessed using a straight leg-lowering test.

with the lumbar extensors or large hip flexors to stabilize the long lever arm of the legs.

Neuromuscular control of the deep core muscles, TA and multifidi, are evaluated with the quality of movement emphasized rather than quantity of muscular strength or endurance time. Unfortunately, no objectifiable manual muscle test exists for either of these important muscles/muscle groups, however, Hides et al.[40] have developed prone and supine tests to evaluate the muscular coordination of the TA and multifidus. The first test for the TA is performed in the prone position with the Stabilizer pressure biofeedback unit placed under the abdomen with the navel in the center and the distal edge of the pad in line with the right and

left anterior superior iliac spines (Figure 5-7). The pressure pad is inflated to 70 mm Hg. It is important to instruct the patient to relax their abdomen fully prior to the start of the test. The patient is then instructed to take a relaxed breath in and out and then draw the abdomen in toward the spine without taking a breath. The patient is asked to hold this contraction for a minimum of 10 seconds with a slow and controlled release. Optimal performance, indicating proper neuromuscular control of the TA, would be a 4–10 mm Hg reduction in the pressure with no pelvic or spinal movement noted. It is important to monitor pelvic and lower extremity positioning as the patient may compensate by putting pressure through their legs or tilting their pelvis to elevate the lower abdomen rather than isolating the TA contraction.

Testing for the TA is also performed in the supine position and relies on palpation and visualization of the lower abdomen. Instructions to the patient remain the same as the prone test and the athletic trainer palpates for bilateral TA contraction just medially and inferiorly to the anterior superior iliac spines and lateral to the rectus abdominus (Figure 5-8). The Stabilizer pad may also be placed under

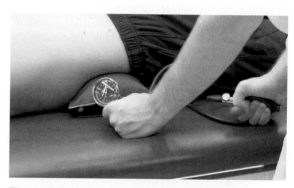

Figure 5-7 Prone Transverse abdominus test.

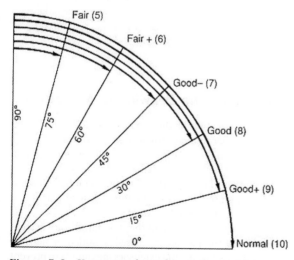

Figure 5-6 Key to muscle grading in the straight-leg lowering test.
Reproduced with permission from Kendall, F.P., McCreary, E.K., Provance P.G., Rodgers, M.M., and Romani, W.A. 2005. *Muscles: Testing and Function*, 5th ed. Baltimore, MD: Lippincott Williams & Wilkins, p. 155.

Fair (5)
Fair + (6)
Good– (7)
Good (8)
Good+ (9)
Normal (10)
90°
75°
60°
45°
30°
15°
0°

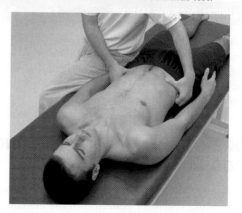

Figure 5-8 Supine Transversus Abdominus test.

the lower lumbar region to monitor if compensation occurs with the pelvis. The pressure reading should remain the same throughout the test. If the pressure reading changes, this indicates that the patient is tilting his/her pelvis anteriorly (pressure decreases) or posteriorly (pressure increases) in an attempt to flatten his/her lower abdomen. The patient is asked to hold this contraction for a minimum of 10 seconds with a slow and controlled release. With a correct contraction of the TA, the athletic trainer feels a slowly developing deep tension in the lower abdominal wall. Incorrect activation of the TA would be evident when the internal oblique dominates and this is detected when a rapid development of tension is palpated or the abdominal wall is pushed out rather than drawn in.

The neuromuscular control of the multifidi are examined with the patient in the prone position and the athletic trainer palpating the level of the multifidus for muscular activation (Figure 5-9). The patient is instructed to breathe in and then out and to hold the breath out while swelling out the muscles under the athletic trainer's fingers. The patient is then asked to hold the contraction while resuming a normal breathing pattern for a minimum of 10 seconds. The athletic trainer palpates the multifidus for symmetrical activation and slow development of muscular activation. This sequence is repeated at the multiple segments in the lumbar spine. Compensation patterns may include anterior or posterior pelvic tilting or elevation of the rib cage in an attempt to swell out the multifidus.

A proper and thorough evaluation of the core muscles will lead the athletic trainer in developing a proper core stabilization program. It is imperative that neuromuscular control of the TA and multifidus precedes all other stabilization exercises. These muscles provide the foundation from which all the other core muscles work.

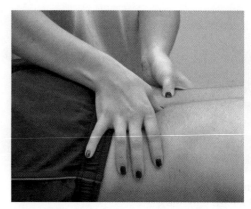

Figure 5-9 Palpating the multifidi for muscular activation.

postures, such as standing or sitting, and progress to very complex tasks, such as high-intensity athletic skills. Patient education is the key to a successful exercise program. The patient must be able to visualize the muscle activation patterns desired and have a high level of body awareness allowing them to activate their core muscles with the proper positioning, neuromuscular control, and level of force generation needed for each individual task.

CLINICAL DECISION MAKING   Exercise 5–6

A golfer has been out of activity for several weeks following a latissimus dorsi strain. As part of his rehabilitation program, you have been progressing him through a core-strengthening program. Describe a level 4 exercise that would be ideal for him.

CLINICAL DECISION MAKING   Exercise 5–5

You have been training a softball player on a core-strengthening program for a week. She has been making improvements, and you think that it is time to progress her. What is your goal, and what parameters should you consider when progressing her?

CORE STABILIZATION TRAINING PROGRAM

As previously noted, the training program must progress in a scientific, systematic pattern with the ultimate goal of training the trunk stabilizers to be active in all phases of functional tasks. These tasks may include simple static

Performing the Drawing-In Maneuver

Muscular activation of the deep core stabilizers (TA and multifidus) coordinated with normal breathing patterns is the foundation for all core exercises. All core stabilization exercises must first start with the concept of the "drawing-in" maneuver (Figure 5-10). Varying opinions[69,81] about the activation of the abdominal muscles during activities exist in the exercise science world.

McGill[69] is a proponent of the abdominal bracing technique where the patient is advised to stiffen or activate both the trunk flexors and extensors maximally to prevent spinal movement. They use the training technique of demonstrating this bracing pattern at the elbow joint. They ask the patient to stiffen their elbow joint by simultaneously activating their elbow flexors and extensors and resisting an external force that attempts to flex their elbow. Once

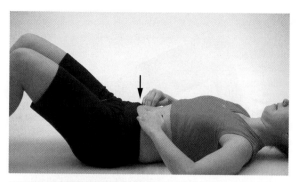

Figure 5-10 The drawing-in maneuver requires a contraction of the transversus abdominus.

the patient has mastered that concept, they apply the same principles to the trunk.

Richardson et al.[81] teach the abdominal hollowing technique where the navel is drawn back toward the spine without spinal movement occurring. This technique does not ask the patients to do a maximal contraction but instead, a submaximal, steady development of muscle activation.

The authors of this chapter have used a teaching technique that incorporates submaximal abdominal hollowing and moderate bracing of the trunk. While standing in front of a mirror, the patients are asked to put their hands on their iliac crests so their fingers rest anteriorly on their transverse abdominals and internal obliques. A good way to state this to the patient is "put your hands on your hips like you are mad." The patient is then instructed to draw their navel back toward their spine without moving their trunk or body while continuing to breathe normally. A good verbal cue is to "make your waist narrow like you are putting on a tight pair of jeans, without sucking in your breath." While in that position the patient is also instructed to not let anyone "push them around" or push them off balance. This helps incorporate the total body bracing technique and the use of the upper and lower extremities to facilitate total body stabilization. This can be referred to as "the power position" or "home base" and these key words may be used when teaching the progression of all core exercises (see Table 5-1 for other teaching cues for proper muscular activation of core muscles). It should be emphasized that proper muscular activation cannot be achieved if the patient is holding the breath.

It should also be noted that the drawing-in maneuver should not be abandoned when the patient is performing other exercises such as weightlifting, walking, or other aerobic tasks such as step aerobics, aqua aerobics, or running.

■ TABLE 5-1 Teaching Cues for Activation of Core Muscles

VERBAL CUES

1. Draw navel back toward spine without moving your spine or tilting your pelvis.
2. Make your waist narrow.
3. Pull your abdomen away from your waistband of your pants.
4. Draw lower abdomen in while simulating zipping up a tight pair of pants.
5. Continue breathing normally while contracting lower abdominals.
6. Tighten pelvic floor.
   a. Women: contract pelvic floor so you do not leak urine.
   b. Men: draw up scrotum as if you are walking in waist deep cold water.

PHYSICAL CUES

1. Use mirror for visual feedback.
2. Put your hands on your waist like you are mad—draw abdomen away from fingertips while still breathing normally.
3. Tactile facilitation.
   a. Use of tape on skin for cutaneous feedback.
   b. String tied snugly around waist.
4. EMG biofeedback unit.
5. Electrical muscular stimulation.
6. Isometric contraction and holding of pelvic floor and hip adductors.

Specific Core Stabilization Exercises

Once the drawing-in maneuver is perfected, neuromuscular control of the TA and multifidus is accomplished in the prone and supine positions as described in the assessment section of this chapter. Then progression of exercises into other positions can take place. Quadriped is a good starting position for the patient to learn and enhance their power position (Figure 5-11). This facilitates the patient keeping their body steady and minimizing trunk movement. The patient is instructed to keep the trunk straight like a tabletop and then draw the stomach up toward the spine (activating the TA and multifidus) while maintaining the normal breathing pattern. This position is held for a minimum 10 seconds and progressed in time to up to 30—60 seconds working on endurance of these trunk muscles. The patient is advised to release the contraction slowly in an eccentric manner and no spinal movement should occur during this release phase. When this position is mastered by the patient and the athletic trainer feels that the patient is ready, the difficulty of the exercise can be progressed, limited only by the capabilities of the patient.

Figures 5-12 through 5-14 illustrate the exercises used in a comprehensive core stabilization training program. Exercises may be broken down into 3 levels in the progressive core stabilization training program: level 1—stabilization (Figure 5-12); level 2—strengthing (Figure 5-13); and level 3—power (Figure 5-14). The patient is started with the exercises at the highest level at which they can maintain stability and optimal neuromuscular control. They are progressed through the program when they achieve mastery of the exercises in the previous level.[1,2,4,l0,12,15, 17,18,22,23,24,25,29,34,39,42,43, 44,45,46,47,48,55,56,62,63,64, 73, 78, 79,90,91]

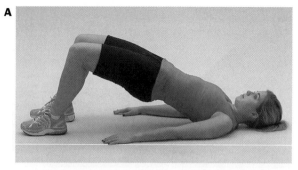

A

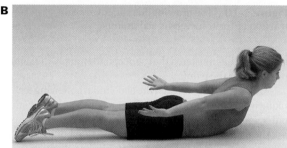

B

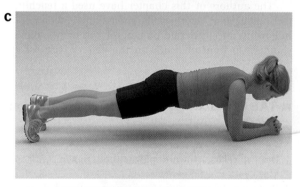

C

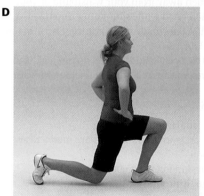

D

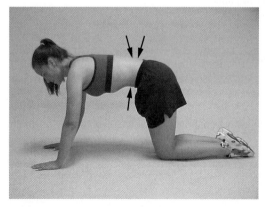

Figure 5-11 Quadriped position for mastering the "drawing-in" maneuver or power position.

Figure 5-12 Level 1 (stabilization) core stability exercises. **A,** Double leg bridging. **B,** Prone cobra. **C,** Human arrow. **D,** Lunge.

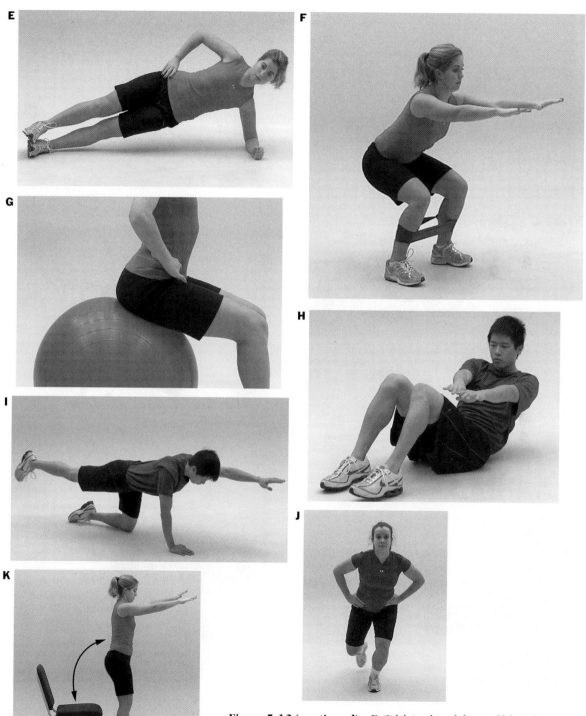

Figure 5-12 (continued)   **E,** Sidelying hip-abdominal lift. **F,** Squats with Theraband. **G,** Pelvic tilts on stability ball. **H,** Three point crunches. **I,** Alternating opposite arm-leg. **J,** Single-leg lunge with abdominal bracing. **K,** Sit to stand with abdominal bracing.

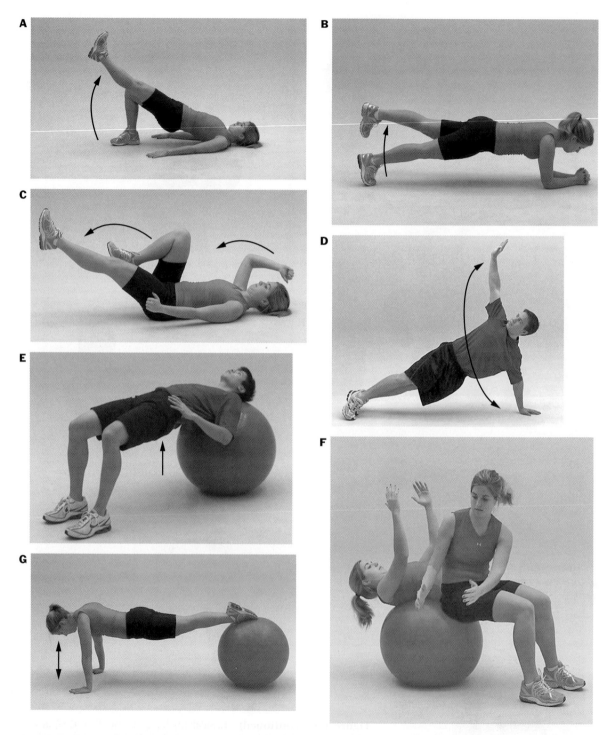

Figure 5-13 Level 2 (Strength) core stability exercises. **A,** Bridge with single-leg extension. **B,** Human arrow with single leg-extension. **C,** Dying bug. **D,** Push-up to side plank. **E,** Bridging on stability ball. **F,** Stability ball diagonal crunches.

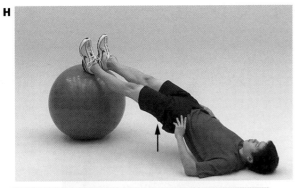

H

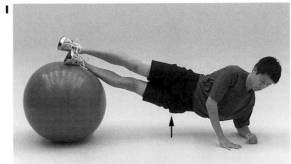

I

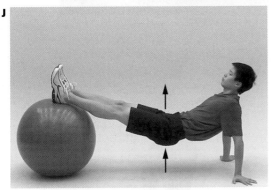

J

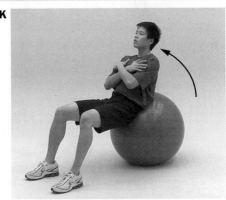

K

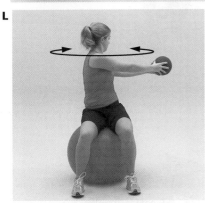

L

Figure 5-13 (continued)
H, Stability ball hip-ups. **I,** Stability ball side plank. **J,** Stability ball pike-ups. **K,** Stability ball crunches. **L,** Stability ball rotation with weighted ball. **M,** Stability ball single arm dumbbell press with rotation. **N,** Stability ball diagonal rotations with weighted ball. **O,** Prone hip extension.

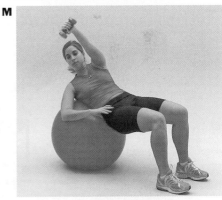

M

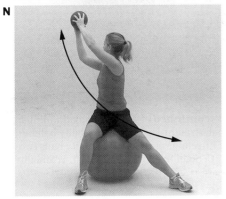

N

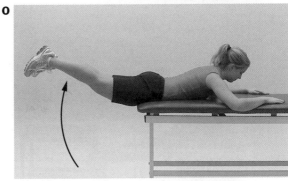

O

P
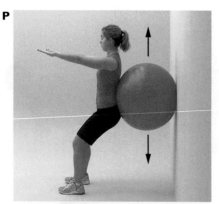

Q
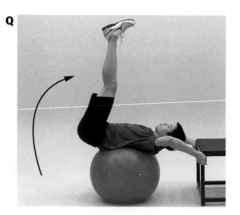

R
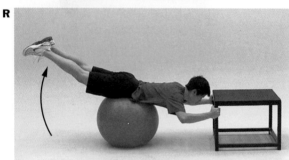

S
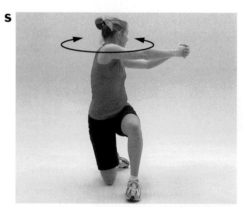

T
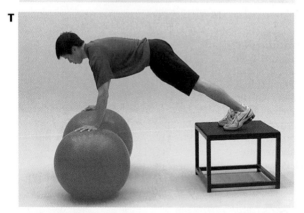

U
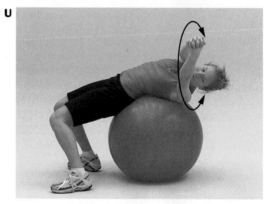

V
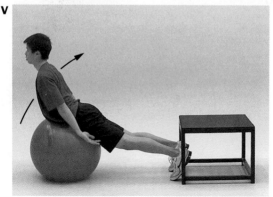

Figure 5-13 (continued)   **P,** Stability ball wall slides. **Q,** Stability ball straight-leg raise. **R,** Stability ball hip extension. **S,** Kneeling rotations. **T,** Stability balls two-arm support. **U,** Stability ball russian twist. **V,** Stability ball prone cobra.

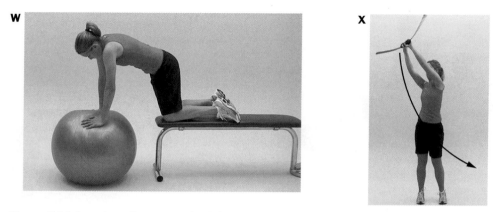

Figure 5-13 (continued)   **W,** Weight shifting on stability ball. **X,** PNF bodyblade.

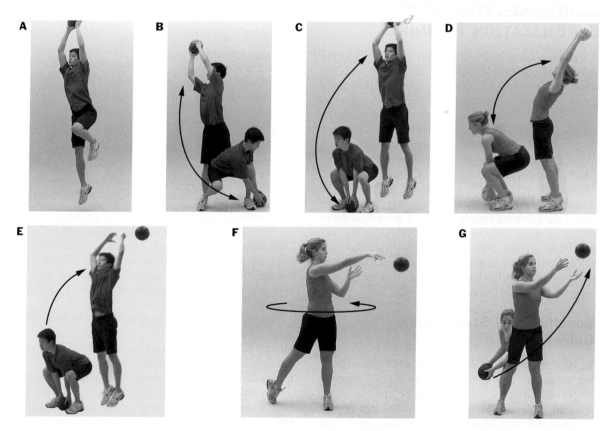

Figure 5-14   Level 3 (Power) core stability exercises. **A,** Weighted ball single-leg jump. **B,** Weighted ball D2 PNF pattern. **C,** Weighted ball double-leg jump. **D,** Ball stand extension. **E,** Overhead weighted ball throw. **F,** Weighted ball one-arm chest pass with rotation. **G,** Weighted ball double-arm rotation toss from squat.

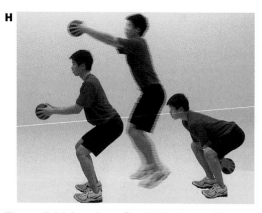

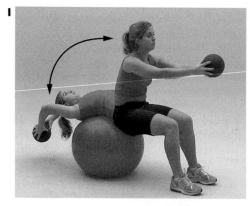

Figure 5-14 (continued) **H** Weighted ball forward jump from squat, **I** Stability ball pullover crunch with weighted ball.

GUIDELINES FOR CORE STABILIZATION TRAINING

A comprehensive core stabilization training program should be systematic, progressive, and functional. The rehabilitation program should emphasize the entire muscle contraction spectrum, focusing on force production (concentric contractions), force reduction (eccentric contractions), and dynamic stabilization (isometric contractions). The core stabilization program should begin in the most challenging environment the individual can control. A progressive continuum of function should be followed to systematically progress the individual. The program should be manipulated regularly by changing any of the following variables: plane of motion, range of motion, loading parameters (physioball, medicine ball, Bodyblade®, power sports trainer, weight vest, dumbbell, tubing), body position, amount of control, speed of execution, amount of feedback, duration (sets, reps, tempo, time under tension), and frequency (Table 5-2).

Specific Core Stabilization Guidelines

When designing a functional core stabilization training program, the athletic trainer should create a proprioceptively-enriched environment and select the appropriate exercises to elicit a maximal training response. The exercises must be safe and challenging, stress multiple planes, incorporate a multisensory environment, be derived from fundamental movement skills, and be activity specific (Table 5-3).

■ **TABLE 5-2**   Program Variation

1. Plane of motion
2. Range of motion
3. Loading parameter
4. Body position
5. Speed of movement
6. Amount of control
7. Duration
8. Frequency

The athletic trainer should follow a progressive functional continuum to allow optimal adaptations.[28,31,36,55] The following are key concepts for proper exercise progression: slow to fast, simple to complex, known to unknown, low force to high force, eyes open to eyes closed, static to dynamic, and correct execution to increased reps/sets/intensity[21,22,28,31,36,55] (Table 5-4).

The goal of core stabilization should be to develop optimal levels of functional strength and dynamic stabilization.[1,10] Neural adaptations become the focus of the program instead of striving for absolute strength gains.[14,28,52,76] Increasing proprioceptive demand by utilizing a multisensory, multimodal (tubing, Bodyblade, physioball, medicine ball, power sports trainer, weight vest, cobra belt, dumbbell) environment becomes more important than increasing the external resistance. The concept of quality before quantity is stressed. Core stabilization training is specifically designed to improve core stabilization and neuromuscular

■ TABLE 5-3   Exercise Selection

1. Safe
2. Challenging
3. Stress multiple planes
4. Proprioceptively enriched
5. Activity specific

■ TABLE 5-4   Exercise Progression

1. Slow to fast
2. Simple to complex
3. Stable to unstable
4. Low force to high force
5. General to specific
6. Correct execution to increased intensity

efficiency. You must be concerned with the sensory information that is stimulating your CNS. If you train with poor technique and neuromuscular control, then you develop poor motor patterns and stabilization.[28,55] The focus of the program must be on function. To determine if the program is functional, answer the following questions:

- Is it dynamic?
- Is it multiplanar ?
- Is it multidimensional?
- Is it proprioceptively challenging?
- Is it systematic?
- Is it progressive?
- Is it based on functional anatomy and science?
- Is it activity specific?[28,31,55]

In summary, the core strengthening program must always start with the drawing-in maneuver that produces neuromuscular control of the TA and multifidus. Abdominal strength is *not* the key, rather, it is abdominal endurance within a stabilized trunk that enhances function and may prevent or minimize injury. The trunk must be dynamic and able to move in multiple directions at various speeds, yet have internal stability that provides a strong base of support in order to support functional mobility and extremity function. The athletic trainer is only limited by his/her own imagination in the development of core stabilization exercises. If the power position is maintained throughout the exercise sequence and the exercise is individualized to the needs of a patient, then it is an appropriate exercise! The key is to integrate individual exercises into functional patterns and simulate the demands of simple tasks and progress to the highest level of skill needed by each individual patient.

Summary

1. Functional kinetic-chain rehabilitation must address each link in the kinetic chain and strive to develop functional strength and neuromuscular efficiency.
2. A core stabilization program should be an integral component for all individuals participating in a closed kinetic-chain rehabilitation program.
3. A core stabilization training program will allow an individual to gain optimal neuromuscular control of the lumbo-pelvic-hip complex and allow the individual with a kinetic-chain dysfunction to return to activity more quickly and safely.
4. The important core muscles do not function as prime movers, rather they function as stabilizers.

5. There are some clinical methods of measuring the function of the TA and multifidus function.
6. Real-time ultrasound is an effective research tool for assessment of core stabilizers.
7. The Stabilizer is a useful adjunct to examination and training of the core.
8. Many possibilities exist for core training progressions. Progression is achieved by changing position, lever arms, resistance, and stability of surfaces.
9. Trunk flexion activities such as the curl and sit-up are not only unnecessary but also may cause injury.

References

1. Aaron, G. 1996. *The use of stabilization training in the rehabilitation of the athlete.* Sports Physical Therapy Home Study Course. LaCrosse, WI: Sports Physical Therapy Section of the American Physical Therapy Association.

2. Akuthota, V., A. Ferreiro, and T. Moore. 2008. Core Stability Exercise Principles. *Current Sports Medicine Reports* 7(1):39.

3. Ashmen K. J., C. B. Swanik, and S. M. Lephart. 1996. Strength and flexibility characteristics of athletes with chronic low back pain. *J Sports Rehab* 5:275–286.

4. Aspden R. M. 1992. Review of the functional anatomy of the spinal ligaments and the erector spinae muscles. *Clin Anat* 5:372–387.

5. Axler, C. T., and S. M. McGill. 1997. Low back loads over a variety of abdominal exercises: Searching for the safest abdominal challenge. *Med Sci Sports Exerc* 29:804–810.

6. Bartelink D. L. 1957. The role of intra-abdominal pressure in relieving the pressure on the lumbar vertebral discs. *J Bone Joint Surg* 39B:718–725.

7. Basmajian, J. 1985. *Muscles alive: Their functions revealed by EMG,* 5th ed. Baltimore, MD: Lippincott Williams & Wilkins.

8. Basmajian, J. 1974. *Muscles Alive.* Baltimore, MD: Lippincott Williams & Wilkins.

9. Beckman, S. M., and T. S. Buchanan. 1995. Ankle inversion and hyper-mobility: Effect on hip and ankle muscle electromyography onset latency. *Arch Phys Med Rehabil* 76:1138–1143.

10. Beim, G., J. L. Giraldo, and D. M. Pincivero, et al. 1997. Abdominal strengthening exercises: A comparative EMG study. *J Sports Rehab* 6:11–20.

11. Biering-Sorenson, F. 1984. Physical measurements as risk indicators for low-back trouble over a one-year period. *Spine* 9:106–119.

12. Blievernicht, J. 1996. *Balance* [Course manual]. Chicago. San Diego, CA: IDEA Health and Fitness Association.

13. Bittenham, D., and G. Brittenham. 1997. *Stronger Abs and Back.* Champaign, IL: Human Kinetics.

14. Bullock-Saxton, J. E. 1997. *Muscles and joint: Inter-relationships with pain and movement dysfunction* [Course manual].

15. Bullock-Saxton, J. E. 1994. Local sensation changes and altered hip muscle function following severe ankle sprain. *Phys Ther* 74:17–23.

16. Bullock-Saxton J. E., V. Janda, and M. Bullock. 1993. Reflex activation of gluteal muscles in walking: An approach to restoration of muscle function for patients with low back pain. *Spine* 5:704–708.

17. Callaghan, J. P., J. L. Gunning, and S. M. McGill. 1978. Relationship between lumbar spine load and muscle activity during extensor exercises. *Phys Ther* 78(1):8–5.

18. Calliet, R. 1962. *Low back pain syndrome.* Oxford: Blackwell.

19. Chaitow, L. 1997. *Muscle energy techniques.* New York: Churchill Livingstone.

20. Chek, P. 1996. *Dynamic medicine ball training* [Correspondence course]. La Jolla, CA: Paul Chek Seminars.

21. Chek, P. 1996 *Swiss ball training* [Correspondence course]. La Jolla, CA: Paul Chek Seminars.

22. Chek, P. 1994. *Scientific back training* [Correspondence course] La Jolla, CA: Paul Chek Seminars.

23. Chek, P. 1992. *Scientific abdominal training* [Correspondence course] La Jolla, CA: Paul Chek Seminars.

24. Creager, C. 1996. *Therapeutic exercise using foam rollers.* Berthoud, CO: Executive Physical Therapy.

25. Cresswell, A. G., H. Grundstrom, and A. Thorstensson. 1992. Observations on intra-abdominal pressure and patterns of abdominal intra-muscular activity in man. *Acta Physiol Scand* 144:409–45. 1992.

26. Cresswell, A. G., L. Oddson, and A. Thorstensson. 1994. The influence of sudden perturbations on trunk muscle activity and intra-abdominal pressure while standing. *Exp Brain Res* 98:336–341.

27. Crisco, J., and M. M. Panjabi. 1991. The intersegmental and multiseg-mental muscles of the lumbar spine. *Spine* 16:793–799.

28. Dominguez, R. H. 1982. *Total body training.* East Dundee, IL: Moving Force Systems.

29. Edgerton, V. R., S. Wolf, and R. R. Roy. 1996. Theoretical basis for patterning EMG amplitudes to assess muscle dysfunction. *Med Sci Sports Exerc* 28:744–751.

30. Finkelstein, M. M. 2002. Medical conditions, medications, and urinary incontinence: Analysis of a population-based survey. *Canadian Family Physician* 48:96–101.

31. Gambetta, V. 1996. *Building the complete athlete* [Course manual]. Chicago. Sarasota, FL: Gambetta Sports Training Systems.

32. Gambetta, V. 1991. *The complete guide to medicine ball training.* Sarasota, FL: Optimum Sports Training.

33. Gracovetsky S., and H. Farfan. 1986. The optimum spine. *Spine* 11:543–573.

34. Gracovetsky, S., H. Farfan, and C. Heuller. 1985. The abdominal mechanism. *Spine* 10:317–324.

35. Grillner, S., J. Nilsson, and A. Thorstensson. 1978. Intra-abdominal pressure changes during natural movements in man. *Acta Physiologica Scandinavica* 103:275–283.

36. Gustavsen, R., and R. Streeck. 1993. *Training therapy: Prophylaxis and rehabilitation.* New York: Thieme.

37. Hall, T., A. David, J. Geere, and K. Salvenson. 1995. Relative recruitment of the abdominal muscles during three levels of exertion during abdominal hollowing. Melbourne, Australia: Australian Physiotherapy Association.

38. Henry, S. M., and K. C. Westervelt. 2005. The use of real-time ultrasound feedback in teaching abdominal hollowing exercises to healthy subjects. *J Orthop Sports Phys Ther* 35:338–345.

39. Hides, J. 2004. Paraspinal mechanism and support of the lumbar spine. In *Therapeutic Exercise for Lumbopelvic Stabilization,* 2nd ed, by Richardson, C., P. Hodges, and J. Hides. Philadelphia, PA: Churchill Livingstone.

40. Hides, J., C. Richardson, and P. Hodges. 2004. Local segmental control. In *Therapeutic Exercise for Lumbopelvic Stabilization,* 2nd ed, by Richardson, C., P. Hodges, and J. Hides. Philadelphia, PA: Churchill Livingstone.

41. Hides, J. A., M. J. Stokes, and M. Saide, et al. 1994. Evidence of lumbar multifidus wasting ipsilateral to symptoms in subjects with acute/subacute low back pain. *Spine* 19:165–177.

42. Hodges, P., A. Kaigle-Holm, and S. Holm, et al. 2003. Intervertebral stiffness of the spine is increased by evoked contraction of transversus abdominis and the diaphragm: In vivo porcine studies. *Spine* 28:2594–2601.

43. Hodges, P. W., and C. A. Richardson. 1997. Contraction of the abdominal muscles associated with movement of the lower limb. *Phys Ther* 77:132.

44. Hodges, P. W., and C. A. Richardson. 1998. Delayed postural contraction of tranverse abdominis in low back pain associated with movement of the lower limb. *J Spinal Disord* 1:46–56.

45. Hodges, P. W., and C. A. Richardson. 1997. Feedforward contraction of transverse abdominis is not influenced by the direction of arm movement. *Exp Brain Res* 114:362–370.

46. Hodges, P. W., and C. A. Richardson. 1996. Inefficient muscular stabilization of the lumbar spine associated with low back pain. *Spine* 21:2640–2650.

47. Hodges, P. W., and C. A. Richardson. 1995. Neuromotor dysfunction of the trunk musculature in low back pain patients. In *Proceedings of the International Congress of the World Confederation of Physical Athletic trainers.* Washington, DC.

48. Hodges, P. W., C. A. Richardson, and G. Jull. 1996. Evaluation of the relationship between laboratory and clinical tests of transversus abdominus function. *Physiother Res Int* 1:30–40.

49. Hodges, P. W., R. R. Sapsford, and H. M. Pengel. 2002. Feedforward activity of the pelvic floor muscles precedes rapid upper limb movements. In *Proceedings of the 7th International Physiotherapy Congress.* Sydney, Australia.

50. Janda, V. 1988. Physical therapy of the cervical and thoracic spine. In *Physical therapy of the cervical and thoracic spine,* Grant, R, ed. New York: Churchill Livingstone.

51. Janda, V. 1986. Muscle weakness and inhibition in back pain syndromes. In *Modern manual therapy of the vertebral column,* by Grieve, G. P. New York: Churchill Livingstone.

52. Janda, V. 1983. *Muscle function testing.* London: Butterworths.

53. Janda V. 1978. Muscles, central nervous system regulation and back problems. In *Neurobiologic mechanisms in manipulative therapy,* Korr, I. M., ed. New York: Plenum.

54. Janda, V., and M. Vavrova. 1990. *Sensory motor stimulation* (video). Brisbane: Body Control Systems.

55. Jesse, J. 1977. *Hidden causes of injury, prevention, and correction for running athletes.* Pasadena: Athletic Press.

56. Jorgensson, A. 1993. The iliopsoas muscle and the lumbar spine. *Australian Physiotherapy* 39:125–132.

57. Jull, G., C. A. Richardson, and M. Comerford. 1991. Strategies for the initial activation of dynamic lumbar stabilization.

In *Proceedings of Manipulative Physioathletic Trainers Association of Australia.* Australia.

58. Jull, G., C. A. Richardson, and C. Hamilton, et al. 1995. *Towards the validation of a clinical test for the deep abdominal muscles in back pain patients.* Australia: Manipulative Physioathletic Trainers Association of Australia.

59. Kendall, F. P. 2005. *Muscles: testing and function,* 5th ed. Baltimore, MD: Lippincott Williams & Wilkins.

60. Kennedy, B. 1980. An Australian program for management of back problems. *Physiotherapy* 66:108–111.

61. Lewit, K. 1988. Muscular and articular factors in movement restriction. *Man Med* 1:83–85.

62. Lewit, K. 1985. *Manipulative therapy in the rehabilitation of the locomotor system.* London: Butterworths.

63. Lewit, K. 1984. Myofascial pain: Relief by post-isometric relaxation. *Arch Phys Med Rehabil* 65:452.

64. Liebenson, C. L. 1996. *Rehabilitation of the spine.* Baltimore: MD: Lippincott Williams & Wilkins.

65. Liebenson, C. L. 1989. Active muscle relaxation techniques. Part I: Basic principles and methods. *J Manipulative Physiol Ther* 12:446–454.

66. Liebenson, C. L. 1990. Active muscle relaxation techniques. Part II: Clinical application. *J Manipulative Physiol Ther* 13(1): 2–6.

67. Mayer, T. G., and R. J. Gatchel 1988. *Functional restoration for spinal disorders: The sports medicine approach.* Philadelphia, PA: Lea & Febiger.

68. Mayer-Posner, J. 1995. *Swiss ball applications for orthopedic and sports medicine.* Denver: Ball Dynamics International.

69. McGill, S. 2004. *Ultimate back fitness and performance.* Waterloo: Wabuno Publishers.

70. McGill, S. M., A. Childs, and C. Liebenson C. 1999. Endurance times for stabilization exercises: Clinical targets for testing and training from a normal database. *Arch Phys Med Rehab* 80:941–944.

71. McGill, S. M., S. Grenier, and M. Bluhm et al. 2003. Previous history of LBP with work loss is related to lingering effects in biomechanical physiological, personal, and psychosocial characteristics. *Ergonomics* 46(7):731–746.

72. Miller, M. I., and J. M. Medeiros 1987. Recruitment of the internal oblique and transversus abdominus muscles on the eccentric phase of the curl-up. *Phys Ther* 67:1213–1217.

73. Morris, J. M., F. Benner and D. B., Lucas 1962. An electromyographic study of the intrinsic muscles of the back in man. *J Anat* 96:509–520.

74. Nachemson, A. 1966. The load on the lumbar discs in different positions of the body. *Clin Orthop* 45:107–122.

75. Norris, C. M. 1993. Abdominal muscle training in sports. *Br J Sports Med* 27:19–27.

76. O'Sullivan, P. E., L. Twomey, and G. Allison 1995. *Evaluation of specific stabilizing exercises in the treatment of chronic low back pain with radiological diagnosis of spondylolisthesis.* Australia: Manipulative Physioathletic Trainers Association of Australia.

77. O'Sullivan, P. E., L. Twomey, and G. Allison, et al. 1997. Altered patterns of abdominal muscle activation in patients with chronic low back pain. *Aust J Physiother* 43:91–98.

78. Panjabi, M. M. 1992. The stabilizing system of the spine. Part I: Function, dysfunction, adaptation, and enhancement. *J Spinal Disord* 5:383–389.

79. Panjabi M. M., D. Tech, and A. A. White 1990. Basic biomechanics of the spine. *Neurosurgery* 7:76–93.

80. Porterfield, J. A., and C. DeRosa 1991. *Mechanical low back pain: Perspectives in functional anatomy.* Philadelphia, PA: Saunders.

81. Richardson, C., P. Hodges, and J. Hides 2004. *Therapeutic exercise for lumbopelvic stabilization,* 2nd ed. Philadelphia, PA: Churchill Livingstone.

82. Richardson, C. A., and G. Jull 1996. Muscle control–pain control. What exercises would you prescribe? *Manual Med* 1:2–10.

83. Richardson, C. A., G. Jull, R. Toppenberg, and M. Comerford 1992. Techniques for active lumbar stabilization for spinal protection. *Aust J Physiother* 38:105–112.

84. Richardson, C. A., C. J. Snijders, J. A. Hides, L. Damen, M. S., Pas, and J. Storm 2002. The relation between the transversus abdominis muscles, sacroiliac joint mechanics, and low back pain. *Spine* 27:399–405.

85. Robinson, R. 1992. The new back school prescription: Stabilization training. Part I. *Occupational Med* 7:17–31.

86. Saal, J. A. 1993. The new back school prescription: Stabilization training. Part II. *Occupational Med* 7:33–42.

87. Saal, J. A. 1989. Nonoperative treatment of herniated disc: An outcome study. *Spine* 14:431–437.

88. Sahrmann, S. 2001. *Diagnosis and treatment of movement impairment syndromes.* Philadelphia, PA: Elsevier Publishing.

89. Sahrmann, S. 1992. Posture and muscle imbalance: Faulty lumbo-pelvic alignment and associated musculolskeletal pain syndromes. *Orthop Div Rev–Can Phys Ther* 12:13–20.

90. Sapsford, R. R., P. W. Hodges, C. A., Richardson, D. H. Cooper, S. J. Markwell, and G. A., Jull 2001. Co-activation of the abdominal and pelvic floor muscles during voluntary exercises. *Neurourol Urodyn* 20:31–42.

91. Snijders, C. J., A. Vleeming, R., Stoekart, J. M. A. Mens, and G. N., Kleinrensink 1995. Biomechanical modeling of sacroiliac joint stability in different postures. *Spine: State Art Rev* 9:419–432.

92. Stokes, M., and A. Young 1984. The contribution of reflex inhibition to arthrogenous muscle weakness. *Clin Sci* 67:7–14.

93. Tesh, K. M., J. Shaw Dunn, and J. H. Evans 1987. The abdominal muscles and vertebral stability. *Spine* 12:501–508.

94. Teyhen, D. S., C. E. Miltenberger, and H. M., Deiters, et al. 2005. The use of ultrasound imaging of the abdominal drawing-in maneuver in subjects with low back pain. *J Orthop Sports Phys Ther* 35:346–355.

95. Thomson, K. D. 1988. On the bending moment capability of the pressurized abdominal cavity during human lifting activity. *Ergonomics* 31:817–828.

96. Warmerdam, A. L. A. 1996. *Arthrokinetic therapy: Manual therapy to improve muscle and joint functioning.* Continuing education course, Marshfield, WI. Port Moody, British Columbia, Canada: Arthrokinetic Therapy and Publishing.

97. Wilke, H. J., S. Wolf, and L. E., Claes 1995. Stability increase of the lumbar spine with different muscle groups: A biomechanical in vitro study. *Spine* 20:192–198.

SOLUTIONS TO CLINICAL DECISION MAKING EXERCISES

5-1 Decreased stabilization endurance in individuals with low back pain with decreased firing of the transversus abdominis, internal oblique, multifidus, and deep erector spinae. Training without proper control of these muscles can lead to improper muscle imbalances and force transmission. Poor core stability can lead to increased intradiscal pressure. Core training will improve the gymnast's posture, muscle balance, and static and dynamic stabilization.

5-2 It could be that she has poor postural control because of a weak core. She probably never regained neuromuscular control of her core following the knee injury. Tennis requires a lot of upper-body movement, so she would probably benefit from core strengthening that would allow her to control her lumbo-pelvic-hip complex while she plays. In choosing her exercises, you should make sure that they are safe and challenging and stress multiple planes that are functional as they are applied to tennis. The exercises should also be proprioceptively enriched and activity-specific.

5-3 Individuals with poor core strength are likely to develop low back pain due to improper muscle stability. The straight leg-lowering test is a good way to assess core strength. The athlete should lie supine on a table with hips flexed to 90 degrees and lower back completely flat against the table. To decrease the lordotic curve, instruct the patient to perform a drawing-in maneuver. The patient then lowers the legs slowly to the table. The test is over when the back starts to arch off of the table. A blood pressure cuff can be used under the low back to observe an increase in the lordotic curve. Someone with a weak core will not be able to maintain the flattened posture for very long while lowering the legs.

5-4 To progress the patient and keep her interested in her rehabilitation program, change her program frequently. Consider these variables as you plan changes: plane of motion, range of motion, loading parameter (Physioballs, tubing, medicine balls, body blades, etc.), body position (from supine to standing), speed of movement, amount of control, duration (sets and reps), and frequency.

5-5 Your ultimate goal with core strengthening is functional strength and dynamic stability. As the athlete progresses, the emphasis should change in these ways: from slow to fast, from simple to complex, from stable to unstable, from low force to high force, from general to specific, and from correct execution to increased intensity. Once the patient has gained awareness of proper muscle firing, encourage her to perform her exercises in a more functional manner. Because activities in most sports require multiplane movement, design her exercises to mimic those requirements.

5-6 Dynamic PNF with a power ball would be ideal for him. The ball will provide a loading parameter, and his range of motion will be functional for the demands of his sport. Adding a twisting component is important so that he is not just training in a single plane of motion prior to swinging his club.

CHAPTER 6

Reestablishing Neuromuscular Control

Scott Lephart
C. Buz Swanik
Freddie Fu
Kellie Huxel

After completion of this chapter, the athletic training student should be able to do the following:

- Explain why neuromuscular control is essential in the rehabilitation process.

- Define proprioception, kinesthesia, neuromuscular control, and stiffness.

- Explain the physiology of articular and tenomuscular mechanoreceptors.

- Describe the afferent and efferent neural pathways.

- Recognize the importance of feedforward and feedback neuromuscular control.

- Identify the various techniques for reestablishing neuromuscular control in both the upper and the lower extremities.

WHY IS NEUROMUSCULAR CONTROL CRITICAL TO THE REHABILITATION PROCESS?

Reestablishing neuromuscular control is a critical component in the rehabilitation of pathological joints. The objective of neuromuscular control activities is to refocus the patient's awareness of peripheral sensations and process these signals into more coordinated motor strategies. This muscle activity serves to protect joint structures from excessive strain and provides a prophylactic mechanism to recurrent injury. Neuromuscular control activities are intended to complement traditional rehabilitation protocols, which encompass the modulation of pain and inflammation, restoration of flexibility, strength, and endurance, as well as psychological considerations.

In the domain of joint motion and position awareness, basic science research has provided insight into the sensory and/or motor characteristics of structures regulating neuromuscular control. Peripheral mechanoreceptors within articular and tenomuscular structures mediate neuromuscular control by conveying joint motion and position sense to the individual. The primary roles of articular structures such as the capsule, ligaments, menisci, and labrum are to stabilize and guide skeletal segments while providing mechanical restraint to abnormal joint movements.[123] However, capsuloligamentous tissue also has a sensory role essential for detecting joint motion and position.[31,58,100]

Tenomuscular receptors contribute to joint motion and position sensation via changes in muscle length, and have been implicated in the regulation of muscle stiffness.[4,55,53,91] Stiffness is the resistance of a muscle or joint to changes in length or position.[55] Therefore increased muscle stiffness, prior to joint loading, is one of the most important mechanisms utilized for dynamic restraint of joints.[101,51,106,110] Recently, the interaction between joint and muscle receptors has received even greater appreciation for contributing to the dynamic restraint system prior to and succeeding joint pathology.[18,31,53]

Injury to articular structures results not only in a mechanical disturbance, but also in a loss of joint sensation. In addition to ligamentous tears, microscopic nerves from peripheral mechanoreceptors may also be damaged; this is referred to as deafferentation.[55,98,103] This partial deafferentation disrupts sensory feedback necessary for reflexive joint stabilization and neuromuscular coordination. There is substantial evidence suggesting that the aberrations in muscle activity subsequent to joint injury are a result of disrupted neural pathways.[10,11,55,78,95,114,121] Therefore, joint pathology not only reduces mechanical stability, it often diminishes the capability of the dynamic restraint system, rendering the joint functionally unstable (Figure 6-1).

The goal of reconstructive surgery is to restore mechanical stability, but evidence strongly supports the reinnervation of graft tissue by peripheral receptors.[92] Therefore surgery, combined with rehabilitation, promotes several neuromuscular characteristics associated with the dynamic restraint system.[73,74] Clinical research has revealed a number of activities that enhance these characteristics and are beneficial to developing neuromuscular control.[16,46,111] To accomplish this, clinicians must identify the peripheral and central neuromuscular characteristics that compensate for mechanical insufficiencies and encourage these adaptations to restore functional stability.

Rehabilitation of the pathological joint should address the preparatory (feed-forward) and reactive (feedback) neuromuscular control mechanisms required for joint stability. The four elements crucial for reestablishing neuromuscular control and functional stability are joint sensation (position, motion, and force), dynamic stability, preparatory and reactive muscle characteristics, and conscious and unconscious functional motor patterns.[106,72]

The following sections will define the sensory receptors and neural pathways that contribute to normal joint stabilization. The theoretical framework for reestablishing neuromuscular control will be presented, followed by specific activities designed to encourage the peripheral, spinal, and cortical adaptations crucial for improving functional stability.

WHAT IS NEUROMUSCULAR CONTROL?

Proprioception refers specifically to conscious and unconscious appreciation of joint position, whereas kinesthesia is the sensation of joint motion or acceleration.[90] The perception of force is an ability to estimate joint loads.[57] These signals are transmitted to the spinal cord via afferent (sensory) pathways. Conscious awareness of joint motion, position, and force is essential for motor learning and the anticipation of movements in sport, while unconscious proprioception modulates muscle function and initiates reflex joint stabilization. The efferent (motor) response to sensory information is termed neuromuscular control.[56] Two motor control mechanisms are involved with interpreting afferent information and coordinating efferent responses.[23,57]

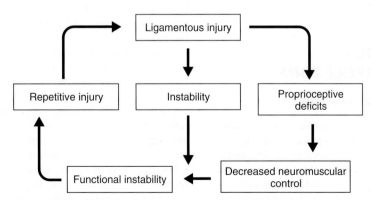

Figure 6-1   Functional stability paradigm depicting the influence of mechanical instability and proprioceptive deficits on neuromuscular control and functional stability, which predisposes the knee to repetitive injury.

Feed-forward neuromuscular control involves planning movements based on sensory information from past experiences.[23,68] The feedback process continuously regulates muscle activity through reflex pathways. Feed-forward mechanisms are responsible for preparatory muscle activity; feedback processes are associated with reactive muscle activity. Electromechanical delay (EMD) is a period of time that elapses between the arrival of a neural impulse (electrical) initiating muscle contraction and the development of force (mechanical). Because of skeletal muscle's orientation and activation characteristics, a diverse array of movement capabilities can be coordinated involving concentric, eccentric, and isometric contractions, while excessive joint motion is restricted. Therefore dynamic restraint is achieved through preparatory and reflexive neuromuscular control.[22,23,35,39,49]

The level of muscle activation, whether it is preparatory or reactive, greatly modifies its stiffness properties.[91,98,51] From a mechanical perspective, muscle stiffness is the ratio in the change of force to the change in length.[4,22,24] In essence, muscles that are more stiff resist stretching episodes more effectively and provide more effective dynamic restraint to joint displacement.[4,85] But, high stiffness would not permit the fast joint motions necessary for physical activity, so muscle stiffness regulation occurs continuously to optimize both joint stability and motion.[118,119] Clinical studies have recently established the importance of muscle stiffness in the dynamic restraint system.[36,44,51,109] In the knee, for example, increases in hamstring muscle activation also significantly increased hamstring stiffness, and there is a moderate correlation between the degree of muscle stiffness in ACL-deficient patients and their functional ability.[85,109] Therefore, efficient regulation of muscle stiffness might embody all of the components in the dynamic restraint system, and thus be vital for restoring functional stability.

THE PHYSIOLOGY OF MECHANORECEPTORS

Articular Mechanoreceptors

The dynamic restraint system is mediated by specialized nerve endings called mechanoreceptors.[38] A mechanoreceptor functions by transducing mechanical deformation of tissue (e.g., stretching, compression) into frequency-modulated neural signals.[38] Increased tissue deformation is coded by an increased afferent discharge rate (action potentials/second) or a rise in the quantity of mechanoreceptors stimulated.[38,41] These signals provide sensory

information concerning internal and external forces acting on the joint. Three morphological types of mechanoreceptors have been identified in joints: Pacinian corpuscles, Meissner corpuscles, and free nerve endings.[31,38,60] These mechanoreceptors are classified as either quick adapting (QA), because they cease discharging shortly after the onset of a stimulus, or slow adapting (SA), because they continue to discharge as long as the stimulus is present.[17,31,38,58,99] In healthy joints, QA mechanoreceptors are believed to provide conscious and unconscious kinesthetic sensations in response to joint movement or acceleration while SA mechanoreceptors provide continuous feedback and thus proprioceptive information relative to joint position.[17,32,38,102] The relative distribution of these receptors can differ between joints; for example, the shoulder has more than the knee, and the joint receptors must be stimulated by considerable loads in order to directly elicit muscle activity.[105] However, sensory organs in the musculotendinous unit largely provide continuous feedback during submaximal loading.

Tenomuscular Mechanoreceptors

Any change in joint position simultaneously alters muscle length and tension. Muscle spindles, embedded within skeletal muscle, detect length and rate of length changes, transmitting these signals to the central nervous system (CNS) through the fastest afferent nerves.[5,18,41] Muscle spindles are also innervated by small motor fibers called gamma efferents.[5,41,71] Having these motor fibers permits the muscle spindle to become more sensitive, if necessary, and accommodates for changes in muscle length while continuously transmitting afferent signals.[5,41,55,53] Muscle spindle afferents project directly on skeletal motoneurons through monosynaptic reflexes.[122] When muscle spindles are stimulated, they elicit a reflex contraction in the agonist muscle.[55,87,122]

Golgi tendon organs (GTO) are also capable of regulating muscle activity and are responsible for monitoring muscle tension or load.[26,50] Located within the tendon and tenomuscular junction, GTOs are force detectors and thus are able to protect the tenomuscular unit by reflexively inhibiting muscle activation when high tension might cause damage. During physical activity, moderate levels of muscle tension may actually reverse this reflex, thus making muscle tension a stimulus to muscle recruitment. Generally, with high muscle tension GTOs would have the opposite effect of muscle spindles by producing a reflex inhibition (relaxation) in the muscle being loaded.[38,50]

NEURAL PATHWAYS OF PERIPHERAL AFFERENTS

Understanding the extent to which articular and tenomuscular sensory information is utilized requires analysis of the reflexive and cortical pathways employed by peripheral afferents. Encoded signals concerning joint motion, position, and force are transmitted from peripheral receptors, via afferent pathways, to the central nervous system (CNS).[25,31] Within the spinal cord, interneurons have a critically important role in providing numerous pathways, via synaptic connections, so that the same information may be transmitted to different parts of the CNS. Ascending pathways (tracts) to the cerebral cortex provide conscious appreciation of proprioception, kinesthesia, and force. Two reflexive pathways couple articular receptors with motor nerves and tenomuscular receptors in the spinal column. A third monosynaptic reflex pathway links the muscle spindles directly with motor nerves.

Sensory information from the periphery is utilized by the cerebral cortex for somatosensory awareness and feed-forward neuromuscular control, whereas balance and postural control are processed at the brain stem.[18,32,41,57] Balance is influenced by the same peripheral afferent mechanism that mediates joint proprioception and is partially dependent upon the inherent ability to integrate joint position sense with vision and the vestibular apparatus. Any disassociation between these three sensory modalities can quickly lead to symptoms of "motion sickness." Balance, therefore, is frequently used to measure sensorimotor integration (e.g., concussions,) and functional joint stability because deficits can result from aberrations in the afferent feedback loop of the lower extremity.

Synapses in the spinal cord link afferent fibers from articular and tenomuscular receptors with efferent motor nerves, constituting the reflex loops between sensory information and motor responses. This reflexive neuromotor link contributes to dynamic stability by utilizing the feedback process for reactive muscular activation.[11,95,105] Interneurons within the spinal column also connect articular receptors and GTOs with large motor nerves innervating muscles and small gamma motor nerves innervating muscle spindles. Johansson[53] contends that articular afferent pathways do not exert as much influence directly on skeletal motoneurons as previously reported, but rather they have more frequent and potent effects on muscle spindles. Muscle spindles, in turn, regulate muscle activation through the monosynaptic stretch reflex. Articular afferents therefore have some influence on the large skeletal motor nerves as well as the spindle receptors, via gamma motor nerves.[53,55]

This sophisticated articular-tenomuscular link has been described as the "final common input." [2,55] The final common input suggests that muscle spindles integrate peripheral afferent information and transmit a final modified signal to the (CNS).[2,55] This feedback loop is responsible for continuously modifying muscle activity during locomotion via the muscle spindle's stretch reflex arc.[48,91] By coordinating reflexive and descending motor commands, muscle stiffness is modified and dynamic stability is maintained.[55,65]

FEED-FORWARD AND FEEDBACK NEUROMUSCULAR CONTROL

The efferent response of muscles transforming neural information into physical energy is termed neuromuscular control.[56] Traditional beliefs about the processing of afferent signals into efferent responses for dynamic stabilization were based on reactive or feedback neuromuscular control pathways.[71] More contemporary theories emphasize the significance of preactivated muscle tension in anticipation of movements and joint loads. Preactivation suggests that prior sensory feedback (experience) concerning the task is utilized to preprogram muscle activation patterns. This process is described as feed-forward neuromuscular control.[22,24,37,68] Feed-forward motor control utilizes advance information about a task, usually from experience, to determine the most coordinated strategy for executing the impending functional task.[23,68] These centrally generated motor commands are responsible for preparatory muscle activity and high-velocity movements.[57]

Preparatory muscle activity serves several functions that contribute to the dynamic restraint system. By increasing muscle activation levels, the stiffness properties of the entire tenomuscular unit are enhanced.[88] This increased muscle activation and stiffness can drastically improve the stretch sensitivity of the muscle spindle system while reducing the electromechanical delay required to develop muscle tension. [19,22,39,49,55,85,88,98] Clinical research has also shown that the stretch reflex can increase muscle stiffness one to three times.[42,79] Heightened stretch sensitivity and stiffness could improve the reactive capabilities of muscle by providing additional sensory feedback and superimposing stretch reflexes onto descending motor commands. [22,54,86]

Whether muscle stiffness increases stretch sensitivity or decreases electromechanical delay, it appears to be crucial for dynamic restraint and functional stability (Figure 6-2). Preactivated muscles therefore can provide quick compensation for external loads and are critical for

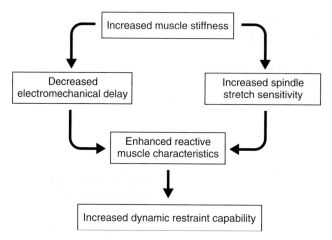

Figure 6-2   Diagram depicting the influence of muscle stiffness on electromechanical delay and muscle spindle sensitivity, which enhances the reactive characteristics of muscle for dynamic joint restraint.

dynamic joint stability.[22, 39] Sensory information about the performance is then used to evaluate the results based on how the brain expected the task to feel, and helps arrange future muscle coordination strategies.

The feedback mechanism of motor control is characterized by numerous reflex pathways continuously adjusting ongoing muscle activity.[12,23,71,87] Information from joint and muscle receptors can reflexively initiate and coordinate muscle activity for motor tasks. This feedback process, however, can result in long conduction delays and is best equipped for maintaining posture and regulating slow stereotyped movements such as walking.[57] The efficacy of reflex-mediated dynamic stabilization is therefore related to the speed and magnitude of joint perturbations. It is unclear what relative contribution feedback-mediated muscle reflexes provide when in vivo loads are placed on joints.

Both feed-forward and feedback neuromuscular control can enhance dynamic stability if the sensory and motor pathways are frequently stimulated. Each time a signal passes through a sequence of synapses, the synapses become more capable of transmitting the same signal.[42,47] When these pathways are "facilitated" regularly, memory of that signal is created and can be recalled to program future movements.[42] Frequent facilitation therefore enhances both the memory about tasks for preprogrammed motor control and reflex pathways for reactive neuromuscular control. Therefore, rehabilitation exercise must be executed with technical precision, repetition, and controlled progression for these physiological adaptations to occur and promote better neuromuscular control.

REESTABLISHING NEUROMUSCULAR CONTROL

Patients who have sustained damage to the articular structures in the upper or lower extremities exhibit distinctive proprioceptive, kinesthetic, and neuromuscular deficits.[6,7,10,11,70,77,74,81,101,102,104,121] Although identifying these abnormalities might be difficult in a clinical setting, a thorough appreciation of the pathoetiology of these conditions is necessary to guide clinicians who are attempting to reestablish neuromuscular control and functional stability. Most researchers believe that disruption of the articular structures results in some level of deafferentation to ligamentous and probably capsular mechanoreceptors.[26,27,70,74,75,102,104] In the acute phase of healing, joint inflammation and pain can compound sensory deficits; however, this cannot account for the chronic deficits in proprioception and kinesthesia associated with pathological joints.[8,60] Research has demonstrated that patients with congenital or pathological joint laxity have diminished capability for detecting joint motion and position.[30,34,104] These proprioceptive and kinesthetic characteristics, coupled with mechanical instability, can lead to functional instability.[71,107]

Developing or reestablishing proprioception, kinesthesia, and neuromuscular control in injured patients will minimize the risk of reinjury. Capsuloligamentous retensioning and reconstruction, coupled with traditional rehabilitation, is one option that appears to restore some kinesthetic awareness, although not equal to that of non-involved limbs.[21,74,92]

The objective of neuromuscular rehabilitation is to develop or reestablish afferent and efferent characteristics that enhance dynamic restraint capabilities with respect to in vivo loads. Four basic elements are crucial to reestablishing neuromuscular control and functional stability: (1) proprioceptive and kinesthetic sensation; (2) dynamic joint stabilization; (3) reactive neuromuscular control; and (4) functional motor patterns.[71] In the pathological joint these dynamic mechanisms are compensatory for the lack of static restraints, and can result in a functionally stable joint.

Several afferent and efferent characteristics contribute to the efficient regulation of these elements and the maintenance of neuromuscular control. These characteristics include the sensitivity of peripheral receptors and facilitation of afferent pathways, muscle stiffness, the onset rate and magnitude of muscle activity, agonist/antagonist coactivation, reflex muscle activation, and discriminatory muscle activation. Specific rehabilitation techniques allow these characteristics to be modified, significantly impacting dynamic stability and function.[10,16,46,52,70,111,120]

Although more prospective clinical research is needed to establish the "best practice" approach in support of the evidence-based medical model, several exercise techniques show promise for inducing beneficial adaptations to these characteristics. The plasticity of the neuromuscular system to change is what permits rapid modifications during rehabilitation that ultimately enhance preparatory and reactive muscle activity.[10,47,50,52,106,108,109,120] The techniques include open- and closed-kinetic-chain activities, balance training, eccentric and high-repetition/low-load exercises, reflex facilitation through reactive or "perturbation" training, stretch-shortening activities, and biofeedback training. Traditional rehabilitation, accompanied by these specific techniques, results in beneficial adaptations to the neuromuscular characteristics responsible for dynamic restraint, enhancing their efficiency for providing a functionally stable joint. It is generally accepted that the rapid performance gains observed within 6–8 weeks of initiating a conditioning program, result from neuromuscular adaptations; however without at least continuous maintenance, these adaptations will disappear.[41,57]

In order to restore dynamic muscle activation necessary for functional stability, one must employ simulated positions of vulnerability that necessitate reactive muscle stabilization. Although there are inherent risks in placing the joint in positions of vulnerability, if this is done in a controlled and progressive fashion, neuromuscular adaptations will occur and subsequently permit the patient to return to competitive situations with confidence that the dynamic mechanisms will protect the joint from subluxation and reinjury.

> **CLINICAL DECISION MAKING**   **Exercise 6–1**
>
> Following a grade 2 ankle sprain and a rehabilitation program to regain strength in the lateral lower leg muscles, your soccer patient continues to sustain repeated inversion ankle injuries during cutting maneuvers. What components of neuromuscular control might be deficient in this patient? What type of rehabilitation exercises should you implement to enhance neuromuscular control?

Neuromuscular Characteristics

Peripheral Afferent Receptors. The foundation for feedback and feed-forward neuromuscular control is based on reliable motion, position, and force information. Altered peripheral afferent information can disrupt motor control and functional stability. Closed-kinetic-chain exercises create axial loads that maximally stimulate articular receptors, especially near the end range of motion, while tenomuscular receptors are excited by all changes in length and tension.[17,38,55,116,117,124] Open-chain activities may require more conscious awareness of limb position because of the non-constrained and freely moving distal segment. Performing open- or closed-chain exercises under weighted conditions increases the level of difficulty and coactivation, which may be used as a training stimulus.[69] Chronic athletic participation can also enhance proprioceptive and kinesthetic acuity by repeatedly facilitating afferent pathways from peripheral receptors. Highly conditioned patients demonstrate greater appreciation of joint kinesthesia and more accurately reproduce limb position than sedentary controls do.[7,75,79] Whether this is a congenital endowment or a training adaptation, greater awareness of joint motion and position can improve feed-forward and feedback neuromuscular control.[75]

Muscle Stiffness. It is evident that muscle stiffness has a significant role in preparatory and reactive dynamic restraint by resisting and absorbing joint loads.[51,82,84,85,110] Therefore exercise modes that optimize muscle stiffness should be encouraged during rehabilitation. Research by Bulbulian and Pousson[14,97] has established that eccentric loading increases muscle tone and stiffness. The GTO receptor is normally associated with muscle inhibition and thus protects the tenomuscular unit from excessive strain. However, chronic overloading of the musculotendinous unit may result in connective tissue proliferation around GTOs that, in effect, desensitizes this mechanoreceptor to muscle tension. If this inhibitor effect can be decreased, then reactive muscle stiffening is facilitated through increased muscle spindle activity.[50] It is also known that during functional activities the GTO inhibition reverses and may actually enhance muscle recruitment.[57] Such evolutions impact both the neuromuscular and the tendinous components of stiffness.[14,35,88,97]

Training techniques that emphasize low loads and high repetitions cause connective tissue adaptations similar to those found with eccentric training. However, increased muscle stiffness resulting from this rehabilitation technique can be attributed to fiber type transition.[35,50,66,67] Slow-twitch fibers have longer crossbridge cycle times and can maintain the prolonged, low-intensity contractions necessary for postural control.[67] In the animal model, Goubel[35] found that low-load/high-repetition training resulted in higher muscle stiffness, compared to strength training. However, Kyrolaninen's[67] analysis of power- and endurance-trained patients inferred that muscle stiffness was greater in the power-trained individuals because the onset of muscle preactivation (EMG) was faster and higher prior to joint loading. It appears that endurance training might enhance stiffness by increasing the baseline motor tone and crossbridge formation time, whereas power training alters the rate and magnitude of muscle tension during preactivation. Both of these adaptations readily adhere to existing principles of progressive rehabilitation, where early strengthening exercises focus on low loads with high repetitions, progressing to shorter, more explosive, sport-specific activities. Research assessing the efficacy of low-load/high-repetition training versus high-load/low-repetition training would be beneficial for optimizing muscle stiffness and functional progression in the injured patient.

Reflex Muscle Activation. Various training modes also cause neuromuscular adaptations that might account for discrepancies in the reflex latency times between power- and endurance-trained patients. Sprint- and/or power-trained individuals have more vigorous reflex responses (tendon-tap) relative to sedentary and endurance-trained samples.[63,64,113] McComas[83] suggests that strength training increases descending (cortical) drive to the large motor nerves of skeletal muscle and the small efferent fibers to muscle spindles, referred to as alpha-gamma coactivation. Increasing both muscle tension and efferent drive to muscle spindles results in a heightened sensitivity to stretch, consequently reducing reflex latencies.[50] Melvill-Jones[86] suggests that the stretch reflexes are superimposed on preprogrammed muscle activity from higher centers, illustrating

the concomitant use of feed-forward and feedback neuromuscular control for regulating preparatory and reactive muscle stiffness. Therefore, preparatory and reactive muscle activation might improve dynamic stability and function if muscle stiffness is enhanced in a mechanically insufficient or reconstructed joint.

A limited number of clinical training studies have been directed at improving reaction times.[10,52,120] Ihara[52] significantly reduced the latency of muscle reactions over a 3-week period by inducing perturbations to patients on unstable platforms. Several other researchers later confirmed this finding with rehabilitation programs designed to improve reflex muscle activation.[10,120] Beard[10] and Wojtyes[120] suggest that agility-type training in the lower extremity produces more desirable muscle reaction times when compared to strength training. This research has significant implications for reestablishing the reactive capability of the dynamic restraint system. Reducing the electromechanical delay between protective muscle activation and joint loading can increase dynamic stability and function. Fitzgerald et al.[28,29] describe a perturbation training program that is dependent on a sense of force-feedback. Patients are exposed to rotatory and translatory movement that progress from predictable perturbations to random, and from small/slow movements to those that are large/fast. Key instruction for the success of the exercises is to match the perturbation but not under-or overreact. This is critical to the concept of optimal stiffness regulation. Overstiffening a muscle/joint complex may provide stability but is not functional while understiffening may permit episodes of "giving way" or "buckling."

Discriminative Muscle Activation. In addition to reactive muscle firing, unconscious control of muscle activity is critical for coordination and balancing joint forces. This is most evident relative to the force couples described for the shoulder complex. Restoring the force couples of agonist and antagonists might initially require conscious, discriminative muscle activation before unconscious control is reacquired. Biofeedback training provides instantaneous sensory feedback concerning specific muscle contractions and can help patients correct errors by consciously altering or redistributing muscle activity.[9,33] The objective of biofeedback training is to reacquire voluntary muscle control and promote functionally specific motor patterns, eventually converting these patterns from conscious to unconscious control[9] (Figure 6-3). Using biofeedback for discriminative muscle control can help eliminate muscle imbalances while reestablishing preparatory and reactive muscle activity for dynamic joint stability.[23,33]

A

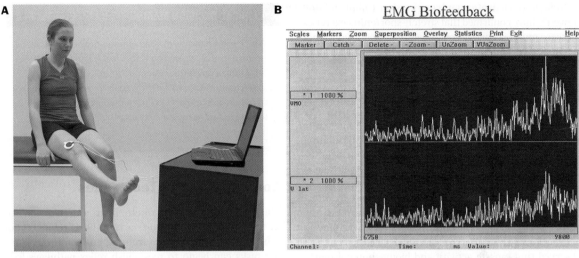

B   EMG Biofeedback

Figure 6-3   Biofeedback training reestablishes discriminative muscle control, eliminating muscle imbalance and promoting functionally specific muscle activation patterns.

Elements for Neuromuscular Control

Proprioception and Kinesthesia. The objective of kinesthetic and proprioceptive training is to restore the neurosensory properties of injured capsuloligamentous structures and enhance the sensitivity of uninvolved peripheral afferents.[78] To what degree this occurs in conservatively managed patients is unknown; however, ligament retensioning and reconstruction coupled with extensive rehabilitation does appear to normalize joint motion and position sense.[8,74,92]

Joint compression is believed to maximally stimulate articular receptors and can be accomplished with closed chain exercises throughout the available ROM.[17,38,55,116,117] Early joint-repositioning tasks enhance conscious proprioceptive and kinesthetic awareness, eventually leading to unconscious appreciation of joint motion and position. Applying a neoprene sleeve or elastic bandage can provide additional proprioceptive and kinesthetic information by stimulating cutaneous receptors[8,94] (Figure 6-4). Exercises that simultaneously involve the noninjured limb may help reestablish conscious awareness of joint position, motion, and load in the injured extremity. To increase the level of difficulty, these exercises can be performed under moderate loads.[69]

Dynamic Stabilization. The objective of dynamic joint stabilization exercises is to encourage preparatory agonist/antagonist coactivation. Efficient coactivation restores the force couples necessary to balance joint forces and increase joint congruency, thereby reducing the loads imparted to the static structures. Dynamic stabilization from muscles requires anticipating and reacting to joint loads. This includes placing the joint in positions of vulnerability where dynamic support is established under controlled conditions. Balance and stretch-shortening exercises both require preparatory and reactive muscle activity through feed-forward and feedback motor control systems, while closed-kinetic-chain exercises are excellent

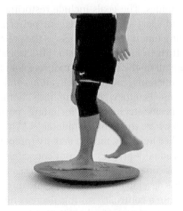

Figure 6-4   Neoprene sleeves stimulate cutaneous receptors, providing additional sensory feedback for joint motion and position awareness.

for inducing coactivation and compression. Chimura[16] and Hewett[45] have confirmed that stretch-shortening exercises increase muscle coactivation and enhance coordination.

Reactive Neuromuscular Control. Reactive neuromuscular training focuses on stimulating the reflex AB pathways from articular and tenomuscular receptors to skeletal muscle. Although preprogrammed muscle stiffness can enhance the reactive capability of muscles by reducing reflex latency time, the objective is to generate joint perturbations that are not anticipated, stimulating reflex stabilization. The efficacy of reactive neuromuscular exercises was demonstrated nearly a decade ago.[52] Persistent use of these reflex pathways can decrease the response time and develop reactive strategies to unexpected joint loads.[41] Furthermore, Caraffa[15] significantly reduced the incidence of knee injuries in soccer players who performed reactive type training. Fitzgerald et al.[28,29] observed that muscle activity and biomechanical markers of gait were normalized in patients who underwent perturbation training after knee injuries. All reactive exercises should induce unanticipated joint perturbations if they are expected to facilitate reflex muscle activation. Reflex-mediated muscle activity is a crucial element in the dynamic restraint mechanism and should complement preprogrammed muscle activity to achieve a functionally stable joint.

Functional Activities. The objective of functional rehabilitation is to return the patient to preinjury activity level while minimizing the risk of reinjury.[107] This may require video analysis and consultation with the coaching staff to identify and correct faulty mechanics or movement techniques. The goals include restoring functional stability and sport-specific movement patterns or skills, then utilizing functional tests to assess the patient's readiness to return to full participation. Functional activities incorporate all of the available resources for stimulating peripheral afferents, muscle coactivation, and reflex and preprogrammed motor control. Emphasis should be placed on sport-specific techniques, including positions and maneuvers where the joint is vulnerable. With repetition and controlled intensity, muscle activity (preparatory and reactive) gradually progresses from conscious to unconscious motor control.[57] Implementing these activities will help patients develop functionally specific movement repertoires within a controlled setting, decreasing the risk of injury upon completion of rehabilitation.

Understanding the afferent and efferent characteristics that contribute to joint sensation, dynamic stabilization, reflex activity, and functional motor pattern is necessary for reestablishing neuromuscular control and functional stability (Table 6-1).

CLINICAL DECISION MAKING   Exercise 6–2

There was an increase in ACL injuries last year on the women's soccer team. You decide to develop a prevention program in an effort to minimize injuries in the upcoming season. What are the main goals of the prevention program with respect to neuromuscular control? What do you feel is the most effective method of training to achieve your goals?

Lower-Extremity Techniques

Many activities that promote neuromuscular control in the lower extremity exist in traditional rehabilitation schemes. Early kinesthetic training and joint repositioning tasks can begin to reestablish reflex pathways from articular afferents to skeletal motor nerves, the muscle spindle system, and cortical motor control centers, while enhancing muscle stiffness increases the stretch sensitivity of tenomuscular receptors. To induce adaptations in muscle stiffness, exercises should be performed with high repetitions and low rest intervals, focusing on the eccentric phase. Increased muscle stiffness and tone will heighten the stretch sensitivity of tenomuscular receptors, providing additional sensory information concerning joint motion and position.

These techniques should focus on individual muscle groups that require attention and progress from no weight to weight-assisted. The use of closed-chain activities is encouraged because they replicate the environment specific to the lower-extremity function. Partial weight bearing, in pools or with unloading devices, simulates the open- and closed-chain environments without subjecting the ankle, knee, or hip to excessive joint loads.[59] The closed-chain nature of these exercises creates joint compression, thus enhancing joint congruency and neurosensory feedback, while minimizing shearing forces on the joints.[93] Early dynamic joint stabilization exercises begin with balance training and partial weight bearing on stable surfaces, progressing to partial weight bearing on unstable surfaces. Balancing on unstable surfaces is initiated once full weight bearing is achieved. Exercises such as "kickers" also require balance and can begin on stable surfaces, progressing to unstable platforms (Figure 6-5).

Slide board training and basic strength exercises can be instituted to stimulate coactivation while increasing muscular force and endurance. Strength exercises focus on eccentric and endurance-type activities in a closed kinetic orientation, further enhancing dynamic stability through

■ TABLE   6-1   The Elements, Rehabilitation Techniques, and Afferent/Efferent Characteristics Necessary for Restoring Proprioception and Neuromuscular Control.

Elements	Rehabilitation Techniques	Afferent/Efferent Characteristics
Proprioception and Kinesthesia	Joint repositioning Functional range of motion Facilitate afferent pathways Axial loading Closed-kinetic-chain exercises	Peripheral receptor sensitivity
Dynamic Stability	Closed-kinetic-chain exercises and translatory forces High-repetition/low-resistance Eccentric loading Stretch-shortening exercises Balance training	Agonist/antagonist coactivation Muscle activation rate and amplitude Peripheral receptor sensitivity Muscle stiffness
Reactive Neuromuscular Control	Reaction to joint perturbation Stretch shortening, plyometrics Balance reacquisition	Reflex facilitation Muscle activation rate and amplitude
Functional Motor Patterns	Biofeedback Sport-specific drills Control-progressive participation	Discriminatory muscle activation Arthrokinematics Coordinated locomotion

increases in preparatory muscle stiffness and reactive characteristics. Eccentric loading is accomplished by activities such as forward and backward stairclimbing or backward downhill walking. Strength and balance exercises can be combined and executed with light external forces to increase the level of difficulty (Figure 6-6).

Biofeedback can also help patients trying to develop agonist/antagonist coactivation during strength exercises. Biofeedback provides additional information concerning muscle activation and encourages voluntary muscle activation by facilitating efferent pathways. Reeducating injured patients through selective muscle activation is

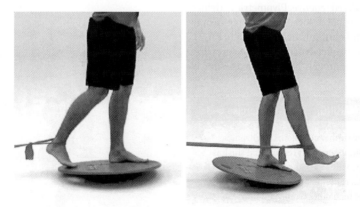

Figure 6-5   "Kickers" use an elastic band fixed to the distal aspect of the involved or uninvolved limb. The patient attempts to balance while executing short kicks with either knee extension or hip flexion. This exercise is most difficult when performed on unstable surfaces.

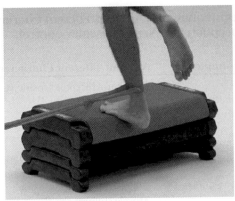
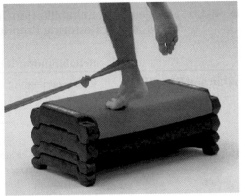

Figure 6-6   Balance and strength exercises are combined by incorporating light external forces and increasing the level of difficulty for balancing while strengthening the muscles required for dynamic stabilization.

necessary for dynamic stabilization and neuromuscular control.

Stretch-shortening exercises are a necessary component for conditioning the neuromuscular apparatus to respond more quickly and forcefully, permitting eccentric deceleration then developing explosive concentric contractions.[1] Stretch-shortening exercises need not be withheld until the late stages of rehabilitation. There is a variety of plyometric activities, and intensity can be controlled by manipulating the load, range of motion or number of repetitions. Stretch-shortening movements require both preparatory and reactive muscle activities along with the related changes in muscle stiffness. This preparatory muscle activation prior to eccentric loading is considered to be preprogrammed, while activation after ground contact is considered reactive. Plyometric activities such as unweighted in a pool or low-impact hopping may commence once weight bearing is achieved (Figure 6-7). Double-leg bounding is an effective intermediate exercise, because the uninvolved limb can be used for assistance.

Stretch-shortening activities are made more difficult with alternate-leg bounding, then single-leg hopping. Subsequent activities such as hopping with rotation, lateral hopping, and hopping onto various surfaces are instituted as tolerated. Plyometric training requires preparatory muscle activation and facilitates reflexive pathways for reactive neuromuscular control.

Rhythmic stabilization exercises should be included during early rehabilitation to enhance lower-extremity neuromuscular coordination and reaction to unexpected joint perturbations. The intensity of rhythmic stabilization is increased by applying greater joint loads and displacements. Foot pass drills are also effective for developing coordinated preparatory and reactive muscle activity; begin with large balls and progress to smaller balls.

CLINICAL DECISION MAKING   **Exercise 6–3**

A female cross-country runner complains of chronic anterior knee pain. Your assessment reveals that she has patellofemoral pain and stiffness with associated hypertrophy of her vastus lateralis and atrophy in the vastus medialis oblique. What modalities would you utilize to correct this muscular imbalance? Discuss the rationale for each modality and how it relates to neuromuscular control.[43]

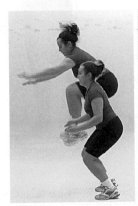
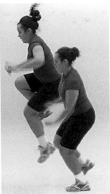

Figure 6-7   Plyometrics begin with double-leg hopping, and progress to single-leg hopping.

Unstable platforms are utilized to manually induce linear and angular perturbations to the joint, altering the patient's center of gravity while the patient attempts to balance (Figure 6-8). These exercises can facilitate adaptations to reflex pathways mediated by peripheral afferents, resulting in reactive muscle activation. Ball tossing can be incorporated in conjunction with balance exercises. This dual tasking creates cognitive loads that may disrupt concentration and help promote reactive adaptations. Walking and running in sand also requires similar reactive muscle activity and can enhance reflexive joint stabilization.

During the later stages of rehabilitation, reactive neuromuscular activity incorporates trampoline hopping. The patient begins by hopping and landing on both feet, progressing to hopping on one foot, and hopping with rotation. The most difficult reactive tasks include hopping while catching a ball, or hopping off of a trampoline onto various landing surfaces such as artificial turf, grass, or dirt.

Functional activities begin with restoring normal gait. Clinicians can give verbal instruction or use a mirror to help patients internalize normal kinematics during the stance and swing phases. This includes backward (retro) walking, which has been shown to further facilitate hamstring activation and balance. If a pool or unloading device is available, crossover walking and figure eights can begin, progressing to jogging and hopping as tolerated. Functional activities during partial weight bearing help restore motor patterns without compromising static restraints. Weight-bearing activities are continued on land with the incorporation of acceleration and deceleration and pivot maneuvers. Drills such as jogging, cutting, and cariocas are initiated, gradually increasing the speed of maneuvers.

The most difficult functional activities are designed to simulate the demands of individual sports and positions and may require input from the coaching staff. Activities such as shuttle runs, carioca crossovers, retro sprinting and forward sprinting are implemented with sport-specific drills such as fielding a ball, receiving a pass, and dribbling a soccer ball. (See Chapter 16)

CLINICAL DECISION MAKING   **Exercise 6–4**

A volleyball player is recovering from an Achilles/gastrocnemius strain. Develop plyometric exercises that can be implemented in each stage of rehabilitation. What would your rationale be for integrating these activities into the patient's rehabilitation? Describe the neuromuscular adaptations that you expect to occur.

Upper Extremity Techniques

Contrary to the lower extremity, the glenohumeral joint lacks inherent stability from capsuloligamentous structures; therefore dynamic mechanisms are even more crucial for maintaining functional stability.[40,115] The difficulty of working with a diverse array of shoulder positions and velocities is compounded by shearing forces associated with manipulating the upper extremity in an open-kinetic-chain environment.[115] Maintaining joint congruency and functional stability requires coordinated muscle activation for dynamic restraint while complex movement repertoires are executed.[74]

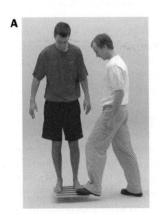
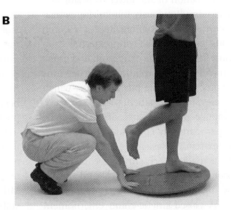

Figure 6-8   An unstable platform promotes reactive muscle activity when a patient attempts to balance and a clinician manually perturbs the platform. **A,** Wobble board. **B,** BAPS board.

Two distinct types of muscle have been identified in the shoulder girdle and are primarily responsible for either stabilization or initiating movement. The orientation and size of the stabilizing muscles, referred to as the rotator cuff, are not suited for creating joint motion but are more capable of steering the humeral head in the glenoid fossa.[74] Larger muscles (primary movers) with insertion sites further from the glenohumeral joint have greater mechanical advantage for initiating joint motion.[74,79] Maintaining proper joint kinematics requires balancing the external forces and internal moments while limiting excessive translation of the humeral head on the glenoid fossa.

Injury to the static structures can result in diminished sensory feedback and altered kinematics of the scapulothoracic and glenohomeral joints. Moreover, failure of the dynamic restraint system exposes the static structures to excessive or repetitive loads, jeopardizing joint integrity and predisposing the patient to reinjury. Surgery is the most effective means of restoring sensorimotor function long-term[3,76,96]; however, this avenue is not always an option. Therefore, developing or restoring neuromuscular control in the upper extremity through rehabilitation exercises is an important component for the eventual return to functional activities. Evidence supporting specific rehabilitation techniques is lacking, but critical review of the scientific literature produces recommendations for implementation to produce best results.

There is general agreement that achieving scapular control early in the rehabilitation program is imperative.[61,89,112] Exercises focusing on scapular retraction as a starting position for all subsequent activities should be incorporated for restoring optimal shoulder complex function and reducing one's risk for secondary injury. To achieve this position, exercises to increase activation of the lower trapezius and serratus anterior while simultaneously minimizing activation of the upper trapezius are appropriate. Recent research suggests the following exercises: sidelying external rotation, sidelying forward flexion, prone extension, and prone horizontal abduction with external rotation.[20] The serratus anterior is also activated during the push-up plus, which can be progressed by elevating the patient's feet.[80]

Activities to enhance proprioceptive and kinesthetic awareness in the upper extremity emulate techniques discussed for the lower extremity. Research advocates use of closed-kinetic-chain activities early in upper extremity rehabilitation to promote afferent feedback and coactivation, which may include weight shifts, table slides, and wall slides.[13,62] A closed-kinetic-chain environment introduces axial loads and muscle coactivation, the resultant joint approximation stimulates capsuloligamentous mechanoreceptors, similar to lower-extremity activi-

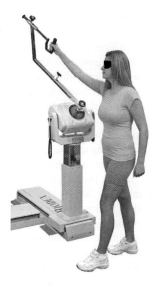

Figure 6-9 Active and passive repositioning activities should be performed in functional positions specific to individual sports.

ties.[74,116] Stretch-shortening (plyometric) exercises in the overhead patient have been shown to improve proprioception. Multiplanar joint repositioning tasks are performed actively and passively to maximize the increased range of motion available in the shoulder. Functional positions, such as overhead throwing, should be incorporated and are more sport-specific (Figure 6-9).

Muscle stiffness can be enhanced by using elastic resistance tubing or a plyoball with an inclined trampoline, concentrating on the eccentric phase, and performing high repetitions with low resistance.[111] These exercises are also well established for strengthening and reconditioning the rotator cuff muscles in functional patterns. To complement elastic tubing exercises, clinicians can utilize commercially available upper-extremity ergometers for endurance training.

Like similar exercises for the lower extremity, dynamic stabilization exercises for the shoulder use unstable platforms to create linear and angular joint displacement, maximally stimulating coactivation. The intensity is controlled by manipulating the degree of joint displacement and loading. Three closed-chain exercises have been described to stimulate coactivation in the shoulder: push-ups, horizontal abduction on a slide board, and tracing circular motions on a slide board with the dominant and nondominant arms[74] (Figure 6-10). These exercises accommodate for the individual's tolerance to joint loads by progressing from a quadruped to a push-up position. Multidirectional slide board exercises also require dynamic stabilization while concomitantly using feed-forward and feedback neuromuscular control. Plyometric exercises with varying ball weights and distances for advancement are also excellent for conditioning preparatory and reactive

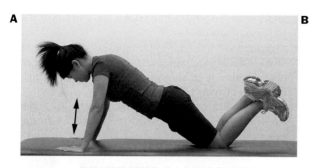

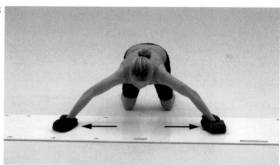

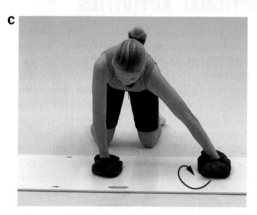

Figure 6-10   Dynamic stabilization exercises for the upper extremity. **A,** Push-ups. **B,** Horizontal abduction on a slide board. **C,** Wax-on wax-off on slide board.

muscle coactivation and can be advanced by increasing the weight of the ball, varying the distance, and introducing multiplanar movements (Figure 6-11).[111]

Reactive neuromuscular characteristics are facilitated by manually perturbing the upper extremity while the patient attempts to maintain a permanent position. During the early phases of rehabilitation, light loads are used with rhythmic stabilization exercises. As the patient progresses, resistance is added to maximize muscle activation (Figure 6-12). Positions where the joint is inherently

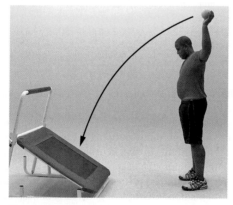

Figure 6-11   Upper-extremity plyometric exercises with a heavy ball require preparatory and reactive muscle activation.

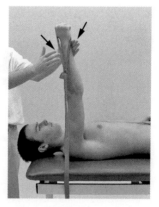

Figure 6-12   Elastic bands are used during rhythmic stabilization exercises to create joint loads and facilitate muscle activation.

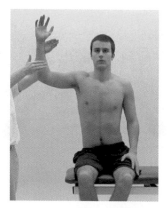

Figure 6-13 Rhythmic stabilization exercises should include simulated positions of vulnerability, promoting neuromuscular adaptations to dynamic stabilization.

unstable must be incorporated, but under controlled intensity (Figure 6-13). Increased joint loads during rhythmic stabilization exercises mimic closed-chain environments and conditions the patient for more difficult reactive drills

---

CLINICAL DECISION MAKING   **Exercise 6–5**

During preparticipation physicals, you note that one of the tennis players has a history of inferior glenohumeral dislocation and, as a result, excessive laxity. The surrounding masculature appears strong, but the patient continues to have sensations of instability. What is the nature of this patient's problem, and what exercises would you use to improve dynamic stability of the rotator cuff muscles? Justify your decision to incorporate these exercises.

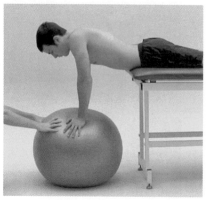

Figure 6-14 Linear displacements produced by a clinician facilitate reflex pathways for dynamic stabilization in the upper extremity.

under weighted conditions on stable surfaces and unstable platforms (Figure 6-14).

Functional training for the upper extremity most often involves developing motor patterns in the overhead position, whether it be shooting a basketball, throwing, or hitting as in volleyball and tennis. However, special considerations are necessary for other sports, like rowing, wrestling, and swimming, which rely heavily on the upper extremity.

FUNCTIONAL ACTIVITIES

Functional activities that involve a combination of strength training, balance, and core stability performed through multiple planes of movement should incorporate the entire kinetic chain, as they need to reproduce the demands of specific events. Beginning with slower velocities and conscious control, activities eventually progress to functional speeds and unconscious control. Technique, rather than speed, should be emphasized to promote the appropriate muscle activation patterns along the kinetic chain and avoid faulty mechanics. Reeducating functional motor patterns involves all of the elements for dynamic restraint and neuromuscular control and will minimize the risk of reinjury upon returning to full participation. Figure 6-15 provides examples of exercises which can be used to enhance neuromuscular control.

CLINICAL DECISION MAKING   **Exercise 6–6**

A wrestler is performing rehabilitation for a grade 2 medial collateral ligament (MCL) sprain. His rehabilitation is in the final stage and you would like to incorporate functional exercises into the protocol. Considering the specific demands related to this sport, develop a progression of functional exercises for this patient's return to full participation.

The speed and complexity of movements in athletic competition requires rapid integration of sensory information by feed-forward and feedback neuromuscular control systems. Although many peripheral, spinal, and cortical elements contribute to the neuromuscular control system, dynamic joint stabilization is contingent upon both cortically programmed preactivation and reflex-mediated muscle activation. Disrupted joint kinematics, muscle activation patterns, and conditioning can contribute to disruption of the dynamic restraint system and must be reestablished for functional stability.

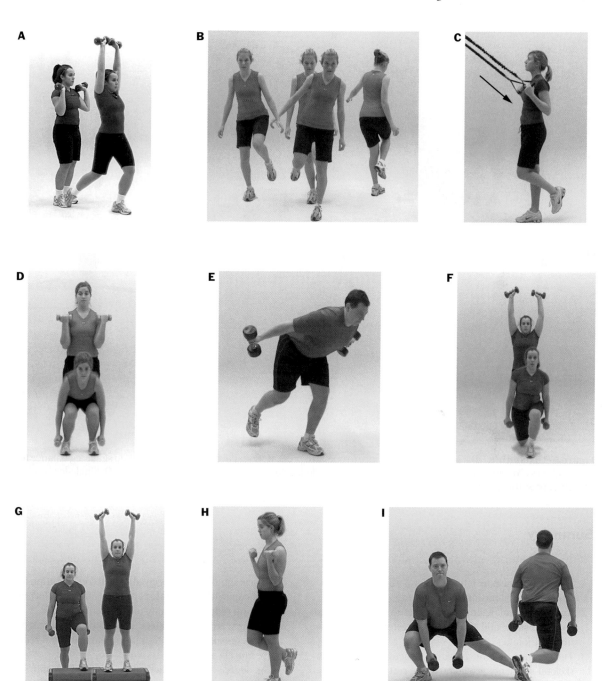

Figure 6-15 Exercises to enhance neuromuscular control. **A**, Two arm push press. **B**, Multiplanar hops to stabilization. **C**, Single leg pulldown using cable or tubing. **D**, Standing dumbbell squat to curl. **E**, Single leg two arm dumbbell cobra. **F**, Dumbbell squat to overhead press. **G**, Stepup double leg balance to overhead press. **H**, Standing single-leg dumbbell bicep curls. **I**, Multiplanar dumbbell lunges.

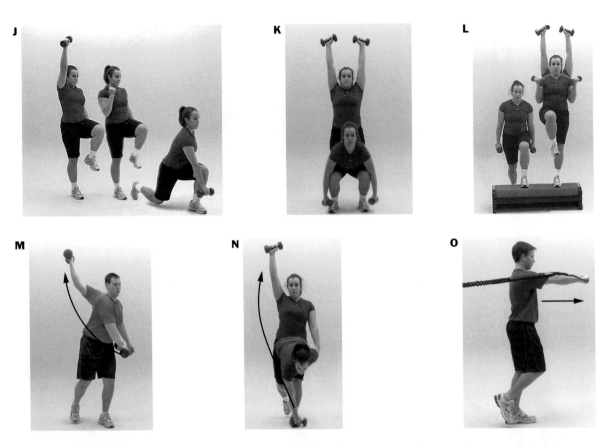

Figure 6-15 (continued) **J**, Front lunge balance to one-arm press. **K**, Squat overhead press. **L**, Stepup single leg balance to overhead press. **M**, Single-leg one-arm dumbbell PNF. **N**, Single-leg Romanian dead lift to overhead press. **O**, Single-leg two-arm chest press using cable.

Summary

1. The efferent response to peripheral afferent information is termed neuromuscular control.
2. Injury to capsuloligamentous structures compromises both the static and the dynamic restraining mechanisms of joints.
3. The primary role of articular structures is to guide skeletal segments providing static restraint, but they also contain mechanoreceptors that mediate the dynamic restraint mechanism.
4. Articular sensations are coupled with information from tenomuscular mechanoreceptors, via cortical and reflex pathways, providing conscious and unconscious appreciation of joint motion and position.
5. Muscle spindles have received special consideration for their capacity to integrate peripheral afferent information and reflexively modify muscle activity.
6. Feed-forward and feedback neuromuscular controls utilize sensory information for preparatory and reactive muscle activity.
7. The degree of muscle activation largely determines a muscle's resistance to stretching or stiffness. Muscles with increased stiffness can assist the dynamic restraint mechanism by resisting excessive joint translation.
8. To reestablish neuromuscular control and functional stability, clinicians may utilize specific rehabilitation techniques—including closed-kinetic-chain activities,

balance training, eccentric and high-repetition/low-load exercises, reflex facilitation through reactive training, stretch-shortening activities, and biofeedback training.

9. Rehabilitative techniques produce adaptations in the sensitivity of peripheral receptors and facilitation of afferent pathways, agonist/antagonist coactivation, muscle stiffness, the onset rate and magnitude of muscle activity, reflex muscle activation, and discriminatory muscle activation.

10. Afferent and efferent characteristics regulate the four elements critical to neuromuscular control and functional stability: proprioception and kinesthesia, dynamic stabilization, reflex muscle activation, and functional motor patterns.

11. Each phase of traditional rehabilitation can incorporate the appropriate activities, emphasizing each of the four elements, according to the individual's tolerance and functional progression. By integrating these elements into the rehabilitation of injured patients, clinicians can maximize the contributions of the dynamic restraint mechanisms to functional stability.

References

1. Abott, J. C., and U. B. Saunders. 1994. Injuries to the ligaments of the knee joint. *Journal of Bone Joint Surgery* December:503–521.

2. Appleberg, B., H. Johansson, M. Hulliger, and P. Sojka. 1986. Actions on motoneurons elicited by electrical stimulation of group III muscle afferent fibers in the hind limb of the cat.: *Journal of Physiology* (London) 375:137–152.

3. Aydin, T., Y. Yildiz, I. Yanmis, C. Yildiz, and T. A. Kalyon. 2001. Shoulder proprioception: A comparison between the shoulder joint in healthy and surgically repaired shoulders. *Arch Orthop Trauma Surg* 121:422–425.

4. Bach, T. M., A. E. Chapman, and T. W., Calvert. 1983. Mechanical resonance of the human body during voluntary oscillations about the ankle joint. *J Biomech* 16:85–90.

5. Barker, D. 1974. The morphology of muscle receptors. In *Handbook of sensory physiology*, Hunt, C. C., ed. Berlin: Springer-Verlag, 191–234.

6. Barrack, R. L., H. B. Skinner, M. E., Brunet, and S. D., Cook. 1983. Joint laxity and proprioception in the knee. *Physician and Sports Medicine* 11:130–135.

7. Barrack, R. L., H. B. Skinner, M. E., Brunet, and S.D., Cook SD. 1984. Joint kinesthesia in the highly trained knee. *J Sports Med Phys Fitness* 24:18–20.

8. Barrett, D. S. 1991. Proprioception and function after anterior cruciate reconstruction. *J Bone Joint Surg Br* 73:833–837.

9. Basmajian, J. V. 1979. *Biofeedback: Principles and practice for clinicians*. Baltimore: Williams & Wilkins.

10. Beard, D. J., C. A. Dodd, H. R. Trundle, and A. H., Simpson. 1994. Proprioception enhancement for anterior cruciate ligament deficiency: A prospective randomised trial of two physiotherapy regimes. *J Bone Joint Surg Br* 76:654–659.

11. Branch, T. P., R. Hunter, and M. Donath. 1989. Dynamic EMG analysis of anterior cruciate deficient legs with and without bracing during cutting. *Am J Sports Med* 17:35–41.

12. Brenner, J., and K. Swanik. 2007. High-risk drinking characteristics in collegiate athletes. *J Am Coll Health.* 56:267–272.

13. Broer M. R. 1993. *Efficiency of Human Movement*. 3rd ed. Philadelphia: W.B. Saunders Co.

14. Bulbulian, R., and D. K. Bowles. 1992. Effect of downhill running on motoneuron pool excitability. *J Appl Physiol* 73:968–973.

15. Caraffa, A., G. Cerulli. M. Proietti, G. Aisa, and A. Rizzo. 1995. Prevention of anterior cruciate ligament in soccer: A prospective controlled study of proprioceptive training. *Knee Surgery Sports Traumatol, Arthroscopy* 4:19–21.

16. Chimura, N. J., K. A. Swanik, C. B. Swanik, and S. V., Straub. 2004. Effects of plyometric training on muscle-activation strategies and performance in female athletes. *J Athl Train* 39:24–31.

17. Clark, F. J., and P. R. Burgess. 1975. Slowly adapting receptors in cat knee joint: Can they signal joint angle? *J Neurophysiol* 38:1448–1463.

18. Clark, F. J., R. C. Burgess, J. W., Chapin, and W. T., Lipscomb. 1985. Role of intramuscular receptors in the awareness of limb position. *J Neurophysiol* 54:1529–1540.

19. Colebatch, J. G., and D. I., McCloskey. 1987. Maintenance of constant arm position or force: Reflex and volitional components in man. *J Physiol* 386:247–261.

20. Cools, A. M., V. Dewitte, F., Lanszweert, D. Notebaert, A. Roets, B. Soetens, B. Cagnie, and E. E. Witvrouw. 2007. Rehabilitation of scapular muscle balance: Which exercises to prescribe? *Am J Sports Med* 35:1744–1751.

21. Corrigan, J. P., W. F. Cashman, and M. P., Brady. 1992. Proprioception in the cruciate deficient knee. *J Bone Joint Surg Br* 74:247–250.

22. Dietz, V., Noth and D., Schmidtbleicher. 1981. Interaction between pre-activity and stretch reflex in human triceps brachii during landing from forward falls. *J Physiol* 311:113–125.

23. Dunn, T. G., S. E. Ponsor, N. Weil, and S. W. Utz. 1986. The learning process in biofeedback: Is it feed-forward or feedback? *Biofeedback Self Regul* 11:143–156.

24. Dyhre-Poulsen, P., E. B. Simonsen, and M. Voigt. 1991. Dynamic control of muscle stiffness and H reflex modulation

during hopping and jumping in man. *J Physiol* 437:287–304.

25. Eccles, R. M., and A. Lindberg. 1959. Synaptic actions in motoneurons by afferents which may evoke the flexion reflex. *Archives of Italian Biology* 1979:199–221.

26. Enoka, R. M. 1994. *Neuromechanical Basis of Kinesiology.* 2nd ed. Champaign, IL: Human Kinetics.

27. Finsterbush, A., and B. Friedman. 1975. The effect of sensory denervation on rabbits' knee joints: A light and electron microscopic study. *J Bone Joint Surg Am* 57:949–956.

28. Fitzgerald, G. K., J. D. Childs, T. M. Ridge, and J. J. Irrgang. 2002. Agility and perturbation training for a physically active individual with knee osteoarthritis. *Phys Ther* 82:372–82.

29. Fitzgerald, G. K., M. J., Axe, and L. Snyder-Mackler. 2000. The efficacy of perturbation training in nonoperative anterior cruciate ligament rehabilitation of physically active individuals. *Phys Ther* 80:128–140.

30. Forwell, L. A., and H. Carnahan. 1996. Proprioception during manual aiming in individuals with shoulder instability and controls. *J Orthop Sports Phys Ther* 23:111–119.

31. Freeman, M. A., and B. Wyke. 1966. Articular contributions to limb muscle reflexes.: The effects of partial neurectomy of the knee-joint on postural reflexes. *Br J Surg* 53:61–68.

32. Gardner, E., F. Latimer, and D. Stiwell. 1949. Central connections for afferent fibers from the knee joint of a cat. *American Journal of Physiology* 159:195–198.

33. Glaros, A. G., and K. Hanson. 1990. EMG biofeedback and discriminative muscle control. *Biofeedback Self Regul* 15:135–143.

34. Glencross, D., and E. Thornton. 1981. Position sense following joint injury. *Journal of Sports Medicine and Physical Fitness.* 1211:23–27.

35. Goubel, F., and J. F. Marini. 1987. Fiber type transition and stiffness modification of soleus muscle of trained rats. *European Journal of Physiology* 410:321–325.

36. Granata, K. P., D. A. Padua, and S. E., Wilson. 2002. Gender differences in active musculoskeletal stiffness: Part II. Quantification of leg stiffness during functional hopping tasks. *J Electromyogr Kinesiol* 12:127–135.

37. Greenwood, R. D. 1976. A view of nineteenth century therapeutics. *J Med Assoc State Ala* 45:25.

38. Grigg, P. 1994. Peripheral neural mechanisms in proprioception. *Journal of Sport Rehabilitation.* 134:1–17.

39. Griller, S. 1972. A role for muscle stiffness in meeting the changing postural and locomotor requirements for force development by ankle extensors. *Acta Physiologica Scandinavia* 1862:92–108.

40. Guanche, C., T. Knatt, M, Solomonow, Y., Lu and R., Baratta. 1995. The synergistic action of the capsule and the shoulder muscles. *Am J Sports Med* 23:301–306.

41. Guyton, A. C. 1981. *Textbook of medical physiology.* 6th ed. Philadelphia: W. B. Saunders.

42. Hagood, S., M. Solomonow, R. Baratta, B. H. Zhou, and R. D'Ambrosia. 1990. The effect of joint velocity on the contribution of the antagonist musculature to knee stiffness and laxity. *Am J Sports Med* 18:182–187.

43. Hamstra-Wright, K. L., C. B. Swanik, T. Y., Ennis, and K. A., Swanik 2005. Joint stiffness and pain in individuals with patellofemoral syndrome. *J Orthop Sports Phys Ther* 35:495–501.

44. Hamstra, K. L., C. B. Swanik, R. T. Tierney, K. C. Huxel, and J. M. Cherubini. 2002. The relationship between muscle tone and dynamic restraint in the physically active. *Journal of Athletic Training* 37:S–41.

45. Hewett, T. E., G. D. Myer, and K. R. Ford. 2005. Reducing knee and anterior cruciate ligament injuries among female athletes. *The Journal of Knee Surgery* 18:82–88.

46. Hewett, T. E., G. D. Myer, and K. R. Ford. 2005. Reducing knee and anterior cruciate ligament injuries among female athletes: A systematic review of neuromuscular training interventions. *J Knee Surg* 8:82–8.

47. Hodgson, J. A., R. R. Roy, R. de Leon, B. Dobkin, and V. R. Edgerton. 1994. Can the mammalian lumbar spinal cord learn a motor task? *Med Sci Sports Exerc* 26:1491–1497.

48. Hoffer, J. A., and S. Andreassen. 1981. Regulation of soleus muscle stiffness in premammillary cats: Intrinsic and reflex components. *J Neurophysiol* 45:267–285.

49. Houk, J. C., P. E. Crago, and W. Z., Rymer. 1981. Function of the dynamic response in stiffness regulation: A predictive mechanism provided by non-linear feedback. London: Macmillan. In *Muscle Receptors and Movement,* Taylor, A., and A. Prochazka, eds.

50. Hutton, R. S., and S. W. Atwater. 1992. Acute and chronic adaptations of muscle proprioceptors in response to increased use. *Sports Med* 14:406–421.

51. Huxel, K. C., C. B. Swanik, K. A. Swanik, A. R. Bartolozzi H. J. Hillstrom, M. R. Sitler, and D. M. Moffit. 2008. Stiffness regulation and muscle-recruitment strategies of the shoulder in response to external rotation perturbations. *J Bone Joint Surg Am* 90:154–162.

52. Ihara, H., and A. Nakayama. 1986. Dynamic joint control training for knee ligament injuries. *Am J Sports Med* 14:309–315.

53. Johansson, H., P. Sjolander, and P. Sojka. 1986. Actions on gamma-motoneurons elicited by electrical stimulation of joint afferent fibres in the hind limb of the cat. *J Physiol* 375:137–152.

54. Johansson, H., P. Sjolander, and P. Sojka. 1991. Receptors in the knee joint ligaments and their role in the biomechanics of the joint. *Crit Rev Biomed Eng* 18:341–368.

55. Johansson, H., P. Sjolander, and P. Sojka 1991. A sensory role for the cruciate ligaments. *Clin Orthop Relat Res* 268:161–178.

56. Jonsson, H., J. Karrholm, and L. G. Elmqvist 1989. Kinematics of active knee extension after tear of the anterior cruciate ligament. *Am J Sports Med* 17:796–802.

57. Kandell, E. R., J. H. Schwartz, and T. M. Jessell. 1996. *Principles of neural science.* 3rd ed. Norwalk, CT: Appleton & Lange.

58. Katonis, P. G., A. P. Assimakopoulos M. V., Agapitos, and E. I. Exarchou. 1991. Mechanoreceptors in the posterior cruciate ligament. *Acta Orthopedica Scandanavia* 62:276–278.

59. Kelsey, D. D., and E. Tyson 1994. A new method of training for the lower extremity using unloading. *J Orthop Sports Phys Ther* 19:218–223.

60. Kennedy, J. C., I. J. Alexander, and K. C. Hayes. 1982. Nerve supply of the human knee and its functional importance. *Am J Sports Med* 10:329–335.
61. Kibler, W. B., J. McMullen, and T. Uhl. 2001. Shoulder rehabilitation strategies, guidelines, and practice. *Orthop Clin North Am* 32:527–538.
62. Kibler, W. B. 2000. Closed kinetic chain rehabilitation for sports injuries. *Phys Med Rehabil Clin N Am* 11:369–384.
63. Koceja, D. M., J. Burke, and G. Kamen. 1991. Organization of segmental reflexes in trained dancers. *Int J Sports Med* 12:285–289.
64. Koceja, D. M., and G. Kamen. 1988. Conditioned patellar tendon reflexes in sprint- and endurance-trained athletes. *Med Sci Sports Exerc* 20:172–177.
65. Kochner, M. S., F. H. Fu, and C. D. Harner. 1994. Neuropathophysiology In *Knee Surgery.* Vol 1. Fu, F. H., and C. D. Harner, eds. Baltimore: Williams & Wilkins.
66. Kovanen, V., H. Suominen, and E. Heikkinen. 1984. Mechanical properties of fast and slow skeletal muscle with special reference to collagen and endurance training. *J Biomech* 17:725–735.
67. Kyrolaninen, H., and P. V. Komi. 1995. The function of neuromuscular system in maximal stretch-shortening cycle exercises: Comparison between power- and endurance-trained athletes. *Journal of Electromyographic Kinesiology* 155:15–25.
68. La Croix, J. M. 1981. The acquisition of autonomic control through biofeedback: The case against an afferent process and a two-process alternative. *Psychophysiology* 1181:573–587.
69. Lamell-Sharp, A. D., C. B. Swanik, and R. T. Tierney. 2002. The effect of variable joint loads on knee joint position and force sensation. *Journal of Athletic Training.* 37(2):S29.
70. Leanderson, J., E. Eriksson, C. Nilsson, and A. Wykman. 1996. Proprioception in classical ballet dancers. A prospective study of the influence of an ankle sprain on proprioception in the ankle joint. *Am J Sports Med* 24:370–374.
71. Leksell, L. 1995. The action potential and excitatory effects of the small ventral root fibers to skeletal muscle. *Acta Physiol Scand* 10(31): S1–84. 10(31):81–84.
72. Lephart, S. M., and T. J. Henry. 1996. The physiological basis for open and closed kinetic chain rehabilitation for the upper extremity. *Journal of Sport Rehabilitation* 156:71–87.
73. Lephart, S. M., M. S. Kocher, F. H. Fu, P. A. Borsa, and C. D. Harner. 1992. Proprioception following ACL reconstruction. *Journal of Sport Rehabilitation* 188–196.
74. Lephart, S. M., J. P. Warner, P. A. Borsa, and F. H. Fu. 1994. Proprioception of the shoulder joint in healthy, unstable, and surgically repaired shoulders. *Journal of Shoulder Elbow Surgery* 134:371–380.
75. Lephart, S. M., J. L. Giraldo, P. A. Borsa, and F. H. Fu. 1996. Knee joint proprioception: A comparison between female intercollegiate gymnasts and controls. *Knee Surg Sports Traumatol Arthrosc.* 4:121–4.
76. Lephart, S. M., J. B. Myers, J. P. Bradley, and F. H. Fu 2002. Shoulder proprioception and function following thermal capsulorraphy. *Arthroscopy* 18:770–778.
77. Lephart, S. M., D. M. Pincivero, J. L. Giraldo, and F. J. Fu. 1997. The role of proprioception in the management and rehabilitation of athletic injuries. *Am J Sports Med* 25:130–7.
78. Lephart, S. M., D. M. Pincivero, and S. L., Rozzi. 1998. Proprioception of the ankle and knee. *Sports Med* 25:149–55.
79. Lieber, R. L., and J. Friden. 1992. Neuromuscular stabilization of the shoulder girdle. In *The shoulder: A balance of mobility and stability,* Matsen F. A., ed. Rosemont, IL: American Academy of Orthopaedic Surgeons 1992:91–106.
80. Ludewig, P. M., M. S. Hoff, E. E. Osowski, S. A. Meschke, and P. J., Rundquist. 2004. Relative balance of serratus anterior and upper trapezius muscle activity during push-up exercises. *Am J Sports Med* 32:484–493.
81. Lynch, S. A., U. Eklund, D. Gottlieb, P. A. Renstrom, and B. Beynnon. 1996. Electromyographic latency changes in the ankle musculature during inversion moments. *Am J Sports Med* 24:362–369.
82. Mair, S. D., A. V. Seaber, R. R. Glisson, and W. E. Garrett, Jr. 1996. The role of fatigue in susceptibility to acute muscle strain injury. *Am J Sports Med* 24:137–143.
83. McComas, A. J. 1994. Human neuromuscular adaptations that accompany changes in activity. *Med Sci Sports Exerc* 26:1498–1509.
84. McNair, P. J., and R. N. Marshall. 1994. Landing characteristics in subjects with normal and anterior cruciate ligament deficient knee joints. *Archives of Physical Medicine and Rehabilitation* 1754:584–589.
85. McNair, P. J., G. A. Wood, and R. N. Marshall. 1992. Stiffness of the hamstring muscles and its relationship to function in anterior cruciate deficient individuals. *Clinical Biomechanics* 172:131–173.
86. Melvill-Jones, G. M., and G. D. Watt. 1971. Observations of the control of stepping and hopping in man. *Journal of Physiology* 219:709–727.
87. Merton, P. A. 1953. Speculations on the servo-control of movement. In *The Spinal Cord,* Wolstenholme, G. E. W., ed. London: Churchill.
88. Morgan, D. L. 1977. Separation of active and passive components of short-range stiffness of muscle. *Am J Physiol,* 232:C45–9.
89. Moseley, J. B., Jr., F. W. Jobe, M. Pink, V. Perry, and V. Tibone, 1992. EMG analysis of the scapular muscles during a shoulder rehabilitation program. *Am J Sports Med* 20:128–134.
90. Mountcastle, V. S. 1980. *Medical Physiology.* 14th ed. St. Louis: Mosby.
91. Nichols, T. R., and J. C. Houk. 1976. Improvement in linearity and regulation of stiffness that results from actions of stretch reflex. *J Neurophysiol* 39:119–142.
92. Ochi M. J. Iwasa, Y. Uchio, N. Adachi, and Y. Sumen. 1999. The regeneration of sensory neurons in the reconstruction of the anterior cruciate ligament. *Journal of Bone and Joint Surgery—British* 81:902–906.
93. Palmitier, R. A., K. N. An, S. G. Scott, and E. Y. Chao. 1991. Kinetic chain exercise in knee rehabilitation. *Sports Med* 11:402–413.

94. Perlau, R., C. Frank, and G. Fick. 1995. The effect of elastic bandages on human knee proprioception in the uninjured population. *Am J Sports Med* 23:251–255.

95. Pope, M. H., R. J. Johnson, D. W. Brown, and C. Tighe. 1979. The role of the musculature in injuries to the medial collateral ligament. *J Bone Joint Surg Am* 61:398–402.

96. Potzl W., L. Thorwesten, C. Gotze, S. Garmann, and D. Steinbeck. 2004. Proprioception of the shoulder joint after surgical repair for instability: A long-term follow-up study. *Am J Sports Med* 32:425–430.

97. Pousson, M., J. Van Hoecke, and F. Goubel. 1990. Changes in elastic characteristics of human muscle induced by eccentric exercise. *J Biomech* 23:343–348.

98. Rack, P. M., and D. R. Westbury. 1974. The short range stiffness of active mammalian muscle and its effect on mechanical properties. *J Physiol* 240:331–350.

99. Schultz, R. A., D. C. Miller, C. S. Kerr, and L. Micheli. 1984. Mechanoreceptors in human cruciate ligaments. A histological study. *J Bone Joint Surg Am* 66:1072–1076.

100. Sherrington, C. S. 1911. *The integrative action of the nervous system.* New Haven: Yale University Press.

101. Sinkjaer, T., and L. Arendt-Nielsen. 1991. Knee stability and muscle coordination in patients with anterior cruciate ligament injuries: An electromyographic approach. *Journal of Electromyographic Kinesiology* 1:209–217.

102. Skinner, H. B., and R. L. Barrack. 1991. Joint position sense in the normal and pathologic knee joint. *Journal of Electromyographic Kinesiology* 1:180–190.

103. Skinner, H. B., R. L. Barrack, S. D. Cook, and R. J. Haddad Jr. 1984. Joint position sense in total knee arthroplasty. *J Orthop Res* 1:276–283.

104. Smith, R. L., and J. Brunolli. 1989. Shoulder kinesthesia after anterior glenohumeral joint dislocation. *Phys Ther* 69:106–112.

105. Solomonow, M., R. Baratta, B. H. Zhou, H. Shoji, W. Bose, C. Beck, and R. D'Ambrosia. 1987. The synergistic action of the anterior cruciate ligament and thigh muscles in maintaining joint stability. *Am J Sports Med* 15:207–13.

106. Swanik, C. B., S. M. Lephart, F. P. Giannantonio, and F. H. Fu. 1997. Reestablishing proprioception and neuromuscular control in the ACL-injured athlete. *Journal of Sports Rehabilitation* 6:182–206.

107. Swanik, C.B., S. M. Lephart, F. P. Giannantonio, and F. H. Fu. 1997. Reestablishing proprioception and neuromuscular control in the ACL-injured athlete. *Journal of Sports Rehabilitation* 6:182–206.

108. Swanik, C. B., S. M. Lephart, J. L. Giraldo, R.G. DeMont, and F. H. Fu. 1999. Reactive muscle firing of anterior cruciate ligament-injured females during functional activities. *Journal of Athletic Training.* 34:121–129.

109. Swanik, C. B., S. M. Lephart, K. A. Swanik, D. A. Stone, and F. H. Fu. 2004. Neuromuscular dynamic restraint in women with anterior cruciate ligament injuries. *Clin Orthop Relat Res* 425:189–99.

110. Swanik, C, Covassin, T, Stearne, D. 2007. The Relationship Between Neurocognitive Function and Noncontact Anterior Cruciate Ligament Injuries. American Journal of Sports Medicine 35(6):943–948.

111. Swanik, K. A., S. M. Lephart, C. B. Swanik, S. P. Lephart, D. A. Stone, and F. H. Fu. 2002. The effects of shoulder plyometric training on proprioception and selected muscle performance characteristics. *J Shoulder Elbow Surg* 11:579–86.

112. Tripp, B. L. 2008. Principles of restoring function and sensorimotor control in patients with shoulder dysfunction. *Clin Sports Med* 27:507–19, x.

113. Upton, A. R. M., and P. F. Radford. 1975. Motorneuron excitability in elite sprinters. In *Biomechanics,* Komi, P. V., ed. Baltimore: University Park, 82–87.

114. Walla, D. J., J. P. Albright, E. McAuley, R. K., Martin, V., Eldridge, and G. El-Khoury. 1985. Hamstring control and the unstable anterior cruciate ligament-deficient knee. *Am J Sports Med* 13:34–9.

115. Warner, J. J. P., S. M. Lephart, and F. H. Fu. 1996. Role of proprioception in pathoetiology of shoulder instability. *Clinical Orthopedics* 330:35–39.

116. Wilk, K. E., C. A. Arrigo, and J. R. Andrews. 1996. Closed and open chain exercises for the upper extremity. *Journal of Sport Rehabilitation* 156:88–102.

117. Wilk, K. E., R. F. Escamilla, G. S., Fleisig, S. W., Barrentine, J. R., Andrews, and M. L. Boyd. 1996. A comparison of tibiofemoral joint forces and electromyographic activity during open and closed kinetic chain exercises. *Am J Sports Med* 24:518–527.

118. Wilson, G. J., G. A. Wood and B. C., Elliott. 1991. Optimal stiffness of series elastic component in a stretch-shorten cycle activity. *J Appl Physiol* 70:825–33.

119. Wilson, G. J., G. A. Wood, and B. C. Elliott. 1991. The relationship between stiffness of the musculature and static flexibility: An alternative explanation for the occurrence of muscular injury. *Int J Sports Med* 12:403–7.

120. Wojtys, E. M., L. V. Huston, P. D. Taylor, and S. D. Bastian. 1996. Neuromuscular adaptations in isokinetic, isotonic, and agility training programs. *Am J Sports Med* 24:187–192.

121. Wojtys, E. M., and L. J. Huston. 1994. Neuromuscular performance in normal and anterior cruciate ligament-deficient lower extremities. *Am J Sports Med* 22:89–104.

122. Wolf, S. L., and R. L. Segal. 1990. Conditioning of the spinal stretch reflex: Implications for rehabilitation. *Phys Ther* 70:652–656.

123. Woo, E., Y. Burns, and L. Johnston. 2003. The effect of task uncertainty on muscle activation patterns in 8–10-year-old children. *Physiother Res Int* 8:143–54.

124. Yack, H. J., C. E. Collins, and T. J. Whieldon. 1993. Comparison of closed and open kinetic chain exercise in the anterior cruciate ligament-deficient knee. *Am J Sports Med* 21:49–54.

SOLUTIONS TO CLINICAL DECISION MAKING EXERCISES

6-1 In addition to strength restoration, rehabilitation should focus on reestablishing neurosensory properties of the injured ligament. Balance, perturbation, and agility exercises should be used to restore proprioception and kinesthesia elements, as well as to enhance reflexive pathways. Closed-kinetic-chain exercises increase joint congruency and neurosensory feedback necessary for reestablishing dynamic stability. Taping or bracing the ankle will provide stability during rehabilitation and practice but also will facilitate additional efferent feedback from cutaneous receptors.

6-2 Prevention programs should concentrate on preparatory and reactive muscle contractions to enhance motor coordination and muscle stiffness of the lower extremity. To achieve these goals, balance, agility, and sports-specific activities should be incorporated into prevention programs. Benefits of balance and agility training are enhanced proprioception, kinesthesia, and reactive muscle activation. Functional activities integrate these neuromuscular elements and should be performed in controlled, isolated movements and progressed to multidirectional complex activities (example: ball dribbling around cones to ball dribbling and cutting against a defender).

6-3 The athletic trainer should recognize that strength and voluntary muscle control of the vastus medialis oblique must be reestablished to achieve balanced coactivation between the vastus lateralis and vastus medialis oblique. Biofeedback training provides sensory feedback, as well as visual and/or auditory encouragement, for selective voluntary muscle control of the vastus medialis oblique.

6-4 Literature supports the use of plyometric training to increase strength and performance. Theories regarding neuromuscular benefits include restoration of functional motor programs, heightened reflexes, and increased proprioceptive awareness. Incorporation of plyometric exercises in the early stages of rehabilitation when the patient is not bearing weight should use elastic tubing for resistance in sitting, supine, and prone positions. As the patient is able to bear more weight, exercises should be progressed from two-legged to one-legged exercises. The range of exercises should be taken into consideration and gradually increased according to the patient's strength and level of pain. Activities that can be easily modified in this manner include forward-to-backward and lateral hopping and jumping maneuvers. Exercises should not be performed at too great a speed—faster movements can harm the healing tissues.

6-5 The rotator cuff muscles are not functioning properly to fulfill their stabilizing role at the glenohumeral joint. Rotator cuff strength should be assessed and imbalances remedied through strengthening and closed-kinetic-chain exercise. Benefits of closed-kinetic-chain exercises are increased joint congruency and enhanced force-couple coactivation. Strength-shortening, or plyometric, exercises promote preparatory and reactive muscle activity, encourage muscle coactivation, and improve proprioception. The importance of proper technique in rehabilitation exercises and sport movements must be addressed. Verbal feedback from the athletic trainer and visual feedback using a mirror can be used to develop proper motor patterns. In this stage of rehabilitation, a coach's critique and information obtained from motion analysis are advantageous and allow the athletic trainer to tailor the patient's protocol to specific needs.

6-6 Functional activities incorporate a variety of stimuli, so that the body must simultaneously integrate and efficiently use multiple elements of neuromuscular control to maintain function and stability. For the wrestler, factors that should be modified to progress from easy to difficult, as well as from isolated to combined, movements are (1) changing levels (e.g., high vs. low body position); (2) lateral movements (i.e., side shuffles); and (3) rational movements (e.g., carioca, pivot). Surface and axial load can be modified to progress the level of difficulty of exercises. A hard, flat surface can be changed to a softer, unstable surface (e.g., foam and mat). Weight vests or belts can be used to increase the axial load, thus enhancing stimulation of articular and tenomuscular receptors. It is also beneficial to receive feedback concerning technique and style from the coaching staff during this stage.

CHAPTER 7

Regaining Postural Stability and Balance

Kevin M. Guskiewicz

After completion of this chapter, the athletic training student should be able to do the following:

- Define and explain the roles of the three sensory modalities responsible for maintaining balance.

- Explain how movement strategies along the closed kinetic chain help maintain the center of gravity in a safe and stable area.

- Differentiate between subjective and objective balance assessment.

- Differentiate between static and dynamic balance assessment.

- Evaluate the effect that injury to the ankle, knee, and head has on balance and postural equilibrium.

- Identify the goals of each phase of balance training, and how to progress the patient through each phase.

- State the differences among static, semidynamic, and dynamic balance-training exercises.

Although maintaining balance while standing may appear to be a rather simple motor skill for able-bodied athletes, this feat cannot be taken for granted in a patient with musculoskeletal dysfunction. Muscular weakness, proprioceptive deficits, and range of motion (ROM) deficits may challenge a person's ability to maintain their center of gravity (COG) within the body's base of support, or in other words, cause them to lose their balance. Balance is the single most important element dictating movement strategies within the closed kinetic chain. Acquisition of effective strategies for maintaining balance is therefore essential for athletic performance. Although balance is often thought of as a static process, it's actually a highly integrative dynamic process involving multiple neurological pathways. While **balance** is the more commonly used term, **postural equilibrium** is a broader term which involves the alignment of joint segments in an effort to maintain the COG within an optimal range of the maximum limits of stability (LOS).

Despite often being classified at the end of the continuum of goals associated with therapeutic exercise,[45] maintenance of balance is a vital component in the rehabilitation of joint injuries which should not be overlooked. Traditionally, orthopedic rehabilitation has placed the emphasis on isolated joint mechanics such as improving ROM and flexibility, and increasing muscle strength and endurance, rather than on afferent information obtained by the joint(s) to be processed by the postural control system. However, research in the area of proprioception and kinesthesia has emphasized the need to train the joint's neural system.[46-50] Joint position sense, proprioception, and kinesthesia are vital to all athletic performance requiring balance. Current rehabilitation protocols should therefore focus on a combination of open- and closed-kinetic-chain exercises. The necessity for a combination of open- and closed-kinetic-chain exercises can be seen during gait (walking or running), as the foot and ankle prepare for heel strike (open chain) and prepare to control the body's COG during mid-stance and toe off (closed chain). This chapter focuses on the postural control system, various balance training techniques, and technological advancements that are enabling sports medicine athletic trainers to assess and treat balance deficits in physically active people.

POSTURAL CONTROL SYSTEM

The athletic trainer must first have an understanding of the postural control system and its various components. The postural control system utilizes complex processes involving both sensory and motor components. Maintenance of postural equilibrium includes sensory detection of body motions, integration of sensorimotor information within the central nervous system (CNS), and execution of appropriate musculoskeletal responses. Most daily activities such as walking, climbing stairs, reaching, or throwing a ball, require static foot placement with controlled balance shifts, especially if a favorable outcome is to be attained. So, balance should be considered both a dynamic and static process. The successful accomplishment of static and dynamic balance is based on the interaction between body and environment.[44] The complexity of this dynamic process can be seen in Figure 7-1. From a clinical perspective, separating the sensory and motor processes of balance means that a person may have impaired balance for one or a combination of two reasons: (1) the position of the center of gravity (COG) relative to the base of support is not accurately sensed; and (2) the automatic movements required to bring the COG to a balanced position are not timely or effectively coordinated.[60]

The position of the body in relation to gravity and its surroundings is sensed by combining visual, vestibular, and somatosensory inputs. Balance movements also involve motions of the ankle, knee, and hip joints, which are controlled by the coordinated actions along the kinetic chain (Figure 7-2). These processes are all vital for producing fluid sport-related movements.

CONTROL OF BALANCE

The human body is a very tall structure balanced on a relatively small base, and its COG is quite high, being just above the pelvis.[78] Many factors enter into the task of controlling balance within the base of support. Balance control involves a complex network of neural connections and centers that are related by peripheral and central feedback mechanisms.[34]

The postural control system operates as a feedback control circuit between the brain and the musculoskeletal system. The sources of afferent information supplied to the postural control system collectively come from visual, vestibular, and somatosensory inputs. The central nervous system's (CNS) involvement in maintaining upright posture can be divided into two components. The first component, **sensory organization,** involves those processes that determine the timing, direction, and amplitude of corrective postural actions based upon information obtained from the vestibular, visual, and somatosensory (proprioceptive) inputs.[56] Despite the availability of multiple sensory inputs, the central nervous system generally relies on only one sense at a time for orientation information. For healthy adults, the preferred sense for balance

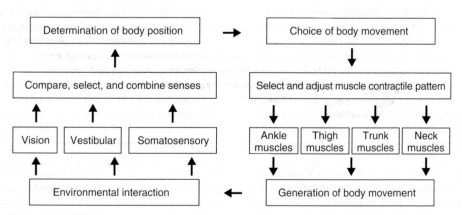

Figure 7-1   Dynamic equilibrium.
Source: Adapted from Allison. L., K. Fuller, R. Hedenberg, et al. 1994. *Contemporary Management of Balance Deficits.* Clackamas, OR: NeuroCom International, with permission.

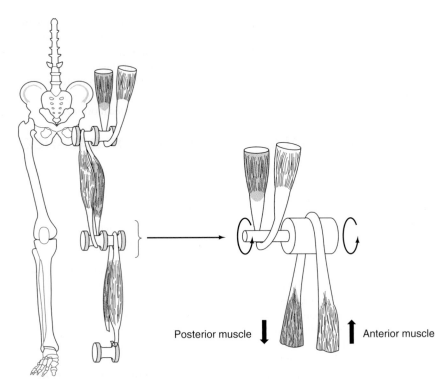

Posterior muscle ↓   ↑ Anterior muscle

Figure 7-2 Paired relationships between major postural musculatures that execute coordinated actions along the kinetic chain to control the center of gravity.

control comes from somatosensory information (i.e., feet in contact with the support surface and detection of joint movement).[37,56] In considering orthopedic injuries, the somatosensory system is of most importance and will be the focus of this chapter.

The second component, **muscle coordination**, is the collection of processes that determine the temporal sequencing and distribution of contractile activity among the muscles of the legs and trunk which generate supportive reactions for maintaining balance. Research suggests that balance deficiencies in people with neurologic problems can result from inappropriate interaction among the three sensory inputs that provide orientation information to the postural control system. A patient may be inappropriately dependent on one sense for situations presenting inter-sensory conflict.[56,70]

From a clinical perspective, stabilization of upright posture requires the integration of afferent information from the three senses, which work in combination and are all critical to the execution of coordinated postural corrections. Impairment of one component is usually compensated for by the remaining two. Often, one of the systems provides

faulty or inadequate information such as different surfaces and/or changes in visual acuity and/or peripheral vision. In this case it is crucial that one of the other senses provides accurate and adequate information so that balance may be maintained. For example, when somatosensory conflict is present such as a moving platform or a compliant foam surface, balance is significantly decreased with the eyes closed as compared to eyes open.

Somatosensory inputs provide information concerning the orientation of body parts to one another and to the support surface.[21,60] **Vision** measures the orientation of the eyes and head in relation to surrounding objects, and plays an important role in the maintenance of balance. On a stable surface, closing the eyes should cause only minimal increases in postural sway in healthy subjects. However, if somatosensory input is disrupted due to ligamentous injury, closing the eyes will increase sway significantly.[12,16,37,38,60] The **vestibular** apparatus supplies information that measures gravitational, linear, and angular accelerations of the head in relation to inertial space. It does not, however, provide orientation information in relation to external objects, and therefore plays only a minor role in the maintenance of balance when the visual and somatosensory systems are providing accurate information.[60]

SOMATOSENSATION AS IT RELATES TO BALANCE

The terms somatosensation, proprioception, kinesthesia, and balance are often used to describe similar phenomena. Somatosensation is a more global term used to describe the proprioceptive mechanisms related to postural control and can accurately be used synonomously. Somatosensation is therefore best defined as a specialized variation of the sensory modality of touch that encompasses the sensation of joint movement (kinesthesia) and joint position (joint position sense).[46,50] As previously discussed, balance refers to the ability to maintain the body's COG within the base of support provided by the feet. Somatosensation and balance work closely, as the postural control system utilizes sensory information related to movement and posture from peripheral sensory receptors (e.g., muscle spindles, GTO, joint afferents, cutaneous receptors). So the question remains, how does proprioception influence postural equilibrium and balance?

Somatosensory input is received from mechanoreceptors, however it is unclear as to whether the tactile senses, muscle spindles, or GTOs are most responsible for controlling balance. Nashner[55] concluded after using electromyography (EMG) responses following platform perturbations, that other pathways had to be involved in the responses they recorded because the latencies were longer than those normally associated with a classic myotatic reflex. The stretch-related reflex is the earliest mechanism for increasing the activation level of muscles about a joint following an externally imposed rotation of the joint. Rotation of the ankles is the most probable stimulus of the myotatic reflex that occurs in many persons. It appears to be the first useful phase of activity in the leg muscles after a change in erect posture.[55] The myotatic reflex can be seen when perturbations of gait or posture automatically evoke functionally directed responses in the leg muscles to compensate for imbalance or increased postural sway.[14,55] Muscle spindles sense a stretching of the agonist, thus sending information along its afferent fibers to the spinal cord. There the information is transferred to alpha and gamma motor neurons that carry information back to the muscle fibers and muscle spindle, respectively, and contract the muscle to prevent or control additional postural sway.[14]

Postural sway was assessed on a platform moving into a "toes-up" and "toes down" position, and a stretch reflex was found in the triceps surae after a sudden ramp displacement into the "toes up" position.[13] A medium latency response (103–118 ms) was observed in the stretched muscle, followed by a delayed response of the antagonistic anterior tibialis muscle (108–124 ms). The investigators also blocked afferent proprioceptive information in an attempt to study the role of proprioceptive information from the legs for the maintenance of upright posture. These results suggested that proprioceptive information from pressure and/or joint receptors of the foot (ischemia applied at ankle) plays an important role in postural stabilization during low frequencies of movement, but is of minor importance for the compensation of rapid displacements. The experiment also included a "visual" component, as subjects were tested with eyes closed, followed by eyes open. Results suggested that when subjects were tested with eyes open, visual information compensated for the loss of proprioceptive input.

Another study[14] used compensatory EMG responses during impulsive disturbance of the limbs during stance on a treadmill to describe the myotatic reflex. Results revealed that during backward movement of the treadmill, ankle dorsiflexion caused the COG to be shifted anteriorly, thus evoking a stretch reflex in the gastrocnemius muscle, followed by weak anterior tibialis activation. In another trial, the movement was reversed (plantar flexion), thus shifting the COG posteriorly and evoking a stretch reflex of the anterior tibialis muscle. Both of these studies suggest that stretch reflex responses help to control the body's COG, and that the vestibular system is unlikely to be directly involved in the generation of the necessary responses.

Elimination of all sensory information from the feet and ankles revealed that proprioceptors in the leg muscles (gastrocnemius and tibialis anterior) were capable of providing sufficient sensory information for stable standing.[20] Researchers speculated that group I or group II muscle spindle afferents, and group Ib afferents from GTOs were the probable sources of this proprioceptive information. The study demonstrated that normal subjects can stand in a stable manner when receptors in the leg muscles are the only source of information about postural sway.

Other studies[5,38] have examined the role of somatosensory information by altering or limiting somatosensory input through the use of platform sway referencing or foam platforms. These studies reported that subjects still responded with well-coordinated movements but the movements were often either ineffective or inefficient for the environmental context in which they were used.

BALANCE AS IT RELATES TO THE CLOSED KINETIC CHAIN

Balance is the process of maintaining the center of gravity (COG) within the body's base of support. Again, the human body is a very tall structure balanced on a relatively small base, and its center of gravity is quite high, being just above the pelvis.[78] Many factors enter into the task of controlling balance within this designated area. One component often overlooked is the role balance plays within the **kinetic chain.** Ongoing debates as to how the kinetic chain should be defined and whether open- or closed-kinetic-chain exercises are best has caused many athletic trainers to lose sight of what is most important. An understanding of the postural control system as well as the theory of the kinetic (segmental) chain about the lower extremity helps conceptualize the role of the chain in maintaining balance. Within the kinetic chain, each moving segment transmits forces to every other segment along the chain, and its motions are influenced by forces transmitted from other segments[10] (see Chapter 12). The act of maintaining equilibrium or balance is associated with the closed kinetic chain, as the distal segment (foot) is fixed beneath the base of support.

The coordination of automatic postural movements during the act of balancing is not determined solely by the muscles acting directly about the joint. Leg and trunk muscles exert indirect forces on neighboring joints through the inertial interaction forces among body segments.[57,58] A combination of one or more strategies (ankle, knee, hip) are used to coordinate movement of the COG back to a stable or balanced position when a person's balance is disrupted by an external perturbation. Injury to any one of the joints or corresponding muscles along the kinetic chain can result in a loss of appropriate feedback for maintaining balance.

BALANCE DISRUPTION

Let's say for example, that a basketball player goes up for a rebound and collides with another player, causing her to land in an unexpected position, therefore compromising her normal balance. In order to prevent a fall from occurring, the body must correct itself by returning the COG to a position within a safer limit of stability (LOS). Afferent mechanoreceptor input from the hip, knee, and ankle joints are responsible for initiating automatic postural responses through the use of one of three possible movement strategies.

Selection of Movement Strategies

Three principle joint systems (ankles, knees, and hips) are located between the base of support and the COG. This allows for a wide variety of postures that can be assumed, while the COG is still positioned above the base of support. As described by Nashner,[60] motions about a given joint are controlled by the combined actions of at least one pair of muscles working in opposition. When forces exerted by pairs of opposing muscle about a joint (e.g., anterior tibialis and gastrocnemius/soleus) are combined, the effect is to resist rotation of the joint relative to a resting position. The degree to which the joint resists rotation is called joint stiffness. The resting position and the stiffness of the joint are each altered independently by changing the activation levels of one or both muscle groups.[39,60] Joint resting position and joint stiffness are by themselves an inadequate basis for controlling postural movements, and it is theorized that the myotatic stretch reflex is the earliest mechanism for increasing the activation level of the muscles of a joint following an externally imposed rotation of the joint.[60]

When a person's balance is disrupted by an external perturbation, movement strategies involving joints of the lower extremity coordinate movement of the COG back to a balanced position. Three strategies (ankle, hip, stepping) have been identified along a continuum.[37] In general, the relative effectiveness of ankle, hip, and stepping strategies in repositioning the COG over the base of support depends on the configuration of the base of support, the COG alignment in relation to the LOS, and the speed of the postural movement.[37,38]

The **ankle strategy** shifts the COG while maintaining the placement of the feet by rotating the body as a rigid mass about the ankle joints. This is achieved by contracting either the gastrocnemius or anterior tibialis muscles to generate torque about the ankle joints. Anterior sway of the body is counteracted by gastrocnemius activity, which pulls the body posteriorly. Conversely, posterior sway of the body is counteracted by contraction of the tibialis anterior. Thus, the importance of these muscles should not be underestimated when designing the rehabilitation program. The ankle strategy is most effective in executing relatively slow COG movements when the base of support is firm and the COG is well within the LOS perimeter. The ankle strategy is also believed to be effective in maintaining a static posture with the COG offset from the center. The thigh and lower trunk muscles contract and thereby resist the destabilization of these proximal joints due to the indirect effects of the ankle muscles on the proximal joints (Table 7-1).

Under normal sensory conditions, activation of ankle musculature is almost exclusively selected to maintain equilibrium. However, there are subtle differences associated with loss of somatosensation and with vestibular dysfunction in terms of postural control strategies. Persons with somatosensory loss appear to rely on their hip musculature

■ **TABLE   7-1**   Function Anatomy of Muscles Involved in Balance Movements

Joint	Extension		Flexion	
	Anatomic	**Function**	**Anatomic**	**Function**
Hip	Paraspinals Hamstrings	Paraspinals Hamstrings Tibialis	Abdominal Quadriceps	Abdominals Quadriceps Gastrocnemius
Knee	Quadriceps	Paraspinals Quadriceps Gastrocnemius	Hamstrings Gastrocnemius	Abdominals Hamstrings Tibialis
Ankle	Gastrocnemius	Abdominals Quadriceps Gastrocnemius	Tibialis	Paraspinals Hamstrings Tibialis

Adapted from Nashner, L.M. 1993. Physiology of Balance. In *Handbook of Balance Function and Testing.* Jacobson, G., C. Newman, and J. Kartush, eds. St. Louis, MO: Mosby, 261–279.

to retain their COG while experiencing forward or backward perturbation or with different support surface lengths.[21]

If the ankle strategy is not capable of controlling excessive sway, the **hip strategy** is available to help control motion of the COG through the initiation of large and rapid motions at the hip joints with antiphase rotation of the ankles. It is most effective when the COG is located near the LOS perimeter, and when the LOS boundaries are contracted by a narrowed base of support. Finally, when the COG is displaced beyond the LOS, a step or stumble (stepping strategy) is the only strategy which can be used to prevent a fall.[58,60]

It is proposed that LOS and COG alignment are altered in individuals exhibiting a musculoskeletal abnormality such as an ankle or knee sprain. For example, weakness of ligaments following acute or chronic sprain about these joints is likely to reduce range of motion therefore shrinking LOS and placing the person at greater risk for a fall with a relatively smaller sway envelope.[58] Pintsaar et al.[67] revealed that impaired function was related to a change from ankle synergy toward hip synergy for postural adjustments among patients with functional ankle instability. This finding, which was consistent with previous results reported by Tropp et al.,[76] suggests that sensory proprioceptive function for the injured patients was affected.

ASSESSMENT OF BALANCE

Several methods of balance assessment have been proposed for clinical use. Many of the techniques have been criticized for offering only subjective ("qualitative")

information measurement of balance rather than an objective ("quantitative") measure.

Subjective Assessment

Prior to the mid 1980s, there were very few methods for systematic and controlled assessment of balance. The assessment of static balance in athletes has traditionally been performed through the use of the standing Romberg Test. This test is performed standing with feet together, arms at the side, and eyes closed. Normally a person can stand motionless in this position, but the tendency to sway or fall to one side is considered a positive Romberg's sign indicating a loss of proprioception.[8] The Romberg Test has, however, been criticized for its lack of sensitivity and objectivity. It is considered to be a rather qualitative assessment of static balance because a considerable amount of stress is required to make the subject sway enough for an observer to characterize the sway.[42]

The use of a quantifiable clinical test battery called the **Balance Error Scoring System (BESS)** is recommended over the standard Romberg test. Three different stances (double, single, and tandem) are completed twice, once while on a firm surface and once while on a piece of medium density foam (balance pad by Airex is recommended) for a total of six trials (Figure 7-3). Patients are asked to assume the required stance by placing their hands on the iliac crests and upon eye closure, the 20-second test begins. During the single leg stances, subjects are asked to maintain the contralateral limb in 20–30 degrees of hip flexion and 40–50 degrees of knee flexion. Additionally,

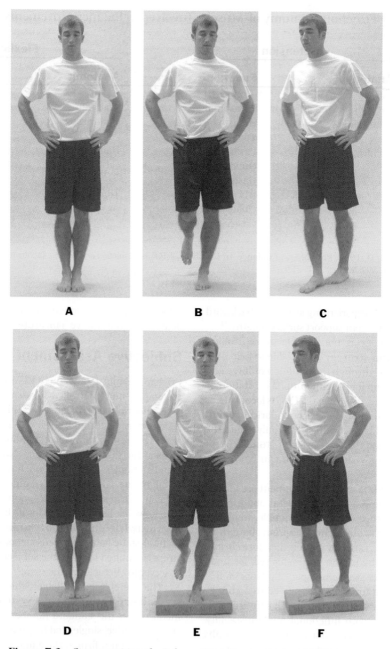

Figure 7-3 Stance positions for Balance Error Scoring System (BESS).
A, Double-leg, firm surface, **B,** Single-leg, firm surface, **C,** Tandem, firm surface,
D, Double-leg, foam surface, **E,** Single-leg, foam surface, **F,** Tandem, foam surface.

the patient is asked to stand quietly and as motionless as possible in the stance position keeping, their hands on the iliac crests and eyes closed. The single-limb stance tests are performed on the non-dominant foot. This same foot is placed toward the rear on the tandem stances. Subjects are told that upon losing their balance, they are to make any necessary adjustments and return to the testing position as quickly as possible. Performance is scored by adding one error point for each error listed in Table 7-2. Trials are considered to be incomplete if the patient is unable to sustain the stance position for longer than 5 seconds during the entire 20-second testing period. These trials are assigned a standard maximum error score of 10. Balance test results during injury recovery are best utilized when compared to baseline measurements, and clinicians working with athletes or patients on a regular basis should attempt to obtain baseline measurements when possible.

Semidynamic and dynamic balance assessment can be performed through functional-reach tests, timed agility tests such as the figure eight test,[15,19,80] carioca, or hop

test,[40,80] Bass Test for Dynamic Balance,[77] timed "T-Band kicks," and timed balance beam walking with the eyes open or closed. The objective in most of these tests is to decrease the size of the base of support, in an attempt to determine a patient's ability to control upright posture while moving. Many of these tests have been criticized for failing to quantify balance adequately, as they merely report the time that a particular posture is maintained, angular displacement, or the distance covered after walking.[6,21,46,60] At any rate, they can often provide the athletic trainer with valuable information about a patient's function and/or return to play capability.

Objective Assessment

Advancements in technology have provided the medical community with commercially available balance systems (Table 7-3) for quantitatively assessing and training static and dynamic balance. These systems provide an easy, practical, and cost-effective method of quantitatively assessing and training functional balance through analysis of postural stability. Thus, the potential exists to assess injured patients and (1) identify possible abnormalities that might be associated with injury; (2) isolate various systems that are affected; (3) develop recovery curves based on quantitative measures for determining readiness to return to activity; and (4) train the injured patient.

Most manufacturers use computer-interfaced forceplate technology consisting of a flat, rigid surface supported on three or more points by independent force-measuring devices. As the patient stands on the forceplate surface, the position of the center of vertical forces exerted on the

■ **TABLE   7-2**   Balance Error Scoring System

Errors

Hands lifted off iliac crests

Opening eyes

Step, stumble, or fall

Moving hip into more than 30 degrees of flexion or abduction

Lifting forefoot or heel

Remaining out of testing position for more than 5 seconds

The BESS score is calculated by adding one error point for each error or any combination of errors occurring during one movement. Error scores from each of the six trials are added for a total BESS score, and higher scores represent poor balance.

■ **TABLE   7-3**   High-Technology Balance Assessment Systems

Static Systems	Dynamic Systems
Chattecx Balance System	Biodex Stability System
EquiTest	Chattecx Balance System
Forceplate	EquiTest
Pro Balance Master	EquiTest with EMG
Smart Balance Master	Forceplate
	Kinesthetic Ability Trainer
	Pro Balance Master
	Smart Balance Master

forceplate over time is calculated (Figure 7-4). The center of vertical force movements provide an indirect measure of postural sway activity.[59] The Kistler and, more recently, Bertec force plates, are used for much of the work in the area of postural stability and balance.[6,17,27,52,54] Manufacturers such as Chattecx Corporation (Hixson, TN) and NeuroCom International, Inc. (Clackamas, OR) have also developed systems with expanded diagnostic and training capabilities that make interpretation of results easier for athletic trainers. Athletic trainers must be aware that the manufacturers often use conflicting terminology to describe various balance parameters, and should consult frequently with the manufacturer to ensure that there is a clear understanding of the measure being taken. These inconsistencies have created confusion in the literature, because what some manufacturers classify as *dynamic balance*, others claim is really *static balance*. Our classification system (see Balance Training section) will hopefully clear up some of the confusion and allow for a more consistent labeling of the numerous balance-related exercises.

Force platforms ideally evaluate four aspects of postural control: steadiness, symmetry, and dynamic stability.

Steadiness is the ability to keep the body as motionless as possible. This is a measure of postural sway. **Symmetry** is the ability to distribute weight evenly between the two feet in an upright stance. This is a measure of center of pressure (COP), center of balance (COB), or center of force (COF), depending which testing system you are using. Although inconsistent with our classification system, **dynamic stability** is often labeled as the ability to transfer the vertical projection of the COG around a stationary supporting base.[27] This is often referred to as a measure of one's perception of their "safe" limits of stability, as their goal is to lean or reach as far as possible without losing one's balance. Some manufacturers measure dynamic stability by assessing a person's postural response to external perturbations from a moving platform in one of four directions: tilting toes up, tilting toes down, shifting medial-lateral (M-L), and shifting anterior-posterior (A-P). Platform perturbation on some systems is unpredictable and determined by the positioning and sway movement of the subject. In such cases, a person's reaction response can be determined (Figure 7-5). Other systems have a more predictable sinusoidal waveform

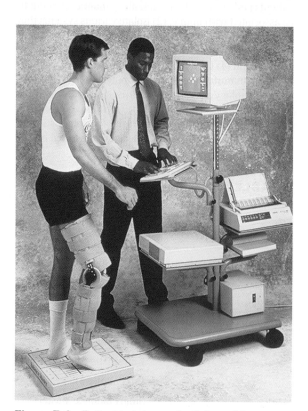

Figure 7-4 Patient training on the Balance Master.

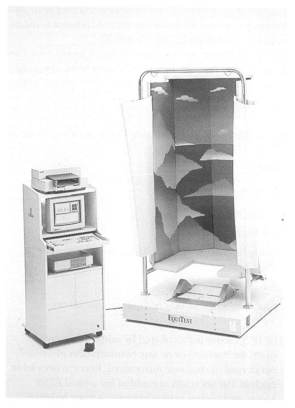

Figure 7-5 EquiTest.

that remains constant regardless of subject positioning (Figure 7-6).

Many of these force platform systems measure the vertical ground reaction force and provide a means of computing the center of pressure (COP). The COP represents the center of the distribution of the total force applied to the supporting surface. The COP is calculated from horizontal moment and vertical force data generated by triaxial force platforms. Center of balance (COB), in the case of the Chattecx Balance System, is the point between the feet where the ball and heel of each foot has 25 percent of the body weight. This point is referred to as the relative weight positioning over the four load cells as measured only by vertical forces. The center of vertical force (COF), on NeuroCom's EquiTest, is the center of the vertical force exerted by the feet against the support surface. In any case (COP, COB, COF), the total force applied to the force platform fluctuates because it includes both body weight and the inertial effects of the slightest movement of the body which occurs even when one attempts to stand motionless. The movement of these force-based

reference points are theorized to vary according to the movement of the body's COG and the distribution of muscle forces required to control posture. Ideally, healthy athletes should maintain their COP very near the A-P and M-L midlines.

Once the COP, COB, or COF is calculated, several other balance parameters can be attained. Deviation from this point in any direction represents a person's postural sway. Postural sway can be measured in various ways, depending on which system is being used. Mean displacement, length of sway path, length of sway area, amplitude, frequency, and direction with respect to the COP can be calculated on most systems. An equilibrium score, comparing the angular difference between the calculated maximum anterior to posterior COG displacements to a theoretical maximum displacement, is unique to NeuroCom International's EquiTest. Sway index (SI), representing the degree of scatter of data about the COB, is unique to the Chattecx Balance System.

Forceplate technology allows for quantitative analysis and understanding of a subject's postural instability. These systems are fully integrated with hardware/software systems for quickly and quantitatively assessing and rehabilitating balance disorders. Most manufacturers allow

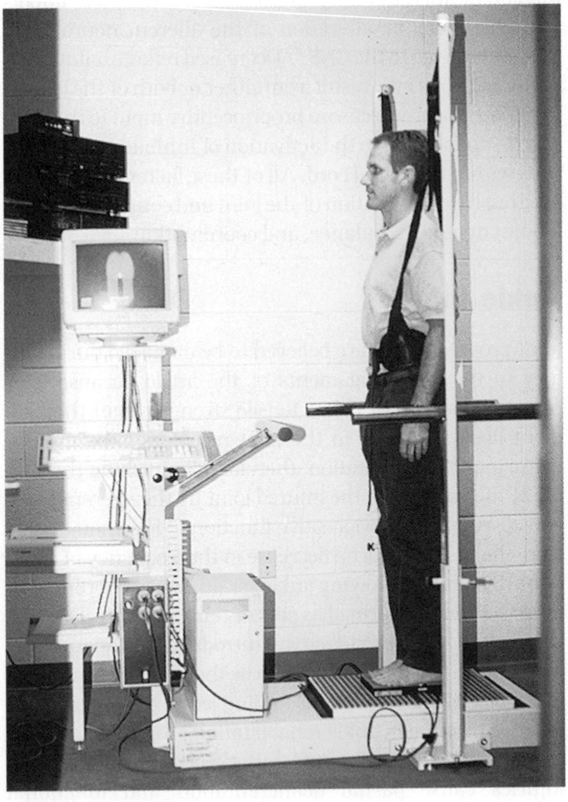

Figure 7-6   Chattecx Balance System.

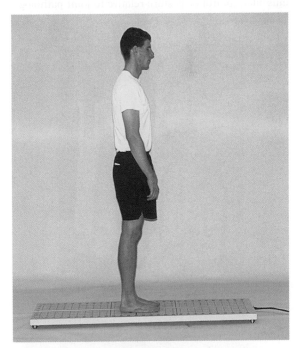

Figure 7-7   Balance Master with accessory 5-foot forceplate.

for both static and dynamic balance assessment in either double or single leg stances, with eyes open or eyes closed. NeuroCom's EquiTest System is equipped with a moving visual surround (wall) that allows for the most sophisticated technology available for isolating and assessing sensory modality interaction.

Long forceplates have been developed by some manufacturers in an attempt to combat criticism that balance assessment is not functional. Inclusion of the long forceplate (Figure 7-7) adds a vast array of dynamic balance exercises for training, such as walking, step-up-and-over, side and crossover steps, hopping, leaping, and lunging. These important return-to-sport activities can be practiced and perfected through the use of the computer's visual feedback.

Biodex Medical Systems (Shirley, NY) manufactures a dynamic multi-axial tilting platform which offers computer-generated data similar to that of a forceplate system. The Biodex Stability System (Figure 7-8) utilizes a dynamic multiaxial platform which allows up to 20 degrees of deflection in any direction. It is theorized that this degree of deflection is sufficient to stress joint mechanoreceptors that provide proprioceptive feedback (at end ranges of motion) necessary for balance control. Athletic trainers can therefore assess deficits in dynamic muscular control of posture relative to joint pathology.

The patient's ability to control the platform's angle of tilt is quantified as a variance from center, as well as degrees of deflection over time, at various stability levels. A large variance is indicative of poor muscle response. Exercises performed on a multiaxial unstable system such as the Biodex are similar to those of the Biomechanical Ankle Platform System (BAPS board) and are especially effective for regaining proprioception and balance following injury to the ankle joint.

INJURY AND BALANCE

It has long been theorized that failure of stretched or damaged ligaments to provide adequate neural feedback in an injured extremity may contribute to decreased proprioceptive mechanisms necessary for maintenance of proper balance. Research has revealed these impairments in individuals with ankle injury[23,31,69] and anterior cruciate ligament (ACL) injury.[4,65] The lack of proprioceptive feedback resulting from such injuries may allow excessive or inappropriate loading of a joint. Furthermore, although the presence of a capsular lesion may interfere with the transmission of afferent impulses from the joint, a more important effect may be alteration of the afferent neural code that is conveyed to the CNS.[82] Decreased reflex excitation of motor neurons may result from either or both of the following events: (a) a decrease in proprioceptive input to the CNS; and (b) an increase in the activation of inhibitory interneurons within the spinal cord. All of these factors may lead to progressive degeneration of the joint and continued deficits in joint dynamics, balance, and coordination.

Ankle Injuries

Joint proprioceptors are believed to be damaged during injury to the lateral ligaments of the ankle because joint receptor fibers possess less tensile strength than the ligament fibers. Damage to the joint receptors is believed to cause joint deafferentation, therefore diminishing the supply of messages from the injured joint up the afferent pathway disrupting proprioceptive function.[24] Freeman et al.[24] were the first to report a decrease in the frequency of functional instability following ankle sprains when coordination exercises were performed as part of rehabilitation. Thus the term *articular deafferentation* was introduced to designate the mechanism that they believed to be the cause of functional instability of the ankle. This finding led to the inclusion of balance training in ankle rehabilitation programs.

Since 1965, Freeman[23] has theorized that if ankle injuries cause partial deafferentation and functional instability, a person's postural sway would be altered

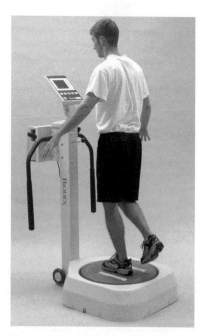

Figure 7-8 Biodex Stability System.

due to a proprioception deficit. While some studies[74,75] have not supported Freeman's theory, other more recent studies using high-tech equipment (forceplate, kinesthesiometer, etc.) have revealed balance deficits in ankles following acute sprains[25,31,66] and/or in ankles with chronic instabilities.[9,22,26,67]

Differences were identified between injured and uninjured ankles in 14 ankle-injured subjects using a computerized strain gauge forceplate.[25] Four of five possible postural sway parameters (standard deviation of the mean center of pressure dispersion, mean sway amplitude, average speed, and number of sway amplitudes exceeding 5 and 10 mm) taken in the frontal plane from a single-leg stance position were reported to discriminate between injured and non-injured ankles. The authors reported that the application of an ankle brace eliminated the differences between injury status when tested on each parameter, therefore improving balance performance. More importantly this study suggests that the stabilometry technique of selectively analyzing postural sway movements in the frontal plane, where the diameter of the supporting area is smallest, leads to higher sensitivity. Because difficulties of maintaining balance after a ligament lesion involves the subtalar axis, it is proposed that increased sway movements of the different body segments would be found primarily in the frontal plane. The authors speculated that this could explain non-significant findings of earlier stabilometry studies[74,75] involving injured ankles.

Orthotic intervention and postural sway was studied in 13 subjects with acute inversion ankle sprains and 12 uninjured subjects under two treatment conditions (orthotic, non-orthotic) and four platform movements (stable, inversion/eversion, plantar flexion/dorsiflexion, medial/lateral perturbations).[31] Results revealed that ankle-injured subjects swayed more than uninjured subjects when assessed in a single-leg test. The analysis also revealed that custom-fit orthotics may restrict undesirable motion at the foot and ankle, and enhance joint mechanoreceptors to detect perturbations and provide structural support for detecting and controlling postural sway in ankle-injured subjects. A similar study[66] reported improvements in static balance for injured subjects while wearing custom-made orthotics.

Studies involving subjects with chronic ankle instabilities[9,22,26,67] indicate that individuals with a history of inversion ankle sprain are less stable in single-limb stance on the involved leg as compared to the uninvolved leg and/or non-injured subjects. Significant differences between injured and uninjured subjects for sway amplitude but not sway frequency using a standard forceplate were revealed.[9] The effect of stance perturbation on frontal plane postural control was tested in three groups of subjects: (1) control (no previous ankle injury); (2) functional ankle instability and 8 week training program; and (3) mechanical instability without functional instability (without shoe, with shoe, with brace and shoe).[67] The authors reported a relative change from ankle to hip synergy at medially directed translations of the support surface on the Neuro-Com EquiTest. The impairment was restored after 8 weeks of ankle disk training. The effect of a shoe and brace did not exceed the effect of the shoe alone. Impaired ankle function was shown to be related to coordination, as subjects changed from ankle toward hip strategies for postural adjustments.

Similarly, researchers[36] reported that lateral ankle joint anesthesia did not alter postural sway or passive joint position sense, but did affect the center of balance position (similar to center of pressure) during both static and dynamic testing. This suggests the presence of an adaptive mechanism to compensate for the loss of afferent stimuli from the region of the lateral ankle ligaments.[36] Subjects tended to shift their center of balance medially during dynamic balance testing and slightly laterally during static balance testing. The authors speculated that center of balance shifting may provide additional proprioceptive input from cutaneous receptors in the sole of the foot or stretch receptors in the peroneal muscle tendon unit, which therefore prevents increased postural sway.

Increased postural sway frequency and latencies are parameters thought to be indicative of impaired ankle joint proprioception.[13,69] Cornwall et al.[9] and Pintsaar et al.,[67] however, found no differences between chronically injured subjects and control subjects on these measures. This raises the question as to whether postural sway was in fact caused by a proprioceptive deficit. Increased postural sway amplitudes in the absence of sway frequencies might suggest that chronically injured subjects recover their ankle joint proprioception over time. Thus, more research is warranted for investigating loss of joint proprioception and postural sway frequency.[9]

In summary, results of studies involving both chronic and acute ankle sprains suggest that increased postural sway and/or balance instability may not be due to a single factor but to disruption of both neurological and biomechanical factors at the ankle joint. Loss of balance may result from abnormal or altered biomechanical alignment of the body, thus affecting the transmission of somatosensory information from the ankle joint. It is possible that observed postural sway amplitudes following injury are a result of joint instability along the kinetic chain, rather than deafferentation. Thus, the orthotic intervention[31,61,62] may have provided more optimal joint alignment.

Knee Injuries

Ligamentous injury to the knee has proven to affect the ability of subjects to accurately detect position.[2,3,4,46,49,50] The general consensus among numerous investigators performing proprioceptive testing is that a clinical proprioception deficit occurs in most patients after an ACL rupture who have functional instability and that this deficit seems to persist to some degree after an ACL reconstruction.[2] Because of the relationships between proprioception (somatosensation) and balance, it has been suggested that the patient's ability to balance on the ACL-injured leg may also be decreased.[4,65]

Studies have evaluated the effects of ACL ruptures on standing balance using forceplate technology, and while some studies have revealed balance deficits,[25,53] others have not.[18,35] Thus, there appear to be conflicting results from these studies depending on which parameters are measured. Mizuta et al.[53] found significant differences in postural sway when measuring center of pressure and sway distance area between 11 functionally stable and 15 functionally unstable subjects who had unilateral ACL-deficient knees. Faculjak et al.[18] however, found no differences in postural stability between 8 ACL-deficient subjects and 10 normal subjects when measuring average latency and response strength on an EquiTest System.

Several potential reasons for this discrepancy exist. First, it has been suggested that there might be a link between static balance and isometric strength of the musculature at the ankle and knee. Isometric muscle strength could therefore compensate for any somatosensory deficit present in the involved knee during a closed-chain static balance test. Second, many studies fail to discriminate between *functionally unstable* ACL-deficient knees and knees which were not *functionally unstable*. This presents a design flaw, especially considering that functionally stable knees would most likely provide adequate balance despite ligamentous pathology. Another suggested reason for not seeing differences between injured knees and uninjured knees on static balance measures could be explained by the role that joint mechanoreceptors play. Neurophysiological studies[28,29,43,46] have revealed that joint mechanoreceptors provide enhanced

---

CLINICAL DECISION MAKING   **Exercise 7–2**

A gymnast recovering from a grade 1 MCL sprain to her right knee is ready to begin her rehabilitation. What factors must first be considered prior to designing her balance exercise program and progression?

---

kinesthetic awareness in the near-terminal range of motion or extremes of motion. Therefore, it could be speculated that if the maximum LOS are never reached during a static balance test, damaged mechanoreceptors (muscle or joint) may not even become a factor. Dynamic balance tests or functional hop tests that involve dynamic balance could challenge the postural control system (ankle strategies are taken over by hip and/or stepping strategies), requiring more mechanoreceptor input. These tests would most likely discriminate between functionally unstable ACL-deficient knees and normal knees.

Head Injury

Neurological status following mild head injury has been assessed using balance as a criterion variable. Athletic trainers and team physicians have long evaluated head injuries with the Romberg tests of sensory modality function to test "balance." This is an easy and effective sideline test; however, the literature suggests there is more to posture control than just balance and sensory modality,[55,56,61,64,72] especially when assessing people with head injury.[30,33] The postural control system, which is responsible for linking brain to body communication, is often affected as a result of mild head injury. Several studies have now identified postural stability deficits in patients up to three days post-injury using commercially available balance systems.[30,33] It appears this deficit is related to a sensory interaction problem, whereby the injured patient fails to use their visual system effectively. This research suggests that objective balance assessment can be used for establishing recovery curves for making return to play decisions in concussed patients. Rehabilitation of concussed patients using balance techniques has yet to be studied.

BALANCE TRAINING

Developing a rehabilitation program that includes exercises for improving balance and postural equilibrium is vital for a successful return to competition from a lower extremity injury. Regardless of whether the patient has sustained a quadriceps strain or an ankle sprain, the injury has caused a disruption at some point between the body's COG and base of support. This is likely to have caused compensatory weight shifts and gait changes along the kinetic chain that have resulted in balance deficits. These deficits may be detected through the use of functional assessment tests and/or computerized instrumentation previously discussed for assessing balance. Having the advanced technology available to quantify balance deficits is an amenity, but not a necessity. Imagination and creativity are often the best tools available to athletic trainers with limited resources who are trying to design balance training protocols.

Because virtually all sport activities involve closed-chain lower extremity function, functional rehabilitation should be performed in the closed kinetic chain. However, ROM, movement speed, and additional resistance may be more easily controlled in the open chain initially. Therefore, adequate, safe function in an open chain may be the first step in the rehabilitation process, but should not be the focus of the rehabilitation plan. The athletic trainer should attempt to progress the patient to functional closed-chain exercises quickly and safely. Depending on severity of injury, this could be as early as one day post-injury.

As previously mentioned, there is a close relationship between somtosensation, kinesthesia, and balance. Therefore, many of the exercises proposed for kinesthetic training are indirectly enhancing balance. Several methods of regaining balance have been proposed in the literature and are included in the most current rehabilitation protocols for ankle[41,73,82] and knee injury.[11,40,51,72,81]

A variety of activities can be used to improve balance, but the athletic trainer should first consider five general rules before beginning:

- The exercises must be safe, yet challenging.
- Stress multiple planes of motion.
- Incorporate a multisensory approach.
- Begin with static, bilateral, and stable surfaces and progress to dynamic, unilateral, and unstable surfaces.
- Progress toward sport-specific exercises.

There are several ways in which the athletic trainer can meet these goals. Balance exercises should be performed in an open area, where the patient will not be injured in the event of a fall. It is best to perform exercises with an assistive device within an arm's reach (e.g., chair, railing, table, wall), especially during the initial phase of rehabilitation. When considering exercise duration for balance exercises, the athletic trainer can use either sets and repetitions or a time-based protocol. The patient can perform 2–3 sets of 15 repetitions and progress to 30 repetitions as tolerated, or perform 10 of the exercises for a 15-second period and progress to 30-second periods later in the program.

CLINICAL DECISION MAKING   **Exercise 7–3**

How can the athletic trainer determine whether a patient is ready to progress to a more challenging balance task and/or balance surface?

Classification of Balance Exercises

Static balance is when the COG is maintained over a fixed base of support (unilateral or bilateral) while standing on a stable surface. Examples of static exercises are a single-leg, double-leg, or tandem-stance Romberg task. *Semidynamic* balance involves one of two possible activities: (1) The person maintains their COG over a fixed base of support while standing on a moving surface (Chattecx Balance System or EquiTest) or unstable surface (Biodex Stability System, BAPS, medium density foam or mini-tramp); or (2) The person transfers their COG over a fixed base of support to selected ranges and/or directions within the LOS while standing on a stable surface (Balance Master's LOS, functional reach tests, mini-squats, or T-Band kicks). *Dynamic* balance involves the maintenance of the COG within the LOS over a moving base of support (feet), usually while on a stable surface. These tasks require the use of a stepping strategy. The base of support is always changing its position, therefore forcing the COG to be adjusted with each movement. Examples of dynamic exercises are walking on a balance beam, step-up-and-over task, or bounding). *Functional* balance tasks are the same as dynamic tasks with the inclusion of sport-specific tasks such as throwing and catching.

Phase I

The progression of activities during this phase should include non-ballistic types of drills. Training for static balance can be initiated once the patient is able to bear weight on the extremity. The patient should first be asked to perform a bilateral 20-second Romberg test on a variety of surfaces, beginning with a hard/firm surface (Figure 7-9).

Once a comfort zone is established, the patient should be progressed to performing unilateral balance tasks on both the involved and uninvolved extremities on a stable surface.

The athletic trainer should make comparisons from these tests to determine the patient's ability to balance bilaterally and unilaterally. It should be noted that even though this is termed static balance, the patient does not remain perfectly motionless. In order to maintain static balance, the patient must make many small corrections at the ankle, hip, trunk, arms, or head as previously discussed (see Selection of Movement Strategies). If the patient is having difficulties performing these activities, they should not be progressed to the next surface. Repetitions of modified Romberg tests can be performed by first using the arms as a counterbalance, then attempting the activity without using the arms. Static balance activities should be

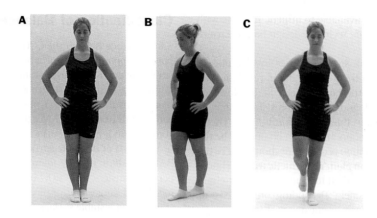

Figure 7-9   Double- and single-leg balance on a stable surface.
A, Double-leg stance. **B,** Double-leg tandem stance. **C,** Single-leg stance.

used as a precurser to more dynamic activities. The general progression of these exercises should be from bilateral to unilateral, with eyes open to eyes closed. The exercises should attempt to eliminate or alter the various sensory information (visual, vestibular, and somatosensory) in order to challenge the other systems. In most orthopedic rehabilitation situations, this is going to involve eye closure and changes in the support surface so the somatosensory system can be overloaded or stressed. This theory is synonymous with the overload principle in therapeutic exercise. Research suggests that balance activities, both with and without visual input, will enhance motor function at the brain stem level.[7.73] However, as the patient becomes more efficient at performing activities involving static balance, eye closure is recommended so that only the somatosensory system is left to control balance.

As improvement occurs on a firm surface, bilateral static balance drills should progress to an unstable surface such as a Tremor box, Dynadisc rocker board on hard surface, Bosu Balance Trainer—flat side up then bubble side up, BAPS board or foam surface (Figure 7-10). The purpose of the different surfaces is to safely challenge the

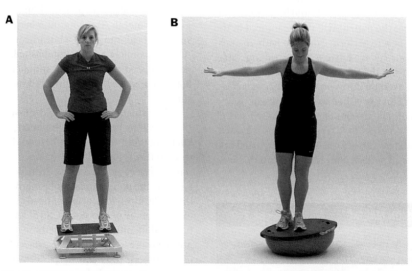

Figure 7-10   Double leg balance on an unstable surface. **A,** Tremor Box. **B,** Bosu Balance Trainer—flat surface.

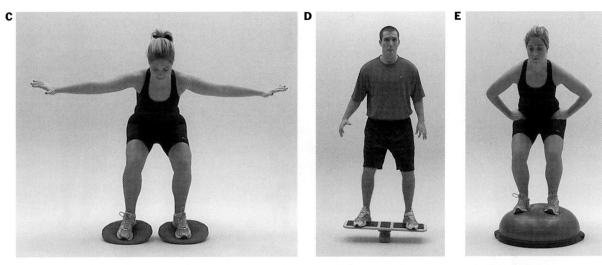

Figure 7-10 (continued) **C,** Dynadiscs. **D,** Extreme Balance Board. **E,** Bosu Balance Trainer—bubble surface.

injured patient, while keeping the patient motivated to rehabilitate the injured extremity. Additionally, the athletic trainer can introduce light shoulder, back, or chest taps in an attempt to challenge the patient's ability to maintain balance (Figure 7-11). Once the control is demonstrated in a bilateral stance, the patient can progress to similar activities using a unilateral stance (Figure 7-12). All of these exercises increase awareness of the location of the COG under a challenged condition, thereby helping to increase ankle strength in the closed kinetic chain. Such training may also increase sensitivity of the muscle

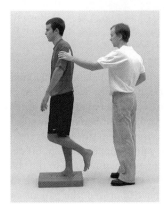

Figure 7-11 An athletic trainer causing perturbations using a shoulder tap is good for transitioning from double-leg balance on an unstable surface to single-leg balance on an unstable surface.

spindle and thereby increase proprioceptive input to the spinal cord, which may provide compensation for altered joint afference.[46]

Although static and semidynamic balance exercises may not be very functional for most sport activities, they are the first step toward regaining proprioceptive awareness, reflex stabilization, and postural orientation. The patient should attempt to assume a functional stance while performing static balance drills. Training in different positions places a variety of demands on the musculotendinous structures about the ankle, knee, and hip joints. For example, a gymnast should practice static balance with the hip in neutral and external rotation, as well as during a tandem stance to mimic performance on a balance beam. A basketball player should perform these drills in the "ready position" on the balls of the feet with the hips and knees slightly flexed. Patients requiring a significant amount of static balance for performing their sport include gymnasts, cheerleaders, and football linemen.[41]

Phase II This phase should be considered the transition phase from static to more dynamic balance activities. Dynamic balance will be especially important for patients who perform activities such as running, jumping, and cutting, which encompasses about 95 percent of all athletes. Such activities require the patient to repetitively lose and gain balance to perform their sport without falling or becoming injured.[41] Dynamic balance activities should only be incorporated into the rehabilitation program once sufficient healing has occurred and the patient has adequate ROM, muscle strength, and endurance. This could

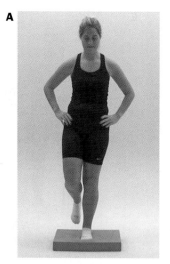

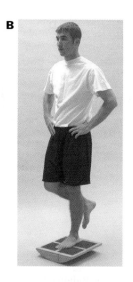

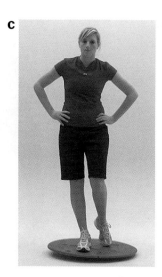

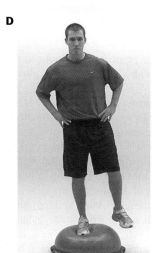

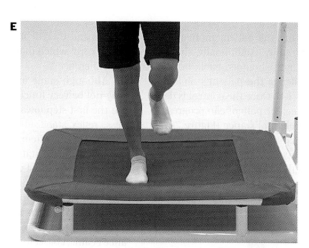

Figure 7-12 Single-leg balance on an unstable surface. **A,** Foam pad. **B,** Rocker Board. **C,** BAPS Board. **D,** Bosu Balance Trainer. **E,** Plyoback.

be as early as a few days post-injury in the case of a grade 1 ankle sprain, or as late as 6 weeks post-surgery in the case of an anterior cruciate reconstruction. Before the athletic trainer progresses the patient to challenging dynamic and sport-specific balance drills, several semidynamic (intermediate) exercises should be introduced.

These semidynamic balance drills involve displacement or perturbation of the COG away from the base of support. The patient is challenged to return and/or steady the COG above the base of support throughout several repetitions of the exercise. Some of these exercises involve a bilateral stance, some involve a unilateral stance, while others involve transferring of weight from one extremity to the other.

The bilateral-stance balance drills include the mini-squat, which is performed with the feet shoulder-width apart and the COG centered over a stable base of support (Figure 7-13A). The trunk should be positioned upright over the legs as the patient slowly flexes the hips and knees into a partial squat—approximately 60 degrees of knee flexion. The patient then returns to the starting position and repeats the task several times. Once ROM, strength, and stability have improved, the patient can progress to a full squat, which approaches 90 degrees knee flexion. These should be performed in front of a mirror so the patient can observe the amount of stability on their return to the extended position. A large stability ball can also be

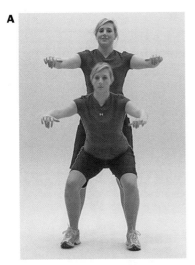 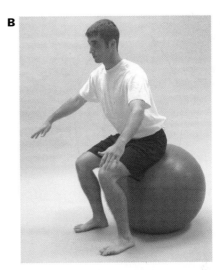

Figure 7-13   Double leg dynamic activities on a stable surface. **A,** Minisquats. **B,** Sit-to-stand from a stability ball.

used to perform sit-to-stand activities (Figure 7-13B). Once the patient reaches a comfort zone, they can perform more challenging variations of these exercises beginning on a stable surface (Figure 7-14) and progressing to weight, cable, or tubing-resisted exercises (Figure 7-15). Rotational maneuvers and weight-shifting exercises on unstable surfaces such as the Bosu, Dynadisc, or foam pad are used to assist the patient in controlling his or her COG during semidynamic movements (Figure 7-16). These exercises are important in the rehabilitation of ankle, knee, and hip injuries, as they help improve weight transfer, COG sway velocity, and left/right weight symmetry. They can be performed in an attempt to challenge anterior-posterior stability or medial-lateral stability.

The athletic trainer has a variety of options for unilateral semidynamic balance exercises. In the progression to more dynamic exercises, the patient should emphasize controlled hip and knee flexion, followed by a smooth return to a stabilization position. Step-ups can be performed either in the sagittal plane (forward step-up) or in the transverse plane (lateral step-up). (Figure 7-17A and B) These drills should begin with the heel of the uninvolved extremity on the floor. Using a 2 count, the patient should shift body weight toward the involved side and use the involved extremity to slowly raise the body onto the step.[73] The involved knee should not be "locked" into full extension. Instead, the knee should be positioned in approximately 5 degrees of flexion, while balancing on the step for 3 seconds. Following the 3 count, the body weight should be shifted toward

the uninvolved side and lowered to the heel of the uninvolved side. Step-up-and-over activities are similar to step-ups, but involve more dynamic transfer of the COG. These should be performed by having the patient both ascend and descend using the involved extremity (Figure 7-17C) or ascend with the involved extremity and descend with the uninvolved extremity forcing the involved leg to support the body on the descend. The athletic trainer can also introduce the patient to more challenging static tasks during this phase. For example, the very popular Thera-Band kicks (T-Band kicks or steamboats) are excellent for improving balance. TheraBand kicks are performed with an elastic material (attached to the ankle of the uninvolved leg) serving as a resistance against a relatively fast kicking motion (Figure 7-17D). The patient's balance on the involved extremity is challenged by perturbations caused by the kicking motion of the uninvolved leg. Four sets of these exercises should be performed, one for each of four possible kicking motions: hip flexion, hip extension, hip abduction, and hip adduction. T-Band kicks can also be performed on foam or a minitramp if additional somatosensory challenges are desired.[72] Single and multiplane lunges can also be used to transition to dynamic activities (Figure 7-17E and F).

The Balance Shoes (Orthopedic Physical Therapy Products, Minneapolis, MN) are another excellent tool for improving the strength of lower extremity musculature and ultimately—improving balance. The shoes allow lower extremity balance and strengthening

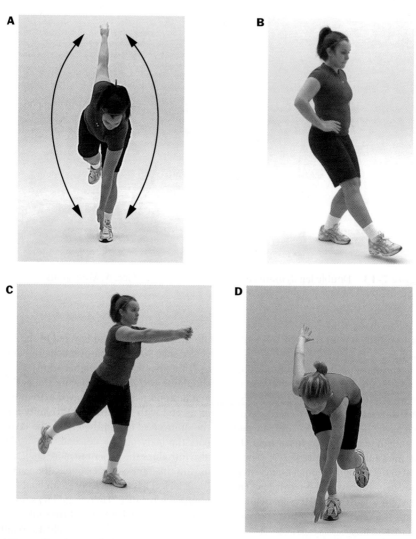

Figure 7-14   Single-leg balance dynamic (multiplane) movements on an stable surface. **A,** Windmill. **B,** Single-leg reach. **C,** Double-arm reach. **D,** Romanian deadlift.

exercises to be performed in a functional, closed-kinetic-chain manner. The shoes consist of a cork sandal with a rubber sole, and a rubber hemisphere similar in consistency to a lacrosse ball positioned under the mid-sole (see Figures 22-28 to 22-34). The design of the sandals essentially creates an individualized perturbation device for each limb that can be utilized in any number of functional activities, ranging from static single-leg stance to dynamic gait activities performed in multiple directions (forward walking, side-stepping, carioca walking, etc.).

Clinical use of the Balance Shoes has resulted in a number of successful clinical outcomes from a subjective standpoint, including treatment of ankle sprains and chronic instability, anterior tibial compartment syndrome, lower leg fractures, and a number of other orthopaedic problems, as well as for enhancement of core stability. Research has revealed that training in the Balance Shoes results in reduced rearfoot motion and improved postural stability in excessive pronators, and that functional activities in the Balance Shoes increase gluteal muscle activity. (See Chapter 22)

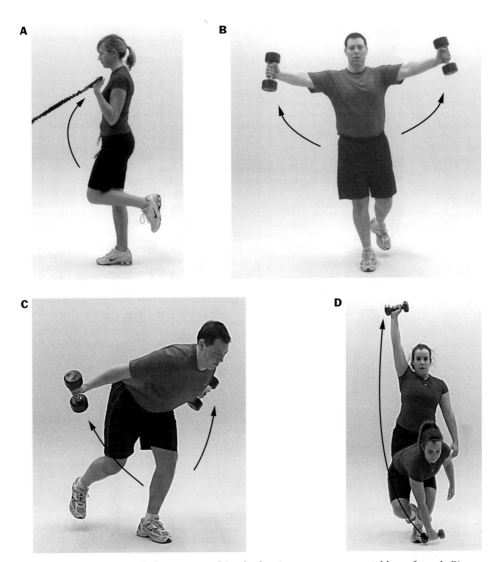

Figure 7-15   Single leg balance-resisted (multiplane) movements on a stable surface. **A,** Bicep curls using cable or tubing. **B,** Dumbbell scaption. **C,** Dumbbell cobra, **D,** Squat touchdown to overhead press.

CLINICAL DECISION MAKING   **Exercise 7–4**

What type of balance exercises would best meet the needs of a tennis player recovering from a grade 2 anterior talo-fibular sprain?

· ·

Phase III   Once the patient can successfully complete the semidynamic exercises presented in Phase II, he or she

should be ready to perform more dynamic and functional types of exercises. The general progression for activities to develop dynamic balance and control is from slow-speed to fast-speed activities, from low-force to high-force activities, and from controlled to uncontrolled activities.[41] In other words, the patient should be working toward sport-specific drills that will allow for a safe return to their respective sport or activity. These exercises will likely differ depending on which sport the person plays. For example, drills to improve lateral

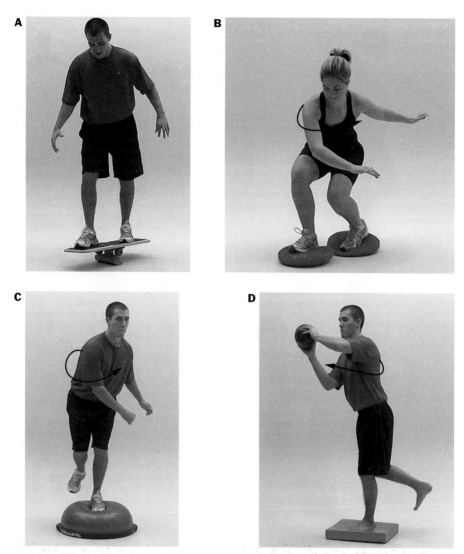

Figure 7-16 Double leg and single leg (multiplane) dynamic balance activities on an unstable surface. **A,** Tandem stance on an Extreme Balance Board. **B,** Standing rotation on Dynadise. **C,** Standing rotation on Bosu Balance Trainer. **D,** Partner throw and catch using a weighted ball while balancing on a foam pad.

weight shifting and sidestepping should be incorporated into a program for a tennis player, while drills to improve jumping and landing are going to be more important for a track athlete who performs the long jump. As previously mentioned, the athletic trainer often needs to use his or her imagination to develop the best protocol for their patient.

Bilateral jumping drills are a good place to begin once the patient has reached Phase III. The patient should begin with jumping or hopping onto a step, or performing butt kicks or tuck jumps, and quickly establishing a stabilized position (Figure 7-18 A–C). A more dynamic exercise involves bilateral jumping either over a line or some object either front to back or side to side. The patient should concentrate on landing on each side of the line as quickly as possible (Figure 7-18D).[72,73] Bilateral dynamic balance exercises should progress to unilateral dynamic balance exercises as quickly as possible during Phase III. At this stage of the rehabilitation, pain and fatigue should not be as much of a

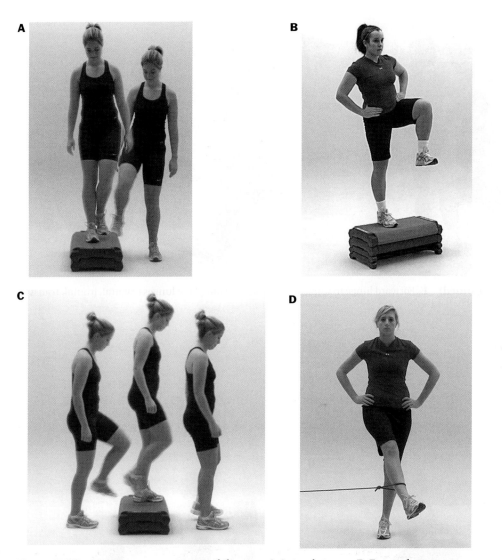

Figure 7-17   Stepping movements to stabilization. **A,** Lateral step up. **B,** Forward step-up to single-leg balance. **C,** Step-up-and-over (alternating lead leg). **D,** Theraband Kicks.

factor. All jumping drills performed bilaterally should now be performed unilaterally, by practicing first on the uninvolved extremity. If additional challenges are needed, a vertical component can be added by having the patient jump over an object such as a box or other suitable object (Figure 7-18E).

As the patient progresses through these exercises, eye closure can be used to further challenge the patient's somatosensation. After mastering these straight plane jumping patterns, the patient can begin diagonal jumping patterns through the use of a cross on the floor formed by two pieces of tape (Figure 7-18F). The intersecting lines create four quadrants that can be numbered and used to perform different jumping sequences such as 1,3,2,4 for the first set and 1,4,2,3 for the second set.[72,73] A larger grid can be designed to allow for longer sequences and longer jumps, both of which require additional strength, endurance, and balance control.

Another good exercise to introduce prior to advancing to Phase III is a balance beam walk, which can be performed against resistance to further challenge the patient (Figure 7-19A). Tubing can be added to dynamic unilateral training exercises. The patient can perform

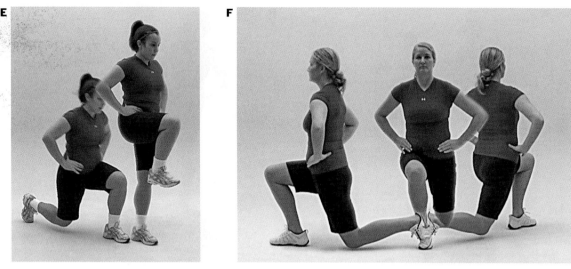

Figure 7-17(continued) **E,** Forward lunge to single-leg balance. **F,** Multiplane lunges (sagittal, frontal, transverse).

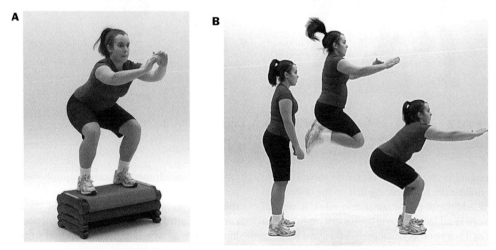

Figure 7-18 Jumping and hopping to stabilization **A,** Forward jump-up to stabilization. **B,** Butt kicks to stabilization.

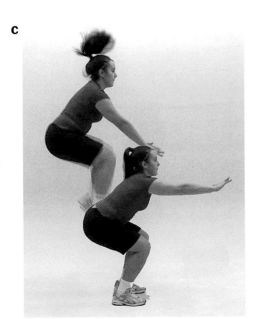

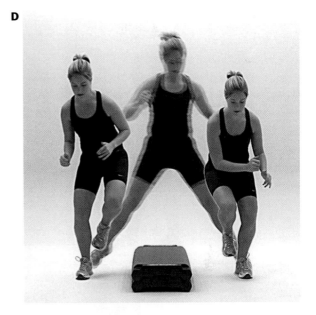

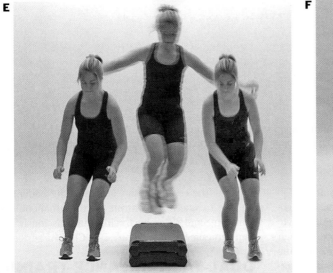

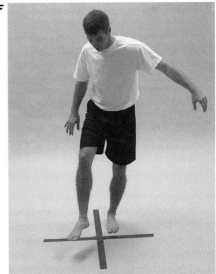

Figure 7-18(continued)   **C,** Tuck jumps to stabilization. **D,** Bidirectional single-leg hop-overs to stabilization. **E,** Bilateral double-leg hop-overs to stabilization. **F,** Diagonal hops to stabilizations.

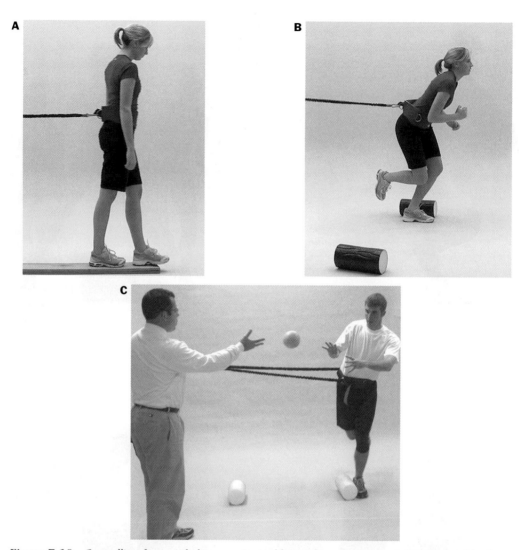

Figure 7-19   Controlling dynamic balance against cable or tubing resistance. **A,** Forward and backward walking on a balance board. **B,** Lateral hopping in the frontal plane. **C,** Throwing and catching a ball during lateral bounding.

stationary running against the tube's resistance, followed by lateral and diagonal bounding exercises. Diagonal bounding, which involves jumping from one foot to another, places greater emphasis on lateral movements. It is recommended that the patient first learn the bounding exercise without tubing, and then attempt the exercise with tubing. A foam roll, towel, or other obstacle can be used to increase jump height and/or distance.[79] (Figure 7-19B) The final step in trying to improve dynamic balance should involve the incorporation of sport-related activities such as throwing and catching a ball. At this

stage of the rehabilitation program, the patient should be able to safely concentrate on the functional activity (catching and throwing), while subconsciously controlling dynamic balance (Figure 7-19C).

DUAL-TASK BALANCE TRAINING AND ASSESSMENT

While the aforementioned balance training and assessment techniques are validated and have proven to be useful in the clinical setting, patients typically function in a

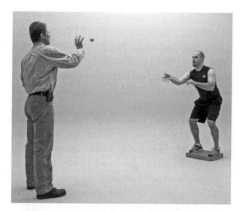

Figure 7-20   Incorporating a cognitive task with sport-specific balance.

more dynamic environment with multiple demands placed upon them concurrently. Participation in sport often requires patients to split their attention between cognitive and dynamic balance tasks. Therefore, a *final progression* for patients recovering from musculoskeletal injury or neurological injury (i.e., concussion) could be the addition of competing motor/coordination and cognitive tasks to assess the patient's performance with these challenges. Though the cognitive and balance demands are unique, the two are linked in that they rely on an individual's system of attention. The attention system should be viewed as independent of the information processing centers of the brain and, like other systems, is able to communicate with multiple systems simultaneously.[68] Evidence has shown the ability to selectively allocate attention between cogni-

tive and balance tasks, but a priority for balance has been demonstrated with increasing difficulty of these tasks.[71]

Once elite athletes progress through the initial phases of the balance exercises, they may reach a point where these dual-task balance exercises can be of benefit. Keeping the patient engaged in his or her rehabilitation program is important, and these added challenges can assist in reproducing the type of demands placed on the patient during more physical activity or competition. In order to better recreate these demands, the systems should be challenged in unison to fully assess the functional limitations of patient, as well as train or rehabilitate these injury-related limitations.

Dual-task exercises must be clearly explained to the patient, so he or she understands the task at hand. The task can be sport specific, and should follow the guidelines previously outlined in this chapter with respect to advancing the exercises using more challenging stances and surfaces.

Incorporating a cognitive task with a sport-specific balance task can be done very easily using different colored balls, and specific rules or instructions provided to the patient. The athletic trainer, standing approximately 15 feet away tosses different colored balls to the patient, who is standing on either a double leg or single leg, and/or firm surface, foam surface, or balance board (Figure 7-20). The patient is told to maintain his balance while catching a blue ball with his *right* hand, red ball with his *left* hand, and yellow ball with *both* hands. This dual task can be difficult initially, but the patient should attempt to work through the increased attention demands while allowing his somatosensory system to subconsciously aid in the maintenance of balance. The complexity can be increased by adding additional rules. For example, the patient can be

A	B	C
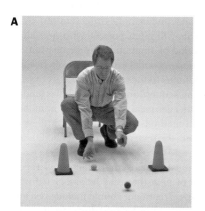	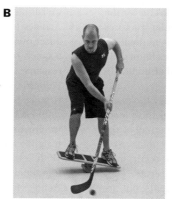	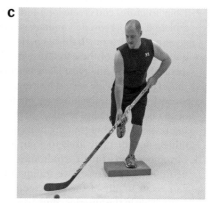

Figure 7-21   Sport-Specific cognitive tasks. **A,** The athletic trainer rolls different colored balls to the patient. **B** and **C,** standing on an unstable surface. The patient must decide where to return the ball while maintaining balance.

instructed to toss the yellow ball back *head high*, blue ball back *waist high*, and to *roll* the yellow ball back.

The exercises can then be made more sport specific. For example, the athletic trainer positions himself about 25 feet from the patient and rolls the different colored balls to the patient standing on either a double leg or single leg, and/or firm surface, foam surface, or balance board (Figure 7-21). A hockey player with a hockey stick is asked to return (aim) the blue ball to the *right* side of the target, the yellow ball to the *center* of the target, and the blue ball to the *left* side of the target.

CLINICAL DECISION MAKING   **Exercise 7–5**

A basketball player has been complaining of feeling pain and laxity upon landing from a rebound. He has no swelling or other signs of an acute injury. What exercises should be introduced to help improve the stability?

CLINICAL VALUE OF HIGH-TECH TRAINING AND ASSESSMENT

The benefit of using the commercially available balance systems is that not only can deficits be detected, but progress can be charted quantitatively through the computer-generated results. For example, NeuroCom's Balance Master (with long forceplate) is capable of assessing a patient's ability to perform coordinated movements essential for sport performance. The system, equipped with a 5-foot-long force platform, is capable of identifying specific components underlying performance of several functional tasks. Exercises are also available on the system that then help to improve the deficits.[62]

Results of a Step-up-and-over test are presented in Figure 7-22. The components which are analyzed in this particular task are: (1) *Lift-Up Index*—quantifies the maximum lifting (concentric) force exerted by the leading leg and is expressed as a percentage of the person's weight; (2) *Movement Time*—quantifies the number of seconds required to complete the task, beginning with initial weight shift to the non-stepping leg and ending with impact of the lagging leg onto the surface; and (3) *Impact Index*—quantifies the maximum vertical impact force (percent of body weight) as the lagging leg lands on the surface.[62]

Research on the clinical applicability of these measures has revealed interesting results. Preliminary observations from two studies in progress suggest that deficits in impact control are a common feature of patients with ACL injuries, even when strength and range of motion of the involved knee are within normal limits. Several other performance assessments are available on this system, including *sit to stand, walk test, step and quick turn, forward lunge, weight bearing/squat,* and *rhythmic weight shift.*

Summary

1. Although some injuries in the region of the lower leg are acute, most injuries seen in an athletic population result from overuse, most often from running.
2. Tibial fractures can create long-term problems for the athlete if inappropriately managed. Fibular fractures generally require much shorter periods for immobilization. Treatment of these fractures involves immediate medical referral and most likely a period of immobilization and restricted weight bearing.
3. Stress fractures in the lower leg are usually the result of the bone's inability to adapt to the repetitive loading response during training and conditioning of the athlete and are more likely to occur in the tibia.
4. Chronic compartment syndromes can occur from acute trauma or repetitive trauma of overuse. They can occur in any of the four compartments, but are most likely in the anterior compartment or deep posterior compartment.
5. Rehabilitation of medial tibial stress syndrome must be comprehensive and address several factors, including musculoskeletal, training, and conditioning, as well as proper shoes and orthotics intervention.
6. Achilles tendinitis will often present with a gradual onset over a period of time and may be resistant to a quick resolution secondary to the slower healing response of tendinous tissue.
7. Perhaps the greatest question after an Achilles tendon rupture is whether surgical repair or cast immobilization is the best method of treatment. Regardless of treatment method, the time required for rehabilitation is significant.
8. With retrocalcaneal bursitis the athlete will report a gradual onset of pain that may be associated with Achilles tendinitis. Treatment should include rest and activity modification in order to reduce swelling and inflammation.

Name:	Doe, John J	Diagnosis:	ACL Tear L Knee	File:	HBM1.QBM
ID:	ATID00001	Operator ID:	Jodi Bower	Date:	03/06/97
DOB:	11/22/55	Referred by:	Dr. Tom Merkle	Time:	6:35:06 PM
Height:	5'11"	Comments:	DOI: 7/4/96; DOS: 7/6/96		

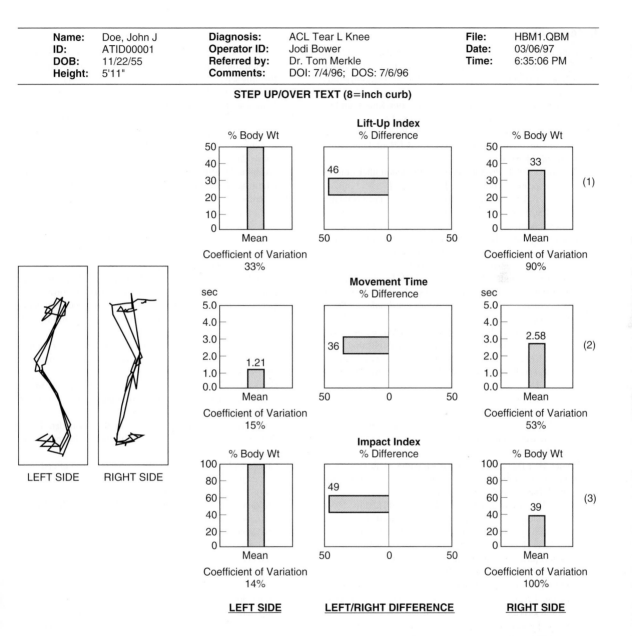

STEP UP/OVER TEXT (8=inch curb)

Figure 7-22   Results from a step-up-and-over protocol on the NeuroCom New Balance Master's long forceplate. Balance master® Version 6.0 and NeuroCom® are registered trademarks of NeuroCom International Inc. Copyright © 1989–1997. All Rights Reserved.

References

1. Balogun, J. A., C.O. Adesinasi, and D.K. Marzouk. 1992. The effects of a wobble board exercise training program on static balance performance and strength of lower extremity muscle. *Physiotherapy Canada* 44:23–30.

2. Barrack, R. L., P. Lund, and H. Skinner. 1994. Knee Joint Proprioception Revisited. *J Sport Rehabil* 3:18–42.

3. Barrack, R. L., H. B. Skinner, and S. L. Buckley. 1989. Proprioception in the anterior cruciate deficient knee. *Am J Sports Med* 17:1–6.

4. Barrett, D. 1991. Proprioception and function after anterior cruciate reconstruction. *J Bone Joint Surg [Br]* 73:833–837.

5. Black, F., C. Wall, and L. Nashner. 1983. Effect of visual and support surface orientations upon postural control in vestibular deficient subjects. *Acta Otolaryngol* 95:199–210.

6. Black, O., C. Wall, H. Rockette, and R. Kitch. 1982. Normal subject postural sway during the Romberg test. *American Journal of Otolaryngology* 3(5):309–318.

7. Blackburn, T., and M. Voight. 1995. Single leg stance: Development of a reliable testing procedure. In *Proceedings of the 12th International Congress of the World Confederation for Physical Therapy.*

8. Booher, J., and G. Thibodeau. 1995. *Athletic Injury Assessment.* St. Louis, MO: Times Mirror/Mosby College Publishing.

9. Cornwall, M., and P. Murrell. 1991. Postural sway following inversion sprain of the ankle. *J American Podiatric Med Assoc* 81:243–247.

10. Davies, G. 1995. The need for critical thinking in rehabilitation. *J Sport Rehabil* 4(1):1–22.

11. DeCarlo, M., T. Klootwyk, and K. Shelbourne. 1997. ACL surgery and accelerated rehabilitation: Revisited. *J Sport Rehabil* 6(2):144–156.

12. Diener, H., J. Dichgans, and B. Guschlbauer, et al. 1986. Role of visual and static vestibular influences on dynamic posture control. *Hum Neurobiol* 5:105–113.

13. Diener, H., J. Dichgans, B. Guschlbauer, and H. Mau. 1984. The significance of proprioception on postural stabilization as assessed by ischemia. *Brain Research* 296:103–109.

14. Dietz, V., G. Horstmann, and W. Berger. 1989. Significance of proprioceptive mechanisms in the regulation of stance. *Progress in Brain Research* 80:419–423.

15. Donahoe, B., D. Turner, and T. Worrell. 1993. The use of functional reach as a measurement of balance in healthy boys and girls ages 5–15. *Physical Therapy* 73(6):S71.

16. Dornan, J., G. Fernie, and P. Holliday. 1978. Visual input: It's importance in the control of postural sway. *Arch Phys Med Rehabil* 59:586–591.

17. Ekdahl, C., G. Jarnlo, and S. Anderson. 1989. Standing balance in healthy subjects: Evaluation of a quantitative test battery on a force platform. *Scandanavian J of Rehabil Med* 21:187–195.

18. Faculjak, P., K. Firoozbakhsh, D. Wausher, and M. McGuire. 1993. Balance characteristics of normal and anterior cruciate ligament deficient knees. *Phys Ther* 73:S22.

19. Fisher, A., S. Wietlisbach, and J. Wilberger. 1988. Adult performance on three tests of equilibrium. *Am J Occupational Ther* 42(1):30–35.

20. Fitzpatrick, R., D. K. Rogers, and D. I. McCloskey. 1994. Stable human standing with lower-limb muscle afferents providing the only sensory input. *J Physiol* 480(2):395–403.

21. Flores, A. 1992. Objective measures of standing balance. *Neurology Report – Am Phys Ther Assoc* 16(1):17–21.

22. Forkin, D. M., C. Koczur, R. Battle, and R. A. Newton. 1996. Evaluation of kinetic deficits indicative of balance control in gymnasts with unilateral chronic ankle sprains. *J Orthop Sports Phys Ther* 23(4):245–250.

23. Freeman, M. 1965. Instability of the foot after injuries to the lateral ligament of the ankle. *J Bone Joint Surg* 47B:678–685.

24. Freeman, M., M. Dean, and I. Hanham. 1965. The etiology and prevention of functional instability of the foot. *J Bone Joint Surg* 47B:669–677.

25. Friden, T., R. Zatterstrom, A. Lindstrand, and U. Moritz. 1989. A stabilometric technique for evaluation of lower limb instabilities. *Am J Sports Med* 17(1):118–122.

26. Garn, S. N., and R. A. Newton. 1988. Kinesthetic awareness in subjects with multiple ankle sprains. *Phys Ther* 68:1667–1671.

27. Goldie, P., T. Bach, and O. Evans. 1989. Force platform measures for evaluating postural control: Reliability and validity. *Arch Phys Med Rehabil* 70:510–517.

28. Grigg, P. 1975. Mechanical factors influencing response of joint afferent neurons from cat knee. *J Neurophysiol* 38:1473–1484.

29. Grigg, P. 1976. Response of joint afferent neurons in cat medial articular nerve to active and passive movements of the knee. *Brain Res* 118:482–485.

30. Guskiewicz, K. M., D.H. Perrin, and B. Gansneder. 1996. Effect of mild head injury on postural stability. *Journal of Athletic Training* 31(4):300–306.

31. Guskiewicz, K. M., and D. H. Perrin. 1996. Effect of orthotics on postural sway following inversion ankle sprain. *J Orthop Sports Phys Ther* 23(5):326–331.

32. Guskiewicz, K. M., and D. H. Perrin. 1996. Research and clinical applications of assessing balance. *J Sport Rehabil* 5:45–63.

33. Guskiewicz, K. M., B.L. Riemann, D. H. Riemann, and L. M. Nashner. 1997. Alternative approaches to the assessment of mild head injury in patients. *Med & Sci in Sport & Exer* 29(7): S213–S221.

34. Guyton, A. 1991. *Textbook of Medical Physiology.* 8th ed. Philadelphia: W.B. Saunders Co.

35. Harrison, E., N. Duenkel, R. Dunlop, and G. Russell. 1994. Evaluation of single-leg standing following anterior cruciate ligament surgery and rehabilitation. *Phys Ther* 74(3):245–252.

36. Hertel, J. N., K. M. Guskiewicz, D. M. Kahler, and D. H. Perrin. 1996. Effect of lateral ankle joint anesthesia on center of balance, postural sway and joint position sense. *J Sport Rehabil* 5:111–119.

37. Horak, F. B., L. M. Nashner, and H.C. Diener. 1990. Postural strategies associated with somatosensory and vestibular loss. *Exp Brain Res* 82:167–177.

38. Horak, F., and L. Nashner. 1986. Central programming of postural movements: Adaptation to altered support surface configurations. *J Neurophysiol* 55:1369–1381.

39. Houk, J. 1979. Regulation of stiffness by skeleto-motor reflexes. *Annual Rev Physiology* 41:99–114.

40. Irrgang, J., and C. Harner. 1997. Recent advances in ACL rehabilitation: Clinical factors. *J Sport Rehab* 6(2):111–124.

41. Irrgang, J., S. Whitney, and E. Cox. 1994. Balance and proprioceptive training for rehabilitation of the lower extremity. *J Sport Rehab* 3:68–83.

42. Jansen, E., R. Larsen, and B. Mogens. 1982. Quantitative Romberg's test: Measurement and computer calculations of postural stability. *Acta Neurol Scand* 66:93–99.

43. Johansson, H., I.J. Alexander, and K.C. Hayes. 1982. Nerve supply of the human knee and its functional importance. *Am J Sports Med* 10:329–335.

44. Kauffman, T. L., L. M. Nashner, and L. K. Allison. 1997. Balance is a critical parameter in orthopedic rehabilitation. *Orthopaedic Phys Ther Clin North America* 6(1):43–78.

45. Kisner, C., and L. A. Colby. 1996. *Therapeutic exercise: Foundations and techniques.* 3rd ed. Philadelphia: F. A. Davis Co.

46. Lephart, S. M. 1993. Re-establishing proprioception, kinesthesia, joint position sense, and neuromuscular control in rehabilitation. In *Rehabilitation Techniques in Sports*, 2nd. ed. W.E. Prentice, ed. St. Louis, MO: Times Mirror Mosby College Publishing, 118–137.

47. Lephart, S. M., and T. J. Henry. 1995. Functional rehabilitation for the upper and lower extremity. *Orthopedic Clin North America* 26(3):579–592.

48. Lephart, S. M., and M. S. Kocher. 1993. The role of exercise in the prevention of shoulder disorders. In *The shoulder: A balance of mobility and stability.* Matsen F. A., F. H. Fu, and R. J. Hawkins, eds. Rosemont, IL: American Academy of Orthopaedic Surgeons, 597–620.

49. Lephart, S. M. M. S. Kocher, and F. H. Fu, et al. 1992. Proprioception following ACL reconstruction. *J Sport Rehabil* 1:186–196.

50. Lephart, S. M., D. Pincivero, J. Giraldo, and F. H. Fu. 1997. The role of proprioception in the management and rehabilitation of athletic injuries. *Am J Sports Med* 25:130–137.

51. Mangine, R., and T. Kremchek. 1997. Evaluation-based protocol of the anterior cruciate ligament. *J Sport Rehab* 6(2):157–181.

52. Mauritz, K., J. Dichgans, and A. Hufschmidt. 1979. Quantitative analysis of stance in late cortical cerebellar atrophy of the anterior lobe and other forms of cerebellar ataxia. *Brain* 102:461–482.

53. Mizuta, H., M. Shiraishi, K. Kubota, K. Kai, and K. Takagi. 1992. A stabilometric technique for evaluation of functional instability in the anterior cruciate ligament deficient knee. *Clin J Sports Med* 2:235–239.

54. Murray, M., A. Seireg, and S. Sepic. 1975. Normal postural stability: Qualitative assessment. *J Bone Joint Surg* 57A(4):510–516.

55. Nashner, L. 1976. Adapting reflexes controlling the human posture. *Exploring Brain Research.* 26:59–72.

56. Nashner, L. 1982. Adaptation of human movement to altered environments. *Trends in Neuroscience* 5:358–361.

57. Nashner, L. 1985. A functional approach to understanding spasticity. In *Electromyography and Evoked Potentials.* Struppler A. and A. Weindl, eds. Berlin: Springer-Verlag, 22–29.

58. Nashner, L. 1989. Sensory, neuromuscular and biomechanical contributions to human balance. In *Balance: Proceedings of the APTA forum*, June 13–15, 1989. Duncan, P. ed. pp. 5–12.

59. Nashner, L. 1993. Computerized Dynamic Posturography. In *Handbook of Balance Function and Testing.* Jacobson G., C. Newman, and J. Kartush, eds. St. Louis, MO:Mosby Year Book, Inc., 280–307.

60. Nashner, L. 1993. Practical Biomechanics and Physiology of Balance. In *Handbook of Balance Function and Testing.* Jacobson, G. C. Newman, and J. Kartush, eds. St. Louis, MO: Mosby Year Book, Inc., 261–279.

61. Nashner, L., F. Black and C. Wall, III. 1982. Adaptation to altered support and visual conditions during stance: Patients with vestibular deficits. *J Neurosci* 2(5):536–544.

62. NeuroCom International, Inc. 1997. The objective quantification of daily life tasks: The NEW Balance Master 6.0 (manual). Clackamas, OR.

63. Newton, R. 1992. Review of tests of standing balance abilities. *Brain Injury* 3:335–343.

64. Norre, M. 1993. Sensory interaction testing in platform posturography. *J Laryngol and Otol* 107:496–501.

65. Noyes, F., S. Barber, and R. Mangine. 1991. Abnormal lower limb symmetry determined by function hop test after anterior cruciate ligament rupture. *Am J Sports Med* 19(5):516–518.

66. Orteza, L., W. Vogelbach, and C. Denegar. 1992. The effect of molded and unmolded orthotics on balance and pain while jogging following inversion ankle sprain. *J Athl Train* 27(1):80–84.

67. Pintsaar, A., J. Brynhildsen, and H. Tropp. 1996. Postural corrections after standardised perturbations of single limp stance: Effect of training and orthotic devices in patients with ankle instability. *Br J Sports Med* 30:151–155.

68. Posner M. I., and S. E. Petersen 1990. The attention system of the human brain. *Annu Rev Neurosci* 1990;13:25–42.

69. Shambers, G.M. 1969. Influence of the fusimotor system on stance and volitional movement in normal man. *Am J Phys Med* 48:225–227.

70. Shumway-Cook, A., and F. Horak. 1986. Assessing the influence of sensory interaction on balance. *Phys Ther* 66(10):1548–1550.

71. Siu K.C., and M. H. Woollacott 2007. Attentional demands of postural control: The ability to selectively allocate information-processing resources. *Gait Posture* 25(1):121–126.

72. Swanik, C.B., S. M. Lephart, F. P. Giannantonio, and F. H. Fu. 1997. Reestablishing proprioception and neuromuscular control in the ACL-injured patient. 6(2):182–206.

73. Tippett, S., and M. Voight. 1995. *Functional progression for sports rehabilitation.* Champaign, IL: Human Kinetics.

74. Tropp, H., J. Ekstrand, and J. Gillquist. 1984. Factors affecting stabilometry recordings of single limb stance. *Am J Sports Med* 12:185–188.

75. Tropp, H., J. Ekstrand, and J. Gillquist. 1984. Stabilometry in functional instability of the ankle and its value in predicting injury. *Med Sci Sports Exerc* 16:64–66.
76. Tropp, H., and P. Odenrick. 1988. Postural control in single limb stance. *J Orthop Res* 6:833–839.
77. Trulock, S. C. 1996. A comparison of static, dynamic and functional methods of objective balance assessment. Master's thesis. Chapel Hill, NC: University of North Carolina,
78. Vander, A., J. Sherman, and D. Luciano. 1990. *Human physiology: The mechanisms of body function.* 5th ed. New York: McGraw-Hill.
79. Voight, M., and G. Cook. 1996. Clinical application of closed kinetic chain exercise. *J. Sport Rehab* 5(1):25–44.
80. Whitney, S. *Clinical and high tech alternatives to assessing postural sway in patients.* Presented at the National Athletic Trainers' Association Annual Meeting, June 11, 1994, Dallas, TX.
81. Wilk, K., N. Zheng, G. Fleisig, J. Andrews, and W. Clancy. 1997. Kinetic chain exercise: Implications for the anterior cruciate ligament patient. *J. Sport Rehab* 6(2):125–143.
82. Wilkerson, G., and J. Nitz. 1994. Dynamic ankle stability: Mechanical and neuromuscular interrelationships. *J. Sport Rehabil* 3:43–57.

SOLUTIONS TO CLINICAL DECISION MAKING EXERCISES

7-1 A preseason baseline score can be obtained on a measure such as the BESS for all athletes, and then used for a postinjury comparison. Because there is such variability within many of the balance measures, it is important to make comparisons only to an athlete's individual baseline measure and not to a normal score. It is best to determine recovery on a measure by using the number of standard deviations (SD) away from the baseline. For example, scores on the BESS that are more than 2 SD or 6 total points would be considered abnormal. Repeated assessments over the course of a rehabilitation progression can be used to determine the effectiveness of the balance exercises.

7-2 The athletic trainer should first ensure that the patient has the necessary pain-free ROM and muscular strength to complete the tasks that are being incorporated into the program. Additionally, for exercises beyond the phase 1 static exercises, the patient must be beyond the acute inflammatory phase of tissue response to injury. Once these factors have been considered, the athletic trainer should focus on developing a protocol that is safe yet challenging, stresses multiple planes of motion, and incorporates a multisensory approach.

7-3 It should be explained to the patient, at the outset, that the goal is to challenge her or his motor control system, to the point that the last two repetitions of each set of exercises should be difficult to perform. When the last two repetitions no longer are challenging to the athlete, he or she should be progressed to the next exercise. This can be determined through subjective information reported from the athlete, as well as the athletic trainer's objective observations. It is very important to provide a variety of exercises and levels of exercises so that the patient maintains a high level of motivation.

7-4 It will be important for the athletic trainer to begin slowly with phase 1 and 2 balance exercises to determine the patient's readiness to move into more dynamic tasks as part of phase 3. The progression outlined in the solution to exercise 7-2 should be followed. However, this is an example of how the athletic trainer can begin to personalize the exercise routine. A tennis player competing at a high level will need to perform a lot of lateral movement along the baseline, therefore necessitating the inclusion of dynamic balance exercises and weight shifts in the frontal plane. Several of the exercises described in this chapter would provide a good starting point for the athletic trainer in accomplishing this goal.

7-5 This patient most likely has a functionally unstable ankle. Research has shown that balance exercises can help improve functional ankle instability. In this situation, the athletic trainer probably can skip phase 1 exercises and move directly to phase 2 and 3 exercises. The athletic trainer should design a program that incorporates challenging unilateral multidirectional exercises involving a multisensory approach (eyes open and eyes closed). The progression should include the progression suggested in this chapter that includes the foam, Bosu Balance Trainer, Dynadisc, BAPS board, Extreme Balance Board, balance beam, and Balance Shoes. Lateral and diagonal hopping exercises will also be a vital part of this protocol. The goal should be to help strengthen the dynamic and static stabilizers surrounding the ankle joint. This should result in rebuilding some of the afferent pathways and ultimately improving ankle joint stability.

CHAPTER 8

Restoring Range of Motion and Improving Flexibility

William E. Prentice

After completing this chapter, the athletic training student should be able to do the following:

- Define flexibility and describe its importance in injury rehabilitation.

- Identify factors that limit flexibility.

- Differentiate between active and passive range of motion.

- Explain the difference between dynamic, static, and proprioceptive neuromuscular facilitation stretching.

- Discuss the neurophysiologic principles of stretching.

- Describe stretching exercises that may be used to improve flexibility at specific joints throughout the body.

- Compare and contrast the various manual therapy techniques including myofascial release, strain/counterstrain, positional release, soft tissue mobilization, and massage that can be used to improve mobility and range of motion.

When injury occurs, there is almost always some associated loss of the ability to move normally. Loss of motion may be due to pain, swelling, muscle guarding, or spasm; inactivity resulting in shortening of connective tissue and muscle; loss of neuromuscular control; or some combination of these factors. Restoring normal range of motion following injury is one of the primary goals in any rehabilitation program.[90] Thus the athletic trainer must routinely include exercise designed to restore normal range of motion to regain normal function.

Flexibility has been defined as the ability to move a joint or series of joints through a full, nonrestricted, pain-free range of motion.[2,3,28,40,46,72,88] Flexibility is dependent on a combination of (1) joint range of motion, which may be limited by the shape of the articulating surfaces and by capsular and ligamentous structures surrounding that joint; and (2) muscle flexibility, or the ability of the musculotendinous unit to lengthen.[102] Flexibility involves the ability of the neuromuscular system to allow for efficient movement of a joint through a range of motion.[3,31,48,52,83,105]

Flexibility can be discussed in relation to movement involving only one joint, such as the knees, or movement involving a whole series of joints, such as the spinal vertebral joints, that must all move together to allow smooth bending or rotation of the trunk. Lack of flexibility in one joint or movement can affect the entire kinetic chain. A person might have good range of motion in the ankles, knees, hips, back, and one shoulder joint but lack normal movement in the other shoulder joint; this is a problem that needs to be corrected before the person can function normally.[11,20]

In this chapter we will concentrate primarily on rehabilitative techniques used to increase the length of the musculotendinous unit and its associated fascia, as well as restricted neural tissue. In addition, a discussion of a variety of manual therapy techniques including myofascial release, strain/counterstrain, positional release therapy (PRT), soft tissue mobilization, and massage as they relate to improving mobility will be included. Joint mobilization and traction techniques used to address tightness in the joint capsule and surrounding ligaments will be discussed in Chapter 13. Loss of the ability to control movement due to impairment in neuromuscular control was discussed in Chapter 6.

IMPORTANCE OF FLEXIBILITY TO THE PATIENT

Maintaining a full, nonrestricted range of motion has long been recognized as essential to normal daily living. Lack of flexibility can also create uncoordinated or awkward movement patterns resulting from lost neuromuscular control. In most patients, functional activities require rela-

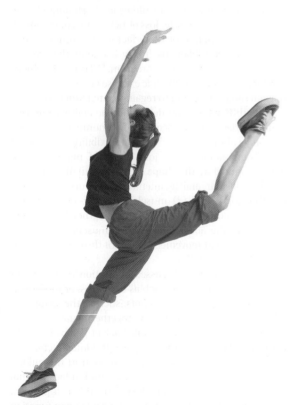

Figure 8-1 Extreme flexibility. Certain dance and athletic activities require extreme flexibility for successful performance.
Source: Prentice, W.E. 2009. *Get fit, stay fit.* New York: McGraw-Hill.

tively "normal" amounts of flexibility. However some sport activities, such as gymnastics, ballet, diving, karate, and especially dance require increased flexibility for superior performance (Figure 8-1).

It has also been generally accepted that flexibility is essential for improving performance in physical activities. However, a review of the evidence-based information in the literature looking at the relationship between flexibility and improved performance is, at best, conflicting and inconclusive.[43,59,104] While many studies done over the years have suggested that stretching improves performance,[11,59,76,111] several recent studies have found that stretching causes decreases in performance parameters such as strength, endurance, power, joint position sense, and reaction times.[9,30,42,43,61,70,83,85,93,106,110]

The same can be said when examining the relationship between flexibility and reducing the incidence of injury. While it is generally accepted that good flexibility reduces the likelihood of injury, a true cause–effect relationship has not been clearly established in the literature.[4,19,76,110]

CLINICAL DECISION MAKING   **Exercise 8–1**

A gymnast is out of practice for 2 weeks because of a stress fracture in her tibia. Why is it essential to incorporate flexibility into the rehabilitation program for this injury?

ANATOMIC FACTORS THAT LIMIT FLEXIBILITY

A number of anatomic factors can limit the ability of a joint to move through a full, unrestricted range of motion. *Muscles* and their tendons, along with their surrounding fascial sheaths, are most often responsible for limiting range of motion. When performing stretching exercises to improve flexibility about a particular joint, you are attempting to take advantage of the highly elastic properties of a muscle. Over time it is possible to increase the elasticity, or the length that a given muscle can be stretched. Persons who have a good deal of movement at a particular joint tend to have highly elastic and flexible muscles.

Connective tissue surrounding the joint, such as ligaments on the joint capsule, can be subject to contractures. Ligaments and joint capsules have some elasticity; however, if a joint is immobilized for a period of time, these structures tend to lose some elasticity and actually shorten. This condition is most commonly seen after surgical repair of an unstable joint, but it can also result from long periods of inactivity.

It is also possible for a person to have relatively slack ligaments and joint capsules. These people are generally referred to as being loose-jointed. Examples of this trait would be an elbow or knee that hyperextends beyond 180 degrees (Figure 8-2). Frequently, there is instability associated with loose-jointedness that can present as great a problem in movement as ligamentous or capsular contractures.

Bony structure can restrict the end point in the range. An elbow that has been fractured through the joint might lay down excess calcium in the joint space, causing the joint to lose its ability to fully extend. However, in many instances we rely on bony prominences to stop movements at normal end points in the range.

Fat can also limit the ability to move through a full range of motion. A person who has a large amount of fat on the abdomen might have severely restricted trunk flexion when asked to bend forward and touch the toes. The fat can act as a wedge between two lever arms, restricting movement wherever it is found.

Skin might also be responsible for limiting movement. For example, a person who has had some type of injury or surgery involving a tearing incision or laceration of the skin, particularly over a joint, will have inelastic scar tissue formed at that site. This scar tissue is incapable of stretching with joint movement.

Over time, skin contractures caused by scarring of ligaments, joint capsules, and musculotendinous units are capable of improving elasticity to varying degrees through stretching. With the exception of bone structure, age, and gender, all the other factors that limit flexibility can be altered to increase range of joint motion.

Neural tissue tightness resulting from acute compression, chronic repetitive microtrauma, muscle imbalances, joint dysfunction, or poor posture can create morphological changes in neural tissues. These changes might include intraneural edema, tissue hypoxia, chemical irritation, or microvascular stasis—all of which could stimulate nociceptors, creating pain. Pain causes muscle guarding and spasm

to protect the inflamed neural structures, and this alters normal movement patterns. Eventually neural fibrosis results, which decreases the elasticity of neural tissue and prevents normal movement within surrounding tissues.[21]

CLINICAL DECISION MAKING   **Exercise 8–2**

Two days after an intense weight-lifting workout, a football player is complaining of quad pain. The athletic trainer determines that the athlete has delayed-onset muscle soreness. The soreness is preventing the athlete from getting a sufficient stretch. What can be done to optimize his stretching?

ACTIVE AND PASSIVE RANGE OF MOTION

Active range of motion, also called *dynamic flexibility*, refers to the degree to which a joint can be moved by a muscle contraction, usually through the midrange of movement. Dynamic flexibility is not necessarily a good indicator of the stiffness or looseness of a joint, because it applies to the ability to move a joint efficiently, with little resistance to motion.[48]

Passive range of motion, sometimes called *static flexibility*, refers to the degree to which a joint can be passively moved to the end points in the range of motion. No muscle contraction is involved to move a joint through a passive range.

When a muscle actively contracts, it produces a joint movement through a specific range of motion.[83,100] However, if passive pressure is applied to an extremity, it is capable of moving farther in the range of motion. It is essential in sports activities that an extremity be capable of moving through a nonrestricted range of motion.[87]

Passive range of motion is important for injury prevention. There are many situations in physical activity in which a muscle is forced to stretch beyond its normal active limits. If the muscle does not have enough elasticity to compensate for this additional stretch, it is likely that the musculotendinous unit will be injured.

Assessment of Active and Passive Range of Motion

Accurate measurement of active and passive range of joint motion is difficult.[50] Various devices have been designed to accommodate variations in the size of the joints, as well as the complexity of movements in articulations that involve more than one joint.[50] Of these devices, the simplest and most widely used is the *goniometer* (Figure 8-3).

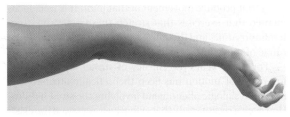

Figure 8-2   Excessive joint motion, such as the hyperextended elbow, can predispose a joint to injury.

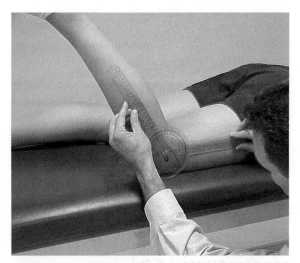

Figure 8-3 Measurement of active knee joint flexion using a goniometer.

A goniometer is a large protractor with measurements in degrees. By aligning the individual arms of the goniometer parallel to the longitudinal axis of the two segments involved in motion about a specific joint, it is possible to obtain reasonably accurate measurement of range of movement. To enhance reliability, standardization of measurement techniques and methods of recording active and passive ranges of motion are critical in individual clinics where successive measurements might be taken by different athletic trainers to assess progress.[49] Table 8-1 provides a list of what would be considered normal active ranges for movements at various joints.

The goniometer has an important place in a rehabilitation setting, where it is essential to assess improvement in joint flexibility to modify injury rehabilitation programs.

In some clinics a digital inclinometer is used instead of a goniometer. An inclinometer is a more precise measuring instrument with high reliability that has most often been used in research settings. Digital inclinometers are affordable and can easily be used to accurately measure range of motion of all joints of the body from complex movements of the spine and large joints of the extremities to the small joints of fingers and toes.

STRETCHING TO IMPROVE MOBILITY

The goal of any effective stretching program should be to improve the range of motion at a given articulation by altering the extensibility of the neuromusculotendinous

■ TABLE 8-1 Active Ranges of Joint Motions

Joint	Action	Degrees Of Motion
Shoulder	Flexion	0–180°
	Extension	0–50°
	Abduction	0–180°
	Medial rotation	0–90°
	Lateral rotation	0–90°
	Flexion	0–90°
Elbow	Flexion	0–160°
Forearm	Pronation	0–90°
	Supination	0–90°
Wrist	Flexion	0–90°
	Extension	0–70°
	Abduction	0–25°
	Adduction	0–65°
Hip	Flexion	0–125°
	Extension	0–15°
	Abduction	0–45°
	Adduction	0–15°
	Medial rotation	0–45°
	Lateral rotation	0–45°
Knee	Flexion	0–140°
Ankle	Plantarflexion	0–45°
	Dorsiflexion	0–20°
Foot	Inversion	0–30°
	Eversion	0–10°

units that produce movement at that joint. It is well documented that exercises that stretch these neuromusculotendinous units and their fascia over time will increase the range of movement possible about a given joint.[41,80]

For many years the efficacy of stretching in improving range of motion has been theoretically attributed to neurophysiologic phenomena involving the stretch reflex. However, a recent study that extensively reviewed the existing literature has suggested that improvements in range of motion resulting from stretching must be explained by mechanisms other than the stretch reflex.[19] Studies reviewed indicate that changes in the ability to tolerate stretch and/or the viscoelastic properties of the stretched muscle are possible mechanisms.

NEUROPHYSIOLOGIC BASIS OF STRETCHING

Every muscle in the body contains various types of mechanoreceptors that, when stimulated, inform the central nervous system of what is happening with that muscle. Two of these mechanoreceptors are important in the stretch reflex: the *muscle spindle* and the *Golgi tendon organ.* Both types of receptors are sensitive to changes in muscle length. The Golgi tendon organs are also affected by changes in muscle tension.

When a muscle is stretched, both the muscle spindles and the Golgi tendon organs immediately begin sending a volley of sensory impulses to the spinal cord. Initially impulses coming from the muscle spindles inform the central nervous system that the muscle is being stretched. Impulses return to the muscle from the spinal cord, causing the muscle to reflexively contract, thus resisting the stretch.[68] The Golgi tendon organs respond to the change in length and the increase in tension by firing off sensory impulses of their own to the spinal cord. If the stretch of the muscle continues for an extended period of time (at least 6 seconds), impulses from the Golgi tendon organs begin to override muscle spindle impulses. The impulses from the Golgi tendon organs, unlike the signals from the muscle spindle, cause a reflex relaxation of the antagonist muscle. This reflex relaxation serves as a protective mechanism that will allow the muscle to stretch through relaxation without exceeding the extensibility limits, which could damage the muscle fibers.[12] This relaxation of the antagonist muscle during contractions is referred to as *autogenic inhibition.*

In any synergistic muscle group, a contraction of the agonist causes a reflex relaxation in the antagonist muscle, allowing it to stretch and protecting it from injury. This phenomenon is referred to as reciprocal inhibition[92] (see Figure 14-2 on p. 301).

EFFECTS OF STRETCHING ON THE PHYSICAL AND MECHANICAL PROPERTIES OF MUSCLE

The neurophysiologic mechanisms of both autogenic and reciprocal inhibition result in reflex relaxation with subsequent lengthening of a muscle. Thus the mechanical properties of that muscle that physically allow lengthening to occur are dictated via neural input.

Both muscle and tendon are composed largely of noncontractile collagen and elastin fibers. Collagen enables a tissue to resist mechanical forces and deformation, whereas elastin composes highly elastic tissues that assist in recovery from deformation.[62]

Collagen has several mechanical and physical properties that allow it to respond to loading and deformation, permitting it to withstand high tensile stress.[103] The mechanical properties of collagen include (1) *elasticity,* which is the capability to recover normal length after elongation; (2) *viscoelasticity,* which allows for a slow return to normal length and shape after deformation, and (3) *plasticity,* which allows for permanent change or deformation. The physical properties include (1) *force-relaxation,* which indicates the decrease in the amount of force needed to maintain a tissue at a set amount of displacement or deformation over time; (2) the *creep response,* which is the ability of a tissue to deform over time while a constant load is imposed; and (3) *hysteresis,* which is the amount of relaxation a tissue has undergone during deformation and displacement. If the mechanical and physical limitations of connective tissue are exceeded, injury results.

Unlike tendon, muscle also has active contractile components that are the actin and myosin myofilaments. Collectively the contractile and noncontractile elements determine the muscle's capability of deforming and recovering from deformation.[112]

Both the contractile and the noncontractile components appear to resist deformation when a muscle is stretched or lengthened. The percentage of their individual contribution to resisting deformation depends on the degree to which the muscle is stretched or deformed and on the velocity of deformation. The noncontractile elements are primarily resistant to the degree of lengthening, while the contractile elements limit high-velocity deformation. The greater the stretch, the more the noncontractile components contribute.[103]

Lengthening of a muscle via stretching allows for viscoelastic and plastic changes to occur in the collagen and elastin fibers. The viscoelastic changes that allow slow deformation with imperfect recovery are not permanent. However, plastic changes, although difficult to achieve, result in residual or permanent change in length due to deformation created by long periods of stretching.

The greater the velocity of deformation, the greater the chance for exceeding that tissue's capability to undergo viscoelastic and plastic change.[112]

EFFECTS OF STRETCHING ON THE KINETIC CHAIN

Joint hypomobility is one of the most frequently treated causes of pain. However, the etiology can usually be traced to faulty posture, muscular imbalances, and abnormal neuromuscular control. Once a particular joint has lost its normal arthrokinematics, the muscles around that joint attempt to minimize the stress at that involved segment. Certain muscles become tight and hypertonic to prevent additional joint translation. If one muscle becomes tight or changes its degree of activation, then synergists, stabilizers, and neutralizers have to compensate, leading to the formation of complex neuromusculoskeletal dysfunctions.

Muscle tightness and hypertonicity have a significant impact on neuromuscular control. Muscle tightness affects the normal length–tension relationships. When one muscle in a force-couple becomes tight or hypertonic, it alters the normal arthrokinematics of the involved joint. This affects the synergistic function of the entire kinetic chain, leading to abnormal joint stress, soft-tissue dysfunction, neural compromise, and vascular/lymphatic stasis. These result in alterations in recruitment strategies and stabilization strength. Such compensations and adaptations affect neuromuscular efficiency throughout the kinetic chain. Decreased neuromuscular control alters the activation sequence or firing order of different muscles involved, and a specific movement is disturbed. Prime movers may be slow to activate, while synergists, stabilizers, and neutralizers substitute and become overactive. When this is the case, new joint stresses will be encountered.[21] For example, if the psoas is tight or hyperactive, then the gluteus maximus will have decreased neural drive. If the gluteus maximus (prime mover during hip extension) has decreased neural drive, then synergists (hamstrings), stabilizers (erector spinae), and neutralizers (piriformis) substitute and become overactive (synergistic dominance). This creates abnormal joint stress and decreased neuromuscular control during functional movements.

Muscle tightness also causes reciprocal inhibition. Increased muscle spindle activity in a specific muscle will cause decreased neural drive to that muscle's functional antagonist. This alters the normal force-couple activity, which in turn affects the normal arthrokinematics of the involved segment. For example, if a patient has tightness or hypertonicity in the psoas, then the functional antagonist (gluteus maximus) can be inhibited (decreased neural drive), causing decreased neuromuscular control. This in turn leads to synergistic dominance—the neuromuscular phenomenon that occurs when synergists compensate for a weak and/or inhibited muscle to maintain force

production capabilities.[21] This process alters the normal force-couple relationships, which in turn creates a chain reaction.

IMPORTANCE OF INCREASING MUSCLE TEMPERATURE PRIOR TO STRETCHING

To most effectively stretch a muscle during a program of rehabilitation, intramuscular temperature should be increased prior to stretching.[75] Increasing the temperature has a positive effect on the ability of the collagen and elastin components within the musculotendinous unit to deform. Also, the capability of the Golgi tendon organs to reflexively relax the muscle through autogenic inhibition is enhanced when the muscle is heated. It appears that the optimal temperature of muscle to achieve these beneficial effects is 39°C, or 103°F. This increase in intramuscular temperature can be achieved either through low-intensity warm-up type exercise or through the use of various therapeutic modalities.[44,91] It is recommended that exercise be used as the primary means for increasing intramuscular temperature.

The use of cold prior to stretching has also been recommended. Cold appears to be most useful when there is some muscle guarding associated with delayed-onset muscle soreness.[82]

CLINICAL DECISION MAKING   **Exercise 8–3**

Following ACL surgery, one of the first goals of rehabilitation is to regain full ROM. How can improvements in knee extension be quantified for day-to-day record keeping?

STRETCHING TECHNIQUES

Stretching techniques for improving flexibility have evolved over the years.[57] The oldest technique for stretching is *dynamic stretching* (ballistic) which makes use of repetitive bouncing motions. A second technique, known as *static stretching*, involves stretching a muscle to the point of discomfort and then holding it at that point for an extended time. This technique has been used for many years. Another group of stretching techniques known collectively as *proprioceptive neuromuscular facilitation* (PNF) techniques, involving alternating contractions and stretches, has also been recommended[58,108] (Figure 8-4). Most recently, emphasis has been on the contribution of *stretching myofascial tissue* as well as *stretching tight neural tissue* in enhancing the ability of the neuromuscular system to efficiently control movement through a full range

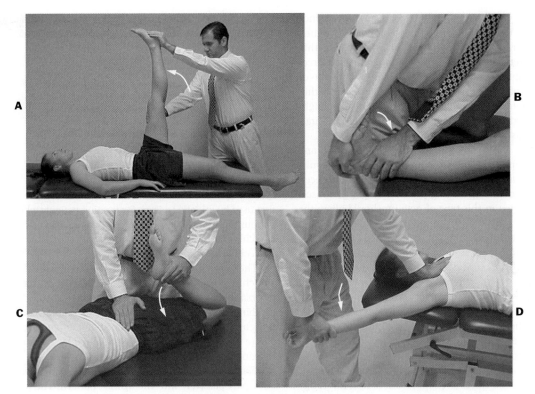

Figure 8-4   Examples of stretching exercises that may be done statically or using a PNF technique. **A,** Hamstrings. **B,** Ankle plantar flexors. **C,** Quadriceps. **D,** Glenohumeral joint extensors.

of motion. Researchers have had considerable discussion about which of these techniques is most effective for improving range of motion, and no clear-cut consensus currently exists.[11,32,41,66,80,86]

Agonist Versus Antagonist Muscles

Before discussing the different stretching techniques, it is essential to define the terms *agonist muscle* and *antagonist muscle.* Most joints in the body are capable of more than one movement. The knee joint, for example, is capable of flexion and extension. Contraction of the quadriceps group of muscles on the front of the thigh causes knee extension, whereas contraction of the hamstring muscles on the back of the thigh produces knee flexion.

To achieve knee extension, the quadriceps group contracts while the hamstring muscles relax and stretch. Muscles that work in concert with one another in this manner are called synergistic muscle groups.[8] The muscle that contracts to produce a movement, in this case the quadriceps, is referred to as the agonist muscle. The muscle being stretched in response to contraction of the agonist

muscle is called the antagonist muscle.[40] In this example of knee extension, the antagonist muscle would be the hamstring group. Some degree of balance in strength must exist between agonist and antagonist muscle groups. This balance is necessary for normal, smooth, coordinated movement, as well as for reducing the likelihood of muscle strain caused by muscular imbalance. Comprehension of this synergistic muscle action is essential to understanding the various techniques of stretching.

CLINICAL DECISION MAKING   **Exercise 8–4**

During a preseason screening, you observe that a rower has only 120 degrees of knee flexion. What are some of the things that might be limiting this motion?

Dynamic Stretching

In dynamic stretching, repetitive contractions of the agonist muscle are used to produce quick stretches of the antagonist muscle.

Over the years, many fitness experts have questioned the safety of the dynamic stretching technique.[47,68] Their concerns have been primarily based on the idea that dynamic stretching creates somewhat uncontrolled forces within the muscle that can exceed the extensibility limits of the muscle fiber, thus producing small microtears within the musculotendinous unit.[35,39,74,112] Certainly this might be true in sedentary individuals or perhaps in individuals who have sustained muscle injuries.

However, many physical activities are dynamic and require a repeated dynamic contraction of the agonist muscle. The antagonist contracting eccentrically to decelerate the dynamic stretching of the antagonist muscle before engaging in this type of activity should allow the muscle to gradually adapt to the imposed demands and reduce the likelihood of injury. Because dynamic stretching is more functional, it should be integrated into a reconditioning program during the later stages of healing when appropriate.

A progressive velocity flexibility program has been proposed that takes the patient through a series of stretching exercises where the velocity of the stretch and the range of lengthening are progressively controlled.[81] The stretching exercises progress from slow static stretching to slow, short, end-range stretching, to slow, full-range stretching, to fast, short, end-range stretching, and to fast, full-range stretching. This program allows the patient to control both the range and the speed with no assistance from an athletic trainer.

Static Stretching

The static stretching technique is another extremely effective and widely used technique of stretching.[52] This technique involves stretching a given antagonist muscle passively by placing it in a maximal position of stretch and holding it there for an extended time. Recommendations for the optimal time for holding this stretched position vary, ranging from as little as 3 seconds to as much as 60 seconds.[48] Several studies have indicated that holding a stretch for 15–30 seconds is the most effective for increasing muscle flexibility.[6,64,67] Stretches lasting longer than 30 seconds seem to be uncomfortable. A static stretch of each muscle should be repeated three or four times. A static stretch can be accomplished by using a contraction of the agonist muscle to place the antagonist muscle in a position of stretch. A passive static stretch requires the use of body weight, assistance from an athletic trainer or partner, or use of a T-bar, primarily for stretching the upper extremity.

CLINICAL DECISION MAKING   **Exercise 8–5**

A freshman high school cross-country runner needs to know how to best stretch on his own. What should he know about how far to go in his stretch and how long he should hold it?

Proprioceptive Neuromuscular Facilitation Stretching Techniques

Proprioceptive neuromuscular facilitation techniques were first used by athletic trainers for treating patients who had various neuromuscular disorders.[58] More recently, PNF stretching exercises have increasingly been used as a stretching technique for improving flexibility.[24,64,71,73]

There are three different PNF techniques used for stretching: contract-relax, hold-relax techniques, and slow reversal-hold-relax.[102] All three techniques involve some combination of alternating isometric or isotonic contractions and relaxation of both agonist and antagonist muscles (a 10-second pushing phase followed by a 10-second relaxing phase).

Contract-relax is a stretching technique that moves the body part passively into the agonist pattern. The patient is instructed to push by contracting the antagonist (the muscle that will be stretched) isotonically against the resistance of the athletic trainer. The patient then relaxes the antagonist while the athletic trainer moves the part passively through as much range as possible to the point where limitation is again felt. This contract-relax technique is beneficial when range of motion is limited by muscle tightness.

Hold-relax is very similar to the contract-relax technique. It begins with an isometric contraction of the antagonist (the muscle that will be stretched) against resistance, combined with light pressure from the athletic trainer to produce maximal stretch of the antagonist. This technique is appropriate when there is muscle tension on one side of a joint and may be used with either the agonist or the antagonist.

Slow reversal-hold-relax, also occasionally referred to as the *contract-relax-agonist-contraction* technique, begins with an isotonic contraction of the agonist, which often limits range of motion in the agonist pattern, followed by an isometric contraction of the antagonist (the muscle that will be stretched) during the push phase. During the relax phase, the antagonists are relaxed while the agonists are contracting, causing movement in the direction of the agonist pattern and thus stretching the antagonist. This technique, like the contract-relax and hold-relax, is useful for increasing range of motion when the primary limiting factor is the antagonistic muscle group.

PNF stretching techniques can be used to stretch any muscle in the body.[11,28,29,34,71,74,79,82,86,102] PNF stretching techniques are perhaps best performed with a partner, although they may also be done using a wall as resistance.

Comparing Stretching Techniques

Although all three stretching techniques discussed to this point have been demonstrated to effectively improve flexibility, there is still considerable debate as to which technique produces the greatest increases in range of movement.[7] The dynamic technique is recommended for anyone who is involved in dynamic activity, despite its potential for causing muscle soreness in the sedentary individual. In physically active individuals, it is unlikely that dynamic stretching will result in muscle soreness.

Static stretching is perhaps the most widely used technique. It is a simple technique and does not require a partner. A fully nonrestricted range of motion can be attained through static stretching over time.

Much research has been done comparing dynamic and static stretching techniques for the improvement of flexibility. Static and dynamic stretching appear to be equally effective in increasing flexibility, and there is no significant difference between the two.[36] However, much of the literature states that with static stretching there is less danger of exceeding the extensibility limits of the involved joints because the stretch is more controlled. Most of the literature indicates that dynamic stretching is apt to cause muscular soreness, especially in sedentary individuals, whereas static stretching generally does not cause soreness and is commonly used in injury rehabilitation of sore or strained muscles.[35,109] Static stretching is likely a much safer stretching technique, especially for sedentary individuals. However, because many physical activities involve dynamic movement, stretching in a warm-up should begin with static stretching followed by dynamic stretching, which more closely resembles the dynamic activity. PNF stretching techniques are capable of producing dramatic increases in range of motion during one stretching session. Studies comparing static and PNF stretching suggest that PNF stretching is capable of producing greater improvement in flexibility over an extended training period.[45,46,82] The major disadvantage of PNF stretching is that a partner is usually required to assist with the stretch, although stretching with an athletic trainer or partner can have some motivational advantages.

How long increases in muscle flexibility can be sustained once stretching stops is debatable.[38,94,113] One study indicated that a significant loss of flexibility was evident after only 2 weeks.[113] It was recommended that flexibility can be maintained by engaging in stretching activities at least once a week. However, to see improvement in flexibility, stretching must be done three to five times per week.[37]

Stretching Neural Structures

The athletic trainer should be able to differentiate between tightness in the musculotendinous unit and abnormal neural tension. The patient should perform both active and passive multiplanar movements that create tension in the neural structures that are exacerbating pain, limiting range of motion, and increasing neural symptoms, including numbness and tingling.[21] For example, the straight leg raising test not only applies pressure to the sacroiliac joint cell but also may indicate a problem in the sciatic nerve (Figure 8-5C). Internally rotating and adducting the hip increases the tension on the neural structures in both the greater sciatic notch and the intervertebral foramen. An exacerbation of pain from 30 degrees to 60 degrees indicates some sciatic nerve involvement. If dorsiflexing the ankle with maximum straight leg raising increases the pain, then the pain is likely due to some nerve root (L3-4, S1-3) or sciatic nerve irritation. Figure 8-5 shows the assessment and stretching positions for neural tension in the median, radial, and sciatic nerves as well as the vertebral nerve roots in the spine.

CLINICAL DECISION MAKING	Exercise 8–6

A coach asks the athletic trainer for recommendations for stretching to help improve the flexibility of his players. What three types of stretches could be recommended, and what are the advantages and disadvantages of each?

SPECIFIC STRETCHING EXERCISES

Chapters 17–24 will include various stretching exercises that may be used to improve flexibility at specific joints or in specific muscle groups throughout the body. The stretching exercises shown in Figure 8-4 provide examples which may be done statically; they may also be done with a partner using a PNF technique. There are many possible variations to each of these exercises.[54] The patient may also perform

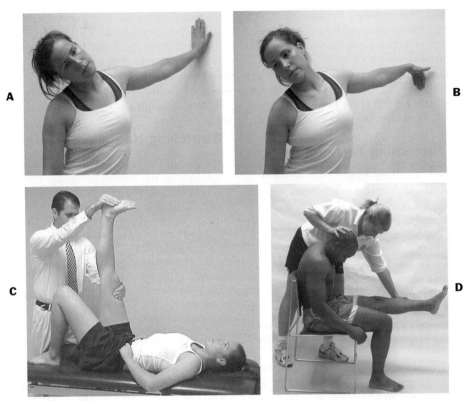

Figure 8-5 Neural tension stretches. **A,** Median nerve. **B,** Radial nerve. **C,** Sciatic nerve. **D,** Slump position.

static stretching exercises using a stability ball (Figure 8-6). The exercises selected are those that seem to be the most effective for stretching of various muscle groups. Table 8-2 provides a list of guidelines and precautions for stretching.

ALTERNATIVE STRETCHING TECHNIQUES

The Pilates Method of Stretching

The Pilates method is a somewhat different approach to stretching for improving flexibility. This method has become extremely popular and widely used among personal fitness trainers, physical therapists, and some athletic trainers. Pilates is an exercise technique devised by German-born Joseph Pilates, who established the first Pilates studio in the United States before World War II. The Pilates method is a conditioning program that improves muscle control, flexibility, coordination, strength, and tone.[10] The basic principles of Pilates exercise are to make the patient more aware of their bodies as single integrated units, to improve body alignment and breathing, and to increase efficiency of movement. Unlike other exercise programs, the Pilates method does not require the repetition of exercises but instead consists of a sequence of carefully performed movements, some of which are carried out on specially designed equipment (Figure 8-7). However, the majority of Pilates exercises are performed on a mat or floor without equipment. (Figure 8-8). Each exercise is designed to stretch and strengthen the muscles involved. There is a specific breathing pattern for each exercise to help direct energy to the areas being worked, while relaxing the rest of the body. The Pilates method works many of the deeper muscles together, improving coordination and balance, to achieve efficient and graceful movement. The goal for the patient is to develop a healthy self-image through the attainment of better posture, proper coordination, and improved flexibility. This method concentrates on body alignment, lengthening

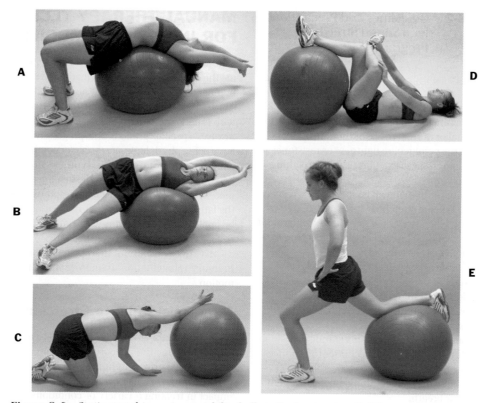

Figure 8-6   Static stretching using a stability ball. **A,** Back extension. **B,** Side stretch. **C,** Latissimus dorsi stretch. **D,** Piriformis stretch. **E,** Quadriceps stretch.

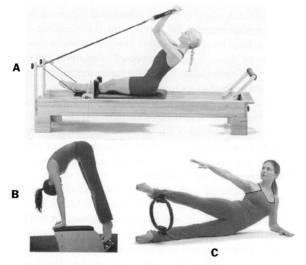

Figure 8-7   Pilates techniques using equipment. **A,** Reformer. **B,** Wunda chair. **C,** Magic ring.

all the muscles of the body into a balanced whole, and building endurance and strength without putting undue stress on the lungs and heart. Pilates instructors believe that problems such as soft-tissue injuries can cause bad posture, which can lead to pain and discomfort. Pilates exercises aim to correct this.

Yoga

Yoga originated in India approximately 6,000 years ago. Its basic philosophy is that most illness is related to poor mental attitudes, posture, and diet. Practitioners of yoga maintain that stress can be reduced through combined mental and physical approaches. Yoga can help an individual cope with stress-induced behaviors like overeating, hypertension, and smoking. Yoga's meditative aspects are believed to help alleviate psychosomatic illnesses. Yoga aims to unite the body and mind to reduce stress. [56] For example, Dr. Chandra Patel, a yoga expert, has found that persons who practice yoga can reduce their blood pressure

■ **TABLE 8-2** **Guidelines and Precautions for a Sound Stretching Program**[96,97]

....

- Warm up using a slow jog or fast walk before stretching vigorously.
- To increase flexibility, the muscle must be stretched within pain tolerances and tissue healing limitations to attain functional or normal range of motion.
- Stretch only to the point where tightness or resistance to stretch, or perhaps some discomfort, is felt. Stretching should not be painful.[1]
- Increases in range of motion will be specific to whatever muscle or joint is being stretched.
- Exercise caution when stretching muscles that surround painful joints. Pain is an indication that something is wrong and should not be ignored.
- Avoid overstretching the ligaments and capsules that surround joints.
- Exercise caution when stretching the low back and neck. Exercises that compress the vertebrae and their discs can cause damage.
- Stretching from a seated rather than a standing position takes stress off the low back and decreases the chances of back injury.
- Be sure to continue normal breathing during a stretch. Do not hold your breath.
- Static and PNF techniques are most often recommended for individuals who want to improve their range of motion.
- Dynamic stretching should be done only by those who are already flexible or accustomed to stretching, and should be done only after static stretching.

....

indefinitely as long as they continue to practice yoga. Yoga involves various body postures and breathing exercises. Hatha yoga uses a number of positions through which the practitioner may progress, beginning with the simplest and moving to the more complex (Figure 8-9). The various positions are intended to increase mobility and flexibility. However, practitioners must use caution when performing yoga positions. Some positions can be dangerous, particularly for someone who is inexperienced in yoga technique.

Slow, deep, diaphragmatic breathing is an important part of yoga. Many people take shallow breaths; however, breathing deeply and fully expanding the chest when inhaling helps lower blood pressure and heart rate. Deep breathing has a calming effect on the body. It also increases production of endorphins.[56]

MANUAL THERAPY TECHNIQUES FOR INCREASING MOBILITY

Following injury, soft tissue loses some of its ability to tolerate the demands of functional loading. A major part of the management of soft-tissue dysfunction lies in promoting soft-tissue adaptation to restore the tissue's ability to cope with functional loading.[53] Specific soft-tissue mobilization involves specific, graded, and progressive application of force using physiologic, accessory, or combined techniques either to promote collagen synthesis, orientation, and bonding in the early stages of the healing process or to promote changes in the viscoelastic response of the tissue in the later stages of healing. Soft-tissue mobilization should be applied in combination with rehabilitation regimes to restore the kinetic control of the tissue.[53]

A variety of manual therapy techniques can be used in injury rehabilitation to improve mobility and range of motion.

Myofascial Release Stretching

Myofascial release is a term that refers to a group of techniques used for the purpose of relieving soft tissue from the abnormal grip of tight fascia.[57] It is essentially a form of stretching that has been reported to have significant impact in treating a variety of conditions.[73] Some specialized training is necessary for the athletic trainer to understand specific techniques of myofascial release.[89] It is also essential to have an in-depth understanding of the fascial system.

Fascia is a type of connective tissue that surrounds muscles, tendons, nerves, bones, and organs. It is essentially continuous from head to toe and is interconnected in various sheaths or planes. Fascia is composed primarily of collagen along with some elastic fibers. During movement the fascia must stretch and move freely. If there is damage to the fascia owing to injury, disease, or inflammation, it will not only affect local adjacent structures but may also affect areas far removed from the site of the injury.[69] Thus it may be necessary to release tightness both in the area of injury and in distant areas. It will tend to soften and release in response to gentle pressure over a relatively long period of time.

Myofascial release has also been referred to as soft-tissue mobilization. Soft-tissue mobilization should not be confused with joint mobilization, although it must be emphasized that the two are closely related.[57] Joint mobilization is used to restore normal joint arthrokinematics, and specific rules exist regarding direction of movement and joint position based on the shape of the articulating surfaces (see

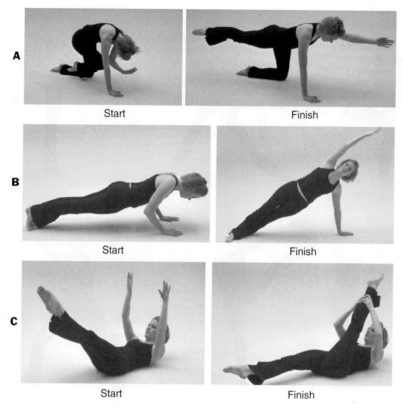

Figure 8-8   Pilates floor exercises. **A,** Alternating arm, opposite-leg extensions. **B,** Push-up to a side plank. **C,** Alternating leg scissors.

Chapter 13). Myofascial restrictions are considerably more unpredictable and may occur in many different planes and directions. Myofascial treatment is based on localizing the restriction and moving into the direction of the restriction, regardless of whether that follows the arthrokinematics of a nearby joint. Thus, myofascial manipulation is considerably more subjective and relies heavily on the experience of the athletic trainer.[69] Myofascial manipulation focuses on large treatment areas, whereas joint mobilization focuses on a specific joint. Releasing myofascial restrictions over a large treatment area can have a significant impact on joint mobility.[73] The progression of the technique is to work from superficial fascial restrictions to deeper restriction. Once more superficial restrictions are released, the deep restrictions can be located and released without causing any damage to superficial tissue. Joint mobilization should follow myofascial release and will likely be more effective once soft-tissue restrictions are eliminated.

As extensibility is improved in the myofascia, elongation and stretching of the musculotendinous unit should be incorporated. In addition, strengthening exercises are recommended to enhance neuromuscular reeducation, which helps promote new, more efficient movement patterns. As freedom of movement improves, postural reeducation may help ensure the maintenance of the less-restricted movement patterns.

Generally, acute cases tend to resolve in just a few treatments. The longer a condition has been present, the longer it will take to resolve. Occasionally, dramatic results will occur immediately after treatment. It is usually recommended that treatment be done at least three times per week.

Myofascial release can be done manually by an athletic trainer or by the patient stretching using a foam roller.[89] Figure 8-10 shows examples of stretching using the foam roller.

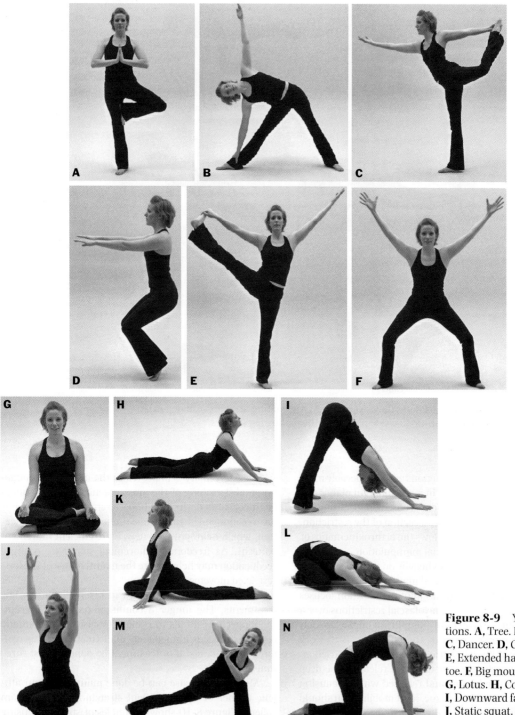

Figure 8-9 Yoga positions. **A,** Tree. **B,** Triangle. **C,** Dancer. **D,** Chair. **E,** Extended hand to big toe. **F,** Big mountain. **G,** Lotus. **H,** Cobra. **I,** Downward facing dog. **J,** Static squat. **K,** Pigeon. **L,** Child. **M,** Runner's lunge with twist. **N,** Cat.

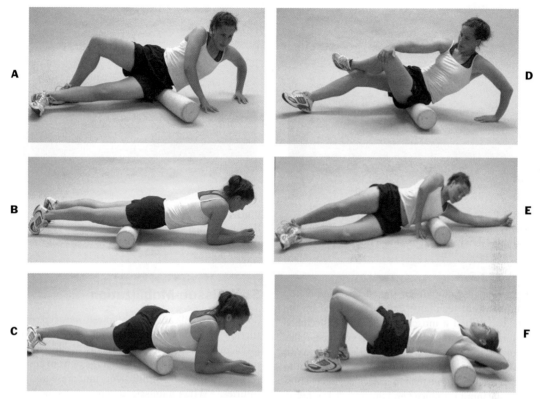

Figure 8-10   Myofascial release stretching using a foam roller. **A,** Tensor fascia latae. **B,** Quadriceps. **C,** Adductors. **D,** Piriformis. **E,** Teres minor. **F,** Thoracic spine.

Strain-Counterstrain Technique

Strain-counterstrain is an approach to decreasing muscle tension and guarding that may be used to normalize muscle function. It is a passive technique that places the body in a position of greatest comfort, thereby relieving pain.[1,55]

In this technique, the athletic trainer locates "tender points" on the patient's body that correspond to areas of dysfunction in specific joints or muscles that are in need of treatment.[99] These tender points are not located in or just beneath the skin, as are many acupuncture points, but instead are deeper in muscle, tendon, ligament, or fascia. They are characterized by tense, tender, edematous spots on the body. They are 1 cm or less in diameter, with the most acute points being 3 mm in diameter, although they may be a few centimeters long within a muscle. There can be multiple points for one specific joint dysfunction. Points might be arranged in a chain, and they are often found in a painless area opposite the site of pain and/or weakness.[55]

The athletic trainer monitors the tension and level of pain elicited by the tender point while moving the patient into a position of ease or comfort. This is accomplished by markedly shortening the muscle.[99] When this position of ease is found, the tender point is no longer tense or tender. When this position is maintained for a minimum of 90 seconds, the tension in the tender point and in the corresponding joint or muscle is reduced or cleared. By slowly returning to a neutral position, the tender point and the corresponding joint or muscle remains pain-free with normal tension. For example, with neck pain and/or tension headaches, the tender point may be found on either the front or back of the patient's neck and shoulders. The athletic trainer will have the patient lie on his/her back and will gently and slowly bend the patient's neck until that tender point is no longer tender. After holding that position for 90 seconds, the athletic trainer gently and slowly returns the neck to its resting position. When that tender point is pressed again, the patient should notice a significant decrease in pain there (Figure 8-11).[99]

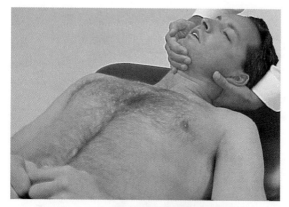

Figure 8-11 Strain-Counterstrain Technique. The body part is placed in a position of comfort for 90 seconds and then slowly moved back to a neutral position.

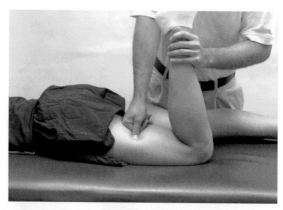

Figure 8-12 The positional release technique places the muscle in a position of comfort with the finger or thumb exerting submaximal pressure on a myofascial trigger point.

The physiologic rationale for the effectiveness of the strain-counterstrain technique can be explained by the stretch reflex.[2] When a muscle is placed in a stretched position, impulses from the muscle spindles create a reflex contraction of the muscle in response to stretch. With strain-counterstrain, the joint or muscle is placed not in a position of stretch but instead in a slack position. Thus, muscle spindle input is reduced and the muscle is relaxed, allowing for a decrease in tension and pain.[2]

Positional Release Therapy

Positional release therapy is based on the strain-counterstrain technique. The primary difference between the two is the use of a facilitating force (compression) to enhance the effect of the positioning.[17,18,90,95]

Like strain-counterstrain, PRT is an osteopathic mobilization technique in which the body part is moved into a position of greatest relaxation.[33] The athletic trainer finds the position of greatest comfort and muscle relaxation for each joint with the help of movement tests and diagnostic tender points. Once located, the tender point is maintained with the palpating finger at a subthreshold pressure. The patient is then passively placed in a position that reduces the tension under the palpating finger producing a subjective reduction in tenderness as reported by the patient. This specific position is adjusted throughout the 90-second treatment period. It has been suggested that maintaining contact with the tender point during the treatment period exerts a therapeutic effect.[17,18] This technique is one of the most effective and gentle methods for the treatment of acute and chronic musculoskeletal dysfunction[90] (Figure 8-12).

Soft Tissue Mobilization

Soft tissue mobilization is a relatively new type of manual therapy that has been developed to correct soft-tissue problems in muscle, tendon, and fascia caused by the formation of fibrotic adhesions that result from acute injury, repetitive or overuse injuries, constant pressure, or tension injuries.[63] When a muscle, tendon, fascia, or ligament is torn (strained or sprained) or a nerve is damaged, the tissues heal with adhesions or scar tissue formation rather than the formation of brand new tissue. Scar tissue is weaker, less elastic, less pliable, and more pain-sensitive than healthy tissue.

These fibrotic adhesions disrupt the normal muscle function, which in turn affects the biomechanics of the joint complex and can lead to pain and dysfunction. Soft tissue mobilization provides a way to diagnose and treat the underlying causes of cumulative trauma disorders that, left uncorrected, can lead to inflammation, adhesions, fibrosis, and muscle imbalances. All of these can result in weak and tense tissues, decreased circulation, hypoxia, and symptoms of peripheral nerve entrapment, including numbness, tingling, burning, and aching.[63] Soft tissue mobilization is a deep-tissue technique used for breaking down scar tissue/adhesions and restoring function and movement.[63] In soft tissue mobilization, the athletic trainer first locates through palpation those adhesions in the muscle, tendon, or fascia that are causing the problem. Once these are located, the athletic trainer traps the affected muscle by applying pressure or tension with the thumb or finger over these lesions in the direction of the fibers. Then the patient is asked to actively move the body part such that the musculature is elongated from a shortened position while the athletic trainer continues to apply tension to the lesion (Figure 8-13). This should be repeated three to five times per treatment session. By breaking up the adhesions, the technique improves the patient's condition by softening and stretching the scar tissue, resulting in increased range of motion, increased strength, and improved circulation, optimizing healing. Treatments tend to be uncomfortable during the movement phases as the scar tissue or adhesions tear apart.[63] This is temporary and subsides almost immediately after the treatment. An important part of soft tissue mobilization is for the patient to heed the athletic trainer's recommendations regarding activity modification, stretching, and exercise.

Graston Technique®

The Graston Technique® is an instrument-assisted soft tissue mobilization that enables clinicians to effectively break down scar tissue and fascial restrictions as well as stretch connective tissue and muscle fibers[36,51] (Figure 8-14). The technique utilizes six hand-held specially-designed stainless steel instruments shaped to fit the contour of the body, to scan an area, locate and then treat the injured tissue that is causing pain and restricting motion.[51] A clinician normally will palpate a painful area looking for usual nodules, restrictive barriers or tissue tensions. The instruments help to magnify existing restrictions and the clinician can feel these through the instruments.[36] Then, the clinician can utilize the instruments to supply precise pressure to break up scar tissue, relieving the discomfort and helping to restore normal function. The instruments, with a narrow surface area at their edge, have the ability to separate fibers.

A specially designed lubricant is applied to the skin prior to utilizing the instrument, allowing the instrument to glide over the skin without causing irritation. Using a cross-friction massage in multiple directions, which involves using the instruments to stroke or rub against the grain of the scar tissue, the clinician creates small amounts of trauma to the affected area.[36] This temporarily causes inflammation in the area, increasing the rate and amount of blood flow in and around the area. The theory is that this process helps initiate and promote the healing process of the affected soft tissues. It is common for the patient to experience some discomfort during the procedure and possibly some bruising. Ice application following the treatment may ease the discomfort. It is recommended that an exercise, stretching, and strengthening program be used in conjunction with the technique to help the injured tissues heal.

Massage

Massage is a mechanical stimulation of the tissues by means of rhythmically applied pressure and stretching (Figure 8-15).[83] Over the years, many claims have been made relative to the therapeutic benefits of massage, but few are based on well-controlled, well-designed studies. Athletic trainers have used massage to increase flexibility and coordination as well as to increase pain threshold; to decrease neuromuscular excitability in the muscle being massaged; to stimulate circulation, thus improving energy transport to the muscle; to facilitate healing and restore joint mobility; and to remove lactic acid, thus alleviating muscle cramps.[83]

How these effects can be accomplished is determined by the specific approaches used with massage techniques

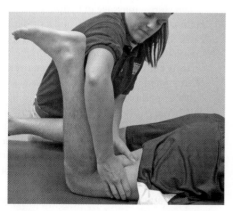
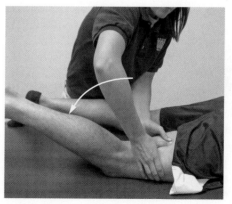

Figure 8-13   Soft tissue mobilization technique. The muscle is elongated from a shortened position while static pressure is applied to the tender point.

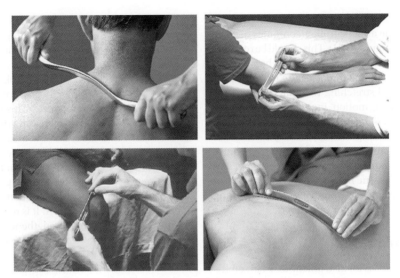

Figure 8-14   The Graston technique uses handheld stainless steel instruments to locate and then separate existing restrictions within a muscle. Source: Courtesy of The Graston Technique®.

and how they are applied. Generally the effects of massage are either *reflexive* or *mechanical*. The effect of massage on the nervous system will differ greatly according to the method employed, the pressure exerted, and the duration of applications. Through the reflex mechanism, sedation is induced. Slow, gentle, rhythmical, and superficial *effleurage* may relieve tension and soothe, rendering the muscles more relaxed. This indicates an effect on sensory and motor nerves locally and some central nervous system response. The mechanical approach seeks to make mechanical or histological changes in myofascial structures through direct force applied superficially.[83]

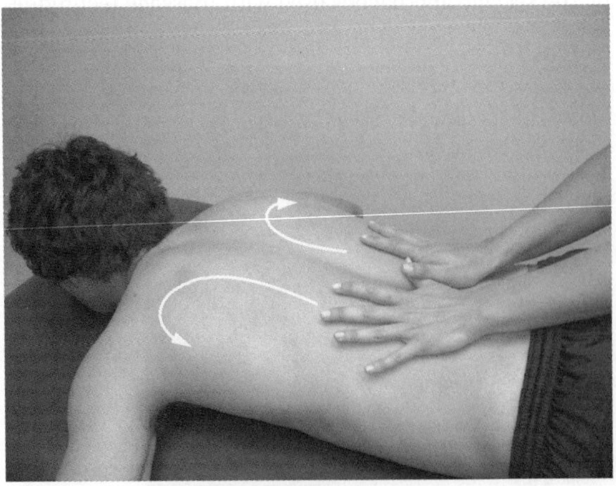

Among the massage techniques used by athletic trainers are the following[83]:

1. *Hoffa massage*—the classic form of massage, strokes include effleurage, petrissage, percussion or tapotement, and vibration.
2. *Friction massage*—used to increase the inflammatory response, particularly in case of chronic tendinitis or tenosynovitis.
3. *Acupressure*—massage of acupuncture and trigger points, used to reduce pain and irritation in anatomical areas known to be associated with specific points.
4. *Connective tissue massage*—a stroking technique used on layers of connective tissue, a relatively new form of treatment in this country, primarily affecting circulatory pathologies.
5. *Myofascial release*—used for the purpose of relieving soft tissue from the abnormal grip of tight fascia.
6. *Rolfing*—a system devised to correct inefficient structure by balancing the body within a gravitational field through a technique involving manual soft-tissue manipulation.
7. *Trager*—attempts to establish neuromuscular control so that more normal movement patterns can be routinely performed.

Figure 8-15   Massage can be an extremely effective technique for improving mobility and range of motion.

Summary

1. Flexibility is the ability of the neuromuscular system to allow for efficient movement of a joint or a series of joints smoothly through a full range of motion.
2. Flexibility is specific to a given joint, and the term *good flexibility* implies that there are no joint abnormalities restricting movement.
3. Flexibility can be limited by muscles and tendons and their fascia, joint capsules or ligaments, fat, bone structure, skin, or neural tissue.
4. *Passive range of motion* refers to the degree to which a joint can be passively moved to the end points in the range of motion. *Active range of motion* refers to movement through the midrange of motion resulting from active contraction.
5. Measurement of joint flexibility is accomplished through the use of a goniometer or an inclinometer.
6. An agonist muscle is one that contracts to produce joint motion, while the antagonist muscle is stretched with contraction of the agonist.
7. Increases in flexibility can be attributed to neurophysiologic adaptations involving the stretch reflex and associated muscle spindles and Golgi tendon organs, changes in the viscoelastic and plastic properties of muscle, adaptations and changes in the kinetic chain, and alterations in intramuscular temperature.
8. Dynamic, static, and PNF techniques have all been used as stretching techniques for improving flexibility.
9. Stretching of tight neural structures and myofascial release stretching are also used to reestablish a full range of motion.
10. Strain-counterstrain is a passive technique that places a body part in a position of greatest comfort to decrease muscle tension and guarding, and to relieve pain.
11. Positional release therapy is similar to strain-counterstrain. Pressure is maintained on a tender point with the body part in a position of comfort for 90 seconds.
12. Soft tissue mobilization is a deep-tissue technique used for breaking down scar tissue and adhesions and restoring function and movement.
13. Massage is the mechanical stimulation of tissue by means of rhythmically applied pressure and stretching. It allows the athletic trainer, as a health care provider, to help a patient overcome pain and relax through the application of the therapeutic massage techniques.

References

1. Alexander, K. M. 1999. Use of strain-counterstrain as an adjunct for treatment of chronic lower abdominal pain. *Phy Ther Case Rep* 2(5):205–208.
2. Allerheiliger, W. 2008. Stretching and warm-up. In *Essentials of strength training and conditioning*, Baechle T, ed. Champaign, IL: Human Kinetics.
3. Alter, M. 2004. *The science of flexibility.* Champaign, IL: Human Kinetics.
4. Andersen, J. C. 2005. Stretching before and after exercise: Effect on muscle soreness and injury risk. *J Athlet Train* 40(3): 218–220.
5. Armiger, P. 2000. Preventing musculotendinous injuries: A focus on flexibility. *Athletic Ther Today* 5(4):20.
6. Bandy, W. D., and J. M. Irion. 1994. The effect of time of static stretch on the flexibility of the hamstring muscles. *Phys Ther* 74: 845–852.
7. Bandy, W. D., J. M. Irion, and M. Briggler. 1998. The effect of static stretch and dynamic range of motion training on the flexibility of the hamstring muscles. *J Orthop Sports Phys Ther* 27(4):295.
8. Basmajian, J. 1984. *Therapeutic exercise*, 4th ed. Baltimore, MD: Lippincott Williams & Wilkins.
9. Behm, D. G., A. Bambury, F. Cahill, and K. Power. 2004. Effect of acute static stretching on force, balance, reaction time, and movement time. *Med Sci Sports Exerc.* 36(8):1397–1402.
10. Bernardo, L. 2007. The effectiveness of Pilates training in healthy adults: An appraisal of the research literature. *Journal of Bodywork and Movement Therapies* 11(2): 106–10.
11. Blahnik, J. 2004. *Full body flexibility.* Champaign, IL: Human Kinetics.
12. Blanke, D. 2002. Flexibility. In *Sports medicine secrets*, Mellion, M., ed. Philadelphia, PA: Hanley & Belfus.
13. Boyle, P. 2004. The effect of static and dynamic stretching on muscle force production. *J Sports Sci* 22(3):273–274.
14. Burke, D. G., C. J. Culligan, and L. E. Holt. 2000. The theoretical basis of proprioceptive neuromuscular facilitation. *J Strength Cond Res* 14(4):496–500.
15. Carter, A. M., S. J. Kinzey, L. F. Chitwood, and J. L. Cole. 2000. Proprioceptive neuromuscular facilitation decreases muscle activity during the stretch reflex in selected posterior thigh muscles. *J Sport Rehab* 9(4):269–278.
16. Chaitlow, L. 2006. *Muscle energy techniques.* Philadelphia, PA: Churchill Livingstone.

17. Chaitlow, L. 2002. *Positional release techniques (advanced soft tissue techniques).* Philadelphia, PA: Churchill Livingstone.

18. Chaitlow, L. 1998. Positional release techniques in the treatment of muscle and joint dysfunction. *Clin Bull Myofascial Ther* 3(1):25–35.

19. Chalmers, G. 2004. Re-examination of the possible role of golgi tendon organ and muscle spindle reflexes in proprioceptive neuromuscular facilitation muscle stretching. *Sports Biomechanics* 3(1):159–183.

20. Chapman, E. A., H. A. deVries, and R. Swezey. 1972. Joint stiffness: Effect of exercise on young and old men. *J Gerontol* 27:218.

21. Clark, M. 2001. *Integrated training for the new millennium.* Calabasas, CA: National Academy of Sports Medicine.

22. Condon, S. A., and R. S. Hutton. 1987. Soleus muscle EMG activity and ankle dorsiflexion range of motion from stretching procedures. *Phys Ther* 67:24–30.

23. Corbin, C., and K. Fox. 1985. Flexibility: The forgotten part of fitness. *J Phys Educ* 16(6):191.

24. Corbin, C., and L. Noble. 1980. Flexibility. *J Phys Educ Rec Dance* 51:23.

25. Corbin, C., and L. Noble. 1985. Flexibility: A major component of physical fitness. In *Implementation of health fitness exercise programs*, Cundiff, D. E., ed. Reston, VA: American Alliance for Health, Physical Education, Recreation and Dance.

26. Cornelius, W., and A. Jackson. 1984. The effects of cryotherapy and PNF on hip extensor flexibility. *J Athlet Train* 19:183–184.

27. Cornelius, W. L., R. W. Hagemann, Jr., and A. W. Jackson. 1988. A study on placement of stretching within a workout. *J Sports Med Phys Fitness* 28(3):234.

28. Cornelius, W. L. 1986. *PNF and other flexibility techniques.* Arlington, VA: Computer Microfilm International. (microfiche; 20 fr.).

29. Cornelius, W. L. 1981. Two effective flexibility methods. *Athlet Train* 16(1):23.

30. Cornwell, A. 1997. The acute effects of passive stretching on active musculotendinous stiffness. *Med Sci Sports Exerc* 29(5), 281.

31. Couch, J. 1982. *Runners world yoga book.* Mountain View, CA: World.

32. Cross, K. M., and T. W. Worrell. 1999. Effects of a static stretching program on the incidence of lower extremity musculotendinous strains. *J Athlet Train* 34(1):11.

33. D'Ambrogio, K., and G. Roth. 1996. *Positional release therapy: Assessment and treatment of musculoskeletal dysfunction.* St. Louis: Mosby/Year Book.

34. Decoster, L., J. Cleland, and C. Altieri. 2005. The effects of hamstring stretching on range of motion: A systematic literature review. *J Orthop Sports Phys Ther* 3(6):377–387.

35. DeLuccio, J. 2006. Instrument assisted soft tissue mobilization utilizing Graston technique: a physical therapist's perspective. *Orthopaedic Physical Therapy Practice* 18(3): 32–4.

36. deVries, H. A. 1962. Evaluation of static stretching procedures for improvement of flexibility. *Res Q* 3:222–229.

37. De Deyne, P. G. 2001. Application of passive stretch and its implications for muscle fibers. *Phys Ther* 81(2):819–827.

38. DePino, G. M., W. G. Webright, and B. L. Arnold. 2000. Duration of maintained hamstring flexibility after cessation of an acute static stretching protocol. *J Athlet Train* 35(1):56.

39. Entyre, B. R., and L. D. Abraham. 1986. Ache-reflex changes during static stretching and two variations of proprioceptive neuromuscular facilitation techniques. *Electroencephalogr Clin Neurophysiol* 63:174–179.

40. Entyre, B. R., and L. D. Abraham. 1988. Antagonist muscle activity during stretching: A paradox reassessed. *Med Sci Sports Exerc* 20:285–289.

41. Entyre, B. R., and E. J. Lee. 1988. Chronic and acute flexibility of men and women using three different stretching techniques. *Res Q Exerc Sport* 59:222–228.

42. Fowles, J. R., D. G. Sale, and J. D. MacDougall. 2000. Reduced strength after passive stretch of the human plantarflexors. *J Appl Physiol* 89(3):1179–1188.

43. Ferreira, G., T. Nunes, and I. Teixeira. 2007. Gains in flexibility related to measures of muscular performance: Impact of flexibility on muscular performance. *Clinical Journal of Sport Medicine* 17(4):276–81.

44. Funk, D., A. M. Swank, K. J. Adams, and D. Treolo. 2001. Efficacy of moist heat pack application over static stretching on hamstring flexibility. *J Strength Cond Res* 15(1):123–126.

45. Godges, J. J., H. MacRae, and C. Longdon, et al. 1989. The effects of two stretching procedures on hip range of motion and joint economy. *J Orthop Sports Phys Ther* 11:350–357.

46. Gribble, P., and W. Prentice. 1999. Effects of static and hold-relax stretching on hamstring range of motion using the Flex-Ability LE 1000. *J Sport Rehab* 8(3):195.

47. Hedrick, A. 2000. Dynamic flexibility training. *Strength Cond J* 22(5):33–38.

48. Herling, J. 1981. It's time to add strength training to our fitness programs. *J Phys Educ Program* 79:17.

49. Heyward, V. H. 2006. Assessing flexibility and designing stretching programs. In *Advanced fitness assessment and exercise prescription*, 4th ed., edited by V. H. Heyward. Champaign, IL: Human Kinetics.

50. Holt, L. E., T. W. Pelham, and D. G. Burke. 1999. Modifications to the standard sit-and-reach flexibility protocol. *J Athlet Train* 34(1):43.

51. Howitt, S. 2006. The conservative treatment of trigger thumb using Graston Techniques and Active Release Techniques. *Journal of the Canadian Chiropractic Association* 50(4): 249–54.

52. Humphrey, L. D. 1981. Flexibility. *J Phys Educ Rec Dance* 52:41.

53. Hunter, G. 1998. Specific soft tissue mobilization in the management of soft tissue dysfunction. *Manual Ther* 3(1):2–11.

54. Ishii, D. K. 1976. Flexibility strexercises for co-ed groups. *Scholastic Coach* 45:31.

55. Jones, L. 1995. *Strain-counterstrain.* Boise, ID: Jones.

56. Kaplan, B., and M. Pierce. 2008. *Yoga for your life: A practice manual of breath and movement for everybody.* New York: Sterling Publishing.

57. Keirns, M., ed. 2000. *Myofascial release in sports medicine.* Champaign, IL: Human Kinetics.

58. Knott, M., and P. Voss. 1985. *Proprioceptive neuromuscular facilitation,* 3rd ed. New York: Harper & Row.

59. Kokkonen, J., and A. Nelson. 2007. Chronic static stretching improves exercise performance. *Medicine and Science in Sports and Exercise* 39(10): 1825–31.

60. Kokkonen, J. E., C. Nelson, and G. Arnold. 1997. Chronic stretching improves sport specific skills. *Med Sci Sports Exerc* 29(5):67.

61. Kokkonen, J. N., A. G. Nelson, and D. A. Arnall. 2001. Acute stretching inhibits strength endurance. *Med Sci Sports Exerc* 35(5):s11.

62. Kubo, K., H. Kanehisa, and T. Fukunaga. 2002. Effect of stretching training on the viscoelastic properties of human tendon structures in vivo. *J Appl Physiol* 92(2):595–601.

63. Leahy, M. 1995. Improved treatments for carpal tunnel and related syndromes. *Chiropractic Sports Med* 9(1):6.

64. Lentell, G., T. Hetherington, and J. Eagan, et al. 1992. The use of thermal agents to influence the effectiveness of a low-load prolonged stretch. *J Orthop Sports Phys Ther* 5:200–207.

65. Liemohn, W. 1988. Flexibility and muscular strength. *J Phys Educ Rec Dance* 59(7):37.

66. Louden, K. L., C. E. Bolier, and K. A. Allison, et al. 1985. Effects of two stretching methods on the flexibility and retention of flexibility at the ankle joint in runners. *Phys Ther* 65:698.

67. Madding, S. W., J. G. Wong, and A. Hallum. 1987. Effects of duration of passive stretching on hip abduction range of motion. *J Orthop Sports Phys Ther* 8:409–416.

68. Mann, D., and C. Whedon. 2001. Functional stretching: Implementing a dynamic stretching program. *Athletic Ther Today* 6(3):10–13.

69. Manheim, C. 2001. *Myofascial release manual.* Thorofare, NJ: Slack.

70. Marek, S., J. Cramer, and L. Fincher. 2005. Acute effects of static and proprioceptive neuromuscular facilitation stretching on muscle strength and power output. *J Athlet Training* 40(2):94–103.

71. Markos, P. D. 1979. Ipsilateral and contralateral effects of proprioceptive neuromuscular facilitation techniques on hip motion and electromyographic activity. *Phys Ther* 59:1366–1373.

72. McAtee, R. 2007. *Facilitated stretching.* Champaign, IL: Human Kinetics.

73. McClellan, E., D. Padua, and W. Prentice. 2000. Effects of myofascial release and static stretching on active range of motion and muscle activity. *J Ath Train* 35(3):329.

74. Moore, M., and R. Hutton. 1980. Electromyographic investigation of muscle stretching techniques. *Med Sci Sports Exerc* 12:322–329.

75. Murphy, P. 1986. Warming up before stretching advised. *Phys Sports Med* 14(3):45.

76. Nelson, R. 2005. An update on flexibility. *Natl Strength Cond Assoc* 27(1): 10–16.

77. Norris, C. 1995. *Flexibility principles and practices.* London: A&C Black.

78. Power, K., D. Behm, F. Cahill, M. Carroll, and W. Young. 2004. An acute bout of static stretching: Effects on force and jumping performance. *Med Sci Sports Exerc* 36(8):1389–1396.

79. Prentice, W. E., and E. Kooima.1986. The use of PNF techniques in rehabilitation of sport-related injury. *Athlet Train* 21(1): 26–31.

80. Prentice, W. E. 1983. A comparison of static stretching and PNF stretching for improving hip joint flexibility. *J Athlet Train* 18:56–59.

81. Prentice WE. A review of PNF techniques—implications for athletic rehabilitation and performance. *Forum Medicum* (51):1–13, 1989.

82. Prentice, W. E. 1982. An electromyographic analysis of heat or cold and stretching for inducing muscular relaxation. *J Orthop Sports Phys Ther* 3:133–140.

83. Prentice, W. 2009. Sports massage. In *Therapeutic modalities in sports medicine and athletic training,* Prentice, W., ed. New York: McGraw-Hill.

83. Rasch, P. 1989. *Kinesiology and applied anatomy.* Philadelphia: Lea & Febiger.

85. Rubini, E., and A. Costa. 2007. The effects of stretching on strength performance. *Sports Medicine* 37(3): 213.

86. Sady, S. P., M. Wortman, and D. Blanke. 1982. Flexibility training: Ballistic, static, or proprioceptive neuromuscular facilitation? *Arch Phys Med Rehab* 63:261–263.

87. Sapega, A. A., T. Quedenfeld, and R. Moyer, et al. 1981. Biophysical factors in range-of-motion exercise. *Phys Sports Med* 9(12):57.

88. Schilling, B. K., and M. H. Stone. 2000. Stretching: Acute effects on strength and power performance. *Strength Cond J* 22(1): 44.

89. Sefton, J. 2004. Myofascial release for athletic trainers, Part 1. *Athletic Therapy Today* 9(1):40.

90. Schiowitz, S. 1990. Facilitated positional release. *J Am Osteopath Assoc* 90(2):145–146, 151–55.

91. Shellock, F., and W. E. Prentice. 1985. Warm-up and stretching for improved physical performance and prevention of sport related injury. *Sports Med* 2:267–278.

92. Shindo, M., H. Harayama, and K. Kondo, et al. 1984. Changes in reciprocal Ia inhibition during voluntary contraction in man. *Exp Brain Res* 53:400–408.

93. Siatras, T., G. Papadopoulos, D. Maeletzi, V. Gerodimos, and P. Kellis. 2003. Static and dynamic acute stretching effect on gymnasts' speed in vaulting. *Ped Ex Sci* 15: 383–391.

94. Spernoga, S. G., T. L. Uhl, B. L. Arnold, B. M. Gansneder. 2001. Duration of maintained hamstring flexibility after a one time, modified hold-relax stretching protocol. *J Athlet Train* 36(1):44–48.

95. Speicher, T. 2006. Top 10 positional release therapy techniques to break the chain of pain, Part 1. *Athletic Therapy Today* 11(5):60.

96. St. George, F. 1997. *The stretching handbook: Ten steps to muscle fitness.* Roseville, IL: Simon & Schuster.

97. Stamford, B. 1994. A stretching primer. *Physician and Sports Medicine* 22(9):85–86.

98. Stone, J. 2000. Myofascial release. *Athlet Ther Today* 5(4):34–35.

99. Stone, J. 2000. Strain-counterstrain. *Athlet Ther Today* 5(6):30.

100. Surburg, P. 1999. Flexibility/range of motion. In *The brockport physical fitness training guide,* Winnick, J. P., ed. Champaign, IL: Human Kinetics.

101. Surburg, P. 1995. Flexibility training program design. In *Fitness programming and physical disability,* Miller, P., ed. Champaign, IL: Human Kinetics.

102. Tanigawa, M. C. 1972. Comparison of the hold relax procedure and passive mobilization on increasing muscle length. *Phys Ther* 52:725.

103. Taylor, D. C., D. E. Brooks, and J. B. Ryan. 1997. Viscoelastic characteristics of muscle: passive stretching versus muscular contractions. *Med Sci Sports Exerc* 29(12):1619–1624.

104. Thacker, S., J. Gilchrist, and D. Stroup. 2004. The impact of stretching on sports injury risk: A systematic review of the literature. *Med Sci Sports Exerc* 36(3):371–378.

105. Tobias, M., and J. P. Sullivan. 1992. *Complete stretching.* New York: Knopf.

106. Van Hatten, B. 2005. Passive versus active stretching. *Phys Ther* 85(1):80.

107. Van Mechelen, P. 1993. Prevention of running injuries by warm-up, cool-down, and stretching. *Am J Sports Med* 21(5):711–719.

108. Voss, D. E., M. K. Lonta, and G. J. Myers. 1985. *Proprioceptive neuro-muscular facilitation: Patterns and techniques,* 3rd ed. Philadelphia, PA: Lippincott Williams & Wilkins.

109. Wessel, J., and A. Wan. 1984. Effect of stretching on intensity of delayed-onset muscle soreness. *J Sports Med* 2:83–87.

110. Winters, M. V., and C. G. Blake, and J. Trost. 2004. Passive versus active stretching of hip flexor muscles in subjects with limited hip extension: A randomized clinical trial. *Phys Ther* 84(9):800–807.

111. Worrell, T., T. Smith, and J. Winegardner. 1994. Effect of hamstring stretching on hamstring muscle performance. *J Orthop Sports Phys Ther* 20(3):154–159.

112. Zachewski, J. 1990. Flexibility for sports. In *Sports physical therapy,* Sanders, B., ed. Norwalk, CT: Appleton & Lange.

113. Zebas, C. J., and M. L. Rivera. 1985. Retention of flexibility in selected joints after cessation of a stretching exercise program. In *Exercise physiology: Current selected research topics,* Dotson, C. O., and J. H. Humphrey, eds. New York: AMS Press.

SOLUTIONS TO CLINICAL DECISION MAKING EXERCISES

8-1 Flexibility is crucial to a gymnast's performance. While she is not training, she must maintain movement at all of her joints so that she does not lose flexibility. Inactivity can cause a shortening of elastic components. This would put her at risk for muscular injury when she resumes her normal activity.

8-2 Applying certain therapeutic modalities, such as ice and/or electrical stimulating currents, can decrease pain and discourage muscle guarding to increase ROM. Delayed-onset muscle soreness will usually begin to subside at about 48 hours following a workout.

8-3 A goniometer can be used to measure the angle between the femur and the fibula, giving you degrees of flexion and extension. To maximize consistency in measurement, it is helpful if the same person takes sequential goniometric measurement.

8-4 The motion might be limited by quadriceps (antagonistic) muscle tightness, tightness of the joint capsule, pathological or damaged bony structure preventing normal accessory motions between the tibia and femur or between the patella and femur, fat/muscle causing tissue approximation, or scar tissue in the anterior portion of the joint.

8-5 A static stretch should be held for about 30 seconds. This allows time for the golgi tendon organs to override the muscle spindles and produce a reflex muscle relaxation. The patient should stretch to the point where tightness or resistance to stretch is felt but it should not be painful. The stretch should be repeated 3 to 5 times.

8-6 Ballistic stretching is dynamic stretching that is useful prior to activity because it is a functional stretch. It mimics activity that will be performed during competition. However, there is some speculation that because it is an uncontrolled stretch, it may lead to injury, especially in sedentary individuals. Static stretching is convenient because it can be done on any muscle and it doesn't require a partner. It is not very functional. PNF stretching will most likely provide the greatest increase in ROM, but it is a little more time consuming and requires a partner.

CHAPTER 9

Regaining Muscular Strength and Endurance

William E. Prentice

After completing this chapter, the athletic training student should be able to do the following:

- Define muscular strength, endurance, and power and discuss their importance in a program of rehabilitation following injury.

- Discuss the anatomy and physiology of skeletal muscle.

- Discuss the physiology of strength development and factors that determine strength.

- Describe specific methods for improving muscular strength.

- Differentiate between muscle strength and muscle endurance.

- Discuss differences between males and females in terms of strength development.

Following all musculoskeletal injuries, there will be some degree of impairment in muscular strength and endurance. For the athletic trainer supervising a rehabilitation program, regaining, and in many instances improving, levels of strength and endurance are critical for discharging and returning the patient to a functional level following injury.

By definition, *muscular strength* is the ability of a muscle to generate force against some resistance. Maintenance of at least a normal level of strength in a given muscle or muscle group is important for normal healthy living. Muscle weakness or imbalance can result in abnormal movement or gait and can impair normal functional movement. Resistance training plays a critical role in injury rehabilitation.

Muscular strength is closely associated with muscular endurance. *Muscular endurance* is the ability to perform repetitive muscular contractions against some resistance for an extended period of time. As we will see later, as muscular strength increases, there tends to be a corresponding increase in endurance. For the average person in the population, developing muscular endurance is likely more important than developing muscular strength because muscular endurance is probably more critical in carrying out the everyday activities of living. This statement becomes increasingly true with age.

CLINICAL DECISION MAKING   Exercise 9–1

A softball pitcher was out for a whole season for rehabilitation following shoulder surgery. Why is it important that she regain all three aspects of muscular fitness?

TYPES OF SKELETAL MUSCLE CONTRACTION

Skeletal muscle is capable of three different types of contraction: *isometric contraction, concentric contraction,* and *eccentric contraction.* An isometric contraction occurs when the muscle contracts to produce tension but there is no change in muscle length. Considerable force can be generated against some immovable resistance even though no movement occurs. In a concentric contraction the muscle shortens in length while tension increases to overcome or move some resistance. In an eccentric contraction, the resistance is greater than the muscular force being produced, and the muscle lengthens while producing tension. Concentric and eccentric contractions are considered dynamic movements.[56]

Recently, *econcentric contraction,* which combines both a controlled concentric and a concurrent eccentric contraction of the same muscle over two separate joints, has been introduced.[19,30] An econcentric contraction is possible only in muscles that cross at least two joints. An example of an econcentric contraction would be a prone, open-kinetic-chain hamstring curl. The hamstrings contract concentrically to flex the knee, while the hip tends to flex eccentrically, lengthening the hamstring. Rehabilitation exercises have traditionally concentrated on strengthening isolated single-joint motions, despite the fact that the same muscle is functioning at a second joint simultaneously. Therefore it has been recommended that the strengthening program includes exercises that strengthen the muscle in the manner in which it contracts functionally. Traditional strength-training programs have been designed to develop strength in individual muscles, in a single plane of motion. However, because all muscles function concentrically, eccentrically, and isometrically in three planes of motion, a strengthening program should be multiplanar, concentrating on all three types of contraction.[15]

FACTORS THAT DETERMINE LEVELS OF MUSCULAR STRENGTH, ENDURANCE, AND POWER

Size of the Muscle

Muscular strength is proportional to the cross-sectional diameter of the muscle fibers. The greater the cross-sectional diameter or the bigger a particular muscle, the stronger it is, and thus the more force it is capable of generating. The size of a muscle tends to increase in cross-sectional diameter with resistance training. This increase in muscle size is referred to as *hypertrophy.*[42] A decrease in the size of a muscle is referred to as *atrophy.*

Number of Muscle Fibers

Strength is a function of the number and diameter of muscle fibers composing a given muscle. The number of fibers is an inherited characteristic; thus a person with a large number of muscle fibers to begin with has the potential to hypertrophy to a much greater degree than does someone with relatively few fibers.[38]

Neuromuscular Efficiency

Strength is also directly related to the efficiency of the nueromuscular system and the function of the motor unit in producing muscular force.[46] As will be noted later in this chapter, initial increases in strength during the first 8 to 10 weeks of a resistance training program can be attributed primarily to increased neuromuscular efficiency.[59] Resistance training will increase neuromuscular efficiency in three ways: there is an increase in the number of motor units being recruited, in the firing rate of each motor unit, and in the synchronization of motor unit firing.[7]

Biomechanical Considerations

Strength in a given muscle is determined not only by the physical properties of the muscle but also by biomechanical factors that dictate how much force can be generated through a system of levers to an external object.[31,38,63]

Position of Tendon Attachment   If we think of the elbow joint as one of these lever systems, we would have the biceps muscle producing flexion of this joint (Figure 9-1). The position of attachment of the biceps muscle on the forearm will largely determine how much force this muscle is capable of generating. If there are two individuals, A and B, and A has a biceps attachment that is closer to the fulcrum (the elbow joint) than B's, then A must produce a greater effort with the biceps muscle to hold the weight at a right angle, because the length of the effort arm will be greater than that for B.

Length–Tension Relationship   The length of a muscle determines the tension that can be generated. By varying the length of a muscle, different tensions can be produced.[31] This length–tension relationship is illustrated in Figure 9-2. At position B in the curve, the interaction of the crossbridges between the actin and myosin myofilaments within the sarcomere is at maximum. Setting

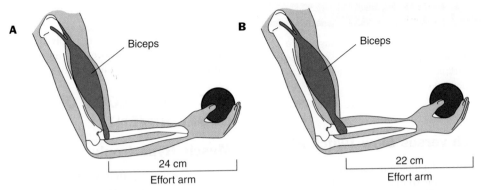

Figure 9-1   The position of attachment of the muscle tendon on the lever arm can affect the ability of that muscle to generate force. **B** should be able to generate greater force than **A** because the tendon attachment on the lever arm is closer to the resistance.

a muscle at this particular length will produce the greatest amount of tension. At position A the muscle is shortened, and at position C the muscle is lengthened. In either case the interaction between the actin and myosin myofilaments through the crossbridges is greatly reduced, thus the muscle is not capable of generating significant tension.

Age

The ability to generate muscular force is also related to age.[4] Both men and women seem to be able to increase strength throughout puberty and adolescence, reaching

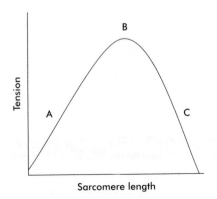

Figure 9-2   The length-tension relation of the muscle. Greatest tension is developed at point B, with less tension developed at points A and C.

a peak around 20 to 25 years of age, at which time this ability begins to level off and in some cases decline. After about age 25, a person generally loses an average of 1 percent of his/her maximal remaining strength each year. Thus at age 65, a person would have only about 60 percent of the strength he/she had at age 25.[45] This loss in muscle strength is definitely related to individual levels of physical activity. People who are more active, or perhaps continue to strength-train, considerably decrease this tendency toward declining muscle strength. In addition to retarding this decrease in muscular strength, exercise can also have an effect in slowing the decrease in cardiorespiratory endurance and flexibility, as well as slowing increases in body fat. Thus strength maintenance is important for all individuals regardless of age for achieving total wellness and good health as well as in rehabilitation after injury.[62]

Overtraining

Overtraining in a physically active patient can have a negative effect on the development of muscular strength. Overtraining is an imbalance between exercise and recovery in which the training program exceeds the body's physiological and psychological limits. Overtraining can result in psychological breakdown (staleness) or physiological breakdown that can involve musculoskeletal injury, fatigue, or sickness. Engaging in proper and efficient resistance training, eating a proper diet, and getting appropriate rest can all minimize the potential negative effects of overtraining.

Fast-Twitch versus Slow-Twitch Fibers

All fibers in a particular motor unit are either **slow-twitch fibers** or **fast-twitch fibers.** Each kind has distinctive metabolic and contractile capabilities.

Slow-Twitch Fibers Slow-twitch fibers are also referred to as *type I* or *slow-oxidative* fibers. They are more resistant to fatigue than fast-twitch fibers; however, the time required to generate force is much greater in slow-twitch fibers.[29] Because they are relatively fatigue resistant, slow-twitch fibers are associated primarily with long-duration, aerobic-type activities.

Fast-Twitch Fibers Fast-twitch fibers are capable of producing quick, forceful contractions but have a tendency to fatigue more rapidly than slow twitch fibers. Fast-twitch fibers are useful in short-term, high-intensity activities, which mainly involve the anaerobic system. Fast-twitch fibers are capable of producing powerful contractions, whereas slow-twitch fibers produce a long-endurance force. There are two subdivisions of fast-twitch fibers. Although both types of fast-twitch fibers are capable of rapid contraction, *type IIa fibers* or *fast-oxidative-glycolytic* fibers are moderately resistant to fatigue, while *type IIb fibers* or *fast-glycolytic* fibers fatigue rapidly and are considered the "true" fast-twitch fibers. Recently, a third group of fast-twitch fibers, *type IIx*, has been identified in animal models. Type IIx fibers are fatigue resistant and are thought to have a maximum power capacity less than that of type IIb but greater than that of type IIa fibers.[45]

Ratio in Muscle Within a particular muscle are both types of fibers, and the ratio of the two types in an individual muscle varies with each person.[32] Muscles whose primary function is to maintain posture against gravity require more endurance and have a higher percentage of slow-twitch fibers. Muscles that produce powerful, rapid, explosive strength movements tend to have a much higher percentage of fast-twitch fibers.

Because this ratio is genetically determined, it can play a large role in determining ability for a given sport activity. Sprinters and weight lifters, for example, have a large percentage of fast-twitch fibers in relation to slow-twitch fibers.[16] Conversely, marathon runners generally have a higher percentage of slow-twitch fibers. The question of whether fiber types can change as a result of training has to date not been conclusively resolved.[10] However, both types of fibers can improve their metabolic capabilities through specific strength and endurance training.[7]

THE PHYSIOLOGY OF STRENGTH DEVELOPMENT

Muscle Hypertrophy

There is no question that resistance training to improve muscular strength results in an increased size, or hypertrophy, of a muscle. What causes a muscle to hypertrophy? A number of theories have been proposed to explain this increase in muscle size.[22]

First, some evidence exists that there is an *increase in the number of muscle fibers (hyperplasia)* due to fibers splitting in response to training.[39] However, this research has been conducted in animals and should not be generalized to humans. It is generally accepted that the number of fibers is genetically determined and does not seem to increase with training.

Second, it has been hypothesized that because the muscle is working harder in resistance training, more blood is required to supply that muscle with oxygen and other nutrients. Thus it is thought that *the number of capillaries is increased.* This hypothesis is only partially correct; no *new* capillaries are formed during resistance training; however, a number of dormant capillaries might become filled with blood to meet this increased demand for blood supply.[45]

A third theory to explain this increase in muscle size seems the most credible. Muscle fibers are composed primarily of small protein filaments, called myofilaments, which are contractile elements in muscle. *Myofilaments* are small contractile elements of protein within the sarcomere. There are two distinct types of myofilaments: thin *actin* myofilaments and thicker *myosin* myofilaments. Fingerlike projections, or crossbridges, connect the actin and myosin myofilaments. When a muscle is stimulated to contract, the crossbridges pull the myofilaments closer together, thus shortening the muscle and producing movement at the joint that the muscle crosses[5] (Figure 9-3).

These *myofilaments increase in size and number* as a result of resistance training, causing the individual muscle fibers to increase in cross-sectional diameter.[58] This increase is particularly present in men, although women will also see some increase in muscle size. More research is needed to further clarify and determine the specific reasons for muscle hypertorphy.

Reversibility   If resistance training is discontinued or interrupted, the muscle will atrophy, decreasing in both strength and mass. Adaptations in skeletal muscle that occur in response to resistance training can begin to reverse in as little as 48 hours. It does appear that consistent exercise of a muscle is essential to prevent reversal of the hypertrophy that occurs due to strength training.

Other Physiological Adaptations to Resistance Exercise

In addition to muscle hypertrophy, there are a number of other physiological adaptations to resistance training.[40] The strength of noncontractile structures, including tendons and ligaments, is increased. The mineral content of bone is increased, thus making the bone stronger and more resistant to fracture. Maximal oxygen uptake is improved when resistance training is of sufficient intensity to elicit heart rates at or above training levels. However, it must be emphasized that these increases are minimal and that if increased maximal oxygen uptake is the goal, aerobic exercise rather than resistance training is recommended. There is also an increase in several enzymes important in aerobic and anaerobic metabolism.[3,25,26] All of these adaptations contribute to strength and endurance.

CLINICAL DECISION MAKING   **Exercise 9-4**

Two football players of the same age have been following the exact same training plan. One is consistently able to perform a hamstring curl using more weight than the other. What could possibly be making him stronger at this task?

TECHNIQUES OF RESISTANCE TRAINING

There are a number of different techniques of resistance training for strength improvement, including isometric exercise, progressive resistive exercise, isokinetic training, circuit training, and plyometric exercise. Regardless of the specific strength-training technique used, the athletic trainer should integrate functional strengthening activities that involve multiplanar, eccentric, concentric, and isometric contractions.

The Overload Principle

Regardless of which of these techniques is used, one basic principle of reconditioning is extremely important. For a muscle to improve in strength, it must be forced to work at a higher level than it is accustomed to. In other words, the muscle must be overloaded. Without overload the muscle will be able to maintain strength as long as training is continued against a resistance to which the muscle is accustomed, but no additional strength gains will be realized. This maintenance of existing levels of muscular strength may be more important in resistance programs that emphasize muscular endurance rather than strength

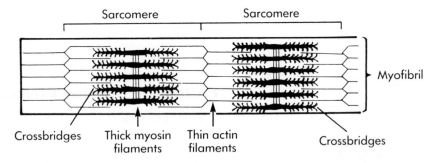

Figure 9-3   Muscles contract when an electrical impulse from the central nervous system causes the myofilaments in a muscle fiber to move closer together.

gains. Many individuals can benefit more in terms of overall health by concentrating on improving muscular endurance. However, to most effectively build muscular strength, resistance training requires a consistent, increasing effort against progressively increasing resistance.[38,56]

Resistive exercise is based primarily on the principles of overload and progression. If these principles are applied, all of the following resistance training techniques will produce improvement of muscular strength over time.

In a rehabilitation setting, progressive overload is limited to some degree by the healing process. If the athletic trainer takes an aggressive approach to rehabilitation, the rate of progression is perhaps best determined by the injured patient's response to a specific exercise. Exacerbation of pain or increased swelling should alert the athletic trainer that their rate of progression is too aggressive.

Isometric Exercise

An *isometric exercise* involves a muscle contraction in which the length of the muscle remains constant while tension develops toward a maximal force against an immovable resistance[6] (Figure 9-4). An isometric contraction provides stabilization strength that helps maintain normal length–tension and force-couple relationships that are critical for normal joint arthrokinematics. Isometric exercises are capable of increasing muscular strength.[54] However, strength gains are relatively specific, with as much as a 20-percent overflow to the joint angle at which training is performed. At other angles, the strength curve drops off dramatically because of a lack of motor activity at that angle. Thus, strength is increased at the specific angle of exertion, but there is no corresponding increase in strength at other positions in the range of motion.

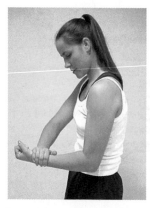

Figure 9-4   Isometric exercises involve contraction against some immovable resistance.

Another major disadvantage of these isometric exercises is that they tend to produce a spike in systolic blood pressure that can result in potentially life-threatening cardiovascular accidents.[29] This sharp increase in systolic blood pressure results from a Valsalva maneuver, which increases intrathoracic pressure. To avoid or minimize this effect, it is recommended that breathing be done during the maximal contraction to prevent this increase in pressure.

The use of isometric exercises in injury rehabilitation or reconditioning is widely practiced. There are a number of conditions or ailments resulting from trauma or overuse that must be treated with strengthening exercises. Unfortunately, these problems can be exacerbated with full range-of-motion resistance exercises. It might be more desirable to make use of positional or functional isometric exercises that involve the application of isometric force at multiple angles throughout the range of motion. Functional isometrics should be used until the healing process has progressed to the point that full-range activities can be performed.

During rehabilitation, it is often recommended that a muscle be contracted isometrically for 10 seconds at a time at a frequency of 10 or more contractions per hour. Isometric exercises can also offer significant benefit in a strengthening program.[64]

There are certain instances in which an isometric contraction can greatly enhance a particular movement. For example, one of the exercises in power weight lifting is a squat. A squat is an exercise in which the weight is supported on the shoulders in a standing position. The knees are then flexed, and the weight is lowered to a three-quarter squat position, from which the lifter must stand completely straight once again.

It is not uncommon for there to be one particular angle in the range of motion at which smooth movement is difficult because of insufficient strength. This joint angle is referred to as a sticking point. A power lifter will typically use an isometric contraction against some immovable resistance to increase strength at this sticking point. If strength can be improved at this joint angle, then a smooth, coordinated power lift can be performed through a full range of movement.

Progressive Resistive Exercise

A second technique of resistance training is perhaps the most commonly used and most popular technique for improving muscular strength in a rehabilitation program. *Progressive resistive exercise* uses exercises that strengthen muscles through a contraction that overcomes some fixed resistance such as with dumbbells, barbells, various exercise machines, or resistive elastic tubing. Progressive resistive exercise uses isotonic, or *isodynamic*, contractions in which force is generated while the muscle is changing in length.

Concentric versus Eccentric Contractions Isotonic contractions can be concentric or eccentric. In performing a bicep curl, to lift the weight from the starting position the biceps muscle must contract and shorten in length. This shortening contraction is referred to as a concentric or positive contraction. If the biceps muscle does not remain contracted when the weight is being lowered, gravity would cause this weight to simply fall back to the starting position. Thus, to control the weight as it is being lowered, the biceps muscle must continue to contract while at the same time gradually lengthening. A contraction in which the muscle is lengthening while still applying force is called an eccentric or negative contraction.

It is possible to generate greater amounts of force against resistance with an eccentric contraction than with a concentric contraction, because eccentric contractions require a much lower level of motor unit activity to achieve a certain force than do concentric contractions. Because fewer motor units are firing to produce a specific force, additional motor units can be recruited to generate increased force. In addition, oxygen use is much lower during eccentric exercise than in comparable concentric exercise. Thus eccentric contractions are less resistant to fatigue than are concentric contractions. The mechanical efficiency of eccentric exercise can be several times higher than that of concentric exercise.[56]

Traditionally, progressive resistive exercise has concentrated primarily on the concentric component without paying much attention to the importance of the eccentric component.[56] The use of eccentric contractions, particularly in rehabilitation of various sport-related injuries, has received considerable emphasis in recent years. Eccentric contractions are critical for deceleration of limb motion, especially during high-velocity dynamic activities.[35] For example, a baseball pitcher relies on an eccentric contraction of the external rotators of the glenohumeral joint to decelerate the humerus, which might be internally rotating at speeds as high as 8000 degrees/second. Certainly, strength deficits or an inability of a muscle to tolerate these eccentric forces can predispose an injury. Thus, in a rehabilitation program the athletic trainer should incorporate eccentric strengthening exercises. Eccentric contractions are possible with all free weights, with the majority of isotonic exercise machines, and with most isokinetic devices. Eccentric contractions are used with plyometric exercise discussed in Chapter 11 and can also be incorporated with functional proprioceptive neuromuscular facilitation (PNF) strengthening patterns discussed in Chapter 14.

In progressive resistive exercise it is essential to incorporate both concentric and eccentric contractions.[33] Research has clearly demonstrated that the muscle should be overloaded and fatigued both concentrically and eccentrically for the greatest strength improvement to occur.[4,22,45] When training specifically for the development of muscular strength, the concentric portion of the exercise should require 1 to 2 seconds, while the eccentric portion of the lift should require 2 to 4 seconds. The ratio of the concentric component to the eccentric component should be approximately 1:2. Physiologically the muscle will fatigue much more rapidly concentrically than eccentrically.

Free Weights versus Exercise Machines Various types of exercise equipment can be used with progressive resistive exercise, including free weights (barbells and dumbbells) or exercise machines such as Cybex, Universal, Paramount, Tough Stuff, Icarian Fitness, King Fitness, Body Solid, Pro-Elite, Life Fitness, Nautilus, BodyCraft, Yukon, Flex, CamBar, GymPros, Nugym, BodyWorks, DP, Soloflex, and Body Master (Figure 9-5). Dumbbells and barbells require the use of iron plates of varying weights that can be easily changed by adding or subtracting equal amounts of weight to both sides of the bar. The exercise machines for the most part have stacks of weights that are lifted through a series of levers or pulleys. The stack of weights slides up and down on a pair of bars that restrict the movement to only one plane. Weight can be increased or decreased simply by changing the position of a weight key.

There are advantages and disadvantages to free weights and machines. The exercise machines are relatively safe to use in comparison with free weights. For example, a bench press with free weights requires a partner to help lift the weight back onto the support racks if the lifter does not have enough strength to complete the lift; otherwise the weight might be dropped on the chest. With the machines the weight can be easily and safely dropped without fear of injury (Figure 9-6).

It is also a simple process to increase or decrease the weight by moving a single weight key with the exercise machines, although changes can generally be made only in increments of 10 or 15 pounds. With free weights, iron plates must be added or removed from each side of the barbell.

The biggest disadvantage in using exercise machines is that with few exceptions the design constraints of the machine allow only single-plane motion, limiting or controlling more functional movements that occur in multiple planes simultaneously.

Anyone who has strength-trained using free weights and exercise machines realizes the difference in the amount of weight that can be lifted. Unlike the machines,

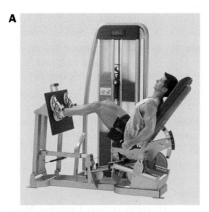

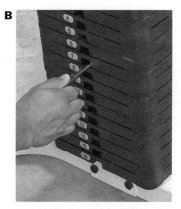

Figure 9-5 Isotonic equipment. **A,** Most exercise machines are isotonic. **B,** Resistance can be easily changed by changing the key in the stack of weights.

free weights have no restricted motion and can thus move in many different directions, depending on the forces applied. With free weights, an element of neuromuscular control on the part of the lifter to stabilize the weight and prevent it from moving in any other direction than vertical will usually decrease the amount of weight that can be lifted.[66]

Surgical Tubing or Theraband   Surgical tubing or Theraband, as a means of providing resistance, has been widely used in rehabilitation (Figure 9-7). The advantage of exercising with surgical tubing or Theraband is that movement can occur in multiple planes simultaneously. Thus exercise can be done against resistance in more functional movement planes. The use of surgical tubing exercise in

CLINICAL DECISION MAKING	Exercise 9–5

A weight lifter has been progressing his maximum bench-press weight. However, he still requires a spotter to get him through the full ROM. He gets "stuck" at about 90 degrees of elbow extension. What can he do to progress through this limitation?

CLINICAL DECISION MAKING	Exercise 9–6

The head athletic trainer wants to buy new equipment for the weight room. What are the advantages and disadvantages to investing in exercise machines rather than free weights?

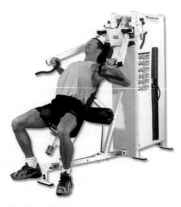

Figure 9-6 Bench press exercise machine with a stack of weights.

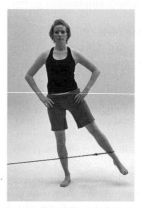

Figure 9-7 Strengthening exercises using surgical tubing are widely used in rehabilitation.

plyometrics and PNF strengthening techniques will be discussed in Chapters 11 and 14. Surgical tubing can be used to provide resistance with the majority of the strengthening exercises shown in Chapters 17 through 23.

Regardless of which type of equipment is used, the same principles of progressive resistive exercise may be applied.

Variable Resistance   One problem often mentioned in relation to progressive resistive exercise reconditioning is that the amount of force necessary to move a weight through a range of motion changes according to the angle of pull of the contracting muscle. It is greatest when the angle of pull is approximately 90 degrees. In addition, once the inertia of the weight has been overcome and momentum has been established, the force required to move the resistance varies according to the force the muscle can produce through the range of motion. Thus it has been argued that a disadvantage of any type of isotonic exercise is that the force required to move the resistance is constantly changing throughout the range of movement. This change in resistance at different points in the range of motion has been labeled *accommodating resistance* or *variable resistance.*

A number of exercise machine manufacturers have attempted to alleviate this problem of changing force capabilities by using a cam in its pulley system. The cam is individually designed for each piece of equipment so that the resistance is variable throughout the movement. The cam is intended to alter resistance so that the muscle can handle a greater load, but at the points where the joint angle or muscle length is mechanically disadvantageous, it reduces the resistance to muscle movement. Whether this design does what it claims is debatable.

Progressive   Resistive   Exercise   Techniques
Perhaps the single most confusing aspect of progressive resistive exercise is the terminology used to describe specific programs.[32] The following list of terms with their operational definitions may help clarify the confusion:

> *Repetitions:* The number of times a specific movement is repeated
> *Repetition maximum (RM):* The maximum number of repetitions at a given weight
> *Set:* A particular number of repetitions
> *Intensity:* The amount of weight or resistance lifted
> *Recovery period:* The rest interval between sets
> *Frequency:* The number of times an exercise is done in a week's period

Recommended Techniques of Resistance Training   Specific recommendations for techniques of improving muscular strength are controversial among athletic

trainers. A considerable amount of research has been done in the area of resistance training relative to (1) the amount of weight to be used; (2) the number of repetitions; (3) the number of sets; and (4) the frequency of training.

A variety of specific programs have been proposed that recommend the optimal amount of weight, number of sets, number of repetitions, and frequency for producing maximal gains in levels of muscular strength. However, regardless of the techniques used, the healing process must dictate the specifics of any strength-training program. Certainly, to improve strength, the muscle must be progressively overloaded. The amount of weight used and the number of repetitions must be sufficient to make the muscle work at higher intensity than it is accustomed to. This factor is the most critical in any resistance training program. The resistance training program must also be designed to ultimately meet the specific competitive needs of the athlete.

Resistance training programs were initially designed by power lifters and body builders. Programs or routines commonly used in training and conditioning include the following:

> *Single set:* One set of 8 to 12 repetitions of a particular exercise performed at a slow speed.
> *Tri-sets:* A group of three exercises for the same muscle group performed using 2 to 4 sets of each exercise with no rest in between.
> *Multiple sets:* Two or three warm-up sets with progressively increasing resistance followed by several sets at the same resistance.
> *Supersets:* Either one set of 8 to 10 repetitions of several exercises for the same muscle group performed one after another, or several sets of 8 to 10 repetitions of two exercises for the same muscle group with no rest in between.
> *Pyramids:* One set of 8 to 12 repetitions with light resistance, then an increase in resistance over 4 to 6 sets until only 1 or 2 repetitions can be performed. The pyramid can also be reversed going from heavy to light resistance.
> *Split routine:* Workouts exercise different muscle groups on successive days. For example, Monday, Wednesday, and Friday might be used for upper body muscles, and Tuesday, Thursday, and Saturday would be used for lower body muscles.
> *Circuit training:* This technique may be useful to the athletic trainer for maintaining or perhaps improving levels of muscular strength or endurance in other parts of the body while the patient allows for healing and reconditioning of an injured body part. Circuit training uses a series of exercise

stations, each of which involves weight training, flexibility, calisthenics, or brief aerobic exercises. Circuits can be designed to accomplish many different training goals. With circuit training the patient moves rapidly from one station to the next, performing whatever exercise is to be done at that station within a specified time period. A typical circuit would consist of 8 to 12 stations, and the entire circuit would be repeated three times.

Circuit training is most definitely an effective technique for improving strength and flexibility. Certainly if the pace or time interval between stations is rapid and if workload is maintained at a high level of intensity with heart rates at or above target training levels, the cardiorespiratory system may benefit from this circuit. However, there is little research evidence that circuit training is very effective in improving cardiorespiratory endurance. It should be, and is most often, used as a technique for developing and improving muscular strength and endurance.[27]

Techniques of Resistance Training Used in Rehabilitation One of the first widely accepted strength development programs to be used in a rehabilitation program was developed by DeLorme and was based on a repetition maximum of 10 (10 RM).[18] The amount of weight used is what can be lifted exactly 10 times (Table 9-1).

Zinovieff proposed the Oxford technique, which, like DeLorme's program, was designed to be used in beginning, intermediate, and advanced levels of rehabilitation.[68] The only difference is that the percentage of maximum was reversed in the three sets (Table 9-2). McQueen's technique[48] differentiates between beginning to intermediate and advanced levels, as in shown in Table 9-3.

Sanders' program (Table 9-4) was designed to be used in the advanced stages of rehabilitation and was based on a formula that used a percentage of body weight to determine starting weights.[56] The following percentages represent median starting points for different exercises:

Barbell squat—45 percent of body weight
Barbell bench press—30 percent of body weight
Leg extension—20 percent of body weight
Universal bench press—30 percent of body weight

TABLE 9-1 DeLorme's Program

Set	Amount of Weight	Repetitions
1	50% of 10 RM	10
2	75% of 10 RM	10
3	100% of 10 RM	10

TABLE 9-2 The Oxford Technique

Set	Amount of Weight	Repetitions
1	100% of 10 RM	10
2	75% of 10 RM	10
3	50% of 10 RM	10

Universal leg extension—20 percent of body weight
Universal leg curl—10 to 15 percent of body weight
Universal leg press—50 percent of body weight
Upright rowing—20 percent of body weight

Knight applied the concept of progressive resistive exercise in rehabilitation. His DAPRE (Daily Adjusted Progressive Resistive Exercise) program (Tables 9-5 and 9-6) allows for individual differences in the rates at which patients progress in their rehabilitation programs.[37]

Berger has proposed a technique that is adjustable within individual limitations (Table 9-7). For any given exercise, the amount of weight selected should be sufficient to allow 6 to 8 RM in each of the three sets, with a recovery period of 60 to 90 seconds between sets. Initial selection of a starting weight might require some trial and error to achieve this 6 to 8 RM range. If at least three sets of 6 RM cannot be completed, the weight is too heavy and should be reduced. If it is possible to do more than three sets of 8 RM, the weight is too light and should be increased.[8] Progression to heavier weights is then determined by the ability to perform at least 8 RM in each of three sets. When progressing weight, an

TABLE 9-3 McQueen's Technique

Set	Amount of Weight	Repetitions
3 (Beginning/intermediate)	100% of 10 RM	10
4–5 (Advanced)	100% of 2–3 RM	2–3

■ **TABLE   9-4**   Sanders' Program

Sets	Amount of Weight	Repetitions
Total of 4 sets (three times per week)	100% of 5 RM	5
Day 1, 4 sets	100% of 5 RM	5
Day 2, 4 sets	100% of 3 RM	5
Day 3, 1 set	100% of 5 RM	5
2 sets	100% of 3 RM	5
2 sets	100% of 2 RM	5

■ **TABLE   9-5**   Knight's DAPRE Program

Set	Amount of Weight	Repetitions
1	50% of RM	10
2	75% of RM	6
3	100% of RM	Maximum
4	Adjusted working weight*	Maximum

*See Table 9-6.

increase of about 10 percent of the current weight being lifted should still allow at least 6 RM in each of three sets.[9]

For rehabilitation purposes, strengthening exercises should be performed on a daily basis initially, with the amount of weight, number of sets, and number of repetitions governed by the injured patient's response to the exercise. As the healing process progresses and pain or swelling is no longer an issue, a particular muscle or muscle group should be exercised consistently every other day. At that point the frequency of weight training should be

■ **TABLE   9-7**   Berger's Adjustment Technique

Sets	Amount of Weight	Repetitions
3	100% of 10 RM	6–8

at least three times per week but no more than four times per week. It is common for serious weight lifters to lift every day; however, they exercise different muscle groups on successive days.

It has been suggested that if training is done properly, using both concentric and eccentric contractions, resistance training is necessary only twice each week. However, this schedule has not been sufficiently documented.

Isokinetic Exercise

An *isokinetic exercise* involves a muscle contraction in which the length of the muscle is changing while the contraction is performed at a constant velocity.[11] In theory, maximal resistance is provided throughout the range of motion by the machine. The resistance provided by the machine will move only at some preset speed, regardless of the torque applied to it by the individual. Thus the key to isokinetic exercise is not the resistance but the speed at which resistance can be moved.

Few isokinetic devices are still available commercially (Figure 9-8). In general, they rely on hydraulic, pneumatic, and mechanical pressure systems to produce this constant velocity of motion. Most isokinetic devices are capable of resisting concentric and eccentric contractions at a fixed speed to exercise a muscle.

■ **TABLE   9-6**   DAPRE Adjusted Working Weight

Number of Repetitions Performed During Third Set	Adjusted Working Weight During Fourth Set	Next Exercise Session
0–2	—5—10 lb	—5–10 lb
3–4	—0–5 lb	Same weight
5–6	Same weight	± 0–10 lb
7–10	± 5–10 lb	± 5–15 lb
11	± 10–15 lb	± 10–20 lb

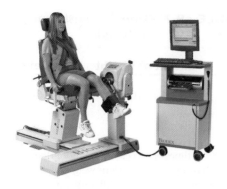

Figure 9-8 The Biodex is an isokinetic device that provides resistance at a constant velocity.

Isokinetics as a Conditioning Tool Isokinetic devices are designed so that regardless of the amount of force applied against a resistance, it can only be moved at a certain speed. That speed will be the same whether maximal force or only half the maximal force is applied. Consequently, in isokinetic training, it is absolutely necessary to exert as much force against the resistance as possible (maximal effort) for maximal strength gains to occur.[11] Maximal effort is one of the major problems with an isokinetic strength-training program.

Anyone who has been involved in a resistance training program knows that on some days it is difficult to find the motivation to work out. Because isokinetic training requires a maximal effort, it is very easy to "cheat" and not go through the workout at a high level of intensity. In a progressive resistive exercise program, the patient knows how much weight has to be lifted for how many repetitions. Thus isokinetic training is often more effective if a partner system is used, primarily as a means of motivation toward a maximal effort. When isokinetic training is done properly with a maximal effort, it is theoretically possible that maximal strength gains are best achieved through the isokinetic training method in which the velocity and force of the resistance are equal throughout the range of motion. However, there is no conclusive research to support this theory.

Whether this changing force capability is a deterrent to improving the ability to generate force against some resistance is debatable. In real life it does not matter whether the resistance is changing; what is important is that an individual develops enough strength to move objects from one place to another.

Another major disadvantage of using isokinetic devices as a conditioning tool is their cost. With initial purchase costs ranging between $50,000 and $80,000 and the necessity of regular maintenance and software upgrades, the use of an isokinetic device for general conditioning or resistance training is, for the most part, unrealistic. Thus isokinetic exercises are primarily used as a diagnostic and rehabilitative tool.

Isokinetics in Rehabilitation Isokinetic strength testing gained a great deal of popularity throughout the 1980s in rehabilitation settings. This trend stems from its providing an objective means of quantifying existing levels of muscular strength and thus becoming useful as a diagnostic tool.[49]

Because the capability exists for training at specific speeds, comparisons have been made regarding the relative advantages of training at fast or slow speeds in a rehabilitation program. The research literature seems to indicate that strength increases from slow-speed training are relatively specific to the velocity used in training. Conversely, training at faster speeds seems to produce a more generalized increase in torque values at all velocities. Minimal hypertrophy was observed only while training at fast speeds, affecting only type II or fast-twitch fibers.[17,52] An increase in neuromuscular efficiency caused by more effective motor unit firing patterns has been demonstrated with slow-speed training.[45]

During the early 1990s, the value of isokinetic devices for quantifying torque values at functional speeds was questioned.

Plyometric Exercise

Plyometric exercise has also been referred to in the literature as reactive neuromuscular training. It is a technique that is being increasingly incorporated into later stages of the rehabilitation program by the athletic trainer. Plyometric training includes specific exercises that encompass a rapid stretch of a muscle eccentrically, followed immediately by a rapid concentric contraction of that muscle to facilitate and develop a forceful explosive movement over a short period of time.[13,20] The greater the stretch put on the muscle from its resting length immediately before the concentric contraction, the greater the resistance the muscle can overcome. Plyometrics emphasize the speed of the eccentric phase. The rate of stretch is more critical than the magnitude of the stretch. An advantage to using plyometric exercises is that they can help to develop eccentric control in dynamic movements.[43]

Plyometric exercises involve hops, bounds, and depth jumping for the lower extremity and the use of medicine balls and other types of weighted equipment for the upper extremity.[12,14] Depth jumping is an example of a plyometric exercise in which an individual jumps to the ground from a specified height and then quickly jumps again as soon as ground contact is made.[53]

Plyometrics tend to place a great deal of stress on the musculoskeletal system. The learning and perfection of specific jumping skills and other plyometric exercises must be technically correct and specific to one's age, activity, physical, and skill development. Plyometric exercise will be discussed in detail in Chapter 11.

CORE STABILIZATION STRENGTHENING

A dynamic core stabilization training program should be a fundamental component of all comprehensive strengthening as well as injury rehabilitation programs.[34,36] The *core* is defined as the lumbo-pelvic-hip complex. The core is where the center of gravity is located and where all movement begins. There are 29 muscles that have their attachment to the lumbo-pelvic-hip complex.

A core stabilization strengthening program can help to improve dynamic postural control, ensure appropriate muscular balance and joint movement around the lumbo-pelvic-hip complex, allow for the expression of dynamic functional strength, and improve neuromuscular efficiency throughout the entire body. Collectively these factors contribute to optimal acceleration, deceleration, and dynamic stabilization of the entire kinetic chain during functional movements. Core stabilization also provides proximal stability for efficient lower extremity movements. Greater neuromuscular control and stabilization strength will offer a more biomechanically efficient position for the entire kinetic chain, therefore allowing optimal neuromuscular efficiency throughout the kinetic chain. This approach facilitates a balanced muscular functioning of the entire kinetic chain.[15]

Many patients develop the functional strength, power, neuromuscular control, and muscular endurance in specific muscles to perform functional activities. However, relatively few patients have developed the muscles required for stabilization. The body's stabilization system has to be functioning optimally to effectively utilize the strength, power, neuromuscular control, and muscular endurance that they have developed in their prime movers. If the extremity muscles are strong and the core is weak, then there will not be enough force created to produce efficient movements. A weak core is a fundamental problem of inefficient movements that leads to injury.[15] Core stabilization techniques were discussed in detail in Chapter 5.

Open- Versus Closed-kinetic-chain Exercises

The concept of the kinetic chain deals with the anatomical functional relationships that exist in the upper and lower extremities. In a weight-bearing position, the lower extremity kinetic chain involves the transmission of forces among the foot, ankle, lower leg, knee, thigh, and hip. In the upper extremity, when the hand is in contact with a weightbearing surface, forces are transmitted to the wrist, forearm, elbow, upper arm, and shoulder girdle.

An *open kinetic chain* exists when the foot or hand is not in contact with the ground or some other surface. In a *closed kinetic chain*, the foot or hand is weight bearing. Movements of the more proximal anatomical segments are affected by these open- versus closed-kinetic-chain positions. For example, the rotational components of the ankle, knee, and hip reverse direction when changing from open- to closed-kinetic-chain activity. In a closed kinetic chain the forces begin at the ground and work their way up through each joint. Also, in a closed kinetic chain forces must be absorbed by various tissues and anatomical structures rather than simply dissipating as would occur in an open chain.

In rehabilitation, the use of closed-chain strengthening techniques has become a treatment of choice for many athletic trainers. Most functional activities involve some aspect of weight bearing with the foot in contact with the ground or the hand in a weightbearing position, so closed-kinetic-chain strengthening activities are more functional than open-chain activities. Therefore rehabilitative exercises should be incorporated that emphasize strengthening of the entire kinetic chain rather than an isolated body segment. Chapter 12 will discuss closed-kinetic-chain activities in detail.

TRAINING FOR MUSCULAR STRENGTH VERSUS MUSCULAR ENDURANCE

Muscular endurance was defined as the ability to perform repeated muscle contractions against resistance for an extended period of time. Most resistance training experts believe that muscular strength and muscular endurance are closely related.[21,50,57] As one improves, there is a tendency for the other to also improve.

It is generally accepted that when resistance training for strength, heavier weights with a lower number of repetitions should be used.[65] Conversely, endurance training uses relatively lighter weights with a greater number of repetitions.

It has been suggested that endurance training should consist of three sets of 10 to 15 repetitions,[9] using the same criteria for weight-selection progression and frequency as recommended for progressive resistive exercise. Thus, suggested training regimens for muscular strength and endurance are similar in terms of sets and numbers of repetitions.[55] Persons who possess great levels of strength tend to also exhibit greater muscular endurance when asked to perform repeated contractions against resistance.[48]

RESISTANCE TRAINING DIFFERENCES BETWEEN MALES AND FEMALES

The approach to strength training is no different for females than for males. However, some obvious physiological differences exist between the genders.

The average female will not build significant muscle bulk through resistance training. Significant muscle hypertrophy is dependent on the presence of the steroidal hormone *testosterone*. Testosterone is considered a male hormone, although all females possess some level of testosterone in their systems. Women with higher testosterone levels tend to have more masculine characteristics, such as increased facial and body hair, a deeper voice, and the potential to develop a little more muscle bulk.[23,50] For the average female, developing large, bulky muscles through strength training is unlikely, although muscle tone can be improved. Muscle tone basically refers to the firmness of tension of the muscle during a resting state.

The initial stages of a resistance training program are likely to rapidly produce dramatic increases in levels of strength.[1] For a muscle to contract, an impulse must be transmitted from the nervous system to the muscle. Each muscle fiber is innervated by a specific motor unit. By overloading a particular muscle, as in weight training, the muscle is forced to work more efficiently. Efficiency is achieved by getting more motor units to fire, thus causing more muscle fibers to contract, which results in a stronger contraction of the muscle. Consequently, both women and men often see extremely rapid gains in strength when a weight-training program is first begun.[28] In females, these initial strength gains, which can be attributed to improved neuromuscular efficiency, tend to plateau, and minimal improvement in muscular strength is realized during a continuing resistance training program. These initial neuromuscular strength gains are also seen in males, although their strength continues to increase with appropriate training.[1] Again, females who possess higher testosterone

levels have the potential to increase their strength further because they are able to develop greater muscle bulk.

Differences in strength levels between males and females are best illustrated when strength is expressed in relation to body weight minus fat. The reduced *strength/body weight ratio* in women is the result of their percentage of body fat. The strength/body weight ratio can be significantly improved through resistance training by decreasing the body fat percentage while increasing lean weight.[45]

The absolute strength differences are considerably reduced when body size and composition are considered. Leg strength can actually be stronger in females than in males, although upper extremity strength is much greater in males.[45]

RESISTANCE TRAINING IN THE ADOLESCENT

The principles of resistance training discussed previously may be applied to adolescents. There are certainly a number of sociological questions regarding the advantages and disadvantages of younger, in particular prepubescent, individuals engaging in rigorous strength-training programs. From a physiological perspective, experts have for years debated the value of strength training in adolescents. Recently, a number of studies have indicated that if properly supervised, adolescents can improve strength, power, endurance, balance, and proprioception; develop a positive body image; improve sport performance; and prevent injuries.[41] A prepubescent child can experience gains in levels of muscle strength without muscle hypertrophy.[51]

An athletic trainer supervising a rehabilitation program for an injured adolescent should certainly incorporate resistive exercise into the program. However, close supervision, proper instruction, and appropriate modification of progression and intensity based on the extent of physical maturation of the individual is critical to the effectiveness of the resistive exercises.[41]

SPECIFIC RESISTIVE EXERCISES USED IN REHABILITATION

Because muscle contractions results in joint movement, the goal of resistance training in a rehabilitation program should be either to regain and perhaps increase the strength of a specific muscle that has been injured or to increase the efficiency of movement about a given joint.[45]

The exercises included throughout Chapters 17 to 24 show exercises for all motions about a particular joint rather than for each specific muscle. These exercises are demonstrated using free weights (dumbbells or bar weights) and some exercise machines. Other strengthening techniques widely used for injury rehabilitation involving isokinetic exercise, plyometrics, core stability training, closed-kinetic-chain exercises, and PNF strengthening techniques will be discussed in greater detail in subsequent chapters.

Summary

1. Muscular strength may be defined as the maximal force that can be generated against resistance by a muscle during a single maximal contraction.
2. Muscular endurance is the ability to perform repeated isotonic or isokinetic muscle contractions or to sustain an isometric contraction without undue fatigue.
3. Muscular endurance tends to improve with muscular strength, thus training techniques for these two components are similar.
4. Muscular strength and endurance are essential components of any rehabilitation program.
5. Muscular power involves the speed with which a forceful muscle contraction is performed.
6. The ability to generate force is dependent on the physical properties of the muscle, neuromuscular efficiency, as well as the mechanical factors that dictate how much force can be generated through the lever system to an external object.
7. Hypertrophy of a muscle is caused by increases in the size and perhaps the number of actin and myosin protein myofilaments, which result in an increased cross-sectional diameter of the muscle.
8. The key to improving strength through resistance training is using the principle of overload within the constraints of the healing process.
9. Five resistance training techniques that can improve muscular strength are isometric exercise, progressive resistive exercise, isokinetic training, circuit training, and plyometric training.
10. Improvements in strength with isometric exercise occur at specific joint angles.
11. Progressive resistive exercise is the most common strengthening technique used by the athletic trainer for rehabilitation after injury.
12. Circuit training involves a series of exercise stations consisting of resistance training, flexibility, and calisthenic exercises that can be designed to maintain fitness while reconditioning an injured body part.
13. Isokinetic training provides resistance to a muscle at a fixed speed.
14. Plyometric exercise uses a quick eccentric stretch to facilitate a concentric contraction.
15. Closed-kinetic-chain exercises might provide a more functional technique for strengthening of injured muscles and joints in the athletic population.
16. Females can significantly increase their strength levels but generally will not build muscle bulk as a result of strength training because of their relative lack of the hormone testosterone.

References

1. Akima, H., H. Takahashi, and S. Y. Kuno. 1999. Early phase adaptations of muscle use and strength to isokinetic training. *Med Sci Sports Exerc* 31(4):588.
2. Allerheiligen, W. 2008. Speed development and plyometric training. In *Essentials of strength training and conditioning*, Baechle, T., ed. Champaign, IL: Human Kinetics.
3. Alway, S. E., D. MacDougall, and G. Sale, et al. 1988. Functional and structural adaptations in skeletal muscle of trained athletess. *J Appl Physiol* 64:1114.
4. Astrand, P. O., and K. Rodahl. 2003. *Textbook of work physiology: Phyiological bases of exercise*. Champaign, IL: Human Kinetics.
5. Baechle, T., ed. 2008. *Essentials of strength training and conditioning*. Champaign, IL: Human Kinetics.
6. Baker, D., G. Wilson, and B. Carlyon. 1994. Generality vs. specificity: A comparison of dynamic and isometric measures of strength and speed-strength. *Eur J Appl Physiol* 68:350–355.
7. Bandy, W., V. Lovelace-Chandler, and B. Bandy et al. 1990. Adaptation of skeletal muscle to resistance training. *J Orthop Sports Phys Ther* 12(6):248–255.
8. Berger, R. 1973. *Conditioning for men*. Boston: Allyn & Bacon.
9. Berger, R. 1962. Effect of varied weight training programs on strength. *Res Q Exerc Sport* 33:168.
10. Booth, F., and D. Thomason. 1999. Molecular and cellular adaptation of muscle in response to exercise: Perspectives of various models. *Physiol Rev* 71:541–585.

11. Brown, L. E. 2000. *Isokinetics in human performance.* Champaign, IL: Human Kinetics.

12. Bruce-Low, S., and D. Smith. 2007. Explosive exercises in sports training: A critical review. *Journal of Exercise Physiology* 10(1):21.

13. Chu, D. 1998. *Jumping into plyometrics.* Champaign, IL: Human Kinetics.

14. Chu, D. 1999. Plyometrics in sports injury rehabilitation and training. *Athlet Ther Today* 4(3):7.

15. Clark, M. 2001. *Integrated training for the new millennium.* Calabasas, CA: National Academy of Sports Medicine.

16. Costill, D., J. Daniels, and W. Evan, et al. 1976. Skeletal muscle enzymes and fiber compositions in male and female track athletes. *J Appl Physiol* 40:149.

17. Coyle, E., D. Feiring, and T. Rotkis et al. 1981. Specificity of power improvements through slow and fast speed isokinetic training. *J Appl Physiol* 51:1437.

18. DeLorme, T., and A. Wilkins 1951. *Progressive resistance exercise.* New York: Appleton-Century-Crofts.

19. Deudsinger, R. H. 1984. Biomechanics in clinical practice. *Phys Ther* 64:1860–1868.

20. Duda, M. 1988. Plyometrics: A legitimate form of power training. *Physician Sports Med* 16:213.

21. Dudley, G. A., and S. J. Fleck. 1987. Strength and endurance training: Are they mutually exclusive? (Review). *Sports Med* 4(2):79.

22. Etheridge, G., and T. Thomas. 1982. Physiological and biomedical changes of human skeletal muscle induced by different strength training programs. *Med Sci Sports Exerc* 14:141.

23. Fahey, T. 2005. *Weight training basics.* St. Louis: McGraw-Hill.

24. Faulkner, J.H. Green, and T. White. 1994. Response and adaptation of skeletal muscle to changes in physical activity. In *Physical activity, fitness, and health,* Bouchard, C., R. Shepard and J. Stephens eds. Champaign, IL: Human Kinetics.

25. Fleck, S. J., and W. J. Kramer. 2004. *Designing resistance training Programs.* Champaign, IL: Human Kinetics.

26. Gabriel, D., and G. Kamen. 2006. Neural adaptation to resistive exercise: Mechanisms and recommendations for training practices. *Sports Medicine* 26(2):133.

27. Gettman, L. 1981. Circuit weight training: A critical review of its physiological benefits. *Physician Sports Med* 9(1):44.

28. Gravelle, B. L., and D. L. Blessing. 2000. Physiological adaptation in women concurrently training for strength and endurance. *J Strength Cond* 14(1):5.

29. Graves, J.E., M. Pollack, and A. Jones, et al. 1989. Specificity of limited range of motion variable resistance training. *Med Sci Sports Exerc* 21:84.

30. Gray, G. W. Ecocentrics—A theoretical model for muscle function (submitted).

31. Harmen, E. 2008. The biomechanics of resistance training. In *Essentials of Strength Training and Conditioning,* Baechle, T., ed. Champaign, IL: Human Kinetics.

32. Hickson, R., C. Hidaka, and C. Foster. 1994. Skeletal muscle fiber type, resistance training and strength-related performance. *Med Sci Sports Exerc* 26:593–598.

33. Hortobagyi, T., and F. I. Katch. 1990. Role of concentric force in limiting improvement in muscular strength. *J Appl Physiol* 68:650.

34. Jones, M., and C. Trowbridge. 1998. Four ways to a safe, effective strength training program. *Athlet Ther Today* 3(2):4.

35. Kaminski, T. W., C. V. Wabbersen, and R. M. Murphy. 1998. Concentric versus enhanced eccentric hamstring strength training: Clinical implications. *J Athlet Train* 33(3):216.

36. King, M. A., 2000. Core stability: Creating a foundation for functional rehabilitation. *Athlet Ther Today* 5(2):6–13.

37. Knight, K., and C. Ingersoll. 2001. Isotonic contractions may be more effective than isometric contractions in developing muscular strength. *Journal of Sport Rehabilitation* 10(2):124.

38. Komi, P. 2003. *Strength and power in sport.* London: Blackwell Scientific.

39. Kraemer, W. 2008. General adaptation to resistance and endurance training programs. In *Essentials of Strength Training and Conditioning,* Baechle, T., ed. Champaign, IL: Human Kinetics.

40. Kraemer, W. J., and N. Ratamess. 2004. Fundamentals of resistance training: Progression and exercise prescription. *Medicine and Science in Sport and Exercise* 36(4):574.

41. Kraemer, W. J., and S.J. Fleck. 2004. *Strength training for young athletes.* Champaign, IL: Human Kinetics.

42. Kraemer, W. J. 2008. General adaptations to resistance and endurance training programs. In *Essentials of strength training and conditioning,* Baechle, T., ed. Champaign, IL: Human Kinetics.

43. Kramer, J., A. Morrow, and A. Leger. 1993. Changes in rowing ergometer, weight lifting, vertical jump and isokinetic performance in response to standard and standard plus plyometric training programs. *Int J Sports Med* 14(8):440–454.

44. Mastropaolo, J. 1992. A test of maximum power theory for strength. *Eur J Appl Physiol* 65:415–420.

45. McArdle, W., F. Katch, and V. Katch. 2006. *Exercise physiology, energy, nutrition, and human performance.* Philadelphia: Lea & Febiger.

46. McComas, A. 1994. Human neuromuscular adaptations that accompany changes in activity. *Med Sci Sports Exerc* 26(12):1498–1509.

47. McGlynn, G. H. 1972. A reevaluation of isometric training. *J Sports Med Phys Fitness* 12:258.

48. McQueen, I. 1954. Recent advance in the techniques of progressive resistance. *Br Med J* 11:11993.

49. Nicholas, J. J. 1989. Isokinetic testing in young nonathletic able-bodied subjects [Review]. *Arch Phys Med Rehabil* 70(3):210.

50. Nygard, C.H., T. Luophaarui, and T. Suurnakki, et al. 1998. Muscle strength and muscle endurance of middle-aged women and men associated to type, duration and intensity of muscular load at work. *Int Arch Occup Environ Health* 60(4):291.

51. Ozmun, J., A. Mikesky, and P. Surburg. 1994. Neuromuscular adaptations following prepubescent strength training. *Med Sci Sports Exerc* 26:514.

52. Pipes, T., and J. Wilmore. 1975. Isokinetic vs. isotonic strength training in adult men. *Med Sci Sports Exerc* 7:262.

53. Radcliffe, J. C. and R. C. Farentinos. 1999. *High-powered plyometrics*. Champaign, IL: Human Kinetics.

54. Rehfeldt, H., G. Caffiber, and H. Kramer, et al. 1989. Force, endurance time, and cardiovascular responses in voluntary isometric contractions of different muscle groups. *Biomed Biochem Acta* 48(5–6):S509.

55. Sale, D., and D. MacDougall. 1986. Specificity in strength training: A review for the coach and athlete *Can J Appl Sports Sci* 6:87.

56. Sanders, M. 1997. Weight training and conditioning. In *Sports Physical Therapy*, Sanders B, ed. Norwalk, CT: Appleton & Lange.

57. Sandler, D. 2005 Speed and strength through plyometrics. In *Sports power*, Sandler, D. Champaign, IL: Human Kinetics.

58. Soest, A., and M. Bobbert. 1993. The role of muscle properties in control of explosive movements. *Biol Cybern* 69:195–204.

59. Staron, R. S., D. L. Karapondo, and W.J. Kreamer. 1994. Skeletal muscle and adaptations during early phase of heavy resistance training in men and women. *J Appl Physiol* 76:1247–1255.

60. Stone, J. 1998. Rehabilitation—speed of movement/muscular power. *Athlet Ther Today* 3(5):10.

61. Stone, J. 1998. Rehabilitation—muscular endurance. *Athlet Ther Today* 3(4):21.

62. Stone, M., and W. Sands. 2006. Maximum strength and strength training–A relationship to endurance? *Strength and Conditioning Journal* 28(3):44.

63. Strauss, R. H., ed. 1991. *Sports medicine*. Philadelphia: WB Saunders.

64. Ulmer, H. W., Knierman, and T. Warlow, et al. 1989. Interindividual variability of isometric endurance with regard to the endurance performance limit for static work. *Biomedical Biochemistry Acta* 48(5–6):S504.

65. Van Etten, L., E. Verstappen, and K. Westerterp. 1994. Effect of body building on weight training induced adaptations in body composition and muscular strength. *Med Sci Sports Exerc* 26:515–521.

66. Weltman, A., and B. Stamford. 1982. Strength training: Free weights vs. machines. *Physician and Sports Medicine* 10:197.

67. Yates, J. W. 1987. Recovery of dynamic muscular endurance. *Eur J Appl Physiol* 56(6):662.

68. Zinovieff, A. 1951. Heavy resistance exercise: The Oxford technique. *Br J Physiol Med* 14:129.

SOLUTIONS TO CLINICAL DECISION MAKING EXERCISES

9-1   She must regain strength to maximize whole-body mechanics for technique and injury prevention. She must regain endurance so that she is sure to make it through a whole game without fatiguing and risking reinjury. And she must restore power so that she can generate speed in her throwing technique.

9-2   Isometric exercise can be performed right away. While in the cast, the athlete can perform muscle contractions that will stimulate blood flow and provide for some maintenance of strength. As soon as the cast is removed, she should perform active concentric and eccentric isotonic contractions until she is strong enough to perform resisted concentric and eccentric exercise with weights or surgical tubing. When planning an isotonic exercise, you should always encourage the athlete to perform the eccentric movement more slowly as it is the stronger movement and will not have a chance to fatigue before the concentric movement does. In athletics it is important to have a strong eccentric component to ensure controlled and balanced movements for good technique and injury prevention.

9-3   Individuals have a particular ratio of fast-twitch to slow-twitch muscle fibers. Those who have a higher ratio of slow-twitch to fast-twitch are better at endurance activities. Because this ratio is genetically determined, it would be surprising if someone who is good at endurance activity could also be good at sprint-type activities.

9-4   The athlete who is able to move more weight probably has a mechanical advantage. If the tendinous insertion of the hamstrings is more distal, a longer lever arm is created and thus less force is required to move the same resistance.

9-5   Doing isometric exercise at that point will help him gain strength for that specific tension point.

9-6   Exercise machines typically are safer and more comfortable. It is easier to change the resistance, and the weight increments are small for easy progressions. Many of the machines utilize some type of cam for accommodating resistance. However, they are expensive and can be used only for one specific joint movement. Dumbbells or free weights are more versatile as well as cheaper. They also implement an additional aspect of training, as it requires neuromuscular control to balance the weight throughout the full range of motion.

CHAPTER 10

Maintaining Aerobic Capacity and Endurance during Rehabilitation

William E. Prentice

After completing this chapter, the athletic training student should be able to do the following:

- Explain the relationships among heart rate, stroke volume, cardiac output, and rate of oxygen use.

- Describe the function of the heart, blood vessels, and lungs in oxygen transport.

- Describe the oxygen transport system and the concept of maximal rate of oxygen use.

- Describe the principles of continuous and interval training and the potential of each technique for improving aerobic activity.

- Describe the difference between aerobic and anaerobic activity.

- Describe the principles of reversibility and detraining.

- Describe caloric threshold goals associated with various stages of exercise programming.

Although strength and flexibility are commonly regarded as essential components in any injury rehabilitation program, often relatively little consideration is given toward maintaining aerobic capacity and cardiorespiratory endurance. When musculoskeletal injury occurs, the patient is forced to decrease physical activity and levels of cardiorespiratory endurance may decrease rapidly. Thus the athletic trainer must design or substitute alternative activities that allow the individual to maintain existing levels of aerobic capacity during the rehabilitation period. Furthermore, the importance of maintaining and improving functional capacity is becoming increasingly evident regardless of musculoskeletal injury. Recent research has demonstrated a reduction in risk for cardiovascular disease associated in improved levels of aerobic capacity. Sandvik et al.[42] reported mortality rates according to fitness quartiles over 16 years of follow-up. The number of deaths in the least fit portion of the study outnumbered the deaths of the most fit by a margin of 61 deaths to 11 deaths from cardiovascular causes.[42] Myers et al. studied 6,213 subjects referred for treadmill testing and concluded that exercise capacity is a more powerful predictor of mortality among men than other established risk factors for cardiovascular disease.[38]

By definition, *cardiorespiratory endurance* is the ability to perform whole-body activities for extended periods of time without undue fatigue.[11,16] The cardiorespiratory system provides a means by which oxygen is supplied to the various tissues of the body. Without oxygen, the cells within the human body cannot possibly function and ultimately death will occur. Thus the cardiorespiratory system is the basic life-support system of the body.[11]

TRAINING EFFECTS ON THE CARDIORESPIRATORY SYSTEM

Basically, transport of oxygen throughout the body involves the coordinated function of four components: heart, blood vessels, blood, and lungs. The improvement of cardiorespiratory endurance through training occurs because of increased capability of each of these four elements in providing necessary oxygen to the working tissues.[48] A basic discussion of the training effects and response to exercise that occur in the heart, blood vessels, blood, and lungs should make it easier to understand why the training techniques discussed later are effective in improving cardiorespiratory endurance.

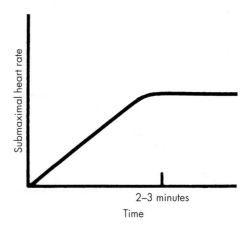

Figure 10-1 For the heart rate to plateau at a given level, 2 to 3 minutes are required.

CLINICAL DECISION MAKING   **Exercise 10–1**

A freshman goalie on the soccer team is not very fit. The coach wants to get her started on a training program to improve her cardiorespiratory endurance. What principles should be considered when designing her program?

Adaptation of the Heart to Exercise

The heart is the main pumping mechanism and circulates oxygenated blood throughout the body to the working tissues. The heart receives deoxygenated blood from the venous system and then pumps the blood through the pulmonary vessels to the lungs, where carbon dioxide is exchanged for oxygen. The oxygenated blood then returns to the heart, from which it exits through the aorta to the arterial system and is circulated throughout the body, supplying oxygen to the tissues.

Heart Rate As the body begins to exercise, the working tissues require an increased supply of oxygen (via transport on red blood cells) to meet the increased demand (cardiac output). Increases in heart rate occur as one response to meet the demand. The heart is capable of adapting to this increased demand through several mechanisms. *Heart rate* shows a gradual adaptation to an increased workload by increasing proportionally to the intensity of the exercise and will plateau at a given level after about 2 to 3 minutes (Figure 10-1). Increases in heart rate produced by exercise are met by a decrease in diastolic filling time. Heart rate parameters change with age, body position, type of exercise, cardiovascular disease, heat and humidity, medications, and blood volume. Conditions that exist in any patient should be taken into consideration

when prescribing exercise to improve aerobic endurance. The commonly used equation to predict maximal heart rate (MHR) is 220–age for healthy men and women. However, the formula has limitations for persons who fall outside the "apparently healthy" classification and should be used with caution. Monitoring heart rate is an indirect method of estimating oxygen consumption.[16] In general, heart rate and oxygen consumption have a linear relationship with exercise intensity. The greater the intensity of the exercise, the higher the heart rate. This relationship is least consistent at very low and very high intensities of exercise (Figure 10-2). During higher-intensity activities, MHR may be achieved before maximum oxygen consumption, which can continue to rise.[35] Because of these

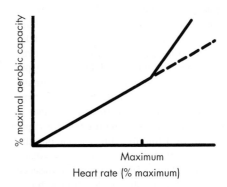

Figure 10-2 Maximum heart rate is achieved at about the same time as maximal aerobic capacity.

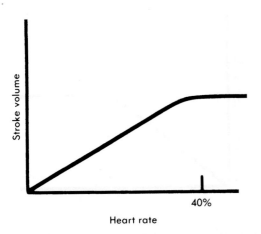

Figure 10-3 Stroke volume plateaus at about 40 percent of maximal heart rate.

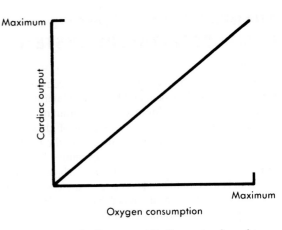

Figure 10-4 Cardiac output limits maximal aerobic capacity.

existing relationships, it should become apparent that the rate of oxygen consumption can be estimated by monitoring the heart rate.[13]

Stroke Volume A second mechanism by which the cardiovascular system is able to adapt to increased demands of cardiac output during exercise is to increase *stroke volume* (the volume of blood being pumped out with each beat). Stroke volume is equal to the difference between end diastolic volume and end systolic volume. Tyical values for stroke volume range from 60 to 100 mL per beat at rest and 100 to 120 mL per beat at maximum.[18] Stroke volume will continue to increase only to the point at which diastolic filling time is simply too short to allow adequate filling. This occurs at about 40 to 50 percent of maximal aerobic capacity or at a heart rate of 110 to 120 beats per minute; above this level, increases in the cadiac output are accounted for by increases in heart rate (Figure 10-3).[12]

Cardiac Output Stroke volume and heart rate collectively determine the volume of blood being pumped through the heart in a given unit of time. Approximately 5 L of blood are pumped through the heart during each minute at rest. This is referred to as the *cardiac output*, which indicates how much blood the heart is capable of pumping in exactly 1 minute. Thus cardiac output is the primary determinant of the maximal rate of oxygen consumption possible (Figure 10-4). During exercise, cardiac output increases to approximately four times that experienced during rest (to about 20 L) in the normal individual and may increase as much as six times in the elite endurance athlete (to about 30 L).

$$\text{Cardiac output} = \text{Stroke volume} \times \text{Heart rate}$$

The aforementioned equation illustrates that any factor that will impact heart rate or stroke volume can either increase or decrease cardiac output. For example, an increase in venous return of blood from working muscle will increase the end diastolic volume. This increased volume will increase stroke volume and, therefore, cardiac output. However, conditions that resist ventricular outflow (high blood pressure) will result in a decrease in cardiac output. Conversely, a condition that would decrease venous return (peripheral artery disease) would decrease stroke volume and attenuate cardiac output.

A commonly reported benefit of aerobic conditioning is a reduced resting heart rate and a reduced heart rate at a standard exercise load. This reduction in heart rate is explained by an increase in stroke volume brought about by increased venous return and to increased contractile conditions in the myocardium. The heart becomes more efficient because it is capable of pumping more blood with each stroke. Because the heart is a muscle, it can hypertrophy, or increase in size and strength due to aerobic exercise, to some extent, but this is in no way a negative effect of training.

Training Effect

Increased stroke volume × Decreased heart rate = Cardiac output

During exercise, females tend to have a 5 to 10 percent higher cardiac output than males do at all intensities. This is likely due to a lower concentration of hemoglobin in the female, which is compensated for during exercise by an increased cardiac output.[51]

Adaptation in Blood Flow The amount of blood flowing to the various organs increases during exercise. However, there is a change in overall distribution of cardiac output; the percentage of total cardiac output to the nonessential organs is decreased, whereas it is increased to active skeletal muscle. Volume of blood flow to the heart muscle or myocardium increases substantially during exercise, even though the percentage of total cardiac output supplying the heart muscle remains unchanged. The increase in flow to skeletal muscle is brought about by withdrawal of sympathetic stimulation to arterioles, and vasodilatation is maintained by intrinsic metabolic control.[40] Trained persons have a higher capillary density than their untrained counterparts to better accommodate the increased supply and demand. In skeletal muscle, there is increased formation of blood vessels or capillaries, although it is not clear whether new ones form or dormant ones simply open up and fill with blood.[44]

The total peripheral resistance is the sum of all forces that resist blood flow within the vascular system. Total peripheral resistance decreases during exercise primarily because of vessel vasodilation in the active skeletal muscles.

Blood Pressure Blood pressure in the arterial system is determined by the cardiac output in relation to total peripheral resistance to blood flow as follows:

$$BP = CO \times TPR,$$

where BP = blood pressure, CO = cardiac output, and TPR = total peripheral resistance.

Blood pressure is created by contraction of the myocardium. Contraction of the ventricles of the heart creates systolic pressure, and relaxation of the heart creates diastolic pressure. Blood pressure is regulated centrally by neural activity on peripheral arterioles and locally by metabolites produced during exercise. During exercise, there is a decrease in total peripheral resistance (via decreased vasoconstriction) and an increase in cardiac output. Systolic pressure increases in proportion to oxygen consumption and cardiac output, while diastolic pressure shows little or no increase.[6] Failure of systolic pressure to increase with increased exercise intensity is considered an abnormal response to exercise and is a general indication to stop an exercise test or session.[1] Blood pressure falls below preexercise levels after exercise and may stay low for several hours. There is general agreement that engaging in consistent aerobic exercise will produce modest reductions in both systolic and diastolic blood pressure at rest as well as during submaximal exercise.[15]

Adaptations in the Blood Oxygen is transported throughout the system, bound to *hemoglobin*. Found in red blood cells, hemoglobin is an iron-containing protein that has the capability of easily accepting or giving up molecules of oxygen as needed. Training for improvement of cardiorespiratory endurance produces an increase in total blood volume, with a corresponding increase in the amount of hemoglobin. The concentration of hemoglobin in circulating blood does not change with training; it may actually decrease slightly.

Adaptation of the Lungs As a result of training, pulmonary function is improved in the trained individual relative to the untrained individual. The volume of air that can be inspired in a single maximal ventilation is increased. The diffusing capacity of the lungs is also increased, facilitating the exchange of oxygen and carbon dioxide. Pulmonary resistance to air flow is also decreased.[33]

CLINICAL DECISION MAKING   **Exercise 10–2**

A lacrosse player sustained a season-ending knee injury at the end of last season. During the off-season he began training for his return to hockey. After several months of training, what physiological changes should be occurring?

MAXIMAL AEROBIC CAPACITY

The maximal amount of oxygen that can be used during exercise is referred to as *maximal aerobic capacity* (exercise physiologists refer to this as $\dot{V}O_2max$). It is considered to be the best indicator of the level of cardiorespiratory endurance. Maximal aerobic capacity is most often presented in terms of the volume of oxygen used relative to body weight per unit of time ($mL \times kg^{-1} \times min^{-1}$).[3]

It is common to see aerobic capacity expressed in metabolic equivalents (METs). Resting oxygen consumption is generally considered to be $3.5 \ mL \times kg^{-1} \times min^{-1}$ or 1 (MET). Therefore, an exercise intensity of 10 METs is equivalent to a $\dot{V}O_2$ of $35 \ mL \times kg^{-1} \times min^{-1}$. A normal maximal aerobic capacity for most collegiate men and women would fall in the range of 35 to $50 \ mL \times kg^{-1} \times min^{-1}$.[35]

Rate of Oxygen Consumption

The performance of any activity requires a certain rate of oxygen consumption, which is about the same for all persons, depending on their present level of fitness. Generally, the greater the rate or intensity of the performance of an

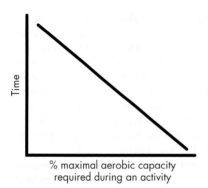

Figure 10-5 The greater the percentage of maximal aerobic capacity required during an activity, the less time an activity can be performed.

activity, the greater will be the oxygen consumption. Each person has his/her own maximal rate of oxygen consumption. The person's ability to perform an activity is closely related to the amount of oxygen required by that activity. This ability is limited by the maximal amount of oxygen the person is capable of delivering into the lungs. Fatigue occurs when insufficient oxygen is supplied to muscles. It should be apparent that the greater the percentage of maximal aerobic capacity required during an activity, the less time the activity may be performed (Figure 10-5).

Three factors determine the maximal rate at which oxygen can be used: (1) external respiration, involving the ventilatory process or pulmonary function; (2) gas transport, which is accomplished by the cardiovascular system (that is, the heart, blood vessels, and blood); and (3) internal respiration, which involves the use of oxygen by the cells to produce energy. Exercise physiologists generally discuss the limiting factors of maximal aerobic capacity based on healthy human subjects in a controlled environment.[4,27] Under these condtions, research presents agreement that the ability to transport oxygen through the heart, lungs, and blood is the limiting factor to the overall rate of oxygen consumption. This indicates that this is not the ability of the mitochondria to consume oxygen that limits $\dot{V}O_2max$. A high maximal aerobic capacity within a person's range indicates that all three systems are working well.

Maximal Aerobic Capacity: An Inherited Characteristic

The maximal rate at which oxygen can be used is a genetically determined characteristic; we inherit a certain range of maximal aerobic capacity, and the more active we are, the higher the existing maximal aerobic capacity will be

within that range.[43,50] Therefore, a training program is capable of increasing maximal aerobic capacity to its highest limit within our range.[50]

Fast-Twitch Versus Slow-Twitch Muscle Fibers The range of maximal aerobic capacity inherited is in a large part determined by the metabolic and functional properties of skeletal muscle fibers. As discussed in detail in Chapter 8, there are two distinct types of muscle fibers, *slow-twitch* or *fast-twitch* fibers, each of which has distinctive metabolic as well as contractile capabilities. Because they are relatively fatigue resistant, slow-twitch fibers are associated primarily with long-duration, aerobic-type activities. Fast-twitch fibers are useful in short-term, high-intensity activities that mainly involve the anaerobic system. In general, if a patient has a high ratio of slow-twitch to fast-twitch muscle fibers, he or she will be able to use oxygen more efficiently and thus will have a higher maximal aerobic capacity.

CLINICAL DECISION MAKING   **Exercise 10–3**

A cyclist wants to know if you can test his maximal aerobic capacity. He says that he has reached a plateau in his training. There hasn't been an increase in his maximal aerobic capacity in about a year. What is your explanation for why this is occurring?

Cardiorespiratory Endurance and Work Ability

Cardiorespiratory endurance plays a critical role in our ability to carry out normal daily activities.[40] Fatigue is closely related to the percentage of maximal aerobic capacity that a particular workload demands.[49] For example, Figure 10-6 presents two people, A and B. A has maximal aerobic capacity of 50 mL/kg per minute, whereas B has a maximal aerobic capacity of only 40 mL/kg per minute. If both A and B are exercising at the same intensity, then A will be working at a much lower percentage of maximal aerobic capacity than B. Consequently, A should be able to sustain his or her activity over a much longer period of time. Everyday activities may be adversely affected if the ability to use oxygen efficiently is impaired. Thus improvement of cardiorespiratory endurance should be an essential component of any conditioning program and must be included as part of the rehabilitation program for the injured patient.[9]

Regardless of the training technique used for the improvement of cardiorespiratory endurance, one principal goal remains the same: *to increase the ability of the cardiorespiratory system to supply a sufficient amount of oxygen*

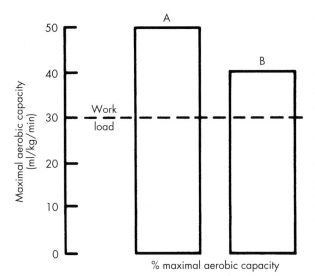

Figure 10-6   Athlete A should be able to work longer than athlete B as a result of a lower percentage use of maximal aerobic capacity.

to working muscles. Without oxygen, the body is incapable of producing energy for an extended period of time.

PRODUCING ENERGY FOR EXERCISE

All living systems need to perform a variety of activities such as growing, generating energy, repairing damaged tissues, and eliminating wastes. All of these activities are referred to as metabolic or cellular *metabolism.*

Muscles are metabolically active and must generate energy to move. Energy is produced from the breakdown of certain nutrients from foodstuffs. This energy is stored in a compound called *adenosine triphosphate* (ATP), which is the ultimate usable form of energy for muscular activity. This ATP is produced in the muscle tissue from blood glucose or glycogen. Fats and proteins can also be metabolized to generate ATP. Glucose not needed immediately can be stored as glycogen in the resting muscle and liver. Stored glycogen in the liver can later be converted back to glucose and transferred to the blood to meet the body's energy needs.[7]

It is important to understand that the intensity and duration of exercise selected as an intervention will have implications on the source of "fuel" to engage in the activity. The fuel is the ATP needed for muscular contraction. Exercise intensity and duration affect the source or pathway that is used to supply the ATP—does the ATP come from the breakdown of circulating blood glucose (glycolysis) or from the Krebs cycle and the electron transport chain (oxidative phosphorization)?

If the combination of duration and intensity is low (40 to 50 percent of $\dot{V}O_2$ max), the body relies more heavily on fats stored in adipose tissue to meet its energy needs. The longer the duration of an activity, the greater the amount of fat used, especially during the later stages of endurance events. During rest and submaximal exertion, both fat and carbohydrates are used to provide energy in approximately a 60- to 40-percent ratio. Carbohydrate must be available to use fat. If glycogen is totally depleted, fat cannot be completely metabolized. Regardless of the nutrient source that produces ATP, it is always available in the cell as an immediate energy source. When all available sources of ATP are used, more must be regenerated for muscular contraction to continue.[8,28]

Various sports activities involve specific demands for energy. For example, sprinting and jumping are high-energy-output activities, requiring a relatively large production of energy for a short time. Long-distance running and swimming, on the other hand, are mostly low-energy-output activities per unit of time, requiring energy production for a prolonged time. Other physical activities demand a blend of both high- and low-energy output. These various energy demands can be met by the different processes in which energy can be supplied to the skeletal muscles.[17]

Anaerobic versus Aerobic Metabolism

Two major energy-generating systems function in muscle tissue: anaerobic and aerobic metabolism. Each of these systems produces ATP.[21] Activities that demand intensive, short-term exercise need ATP that is rapidly available and metabolized to meet energy needs. After a few seconds of intensive exercise, however, the small stores of ATP are used up. The body then utilizes stored glycogen as an energy source. Glycogen can be broken down to supply glucose, which is then metabolized within the muscle cells to generate ATP for muscle contractions.[35]

Glucose can be metabolized to generate small amounts of ATP energy without the need for oxygen. This energy system is referred to as *anaerobic metabolism* (occurring in the absence of oxygen). As exercise continues, the body has to rely on a more complex form of carbohydrate and fat metabolism to generate ATP. This second energy system requires oxygen and is therefore referred to as *aerobic metabolism* (occurring in the presence of oxygen). The aerobic system of producing energy generates considerably more ATP than the anaerobic one.

In most activities, both aerobic and anaerobic systems function simultaneously. The degree to which the two major energy systems are involved is determined by the intensity and duration of the activity.[47] If the intensity of the activity is such that sufficient oxygen can be supplied to meet the demands of working tissues, the activity is considered to be *aerobic*. Conversely, if the activity is of high-enough intensity or the duration is such that there is insufficient oxygen available to meet energy demands, the activity becomes *anaerobic*.[51]

Excess Postexercise Oxygen Consumption (Oxygen Deficit)   As the intensity of the exercise increases and insufficient amounts of oxygen are available to the tissues, an oxygen deficit is incurred. Oxygen deficit occurs in the beginning of exercise (within the first 2 or 3 minutes) when the oxygen demand is greater than the oxygen supplied. It was been hypothesized that this oxygen debt is caused by lactic acid produced during anaerobic activity and this debt must be "paid back" during the postexercise period. However, there is presently a different rationale for this oxygen deficit, which is currently referred to as "excess postexercise oxygen consumption." It is theoretically caused by disturbances in mitochondrial function from an increase in temperature.[35]

TECHNIQUES FOR MAINTAINING CARDIORESPIRATORY ENDURANCE

There are several different training techniques that may be incorporated into a rehabilitation program through which cardiorespiratory endurance can be maintained. Certainly, a primary consideration for the athletic trainer would be whether the injury involves the upper or lower extremity. With injuries that involve the upper extremity, weight-bearing activities can be used, such as walking, running, stair climbing, and modified aerobics. However, if the injury is to the lower extremity, alternative non-weightbearing activities, such as swimming or stationary cycling, may be necessary. The goal of the athletic trainer is to try to maintain cardiorespiratory endurance throughout the rehabilitation process.

The principles of the training techniques discussed next can be applied with running, cycling, swimming, stair climbing, or any other activity designed to maintain levels of cardiorespiratory fitness.

Continuous Training

Continuous training involves the following considerations:

The frequency of the activity
The intensity of the activity
The type of activity
The time (duration) of the activity

Frequency of Training   The American College of Sports Medicine (ACSM) recommends that the average person engage in three to five exercise sessions per week.[1] A competitive athlete should be prepared to train as often as six times per week. Everyone should take off at least 1 day per week to give damaged tissues a chance to repair themselves.

Intensity of Training   The intensity of exercise is also a critical factor, though recommendations regarding training intensities vary.[24] This statement is particularly true in the early stages of training, when the body is forced to make a lot of adjustments to increased workload demands. The ACSM guidelines regarding intensity of exercise recommend the following: 55/65- to 90-percent of MHR, or 40/50- to 85-percent of maximum oxygen uptake reserve ($\dot{V}O_2R$) or MHR reserve (HRR). HRR and $\dot{V}O_2R$ are calculated from the difference between resting and maximum heart rate and resting and maximum $\dot{V}O_2$, respectively. To estimate training intensity, a percentage of this value is added to the resting heart rate and/or resting $\dot{V}O_2$ and is expressed as a percentage of HRR or $\dot{V}O_2R$. The lower intensity values (i.e., 40- to 49-percent of $\dot{V}O_2R$ or HRR and 55- to 64-percent of MHR) are most applicable to individuals who are quite unfit. These intensities require the athletic trainer to either know the person's maximal values or use a prediction equation to estimate these intensities. A great rule of thumb is to always go with actual data over prediction data when available. There are many limitations to prediction equations. Due to the linear relationship between heart rate, oxygen consumption, and exercise intensity, it becomes a relatively simple process to identify a specific workload (pace) that will make the heart rate plateau at the desired level.[46] By monitoring heart rate, we know whether the pace is too fast or too slow to achieve the desired range of intensity.[31] Prior to selecting an exercise intensity, the athletic trainer should consider several factors. These include current level of fitness, medications, cardiovascular risk profile, individuals likes and dislikes, and patient goals and objectives.[1]

Monitoring Heart Rate.   There are several methods to measure heart rate response during exercise. These include, but are not limited to, palpation of the heart rate at the radial or carotid artery, pulse oximetry, telemetry (heart rate monitors), or via electrocardiography (ECG). One of the easiest methods is to palpate the radial artery. This assessment can be done by the patient or the athletic trainer. The carotid artery is simple to find, especially during exercise. However, there are pressure receptors located in the carotid artery that, if subjected to hard pressure from the two fingers, will slow down the heart rate, giving a false indication of exactly what the heart rate is. Thus the pulse at the radial artery proves the most accurate measure of heart rate. Regardless of where the heart rate is taken, it should be recorded prior to exercise, during exercise to ensure target intensities, and monitored following exercise to ensure recovery. Another factor must be considered when measuring heart rate during exercise. The patient is trying to elevate heart rate to a specific target rate and maintain it at that level during the entire workout.[22] Heart rate can be increased or decreased by speeding up or slowing down the pace. Based on the fact that heart rates will attain a steady state or plateau to a prescribed work rate in 2 to 3 minutes, the athletic trainer should allow sufficient time prior to assessment of heart rate. Thus the patient should be actively engaged in the workout for 2 to 3 minutes before measuring pulse.[53]

There are several formulas that will easily allow the athletic trainer to identify a target training heart rate.[39] Exact determination of MHR involves exercising a patient at a maximal level and monitoring the heart rate using an ECG. This process is difficult outside of a laboratory. However, an approximate estimate of MHR for both males and females in the population is thought to be about 220 beats per minute.[41] MHR is related to age. With aging, MHR decreases.[32] So as previously mentioned, a relatively simple estimate of MHR would be MHR = 220–age. For a 40-year-old patient, MHR would be about 180 beats per minute (220–40 = 180). If you are interested in working at 70 percent of your maximal heart rate, the target heart rate can be calculated by multiplying $0.7 \times (220\text{–age})$. The intensity range of 70 to 85 percent of MHR approximates 55 to 75 percent of $\dot{V}O_2max$. Again using a 40-year-old person as an example, a target heart rate would be 126 beats per minute $(0.7 \times [220\text{—}40] = 126)$.

Another commonly used formula that takes into account your current level of fitness is the Karvonen equation, sometimes referred to as the *heart rate reserve* method.[25,29]

$$\text{Target training HR} = \text{Resting HR} + (0.6 [\text{Maximum} - \text{Resting HR}])$$

Resting heart rate generally falls between 60 and 80 beats per minute. According to the Karvonen equation, a 40-year-old patient with a resting pulse of 70 beats per minute would have a target training heart rate of 136 beats per minute $(70 + 0.6 [180 - 70] = 136)$.

Regardless of the formula used, to see minimal improvement in cardiorespiratory endurance, the patient must train with the heart rate elevated to at least 60 percent of its maximal rate.[1,23,30] Exercising at a 70-percent level is considered moderate, because activity can be continued for a long period of time with little discomfort and still produce a training effect.[36] In a trained individual, it is not difficult to sustain a heart rate at the 85-percent level.[14]

Rating of Perceived Exertion.   Rating of perceived exertion (RPE) can be used in addition to monitoring heart rate to indicate exercise intensity.[5] During exercise, individuals are asked to rate subjectively on a numerical scale from 6 to 20 exactly how they feel relative to their level of exertion (Table 9-1). More intense exercise that requires a higher level of oxygen consumption and energy expenditure is directly related to higher subjective ratings of perceived exertion. Over a period of time, patients can be taught to exercise at a specific RPE that relates directly to more objective measures of exercise intensity.[20,37]

Type of Exercise   The type of activity used in continuous training must be aerobic. Aerobic activities are activities that generally involve repetitive, whole-body, large-muscle movements that are rhythmical in nature and use large amounts of oxygen, elevate the heart rate, and maintain it at that level for an extended period of time. Examples of aerobic activities are walking, running, jogging, cycling, swimming, rope skipping, stepping, aerobic dance exercise, rollerblading, and cross-country skiing.

The advantage of these aerobic activities as opposed to more intermittent activities, such as racquetball, squash, basketball, or tennis, is that aerobic activities are easy to regulate in intensity by either speeding up or slowing

■ **TABLE   9-1   Rating of Perceived Exertion**

Scale	Verbal Rating
6	
7	Very, very light
8	
9	Very light
10	
11	Fairly light
12	
13	Somewhat hard
14	
15	Hard
16	
17	Very hard
18	
19	Very, very hard
20	

Source: Borg, G.A. 1982. Psychophysical basis of perceived exertion. *Med Sci Sports Exerc* 14:377.

down the pace.[34] Because we already know that a given intensity of the workload elicits a given heart rate, these aerobic activities allow us to maintain heart rate at a specified or target level. Intermittent activities involve variable speeds and intensities that cause the heart rate to fluctuate considerably. Although these intermittent activities will improve cardiorespiratory endurance, they are much more difficult to monitor in terms of intensity. It is important to point out that any type of activity, from gardening to aerobic exercise, can improve fitness.[39]

Time (Duration)   For minimal improvement to occur, the patient must participate in at least 20 minutes of continuous activity with the heart rate elevated to its working level. The ACSM recommends duration of training to be 20 to 60 minutes of continuous or intermittent (minimum of 10-minute bouts accumulated throughout the day) aerobic activity. Duration will vary with the intensity of the activity. Lower-intensity activity should be conducted over a longer period of time (30 minutes or more). Patients training at higher levels of intensity should train at least 20 minutes or longer because of the importance of "total fitness" and that it is more readily attained with exercise sessions of longer duration, and because of the potential hazards and adherence problems associated with high-intensity activity, moderate-intensity activity of longer duration is recommended for adults not training for athletic competition.

Generally, the greater the duration of the workout, the greater the improvement in cardiorespiratory endurance.

CLINICAL DECISION MAKING   **Exercise 10–4**

Your ice hockey players have been fatiguing early in the game. What type of training will best help them improve their fitness specifically for their sport?

Interval Training

Unlike continuous training, *interval training* involves activities that are more intermittent. Interval training consists of alternating periods of relatively intense work and active recovery. It allows for performance of much more work at a more intense workload over a longer period of time than if working continuously. We have stated that it is most desirable in continuous training to work at an intensity of about 60- to 80-percent of maximal heart rate. Obviously, sustaining activity at a relatively high intensity over a 20-minute period would be extremely difficult. The advantage of interval training is that it allows work at this 80-percent

or higher level for a short period of time followed by an active period of recovery during which you may be working at only 30- to 45-percent of MHR. Thus the intensity of the workout and its duration can be greater than with continuous training.

There are several important considerations in interval training. The training period is the amount of time in which continuous activity is actually being performed, and the recovery period is the time between training periods. A set is a group of combined training and recovery periods, and a repetition is the number of training/recovery periods per set. Training time or distance refers to the rate or distance of the training period. The training/ recovery ratio indicates a time ratio for training versus recovery.

An example of interval training would be a patient exercising on a stationary bike. An interval workout would involve 10 repetitions of pedaling at a maximum speed for 20 seconds followed by pedaling at 40-percent of maximum speed for 90 seconds. During this interval training session, heart rate would probably increase to 85- to 95-percent of maximal level while pedaling at maximum speed and should probably fall to the 35- to 45-percent level during the recovery period.

Older adults should exercise some caution when using interval training as a method for improving cardiorespiratory endurance. The intensity levels attained during the active periods may be too high and create undue risk for the older adult.

CLINICAL DECISION MAKING   **Exercise 10–5**

In an interval workout, at what intensities should an athlete work during the work period and during the active recovery period?

COMBINING CONTINUOUS AND INTERVAL TRAINING

As indicated previously, most physical activities involve some combination of aerobic and anaerobic metabolism.[52] Continuous training is generally done at an intensity level that primarily uses the aerobic system. In interval training, the intensity is sufficient to necessitate a greater percentage of anaerobic metabolism.[19] Therefore for the physically active patient, the athletic trainer should incorporate both training techniques into a rehabilitation program to maximize cardiorespiratory fitness.

CALORIC THRESHOLDS AND TARGETS

The interplay between the duration, intensity, and frequency of exercise creates a caloric expenditure from exercise sessions. The amount of caloric expenditure is important to a wide range of patients including those interested in weight loss as well as those under very strenuous training regimens. General acceptance exists such that the health benefits and training changes associated with exercise programs are related to the total amount of work (indicated by caloric expenditure) completed during training.[1] These caloric thresholds may be different to elicit improvements in VO_2max, weight loss, or risk of premature chronic disease. The ACSM recommends a range of 150 to 400 calories of energy expenditure per day in exercise or physical activity. Expenditure of 1000 kilocalories per week should be the initial goal for those not previously engaged in regular activity. Patients should be moved toward the upper end of the recommendation (300 to 400 kcal per day) to obtain optimal fitness. The estimation of caloric expenditure is easily accomplished using the METs associated with a given activity and the formula[1]:

$$(MET \times 3.5 \times body\ weight\ in\ Kg) / 200 = kcal/min$$

Numerous charts and tables exist that estimate activities in terms of intensity requirements expressed in METs. If a weekly goal of 1000 kcal is established for a 70-kg person at an intensity of 6 METs, the caloric expenditure would be calculated as follows:

$$(6 \times 3.5 \times 70kg) / 200 = kcal/min$$

At an exercise intensity of 6 METs, the patient would need to exercise 136 minutes to achieve the 1000 kcal goal. If the patient wants to exercise 4 days each week, 34 minutes of exercise will be required per day.

The primary goal of weight loss is to consume or burn more calories than are taken in (eaten). The calories used during exercise can be added to the calories cut from the diet to calculate total caloric deficit needed to create weight loss. The aforementioned patient could reduce his/her caloric intake by 400 kcals each day. This will total 2800 kcal that have been restricted from the diet. These calories are then added to the 1000 kcal used for exercise. A pound of fat is equivalent to 3500 kcal. The combination of reduced caloric intake and increased use of kcal for exercise in the example is 3800 kcals, or slightly more than 1 pound of weight loss in 1 week.

DETRAINING

Physical training promotes a wide range of physiologic changes. These include increased size and number of mitochondria, increased capillary bed density, changes in resting and exercise heart rate, blood pressure, myocardial oxygen consumption, and improved VO_2 max, to mention a few. It would seem logical that if the stimulus (exercise) is removed, these changes will dissipate. Long periods of inactivity are associated with the reversal of the aforementioned changes. Improvements may be lost in as little as 12 days to as long as several months to see a complete reversal of changes.

Summary

1. The athletic trainer should routinely incorporate activities that will help maintain levels of cardiorespiratory endurance into the rehabilitation program.
2. Cardiorespiratory endurance involves the coordinated function of the heart, lungs, blood, and blood vessels to supply sufficient amounts of oxygen to the working tissues.
3. The best indicator of how efficiently the cardiorespiratory system functions is the maximal rate at which oxygen can be used by the tissues.
4. Heart rate is directly related to the rate of oxygen consumption. It is therefore possible to predict the intensity of the work in terms of a rate of oxygen use by monitoring heart rate.
5. Aerobic exercise involves an activity in which the level of intensity and duration is low enough to provide a sufficient amount of oxygen to supply the demands of the working tissues.
6. In anaerobic exercise, the intensity of the activity is so high that oxygen is being used more quickly than it can be supplied; thus an oxygen debt is incurred that must be repaid before working tissue can return to its normal resting state.
7. Continuous or sustained training for maintenance of cardiorespiratory endurance involves selecting an activity that is aerobic in nature and training at least three times per week for a time period of no less than

20 minutes with the heart rate elevated to at least 60-percent of maximal rate.

8. Interval training involves alternating periods of relatively intense work followed by active recovery periods. Interval training allows performance of more work at a relatively higher workload than continuous training.

9. Aerobic exercise is a very powerful tool when considering the decreased mortality and morbidity associated with improvements in functional capacity. The athletic trainer with a working knowledge of the principles of exercise prescription and testing is best capable of ensuring the safety and effectiveness of interventions.

References

1. Armstrong, L., P. Bubaker, and M. Whaley. 2005. *ACSM's guidelines for exercise testing and prescription.* Philadelphia: Lippincott Williams & Wilkins.

2. Åstrand, P.O., and K. Rodahl. 2003. *Textbook of work physiology: physiological basis of exercise.* Champaign, IL: Human Kinetics.

3. Åstrand, P.O. 1954. Åstrand-rhyming nomogram for calculation of aerobic capacity from pulse rate during submaximal work. *J Appl Physiol* 7:218.

4. Bassett, D., and E. Howley. 2000. Limiting factors for maximal oxygen uptake and determinants of endurance performance. *Med Sci Sports Exerc* 32:70–84.

5. Borg, G.A. 1982. Psychophysical basis of perceived exertion. *Med Sci Sports Exerc* 14:377.

6. Brooks, G., T. Fahey, and T. White. 2004. *Exercise physiology: Human bioenergetics and its applications.* New York: McGraw-Hill.

7. Brooks, G., and J. Mercier. 1994. The balance of carbohydrate and lipid utilization during exercise: The crossover concept. *J App Physiol* 76:2253–2261.

8. Cerretelli, P. 1992. Energy sources for muscle contraction. *Sports Med* 13:S106–S110.

9. Chillag, S.A. 1986. Endurance patients: Physiologic changes and nonorthopedic problems [Review]. *South Med J* 79:1264.

10. Convertino, V.A. 1987. Aerobic fitness, endurance training, and orthostatic intolerance [Review]. *Exerc Sport Sci Rev* 15:223.

11. Cooper, K.H. 1985. *The aerobics program for total well-being.* New York: Bantam Books.

12. Cox, M. 1991. Exercise training programs and cardiorespiratory adaptation. *Clin Sports Med* 10:19–32.

13. deVries, H. 1993. *Physiology of exercise for physical education and athletics.* St. Louis: McGraw-Hill.

14. Dicarlo, L., P. Sparling, and M. Millard-Stafford. 1991. Peak heart rates during maximal running and swimming: Implications for exercise prescription. *Int J Sports Ed* 12:309–312.

15. Durstein, L., R. Pate, and D. Branch. 2005. Cardiorespiratory responses to acute exercise. In *American College of Sports Medicine: Resource manual for guidelines for exercise testing and prescription.* Philadelphia: Lippincott, Williams, & Wilkins.

16. Fahey, T., ed. 1995. *Encyclopedia of sports medicine and exercise physiology.* New York: Garland.

17. Fox, E., R. Bowers, and M. Foss. 1981. *The physiological basis of physical education and athletics.* Philadelphia: Saunders.

18. Franklin, B. 2005. Cardiorespiratory responses to acute exercise. In *American College of Sports Medicine: Resource manual for guidelines for exercise testing and prescription,* 4th ed. Philadelphia: Lippincott Williams & Wilkins.

19. Gaesser, G.A., and L. A. Wilson. 1988. Effects of continuous and interval training on the parameters of the power–endurance time relationship for high-intensity exercise. *Int J Sports Med* 9:417.

20. Glass, S., M. Whaley, and M. Wegner. 1991. A comparison between ratings of percieved exertion among standard protocols and steady state running. *Int J Sports Ed* 12:77–82.

21. Green, J., and A. Patla A. 1992. Maximal aerobic power: Neuromuscular and metabolic considerations. *Med Sci Sport Exerc* 24:38–46.

22. Greer, N., and F. Katch. 1982. Validity of palpation recovery pulse rate to estimate exercise heart rate following four intensities of bench step exercise. *Res Q Exerc Sport* 53:340.

23. Hage, P. 1982. Exercise guidelines: Which to believe? *Phys Sports Med* 10:23.

24. Hawley, J., K. Myburgh, and T. Noakes. 1995. Maximal oxygen consumption: A contemporary perspective. In *Encyclopedia of sports medicine and exercise physiology,* Fahey, T., ed. New York: Garland.

25. Hickson, R.C., C. Foster, and M. Pollac, et al. 1985. Reduced training intensities and loss of aerobic power, endurance, and cardiac growth. *J Appl Physiol* 58:492.

26. Hill, A., C. Long, and H. Lupton. 1924. Muscular exercise: Lactic acid and the supply and utilization of oxygen, Parts VII–VIII. *Proc Roy Soc B* 97:155–176.

27. Hill, A., and H. Lupton. 1923. Muscular exercise: Lactic acid and the supply and utilization of oxygen. *Q J Med* 16:135–171.

28. Honig, C., R. Connett, and T. Gayeski. 1992. O_2 transport and its interaction with metabolism. *Med Sci Sports Exerc* 24:47–53.

29. Karvonen, M.J., E. Kentala, and D. Mustala. 1957. The effects of training on heart rate: A longitudinal study. *Ann Med Exp Biol* 35:305.

30. Koyanagi, A., K. Yamamoto, and K. Nishijima. Recommendation for an exercise prescription to prevent coronary heart disease. *Ed Syst* 17:213–217.

31. Levine, G., and G. Balady. 1993. The benefits and risks of exercise testing: The exercise prescription. *Adv Intern Ed* 38:57–79.

32. Londeree, B., and M. Moeschberger. 1982. Effect of age and other factors on maximal heart rate. *Res Q Exerc Sport* 53:297.

33. MacDougall, D., and D. Sale. 1981. Continuous vs. interval training: A review for the patient and coach. *Can J Appl Sport Sci* 6:93.

34. Marcinik, E.J., K. Hogden, and K. Mittleman, et al. 1985. Aerobic/calisthenic and aerobic/circuit weight training programs for Navy men: A comparative study. *Med Sci Sports Exerc* 17:482.

35. McArdle, W., F. Katch, and V. Katch. 2006. *Exercise physiology, energy, nutrition, and human performance.* Philadelphia: Lippincott Williams & Wilkins.

36. Mead, W., and R. Hartwig. 1981. Fitness evaluation and exercise prescription. *Fam Pract* 13:1039.

37. Monahan, T. 1988. Perceived exertion: An old exercise tool finds new applications. *Phys Sports Med* 16:174.

38. Myers, J., M. Praksah, V. Froelicher, D. Do, S. Partington, and J. Atwood. 2002. Exercise capacity and mortality among men referred for exercise testing. *N Engl J Med* 346 (11):793–8041.

39. Pate, R., M. Pratt, and S. Blair. 1995. Physical activity and public health: A recommendation from the CDC and ACSM. *JAMA* 273:402–407.

40. Powers, S. 2005. Fundamentals of exercise metabolism. In *Resource manual for guidelines for exercise testing and prescription,* 4th ed, American College of Sports Medicine. Philadelphia: Lippincott, Williams & Wilkins.

41. Rowland, T.W., and G.M. Green. 1989. Anaerobic threshold and the determination of training target heart rates in premenarcheal girls. *Pediatr Cardiol* 10:75.

42. Sandvik, L., J. Erikssen, E. Thaulow, G. Erikssen, R. Mundal, and K. Rodahl. Physical fitness as a predictor of mortality among healthy, middle-aged Norwegian men. *N Engl J Med* 328:533–537.

43. Saltin, B., and S. Strange. 1992. Maximal oxygen uptake: Old and new arguments for a cardiovascular limitation. *Med Sci Sports Exerc* 24:30–37.

44. Smith, M., and J. Mitchell. 2005. Cardiorespiratory adaptations to exercise training. In *Resource manual for guidelines for exercise testing and prescription,* 4th ed, American College of Sports Medicine. Philadelphia: Lippincott, Williams & Wilkins.

45. Stachenfeld, N., M. Eskenazi, and G. Gleim. 1992. Predictive accuracy of criteria used to assess maximal oxygen consumption. *Am Heart J* 123:922–925.

46. Swain, D., K. Abernathy, and C. Smith. 1994. Target heart rates for the development of cardiorespiratory fitness. *Med Sci Sports Exerc* 26:112–116.

47. Vago, P., M. Mercier, and M. Ramonatxo, et al. 1987. Is ventilatory anaerobic threshold a good index of endurance capacity? *Int J Sports Med* 8:190.

48. Wagner, 1991. P. Central and peripheral aspects of oxygen transport and adaptations with exercise. *Sports Med* 11:133–142.

49. Weltman, A., J. Weltman, and R. Ruh, et al. 1989. Percentage of maximal heart rate reserve, and $\dot{V}O_2$ peak for determining endurance training intensity in sedentary women [Review]. *Int J Sports Med* 10:212.

50. Weymans, M., and T. Reybrouck. 1989. Habitual level of physical activity and cardiorespiratory endurance capacity in children. *Eur J Appl Physiol* 58:803.

51. Williford, H., M. Scharff-Olson, and D. Blessing. 1993. Exercise prescription for women: Special considerations. *Sports Ed* 15:299–311.

52. Wilmore, J., and D. Costill. 2008. *Physiology of sport and exercise.* Champaign, IL: Human Kinetics.

53. Zhang, Y., M. Johnson, and N. Chow. 1991. Effect of exercise testing protocol on parameters of aerobic function. *Med Sci Sports Exerc* 23:625–630.

SOLUTIONS TO CLINICAL DECISION MAKING EXERCISES

10-1 Frequency, intensity, type, and time. All of these should be specific to the demands of her sport. For example, she would benefit more from interval training than endurance as she performs in short bursts during a game. Her exercise should also incorporate flexibility and agility activities that would enhance her functional performance in the goal.

10-2 He should have a marked decrease in resting heart rate and blood pressure. This is due in part to an increase in stroke volume and cardiac output. He should have a decreased body fat percentage as resting metabolic rate increases, encouraging energy expenditure.

10-3 He might be reaching his maximum aerobic capacity. Everyone has a limited inherited range of aerobic capacity. Once an athlete reaches the upper end of that range, it is unlikely that additional significant improvement will occur.

10-4 Interval training, because the sport requires quick sprints interrupted by short recovery periods.

10-5 They should be working at 85- to 90-percent of their maximum heart rate during the work period and at 35- to 45 percent of their maximum heart rate during the active recovery period.

The Tools of Rehabilitation

CHAPTER 11

Plyometrics in Rehabilitation

Steve Tippett
Michael Voight

After completion of this chapter, the athletic training student should be able to do the following:

- Define plyometric exercise and identify its function in a rehabilitation program.

- Assess the mechanical, neurophysiological, and neuromuscular control mechanisms involved in plyometric training.

- Review how biomechanical evaluation, stability, dynamic movement, and flexibility should be assessed before beginning a plyometric program.

- Explain how a plyometric program can be modified by changing intensity, volume, frequency, and recovery.

- Discuss how plyometrics can be integrated into a rehabilitation program.

- Recognize the value of different plyometric exercises in rehabilitation.

WHAT IS PLYOMETRIC EXERCISE?

In sports training and rehabilitation of athletic injuries, the concept of specificity has emerged as an important parameter in determining the proper choice and sequence of exercise in a training program. The jumping movement is inherent in numerous sport activities such as basketball, volleyball, gymnastics, and aerobic dancing. Even running is a repeated series of jump-landing cycles. Therefore jump training should be used in the design and implementation of the overall training program.

Peak performance in sport requires technical skill and power. Skill in most activities combines natural athletic ability and learned specialized proficiency in an activity. Success in most activities is dependent upon the speed at which muscular force or power can be generated. Strength and conditioning programs throughout the years have attempted to augment the force production system to maximize the power generated. Because power combines strength and speed, it can be increased by increasing the amount of work or force that is produced by the muscles or by decreasing the amount of time required to produce the force. Although weight training can produce increased gains in strength, the speed of movement is limited. The amount of time required to produce muscular force is an important variable for increasing the power output. A form of training that attempts to combine speed of movement with strength is plyometrics.

The roots of plyometric training can be traced to eastern Europe, where it was known simply as jump training. The term *plyometrics* was coined by American track and field coach Fred Wilt.[46] The development of the term is confusing. *Plyo-* comes from the Greek word plythein, which means "to increase." *Plio* is the Greek word for "ore," and *metric* literally means "to measure." Practically, plyometrics is defined as a quick, powerful movement involving prestretching the muscle and activating the stretch-shortening cycle to produce a subsequently stronger concentric contraction. It takes advantage of the length-shortening cycle to increase muscular power.

In the late 1960s and early 1970s when the Eastern Bloc countries began to dominate sports requiring power, their training methods became the focus of attention. After the 1972 Olympics, articles began to appear in coaching magazines outlining a strange new system of jumps and bounds that had been used by the Soviets to increase speed. Valery Borzov, the 100-meter gold medalist, credited plyometric exercise for his success. As it turns out, the Eastern Bloc countries were not the originators of plyometrics, just the organizers. This system of hops and jumps has been used by American coaches for years as a method of conditioning. Both rope jumping and bench hops have been used to improve quickness and reaction times. The organization of this training method has been credited to the legendary Soviet jump coach Yuri Verhoshanski, who during the late 1960s began to tie this method of miscellaneous hops and jumps into an organized training plan.[40]

The main purpose of plyometric training is to heighten the excitability of the nervous system for improved reactive ability of the neuromuscular system.[43] Therefore, any type of exercise that uses the myotatic stretch reflex to produce a more powerful response of the contracting muscle is plyometric in nature. All movement patterns in both athletics and activities of daily living (ADL) involve repeated stretch-shortening cycles. Picture a jumping athlete preparing to transfer forward energy to upward energy. As the final step is taken before jumping, the loaded leg must stop the forward momentum and change it into an upward direction. As this happens, the muscle undergoes a lengthening eccentric contraction to decelerate the movement and prestretch the muscle. This prestretch energy is then immediately released in an equal and opposite reaction, thereby producing kinetic energy. The neuromuscular system must react quickly to produce the concentric shortening contraction to prevent falling and produce the upward change in direction. Most elite athletes will naturally exhibit with great ease this ability to use stored kinetic energy. Less gifted athletes can train this ability and enhance their production of power. Consequently, specific functional exercise to emphasize this rapid change of direction must be used to prepare patients and athletes for return to activity. Because plyometric exercises train specific movements in a biomechanically accurate manner, the muscles, tendons, and ligaments are all strengthened in a functional manner.

Most of the literature to date on plyometric training has been focused on the lower quarter. Because all movements in athletics involve a repeated series of stretch-shortening cycles, adaptation of the plyometric principles can be used to enhance the specificity of training in other sports or activities that require a maximum amount of muscular force in a minimal amount of time. Whether the athlete is jumping or throwing, the musculature around the involved joints must first stretch and then contract to produce the explosive movement. Because of the muscular demands during the overhead throw, plyometrics have been advocated as a form of conditioning for the overhead throwing athlete.[42,45] Although the principles are similar, different forms of plyometric exercises should be applied to the upper extremity to train the stretch-shortening cycle. Additionally, the intensity of the upper extremity plyometric program is usually less than that of the lower extremity, due to the smaller muscle mass and type of muscle function of the upper extremity compared to the lower extremity.

The role of the core muscles of the abdominal region and the lumbar spine in providing a vital link for stability and power cannot be overlooked. Plyometric training for these muscles can be incorporated in isolated drills as well as functional activities.

BIOMECHANICAL AND PHYSIOLOGICAL PRINCIPLES OF PLYOMETRIC TRAINING

The goal of plyometric training is to decrease the amount of time required between the yielding eccentric muscle contraction and the initiation of the overcoming concentric contraction. Normal physiological movement rarely begins from a static starting position but rather is preceded by an eccentric prestretch that loads the muscle and prepares it for the ensuing concentric contraction.[11] The coupling of this eccentric-concentric muscle contraction is known as the stretch-shortening cycle. The physiology of this stretch-shortening cycle can be broken down into two components: proprioceptive reflexes and the elastic properties of muscle fibers. These components work together to produce a response, but they will be discussed separately for the purpose of understanding.

Mechanical Characteristics

The mechanical characteristics of a muscle can best be represented by a three-component model (Figure 11-1). A contractile component (CC), series elastic component (SEC), and parallel elastic component (PEC) all interact to produce a force output. Although the CC is usually the focal point of motor control, the SEC and PEC also play an

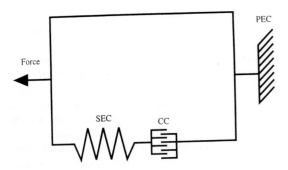

Figure 11-1   Three-component model.

important role in providing stability and integrity to the individual fibers when a muscle is lengthened. During this lengthening process, energy is stored within the musculature in the form of kinetic energy.

When a muscle contracts in a concentric fashion, most of the force that is produced comes from the muscle fiber filaments sliding past one another. Force is registered externally by being transferred through the SEC. When eccentric contraction occurs, the muscle lengthens like a spring. With this lengthening, the SEC is also stretched and allowed to contribute to the overall force production. Therefore the total force production is the sum of the force produced by the CC and the stretching of the SEC. An analogy would be the stretching of a rubber band. When a stretch is applied, potential energy is stored and applied as it returns to its original length when the stretch is released. Significant increases in concentric muscle force production have been documented when immediately preceded by an eccentric contraction.[2,4,9] This increase might be partly due to the storage of elastic energy, because the muscles are able to use the force produced by the SEC. When the muscle contracts in a concentric manner, the elastic energy that is stored in the SEC can be recovered and used to augment the shortening contraction. The ability to use this stored elastic energy is affected by three variables: time, magnitude of stretch, and velocity of stretch.[23] The concentric contraction can be magnified only if the preceding eccentric contraction is of short range and performed quickly without delay.[2,4,9] Bosco and Komi proved this concept experimentally when they compared damped versus undamped jumps.[4] Undamped jumps produced minimal knee flexion upon landing and were followed by an immediate rebound jump. With damped jumps, the knee flexion angle increased significantly. The power output was much higher with the undamped jumps. The increased knee flexion seen in the damped jumps decreased elastic behavior of the muscle, and the potential elastic energy

stored in the SEC was lost as heat. Similar investigations produced greater vertical jump height when the movement was preceded by a countermovement as opposed to a static jump.[2,5,6,29]

The type of muscle fiber involved in the contraction can also affect storage of elastic energy. Bosco et al. noted a difference in the recoil of elastic energy in slow-twitch versus fast-twitch muscle fibers.[7] This study indicates that fast-twitch muscle fibers respond to a high-speed, small amplitude prestretch. The amount of elastic energy used was proportional to the amount stored. When a long, slow stretch is applied to muscle, slow- and fast-twitch fibers exhibit a similar amount of stored elastic energy; however, this stored energy is used to a greater extent with the slow-twitch fibers. This trend would suggest that slow-twitch muscle fibers might be able to use elastic energy more efficiently in ballistic movement characterized by long and slow prestretching in the stretch-shortening cycle.

Neurophysiological Mechanisms

The proprioceptive stretch reflex is the other mechanism by which force can be produced during the stretch-shortening cycle.[10] Mechanoreceptors located within the muscle provide information about the degree of muscular stretch. This information is transmitted to the central nervous system and becomes capable of influencing muscle tone, motor execution programs, and kinesthetic awareness. The mechanoreceptors that are primarily responsible for the stretch reflex are the Golgi tendon organs and muscle spindles.[31] The muscle spindle is a complex stretch receptor that is located in parallel within the muscle fibers. Sensory information regarding the length of the muscle spindle and the rate of the applied stretch is transmitted to the central nervous system. If the length of the surrounding muscle fibers is less than that of the spindle, the frequency of the nerve impulses from the spindle is reduced. When the muscle spindle becomes stretched, an afferent sensory response is produced and transmitted to the central nervous system. Neurological impulses are in turn sent back to the muscle, causing a motor response. As the muscle contracts, the stretch on the muscle spindle is relieved, thereby removing the original stimulus. The strength of the muscle spindle response is determined by the rate of stretch.[31] The more rapidly the load is applied to the muscle, the greater the firing frequency of the spindle and resultant reflexive muscle contraction.

The Golgi tendon organ lies within the muscle tendon near the point of attachment of the muscle fiber to the tendon. Unlike the facilitory action of the muscle spindle, the Golgi tendon organ has an inhibitory effect on the muscle by contributing to a tension-limiting reflex. Because the Golgi tendon organs are in series alignment with the contracting muscle fibers, they become activated with tension or stretch within the muscle. Upon activation, sensory impulses are transmitted to the central nervous system. These sensory impulses cause an inhibition of the alpha motor neurons of the contracting muscle and its synergists, thereby limiting the amount of force produced. With a concentric muscle contraction, the activity of the muscle spindle is reduced because the surrounding muscle fibers are shortening. During an eccentric muscle contraction, the muscle stretch reflex generates more tension in the lengthening muscle. When the tension within the muscle reaches a potentially harmful level, the Golgi tendon organ fires, thereby reducing the excitation of the muscle. The muscle spindle and Golgi tendon organ systems oppose each other, and increasing force is produced. The descending neural pathways from the brain help to balance these forces and ultimately control which reflex will dominate.[34]

The degree of muscle fiber elongation is dependent upon three physiological factors. Fiber length is proportional to the amount of stretching force applied to the muscle. The ultimate elongation or deformation is also dependent upon the absolute strength of the individual muscle fibers. The stronger the tensile strength, the less elongation that will occur. The last factor for elongation is the ability of the muscle spindle to produce a neurophysiological response. A muscle spindle with a low sensitivity level will result in a difficulty in overcoming the rapid elongation and therefore produce a less powerful response. Plyometric training will assist in enhancing muscular control within the neurological system.[10]

The increased force production seen during the stretch-shortening cycle is due to the combined effects of the storage of elastic energy and the myotatic reflex activation of the muscle.[4,2,5,8,9,30,36] The percentage of contribution from each component is unknown.[5] The increased amount of force production is dependent upon the time frame between the eccentric and concentric contractions.[9] This time frame can be defined as the amortization phase.[15] The amortization phase is the electromechanical delay between eccentric and concentric contraction during which time the muscle must switch from overcoming work to acceleration in the opposite direction. Komi found that the greatest amount of tension developed within the muscle during the stretch-shortening cycle occurred during the phase of muscle lengthening just before the concentric contraction.[28] The conclusion from this study was that an increased time in the amortization phase would lead to a decrease in force production.

Physiological performance can be improved by several mechanisms with plyometric training. Although there has been documented evidence of increased speed of the stretch reflex, the increased intensity of the subsequent muscle contraction might be best attributed to better recruitment of additional motor units.[13,21] The force-velocity relationship states that the faster a muscle is loaded or lengthened eccentrically, the greater the resultant force output. Eccentric lengthening will also place a load on the elastic components of the muscle fibers. The stretch reflex might also increase the stiffness of the muscular spring by recruiting additional muscle fibers.[13,21] This additional stiffness might allow the muscular system to use more external stress in the form of elastic recoil.[13]

Another possible mechanism by which plyometric training can increase the force or power output involves the inhibitory effect of the Golgi tendon organs on force production. Because the Golgi tendon organ serves as a tension-limiting reflex, restricting the amount of force that can be produced, the stimulation threshold for the Golgi tendon organ becomes a limiting factor. Bosco and Komi have suggested that plyometric training can desensitize the Golgi tendon organ, thereby raising the level of inhibition.[4] If the level of inhibition is raised, a greater amount of force production and load can be applied to the musculoskeletal system.

CLINICAL DECISION MAKING   **Exercise 11–1**

A high school female basketball player is engaged in an off-season conditioning program that involves box jumps and depth jumps. As a result of these activities in conjunction with a running program to enhance cardiovascular fitness, she now complains of unilateral parapatellar pain. The knee pain is significant enough that she cannot take part in the plyometric program. The coach feels the athlete needs to address both her conditioning and her power training, and wants to know what can be done to improve the athlete's performance but not increase the knee pain. How can you help?

Neuromuscular Coordination

The last mechanism in which plyometric training might improve muscular performance centers around neuromuscular coordination (see Chapter 6). The speed of muscular contraction can be limited by neuromuscular coordination. In other words, the body can move only within a set speed range, no matter how strong the muscles are.

Training with an explosive prestretch of the muscle can improve the neural efficiency, thereby increasing neuromuscular performance. Plyometric training can promote changes within the neuromuscular system that allow the individual to have better control of the contracting muscle and its synergists, yielding a greater net force even in the absence of morphological adaptation of the muscle. This neural adaptation can increase performance by enhancing the nervous system to become more automatic.

In summary, effective plyometric training relies more on the rate of stretch than on the length of stretch. Emphasis should center on the reduction of the amortization phase. If the amortization phase is slow, the elastic energy is lost as heat and the stretch reflex is not activated. Conversely, the quicker the individual is able to switch from yielding eccentric work to overcoming concentric work, the more powerful the response.

PROGRAM DEVELOPMENT

Specificity is the key concept in any training program. Sport-specific activities should be analyzed and broken down into basic movement patterns. These specific movement patterns should then be stressed in a gradual fashion, based upon individual tolerance to these activities. Development of a plyometric program should begin by establishing an adequate strength base that will allow the body to withstand the large stress that will be placed upon it. A greater strength base will allow for greater force production due to increased muscular cross-sectional area. Additionally, a larger cross-sectional area can contribute to the SEC and subsequently store a greater amount of elastic energy.

Plyometric exercises can be characterized as rapid eccentric loading of the musculoskeletal complex.[13] This type of exercise trains the neuromuscular system by teaching it to more readily accept the increased strength loads.[3] Also, the nervous system is more readily able to react with maximal speed to the lengthening muscle by exploiting the stretch reflex. Plyometric training attempts to fine-tune the neuromuscular system, so all training programs should be designed with specificity in mind.[33] This goal will help to ensure that the body is prepared to accept the stress that will be placed upon it during return to function.

Plyometric Prerequisites

Biomechanical Examination. Before beginning a plyometric training program, a cursory biomechanical examination and a battery of functional tests should be performed to identify potential contraindications or precautions. Lower-quarter biomechanics should be sound to help ensure a stable base of support and normal force transmission. Biomechanical abnormalities of the lower quarter are not contraindications for plyometrics but can contribute to stress failure-overuse injury if not addressed. Before initiating plyometric training, an adequate strength base of the stabilizing musculature must be present. Functional tests are very effective to screen for an adequate strength base before initiating plyometrics. Poor strength in the lower extremities will result in a loss of stability when landing and also increase the amount of stress that is absorbed by the weightbearing tissues with high-impact forces, which will reduce performance and increase the risk of injury. The Eastern Bloc countries arbitrarily placed a one-repetition maximum in the squat at 1.5 to 2 times the individual's body weight before initiating lower-quarter plyometrics.[3] If this were to hold true, a 200-pound individual would have to squat 400 pounds before beginning plyometrics. Unfortunately, not many individuals would meet this minimal criteria. Clinical and practical experience has demonstrated that plyometrics can be started without that kind of leg strength.[13] A simple functional parameter to use in determining whether an individual is strong enough to initiate a plyometric training program has been advocated by Chu.[14] Power squat testing with a weight equal to 60 percent of the individual's body weight is used. The individual is asked to perform five squat repetitions in 5 seconds. If the individual cannot perform this task, emphasis in the training program should again center on the strength-training program to develop an adequate base.

CLINICAL DECISION MAKING   **Exercise 11–2**

A college track sprinter has been instructed by her strength coach to begin off-season plyometrics consisting of box jumps and high stepping drills. The patient suffered a second-degree upper hamstring strain during the last half of track season and is reluctant to start the plyometric program. What can be done to prevent this injury from recurring?

Because eccentric muscle strength is an important component to plyometric training, it is especially important to ensure an adequate eccentric strength base is present. Before an individual is allowed to begin a plyometric regimen, a program of closed-chain stability training that focuses on eccentric lower-quarter strength should be initiated. In addition to strengthening in a functional manner, closed-chain weightbearing exercises also allow the individual to use functional movement patterns. The same holds true for adequate upper-extremity strength prior to initiating an upper-extremity plyometric program. Closed-chain activities such as wall push-ups, traditional push-ups and their modification, as well as functional tests can be utilized to ascertain readiness for upper-extremity plyometrics.[24,37,38] Once cleared to participate in the plyometric program, precautionary safety tips should be adhered to.

Stability Testing.   Stability testing before initiating plyometric training can be divided into two subcategories: static stability and dynamic movement testing. Static stability testing determines the individual's ability to stabilize and control the body. The muscles of postural support must be strong enough to withstand the stress of explosive training. Static stability testing (Figure 11-2) should begin with simple movements of low motor complexity and progress to more difficult high motor skills. The basis for lower-quarter stability centers around single-leg strength. Difficulty can be increased by having the individual close his or her eyes. The basic static tests are one-leg standing and single-leg quarter squats that are held for 30 seconds. An individual should be able to perform one-leg standing for 30 seconds with eyes open and closed before the initiation of plyometric training. The individual should be observed for shaking or wobbling of the extremity joints. If there is more movement of a weightbearing joint in one direction than the other, the musculature producing the movement in the opposite direction needs to be assessed for specific weakness. If weakness is determined, the individual's program should be limited and emphasis placed on isolated strengthening of the weak muscles. For dynamic jump exercises to be initiated, there should be no wobbling of the support leg during the quarter knee squats.

After an individual has satisfactorily demonstrated both single-leg static stance and a single-leg quarter squat,

more dynamic tests of eccentric capabilities can be initiated. Once an individual has stabilization strength, the concern shifts toward developing and evaluating eccentric strength. The limiting factor in high-intensity, high-volume plyometrics is eccentric capabilities. Eccentric strength can be assessed with stabilization jump tests. If an individual has an excessively long amortization phase or a slow switching from eccentric to concentric contractions, the eccentric strength levels are insufficient.

Dynamic Movement Testing.   Dynamic movement testing will assess the individual's ability to produce explosive, coordinated movement. Vertical or single-leg jumping for distance can be used for the lower quarter. Researchers have investigated the use of single-leg hop for distance and a determinant for return to play after knee injury. A passing score on their test is 85 percent in regard to symmetry. The involved leg is tested twice, and the average between the two trials is recorded. The noninvolved leg is tested in the same fashion, and then the scores of the noninvolved leg are divided by the scores of the involved leg and multiplied by 100. This provides the symmetry index score. Another functional test that can be used to determine whether an individual is ready for plyometric training is the ability to long jump a distance equal to the individual's height.

In the upper quarter, the medicine ball toss is used as a functional assessment. The seated chest pass is used as a measure of upper body power. To perform this test, the patient sits tall with their back against the back rest of a chair. While holding onto a medicine ball (4kg for men and 2kg for women and juniors), the patient tries to chest pass the ball as far as possible keeping their back in contact with the chair. This should be repeated until the longest pass has been measured. Use the distance from where the ball bounces to the patient's chest as the distance. As can be seen in Table 11-1, under 17 feet for men and under 15 feet for women is an indicator of power weakness.

The sit-up-and-throw test is a great test to assess abdominal and lat power. The sit-up evaluates core power while the overhead throw evaluates the lat and trunk power. To perform this test, the patient lies supine with their knees bent and feet flat on the ground while holding onto a medicine ball with both hands (4kg for men and 2kg for women and juniors), with the ball directly over their head like a soccer throw in. Next have them try to sit up and throw the ball as far as possible. This should be repeated until the longest pass has been measured. Use the distance from where the ball bounces to the patient's chest as the distance. As can be seen in Table 11-2, under 17 feet for men and under 15 feet for women is an indicator of power weakness.

Plyometric Static Stability Testing

- Single-Leg Stance — 30 sec
  - Eyes open
  - Eyes closed

- Single-Leg 25% Squat — 30 sec
  - Eyes open
  - Eyes closed

- Single-Leg 50% Squat — 30 sec
  - Eyes open
  - Eyes closed

Figure 11-2   Static stability testing.

■ **TABLE   11-1** Seated Chest Pass Test (feet)

Female	Excellent	Good	Average	Needs Work
Adult	>21'	17–21'	15–17'	<15'
Junior (<16)	>19'	16–19'	14–16'	<14'
Male	**Excellent**	**Good**	**Average**	**Needs Work**
Adult	>24'	20–24'	17–20'	<17'
Junior (<16)	>20'	18–20'	15–18'	<15'

■ **TABLE   11-2** Sit Up and Throw Test (feet)

Female	Excellent	Good	Average	Needs Work
Adult	>21'	17–21'	15–17'	<15'
Junior (<16)	>19'	16–19'	14–16'	<14'
Male	**Excellent**	**Good**	**Average**	**Needs Work**
Adult	>24'	20–24'	17–20'	<17'
Junior (<16)	>20'	18–20'	15–18'	<15'

Flexibility. Another important prerequisite for plyometric training is general and specific flexibility, because a high amount of stress is applied to the musculoskeletal system. Therefore all plyometric training sessions should begin with a general warm-up and flexibility exercise program. The warm-up should produce mild sweating.[26] The flexibility exercise program should address muscle groups involved in the plyometric program and should include static and short dynamic stretching techniques.[25]

Plyometric Prerequisites Summary. When the individual can demonstrate static and dynamic control of their body weight with single-leg squats or adequate medicine ball throws for the upper extremity and core, low-intensity in-place plyometrics can be initiated. Plyometric training should consist of low-intensity drills and progress slowly in deliberate fashion. As skill and strength foundation increase, moderate-intensity plyometrics can be introduced. Mature patients with strong weight-training backgrounds can be introduced to ballistic-reactive plyometric exercises of high intensity.[14] Once the individual has been classified as beginner, intermediate, or advanced, the plyometric program can be designed and initiated.

PLYOMETRIC PROGRAM DESIGN

As with any conditioning program, the plyometric training program can be manipulated through training variables: direction of body movement, weight of the individual, speed of the execution, external load, intensity, volume, frequency, training age, and recovery.

Direction of Body Movement Horizontal or forward body movement is less stressful than vertical movement due to the impact of loading. This is dependent upon the weight of the patient and the technical proficiency demonstrated during the jumps.

CLINICAL DECISION MAKING   **Exercise 11–3**

The coach of a junior football league team (ages 10 and 11) wants to institute a plyometric conditioning program for the team. The coach has met some resistance from concerned parents regarding the intensity of this type of training. A meeting with the parents has been scheduled and the coach wants you to discuss plyometric training with them. What things should the athletic trainer address in this meeting?

Weight of the Patient   The heavier the patient, the greater the training demand placed on the patient. What might be a low-demand in-place jump for a lightweight patient might be a high-demand activity for a heavyweight patient.

Speed of Execution of the Exercise   Increased speed of execution on exercises like single-leg hops or alternate-leg bounding raises the training demand on the individual.

External Load   Adding an external load can significantly raise the training demand. Do not raise the external load to a level that will significantly slow the speed of movement.

Intensity   Intensity can be defined as the amount of effort exerted. With traditional weight lifting, intensity can be modified by changing the amount of weight that is lifted. With plyometric training, intensity can be controlled by the type of exercise that is performed. Double-leg jumping is less stressful than single-leg jumping. As with all functional exercise, the plyometric exercise program should progress from simple to complex activities. Intensity can be further increased by altering the specific exercises. The addition of external weight or raising the height of the step or box will also increase the exercise intensity.[22]

Volume   Volume is the total amount of work that is performed in a single workout session. With weight training, volume would be recorded as the total amount of weight that was lifted (weight times repetitions). Volume of plyometric training is measured by counting the total number of foot contacts. The recommended volume of foot contacts in any one session will vary inversely with the intensity of the exercise. A beginner should start with low-intensity exercise with a volume of approximately 75 to 100 foot contacts. As ability is increased, the volume is increased to 200 to 250 foot contacts of low to moderate intensity.

Frequency   Frequency is the number of times an exercise session is performed during a training cycle. With weight training, the frequency of exercise has typically been three times weekly. Unfortunately, research on the frequency of plyometric exercise has not been conducted. Therefore the optimum frequency for increased performance is not known. It has been suggested that 48 to 72 hours of rest are necessary for full recovery before the next training stimulus.[14] Intensity, however, plays a major role in determining the frequency of training. If an adequate recovery period does not occur, muscle fatigue will result with a corresponding increase in neuromuscular reaction times. The beginner should allow at least 48 hours between training sessions.

Training Age   Training age is the number of years an individual has been in a formal training program. At younger training ages the overall training demand should be kept low. Prepubescent and pubescent individuals of both genders are engaged in more intense physical training programs. Many of these programs contain plyometric drills. Because youth sports involve plyometric movements, training for these sports should also involve plyometric activities. The literature does not have long-term data looking at the effects of plyometric activities on human articular cartilage and long-bone growth. Research demonstrates that plyometric training does indeed result in strength gains in prepubescent individuals, and that plyometric training may in fact contribute to increased bone mineral content in young females.[18,47]

Recovery   Recovery is the rest time used between exercise sets. Manipulation of this variable will depend on whether the goal is to increase power or muscular endurance. Because plyometric training is anaerobic in nature, a longer recovery period should be used to allow restoration of metabolic stores. With power training, a work/rest ratio of 1:3 or 1:4 should be used. This time frame will allow maximal recovery between sets. For endurance training, this work/rest ratio can be shortened to 1:1 or 1:2. Endurance training typically uses circuit training, where the individual moves from one exercise set to another with minimal rest in between.

The beginning plyometric program should emphasize the importance of eccentric versus concentric muscle contractions. The relevance of the stretch-shortening cycle with decreased amortization time should be stressed. Initiation of lower-quarter plyometric training begins with low-intensity in-place and multiple-response jumps. The individual should be instructed in proper exercise technique. The feet should be nearly flat in all landings, and the individual should be encouraged to "touch and go." An analogy would be landing on a hot bed of coals. The goal is to reverse the landing as quickly as possible, spending only a minimal amount of time on the ground.

CLINICAL DECISION MAKING   **Exercise 11–4**

During the off-season, a college lineman has set personal goals to increase his weight from his present playing weight of 270 pounds to 290 pounds. He also wants to improve his quickness off the line. He is engaged in traditional strength training and an aerobic program, and he wants to add plyometrics to the program. Is his body weight a contraindication for a plyometric program?

Success of the plyometric program will depend on how well the training variables are controlled, modified, and manipulated. In general, as the intensity of the exercise is increased, the volume is decreased. The corollary to this is that as volume increases, the intensity is decreased. The overall key to successfully controlling these variables is to be flexible and listen to what the individual's body is telling you. The body's response to the program will dictate the speed of progression. Whenever in doubt as to the exercise intensity or volume, it is better to underestimate to prevent injury.

Before implementing a plyometric program, the athletic trainer should assess the type of patient that is being rehabilitated and whether plyometrics are suitable for that individual. In most cases, plyometrics should be used in the latter phases of rehabilitation, starting in the advanced strengthening phase once the patient has obtained an appropriate strength base.[36,38] When utilizing plyometric training in the uninjured population, the application of plyometric exercise should follow the concept of periodization.[43] The concept of periodization refers to the year-round sequence and progression of strength training, conditioning, and sport-specific skills.[45] There are four specific phases in the year-round periodization model: the competitive season, postseason training, the preparation phase, and the transitional phase.[43] Plyometric exercises should be performed in the latter stages of the preparation phase and during the transitional phase for optimal results and safety. To obtain the benefits of a plyometric program, the individual should (1) be well conditioned with sufficient strength and endurance; (2) exhibit athletic abilities; (3) exhibit coordination and proprioceptive abilities; and (4) be free of pain from any physical injury or condition.

It should be remembered that the plyometric program is not designed to be an exclusive training program for the individual. Rather, it should be one part of a well-structured training program that includes strength training, flexibility training, cardiovascular fitness, and sport-specific training for skill enhancement and coordination. By combining the plyometric program with other training techniques, the effects of training are greatly enhanced.

GUIDELINES FOR PLYOMETRIC PROGRAMS

The proper execution of the plyometric exercise program must continually be stressed. A sound technical foundation from which higher-intensity work can build should be established. It must be remembered that jumping is a continuous interchange between force reduction and force production. This interchange takes place throughout the entire body: ankle, knee, hip, trunk, and arms. The timing and coordination of these body segments yields a positive ground reaction that will result in a high rate of force production.[16]

CLINICAL DECISION MAKING   **Exercise 11–5**

A teenage amateur female swimmer swims distance freestyle events and has generalized ligamentous laxity. Over the course of the previous season she complained of shoulder pain. Her pain was accompanied by increased times in all of her events. Her physician diagnosed her with multidirectional instability and secondary shoulder impingement syndrome. The physician wants the patient to begin a plyometric program. How will you incorporate plyometrics into the training program?

As the plyometric program is initiated, the individual must be made aware of several guidelines.[43] Any deviation from these guidelines will result in minimal improvement and increased risk for injury. These guidelines include the following:

1. Plyometric training should be specific to the individual goals of the individual. Activity-specific movement patterns should be trained. These sport-specific skills should be broken down and trained in their smaller components and then rebuilt into a coordinated activity-specific movement pattern.
2. The quality of work is more important than the quantity of work. The intensity of the exercise should be kept at a maximal level.
3. The greater the exercise intensity level, the greater the recovery time.
4. Plyometric training can have its greatest benefit at the conclusion of the normal workout. This pattern will best replicate exercise under a partial-to-total fatigue environment that is specific to activity. Only low- to medium-stress plyometrics should be used at the conclusion of a workout, because of the increased potential of injury with high-stress drills.
5. When proper technique can no longer be demonstrated, maximum volume has been achieved and the exercise must be stopped. Training improperly or with fatigue can lead to injury.
6. The plyometric training program should be progressive in nature. The volume and intensity can be modified in several ways:
   a. Increase the number of exercises.
   b. Increase the number of repetitions and sets.
   c. Decrease the rest period between sets of exercise.
7. Plyometric training sessions should be conducted no more than three times weekly in the preseason phase of training. During this phase, volume should prevail.

During the competitive season, the frequency of plyometric training should be reduced to twice weekly, with the intensity of the exercise becoming more important.

8. Dynamic testing of the individual on a regular basis will provide important progression and motivational feedback.

9. In addition to proper technique and exercise dosage, proper equipment is also required. Equipment should allow for the safe performance of the activity, landing surfaces should be even and allow for as much shock absorption as possible, and footwear should provide adequate shock absorption and forefoot support.

The key element in the execution of proper technique is the eccentric or landing phase. The shock of landing from a jump is not absorbed exclusively by the foot but rather is a combination of the ankle, knee, and hip joints all working together to absorb the shock of landing and then transferring the force.

INTEGRATING PLYOMETRICS INTO THE REHABILITATION PROGRAM: CLINICAL CONCERNS

When used judiciously, plyometrics are a valuable asset in the sports rehabilitation program. Clinical plyometrics should involve loading of the healing tissue. These activities may include (1) medial/lateral loading; (2) rotational loading; and (3) shock absorption/deceleration loading.

CLINICAL DECISION MAKING   **Exercise 11–6**

A professional soccer player sustained an Achilles tendon rupture 10 weeks ago. The tendon was surgically repaired. The patient was in a brace that was gradually adjusted to allow full weight bearing and dorsiflexion to neutral in the brace. He has been out of the brace completely and walking without a limp for 2 weeks. He wants to begin a jumping and hopping program to increase strength and power in the calf. What type of guidelines should be employed to safely begin these activities?

Medial/Lateral Loading

Virtually all sporting activities involve cutting maneuvers. Inherent to cutting activities is adequate function in the medial and lateral directions. A plyometric program designed to stress the individual's ability to accept weight on the involved lower extremity and then perform cutting activities off that leg is imperative. Individuals who have suffered sprains to the medial or lateral capsular and ligamentous complex of the ankle and knee, as well as the hip abductor/adductor and ankle invertor/evertor muscle strains, are candidates for medial/lateral plyometric loading. Medial/lateral loading drills should be implemented following injury to the medial soft tissue around the knee after a valgus stress. By gradually imparting progressive valgus loads, tissue tensile strength is augmented.[48] In the rehabilitation setting, bilateral support drills can be progressed to unilateral valgus loading efforts. Specifically, lateral jumping drills are progressed to lateral hopping activities. However, the medial structures must also be trained to accept greater valgus loads sustained during cutting activities. As a prerequisite to full-speed cutting, lateral bounding drills should be performed. These efforts are progressed to activities that add acceleration, deceleration, and momentum. Lateral sliding activities that require the individual to cover a greater distance can be performed on a slide board. If a slide board is not available, the same movement pattern can be stressed with plyometrics.

Rotational Loading

Because rotation in the knee is controlled by the cruciate ligaments, menisci, and capsule, plyometric activities with a rotational component are instrumental in the rehabilitation program after injury to any of these structures. As previously discussed, care must be taken not to exceed healing time constraints when using plyometric training.

Shock Absorption (Deceleration Loading)

Perhaps some of the most physically demanding plyometric activities are shock absorption activities that place a tremendous amount of stress upon muscle, tendon, and articular cartilage. As previously stated, the majority of lower-quarter sport function occurs in the closed kinetic chain. Lower-extremity plyometrics are an effective functional closed-chain exercise that can be incorporated into the rehabilitation program. Through the eccentric prestretch, plyometrics place added stress on the tendinous portion of the contractile unit. Eccentric loading is beneficial in the management of tendinitis.[44] Through a gradually progressed eccentric loading program, healing tendinous tissue is stressed, yielding an increase in ultimate tensile strength. This eccentric load can be applied through jump-down exercises (See Figure 11-6).

Therefore, in the final preparation for a return to sports involving repetitive jumping and hopping, shock absorption drills should be included in the rehabilitation program. One way to prepare the individual for shock absorption drills is to gradually maximize the effects of gravity, such as beginning in a gravity-minimized position and progressing to performance against gravity. Popular activities to minimize gravity include water activities or assisted efforts through unloading jumps and hops in the supine position on a leg press or similar device.

SPECIFIC PLYOMETRIC EXERCISES

Plyometric drills can be categorized into (1) weighted ball toss plyometric exercises (Figure 11-3); (2) dynamic weighted ball plyometric exercises (Figure 11-4); (3) in-place jumping plyometric exercises (Figure 11-5) that involve activities that can be performed in essentially the same or small amount of space; and (4) depth jumping and bounding plyometric exercises (Figure 11-6) that may involve jumping down from a predetermined height and performing a vari-

ety of activities upon landing or activities that occur across a given distance. In-place jumping drills (bilateral activities) can be progressed to hopping (unilateral activities). Chapters 17 through 24 have additional region-specific plyometric exercises commonly used in rehabilitation.

The exercises in Figures 11-3 through 11-6 are a good starting point from which to develop a clinical plyometric program. Manipulations of volume, frequency, and intensity can advance the program appropriately. Proper progression is of prime importance when using plyometrics in the rehabilitation program. These progressive activities are reinjuries waiting to happen if the progression does not allow for adequate healing or development of an adequate strength base.[32] A close working relationship fostering open communication and acute observation skills is vital in helping ensure that the program is not overly aggressive.

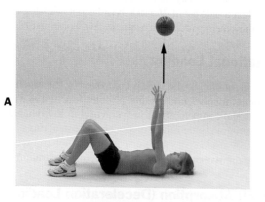

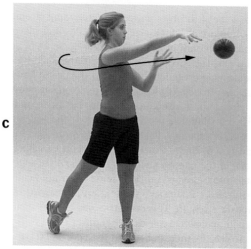

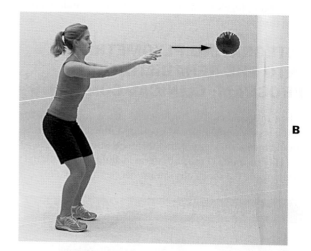

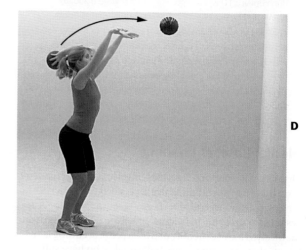

Figure 11-3 Weighted ball toss plyometric exercises. **A,** Supine toss. **B,** Two-arm chest pass. **C,** One-arm chest pass with rotation. **D,** Soccer throw.

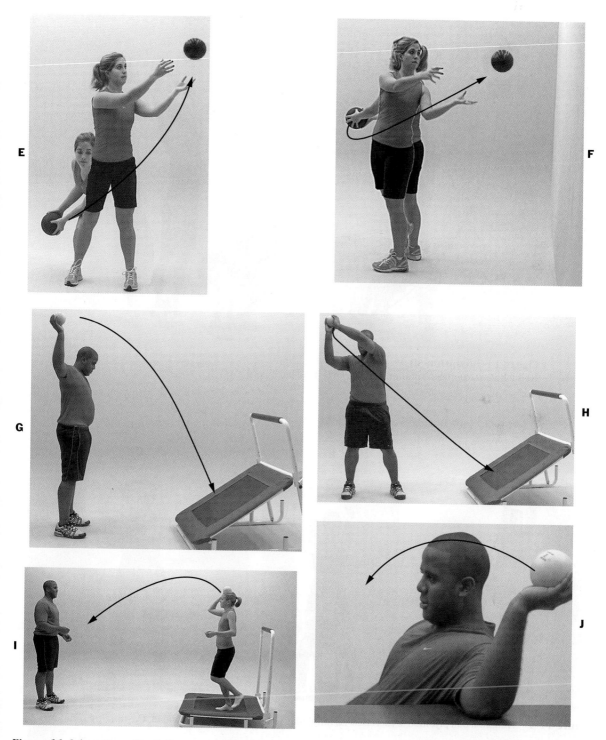

Figure 11-3 (continued)   **E,** Two-arm rotation toss from squat. **F,** Reverse toss with rotation. **G,** Plyoback standing single-arm toss. **H,** Plyoback two-arm toss with rotation. **I,** Plyoback single-leg partner ball toss. **J,** Single-arm ball throw.

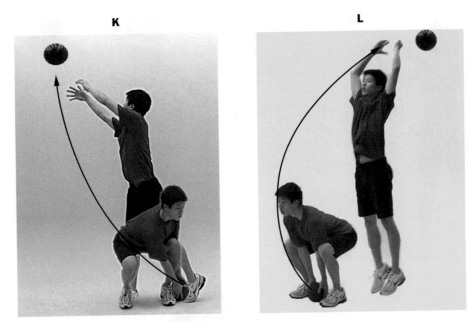

Figure 11-3 (continued)
K, Backward extension rotation toss. **L,** Overhead backward toss.

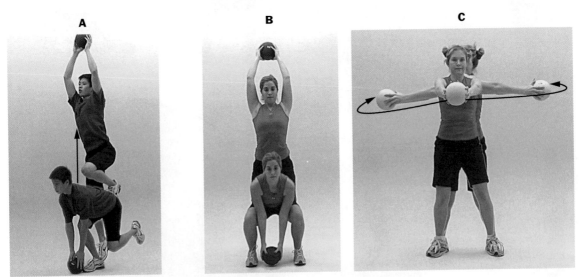

Figure 11-4 Weighted ball plyometric exercises. **A,** Single-leg jump. **B,** Squat to overhead. **C,** Standing rotations.

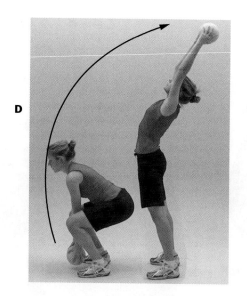

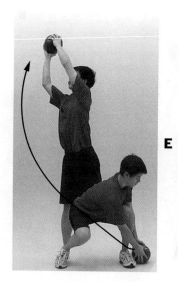

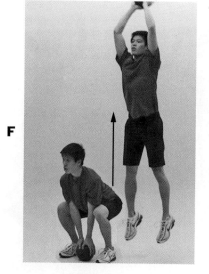

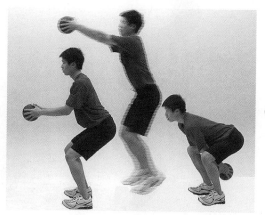

Figure 11-4 (continued)   **D,** Standing extension. **E,** D2 PNF pattern. **F,** Double-leg jump. **G,** Forward jump from squat.

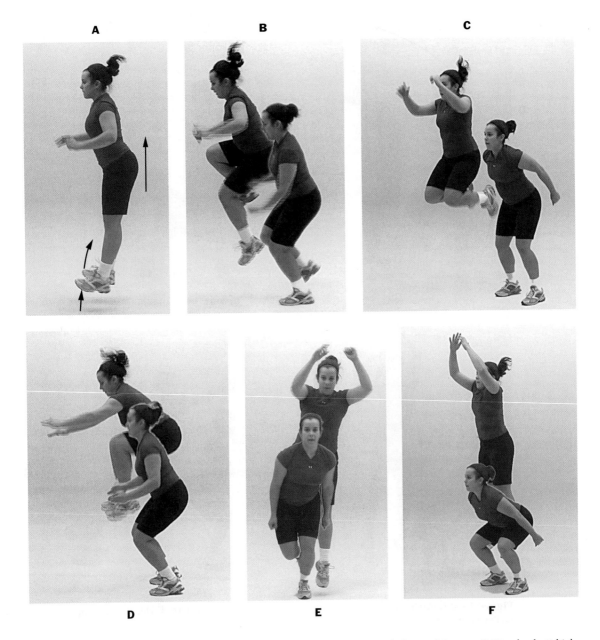

Figure 11-5 In-place jumping plyometric exercises. **A,** Ankle jumps. **B,** Single-leg tuck jumps. **C,** Two-leg butt kicks. **D,** Two-leg tuck jumps. **E,** Single-leg hops. **F,** Squat jumps.

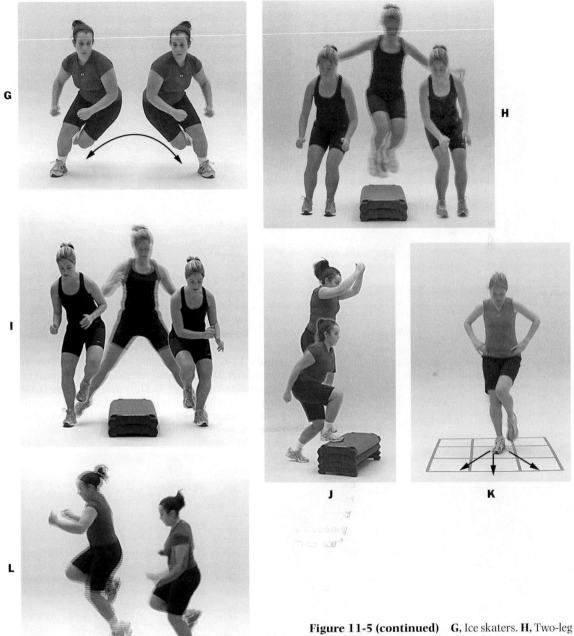

Figure 11-5 (continued)   G, Ice skaters. **H,** Two-leg lateral hop-overs. **I,** Single-leg lateral hop-overs. **J,** Alternate-leg power step-ups. **K,** Single-leg shark skill test. **L,** Single-leg short hurdle jump.

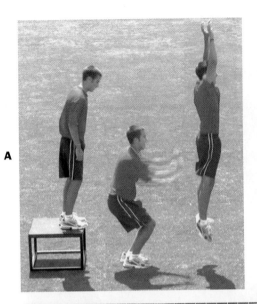

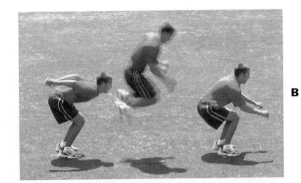

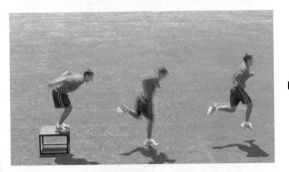

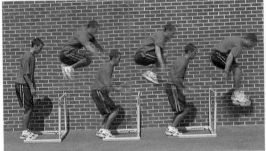

A

B

C

D

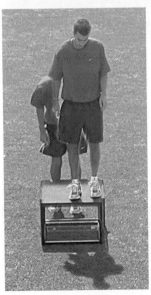

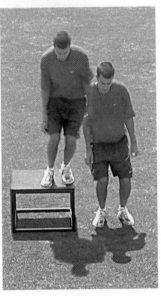

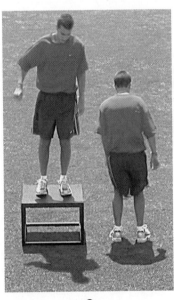

Figure 11-6 Depth jumping and bounding plyometric exercises. **A,** Depth jump to vertical jump. **B,** Repeat two-leg standing long jumps. **C,** Three-hurdle jumps. **D,** Depth jump to bounding. **E,** Box jumps up and down sagittal plane. **F,** Box jumps up and down frontal plane. **G,** Box jumps up and down transverse plane.

E

F

G

Summary

1. Although the effects of plyometric training are not yet fully understood, it still remains a widely used form of combining strength with speed training to functionally increase power. While the research is somewhat contradictory, the neurophysiological concept of plyometric training is on a sound foundation.
2. A successful plyometric training program should be carefully designed and implemented after establishing an adequate strength base.
3. The effects of this type of high-intensity training can be achieved safely if the individual is supervised by a knowledgeable person who uses common sense and follows the prescribed training regimen.
4. The plyometric training program should use a large variety of different exercises, because year-round training often results in boredom and a lack of motivation.
5. Program variety can be manipulated with different types of equipment or kinds of movement performed.
6. Continued motivation and an organized progression are the keys to successful training.
7. Plyometrics are also a valuable asset in the rehabilitation program after a sport injury.
8. Used after both upper- and lower-quarter injury, plyometrics are effective in facilitating joint awareness, strengthening tissue during the healing process, and increasing sport-specific strength and power.
9. The most important considerations in the plyometric program are common sense and experience.

References

1. Adams, T. 1984. An investigation of selected plyometric training exercises on muscular leg strength and power. *Track and Field Quarterly Review* 84(1): 36–40.
2. Asmussen, E., and F. Bonde-Peterson. 1974. Storage of elastic energy in skeletal muscles in man. *Acta Physiologica Scandinavia* 91:385.
3. Bielik, E., D. Chu, F. Costello, et al. 1986. Roundtable: 1. Practical considerations for utilizing plyometrics. *National Strength and Conditioning Association Journal* 8:14.
4. Bosco, C., and P. V. Komi. 1979. Potentiation of the mechanical behavior of the human skeletal muscle through prestretching. *Acta Physiologica Scandinavia* 106:467.
5. Bosco, C., and P. V. Komi. 1982. Muscle elasticity in athletes. In *Exercise and sports biology*, edited by P. V. Komi. Champaign, IL: Human Kinetics.
6. Bosco, C., J. Tarkka, and P. V. Komi. 1982. Effect of elastic energy and myoelectric potentiation of triceps surae during stretch-shortening cycle exercise. *International Journal of Sports Medicine* 2:137.
7. Bosco, C., J. Tihanyia, and P. V. Komi, et al. 1987. Store and recoil of elastic energy in slow and fast types of human skeletal muscles. *Acta Physiologica Scandinavia* 16:343.
8. Cavagna, G. A., B. Dusman, and R. Margaria. 1968. Positive work done by a previously stretched muscle. *Journal of Applied Physiology* 24:21.
9. Cavagna, G., F. Saibene, and R. Margaria. 1965. Effect of negative work on the amount of positive work performed by an isolated muscle. *Journal of Applied Physiology* 20:157.
10. Chimera, N., K. Swanik, and C. Swanik. 2004. Effects of plyometric training on muscle-activation strategies and performance in female athletes. *Journal of Athletic Training* 39(1):24–31.
11. Chmielewski T., G. Myer, and D. Kauffman. 2006. Plyometric exercise in the rehabilitation of athletes: Physiological responses and clinical application. *Journal of Orthopaedic & Sports Physical Therapy* 36(5):308–319.
12. Chu, D. 1984. Plyometric exercise. *National Strength and Conditioning Association Journal* 6:56.
13. Chu, D. 1989. Conditioning/plyometrics. Paper presented at 10th Annual Sports Medicine Team Concept Conference, San Francisco, December.
14. Chu, D. 1992. *Jumping into plyometrics*. Champaign, IL: Leisure Press.
15. Chu, D., and L. Plummer. 1984. The language of plyometrics. *National Strength and Conditioning Association Journal* 6:30.
16. Cissik, J. 2004. Plyometric Fundamentals. *NSCA's Performance Training Journal* 3(2):9–13.
17. Curwin, S., and W. D. Stannish. 1984. *Tendinitis: Its etiology and treatment*. Lexington, MA: Collamore Press.
18. Diallo, O., E. Dore, and P. Duchercise, et al. 2001. Effects of plyometric training followed by a reduced training programme on physical performance in prepubescent soccer players. *Journal of Sports Medicine and Physical Fitness* 41:342–48.
19. Dunsenev, C. I. 1979. Strength training for jumpers. *Soviet Sports Review* 14:2.
20. Dunsenev, C. I. 1982. Strength training of jumpers. *Track and Field Quarterly* 82:4.
21. Ebben, W., C. Simenz, and R. Jensen. 2008. Evaluation of plyometric intensity using electromyography. *Journal of Strength & Conditioning Research* 22(3):861.

22. Ebben, W. 2007. Practical Guidelines for Plyometric Intensity. *NSCA's Performance Training Journal* 6(5):12.

23. Enoka, R. M. 1989. *Neuromechanical basis of kinesiology.* Champaign, IL: Human Kinetics.

24. Goldbeck, T., and G. Davies. 2000. Test-retest reliability of the closed chain upper extremity stability test: A clinical field test. *Journal of Sport Rehabilitation* 9:35–45.

25. Javorek, I. 1989. Plyometrics. *National Strength and Conditioning Association Journal* 11:52.

26. Jensen, C. 1975. Pertinent facts about warming. *Athletic Journal* 56:72.

27. Katchajov, S., K. Gomberaze, and A. Revson. 1976. Rebound jumps. *Modern Athlete and Coach* 14(4):23.

28. Komi, P. V. 1984. Physiological and biomechanical correlates of muscle function: Effects of muscle structure and stretch shortening cycle on force and speed. In *Exercise and sports sciences review,* edited by Terjung. Lexington, MA: Collamore Press.

29. Komi, P. V., and C. Bosco. 1978. Utilization of stored elastic energy in leg extensor muscles by men and women. *Medicine and Science in Sports and Exercise* 10(4): 261.

30. Komi, P. V., and E. Buskirk. 1972. Effects of eccentric and concentric muscle conditioning on tension and electrical activity of human muscle. *Ergonomics* 15:417.

31. Lundon, P. 1985. A review of plyometric training. *National Strength and Conditioning Association Journal* 7:69.

32. Pretz. R. 2006. Plyometric exercises for overhead-throwing athletes. *Strength & Conditioning Journal* 28(1):36.

33. Rach, P. J., M. D. Grabiner, and R. J. Gregor, et al. 1989. *Kinesiology and applied anatomy.* 7th ed. Philadelphia: Lea & Febiger.

34. Rowinski, M. 1988. *The role of eccentric exercise.* Biodex Corp, Pro Clinica.

35. Shiner, J., T. Bishop, and A. Cosgarea. 2005. Integrating low-intensity plyometrics into strength and conditioning programs. *Strength & Conditioning.* 27(6):10.

36. Thomas, D.W. 1988. Plyometrics—More than the stretch reflex. *National Strength and Conditioning Association Journal* 10:49.

37. Tippett, S. 1992. Closed chain exercise. *Orthopaedic Physical Therapy Clinics of North America* 1:253–67.

38. Tippett, S., and M. Voight. 1995. *Functional progressions for sport rehabilitation.* Champaign, IL: Human Kinetics.

39. Verhoshanski, Y. 1969. Are depth jumps useful? *Yesis Review of Soviet Physical Education and Sport* 4:74–79.

40. Verhoshanski, Y., and G. Chornonson. 1967. Jump exercises in sprint training. *Track and Field Quarterly* 9:1909.

41. Verkhoshanski, Y. 1969. Perspectives in the improvement of speed-strength preparation of jumpers. *Yesis Review of Soviet Physical Education and Sports* 28–29.

42. Voight, M., and D. Bradley. 1994. Plyometrics. In *A compendium of isokinetics in clinical usage and rehabilitation techniques,* 4th ed., edited by G. J. Davies. Onalaska, WI: S & S.

43. Voight, M., and P. Draovitch. 1991. Plyometrics. In *Eccentric muscle training in sports and orthopedics,* edited by M. Albert. New York: Churchill Livingstone.

44. Von Arx, F. 1984. Power development in the high jump. *Track Technique* 88:2818–19.

45. Wilk, K. E., M. L. Voight, M. A. Keirns, V. Gambetta, J. Andrews, and C. J. Dillman. 1993. Stretch-shortening drills for the upper extremities: Theory and clinical application. *Journal of Orthopaedic and Sports Physical Therapy* 17:225–39.

46. Wilt, F. 1975. Plyometrics—What it is and how it works. *Athletic Journal* 55b:76.

47. Witzke, K., and C. Snow. 2000. Effects of plyometric jump training on bone mass in adolescent girls. *Medicine and Science in Sports and Exercise* 32:1051–57.

48. Woo, S. L., M. Inoue, and E. McGurk-Burleson, et al. 1987. Treatment of the medial collateral ligament injury: Structure and function of canine knees in response to differing treatment regimens. *American Journal of Sports Medicine* 15(1): 22–29.

SOLUTIONS TO CLINICAL DECISION MAKING EXERCISES

11-1 Although the patient is in the off-season and actual performance is not jeopardized, her overall activity level must be adjusted to allow for pain-free performance of her conditioning program. The intensity of the plyometric program must be adjusted. Instead of box jumps and depth jumps, the patient should regress to beginner skills such as in-place jumping (both legs) and progress to unilateral activities as tolerated. If these activities cause pain, the plyometric program should be discontinued until symptoms improve. At the heart of the patient's problem may be underlying biomechanical concerns that predispose her to knee pain. A thorough assessment of her lower-extremity biomechanics, flexibility, and strength should be performed. Core strength and stability of the low back and hips must be assessed. Assessment of the patellofemoral joint must also be performed. Appropriate interventions to address any dysfunction must be included as a vital prerequisite prior to advancing the plyometric program.

11-2 As the high-stepping drills involve hip flexion, care must be taken in performing these drills. There is a good chance that the initial injury occurred with hip flexion and knee extension while sprinting, so reintroducing the patient to these positions is an absolute must in the rehabilitation program. A gradual return to these activities is essential to maximize strength without reinjury. Symmetrical flexibility of the hamstrings is a must. Single-joint concentric and eccentric strengthening should be performed without pain to the point of symmetry with the opposite side. When she has an adequate strength and flexibility base, she can begin bilateral and then unilateral plyometric leg-press activities (with less-than-body-weight resistance) on the Shuttle, followed by weightbearing beginner plyometrics (jumping and hopping). Emphasize activities involving degrees of hip flexion similar to the amount of hip flexion involved in sprinting. When these activities are tolerated well, the patient can then begin high-knee running drills, box jumps, and depth jumps.

11-3 Plyometrics have been shown to be beneficial in producing strength gains in individuals of this age. Plyometrics certainly can enhance anaerobic conditioning as well. Plyometrics, however, are but one component of the entire conditioning program. Proper attention should also be given to safe strength training, flexibility, aerobic conditioning, as well as proper football techniques and protective equipment. There are no long-term data to show that plyometrics are detrimental to the adolescent and many of the activities inherent to football are plyometric in nature. Keep the plyometric activities at the beginner phase and use the beginner skills to develop an adequate strength base. Stress correct form and technique. Watch for substitutions of movement and progress to intermediate activities if and when the athletes demonstrate correct performance of the beginner skills. Finally, because the athletes are in the playing season, frequency of plyometrics should be minimized.

11-4 Individuals of all sizes can safely take part in plyometrics if they have an adequate strength base. Chances are that this individual is familiar with plyometric training already, so technique and progression should not be an issue. As the individual gains weight, however, the relative load on his weightbearing joints increases. His exercise dosage should reflect his change in weight. Adequate closed-chain strength must increase to support the additional weight prior to plyometrics. After he has made appropriate gains in controlled closed-chain strengthening (leg press, squats), plyometrics can be introduced and progressed. It is equally important that the individual's weight gain be fat-free weight with proper attention given to sound nutritional guidelines.

11-5 Of all sporting activities, swimming might be the one with the least amount of eccentric muscle activity. This does not mean that plyometric training to develop power is not important. Plyometrics for the swimmer should include lower-extremity work for starts and turns, as well as trunk plyometrics for power in the water. Upper-extremity plyometrics in this patient may be problematic due to her shoulder instability. Be sure that she has adequate strength in her scapular stabilizers as well as proper posture to minimize an anterior glenoid. Combinations of abduction, horizontal abduction, and external rotation common in plyometrics involving throwing motions might apply excessive stress in an anterior direction. Activities involving horizontal adduction as well as weightbearing activities in a prone or quadruped position may apply excessive stress in a posterior direction. Try to keep activities bilateral and symmetrical. Emphasize scapular retraction, and try to have the patient keep and attempt to maintain scapular stability.

11-6 Obviously, plyometrics can be used to facilitate strength gain in the entire lower extremity. However, excessive stress to the healing tendon can be detrimental in terms of tendinitis, tendinosis, and possibly even re-rupture. Plyometrics should not even be considered until the patient is able to demonstrate normal strength (symmetrical unilateral toe raises), symmetrical gastrocnemius-soleus flexibility, as well as pain-free and substitution-free gait. Only after attaining these goals should plyometrics be instituted. The program should begin with bilateral nonsupport activities and progress to unilateral nonsupport activities. Loads with less than body weight on the Shuttle are an effective precursor to weightbearing activities.

CHAPTER 12

Open- versus Closed-Kinetic-Chain Exercise in Rehabilitation

William E. Prentice

After completing this chapter, the athletic training student should be able to do the following:

- Differentiate between the concepts of an open kinetic chain and a closed kinetic chain.

- Contrast the advantages and disadvantages of using open- versus closed-kinetic-chain exercise.

- Recognize how closed-kinetic-chain exercises can be used to regain neuromuscular control.

- Analyze the biomechanics of closed-kinetic-chain exercise in the lower extremity.

- Compare how both open- and closed-kinetic-chain exercises should be used in rehabilitation of the lower extremity.

- Identify the various closed-kinetic-chain exercises for the lower extremity.

- Examine the biomechanics of closed-kinetic-chain exercises in the upper extremity.

- Explain how closed-kinetic-chain exercises are used in rehabilitation of the upper extremity.

- Recognize the various types of closed-kinetic-chain exercises for the upper extremity.

Over the years, the concept of **closed-kinetic-chain exercise** has received considerable attention as a useful and effective technique of rehabilitation, particularly for injuries involving the lower extremity.[81] The ankle, knee, and hip joints constitute the kinetic chain for the lower extremity. When the distal segment of the lower extremity is stabilized or fixed, as is the case when the foot is weight bearing on the ground, the kinetic chain is said to be closed. Conversely, in an **open kinetic chain,** the distal segment is mobile and not fixed. Traditionally, rehabilitation strengthening protocols have used open-kinetic-chain exercises such as knee flexion and extension on a knee machine.

Closed-kinetic-chain exercises are used more often in rehabilitation of injuries to the lower extremity, but they are also useful in rehabilitation protocols for certain upper-extremity activities. For the most part, the upper extremity functions in an open kinetic chain with the hand moving freely. But there are a number of activities in which the upper extremity functions in a closed kinetic chain.

Despite the recent popularity of closed-kinetic-chain exercises, it must be stressed that both open- and closed-kinetic-chain exercises have their place in the rehabilitative process.[21] This chapter will attempt to clarify the role of both open- and closed-kinetic-chain exercises in that process.

CONCEPT OF THE KINETIC CHAIN

The concept of the kinetic chain was first proposed in the 1970s and initially referred to as the *link system* by mechanical engineers.[69] In this link system, pin joints connect a series of overlapping, rigid segments (Figure 12-1). If both ends of this system are connected to an immovable frame, there is no movement of either the proximal or the distal end. In this closed link system, each moving body segment receives forces from, and transfers forces to, adjacent body segments and thus either affects or is affected by the motion of those components.[29] In a closed link system, movement at one joint produces predictable movement at all other joints.[69] In reality, this type of closed link system does not exist in either the upper or the lower extremity. However, when the distal segment in an extremity (that is, the foot or hand) meets resistance or is fixed, muscle recruitment patterns and joint movements are different than when the distal segment moves freely.[69] Thus, two systems—a closed system and an open system—have been proposed.

Whenever the foot or the hand meets resistance or is fixed, as is the case in a closed kinetic chain, movement of the more proximal segments occurs in a predictable pattern. If the foot or hand moves freely in space as in an open kinetic chain, movements occurring in other segments within the chain are not necessarily predictable.[13]

To a large extent, the term *closed-kinetic-chain exercise* has come to mean "weightbearing exercise." However, although all weightbearing exercises involve some elements of closed-kinetic-chain activities, not all closed-kinetic-chain activities are weight bearing.[67]

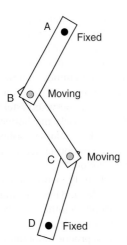

Figure 12-1   If both ends of a link system are fixed, movement at one joint produces predictable movement at all other joints.

Muscle Actions in the Kinetic Chain

Muscle actions that occur during open-kinetic-chain activities are usually reversed during closed-kinetic-chain activities. In open-kinetic-chain exercise, the origin is fixed and muscle contraction produces movement at the insertion. In closed-kinetic-chain exercise, the insertion is fixed and the muscle acts to move the origin. Although this may be important biomechanically, physiologically the muscle can lengthen, shorten, or remain the same length, and thus it makes little difference whether the origin or insertion is moving in terms of the way the muscle contracts.

Concurrent Shift in a Kinetic Chain

The concept of the *concurrent shift* applies to biarticular muscles that have distinctive muscle actions within the kinetic chain during weightbearing activities.[39] For example, in a closed kinetic chain simultaneous hip and knee extension occur when a person stands from a seated position. To produce this movement, the rectus femoris shortens across the knee while it lengthens across the hip. Conversely, the hamstrings shorten across the hip and simultaneously lengthen across the knee. The resulting concentric and eccentric contractions at opposite ends of the muscle produce the concurrent shift. This type of contraction occurs during functional activities including walking, stair climbing, and jumping and cannot be reproduced by isolated open-kinetic-chain knee flexion and extension exercises.[39]

The concepts of the reversibility of muscle actions and the concurrent shift are hallmarks of closed-kinetic-chain exercises.[67]

ADVANTAGES AND DISADVANTAGES OF OPEN- VERSUS CLOSED-KINETIC-CHAIN EXERCISES

Open- and closed-kinetic-chain exercises offer distinct advantages and disadvantages in the rehabilitation process. The choice to use one or the other depends on the desired treatment goal. Characteristics of closed-kinetic-chain exercises include increased joint compressive forces, increased joint congruency (and thus stability) decreased shear forces, decreased acceleration forces, large resistance forces, stimulation of proprioceptors, and enhanced dynamic stability—all of which are associated with weight bearing. Characteristics of open-kinetic-chain exercises include increased acceleration forces, decreased resistance forces, increased distraction and rotational forces, increased deformation of joint and muscle mechanoreceptors, concentric acceleration and eccentric deceleration forces, and promotion of functional activity. These are typical of non-weightbearing activities.[46]

From a biomechanical perspective, it has been suggested that closed-kinetic-chain exercises are safer and produce stresses and forces that are potentially less of a threat to healing structures than open-kinetic-chain exercises.[62] Coactivation or co-contraction of agonist and antagonist muscles must occur during normal movements to provide joint stabilization. Co-contraction, which occurs during closed-kinetic-chain exercise, decreases the shear forces acting on the joint, thus protecting healing soft tissue structures that might otherwise be damaged by open-chain exercises.[29] Additionally, weightbearing activity increases joint compressive forces, further enhancing joint stability.

It has also been suggested that closed-kinetic-chain exercises, particularly those involving the lower extremity, tend to be more functional than open-kinetic-chain exercises because they involve weightbearing activities.[79] The majority of activities performed in daily living, such as walking, climbing, and rising to a standing position, as well as in most sport activities, involve a closed-kinetic-chain system. Because the foot is usually in contact with the ground, activities that make use of this closed system are said to be more functional. With the exception of a kicking movement, there is no question that closed-kinetic-chain exercises are more activity specific, involving exercise that more closely approximates the desired activity. For example, knee extensor muscle strength in a closed kinetic chain is more closely related to jumping ability than knee extensor strength in a closed kinetic chain.[8] In a clinical setting, specificity of training must be emphasized to maximize carryover to functional activities.[67]

With open-kinetic-chain exercises, motion is usually isolated to a single joint. Open-kinetic-chain activities may include exercises to improve strength or range of motion.[34] They may be applied to a single joint manually, as in proprioceptive neuromuscular facilitation or joint mobilization techniques, or through some external resistance using an exercise machine. Isolation-type exercises typically use a contraction of a specific muscle or group of muscles that produces usually single plane and occasionally multiplanar movement.[32] Isokinetic exercise and testing is usually done in an open kinetic chain and can provide important information relative to the torque production capability of that isolated joint.[4]

When there is some dysfunction associated with injury, the predictable pattern of movement that occurs

during closed-kinetic-chain activity might not be possible due to pain, swelling, muscle weakness, or limited range of motion. Thus, movement compensations result that interfere with normal motion and muscle activity. If only closed-kinetic-chain exercise is used, the joints proximal or distal to the injury might not show an existing deficit. Without using open-kinetic-chain exercises that isolate specific joint movements, the deficit might go uncorrected, thus interfering with total rehabilitation.[19] The athletic trainer should use the most appropriate open- or closed-kinetic-chain exercise for the given situation.

Closed-kinetic-chain exercises use varying combinations of isometric, concentric, and eccentric contractions that must occur simultaneously in different muscle groups, creating multiplanar motion at each of the joints within the kinetic chain. Closed-kinetic-chain activities require synchronicity of more complex agonist and antagonist muscle actions.[27]

CLINICAL DECISION MAKING   **Exercise 12–1**

Following an ACL, surgery, an athletic trainer is ready to incorporate some closed-chain exercise into the rehabilitation program. What are some of the options, and what are advantages of each?

USING CLOSED-KINETIC-CHAIN EXERCISES TO REGAIN NEUROMUSCULAR CONTROL

In Chapter 6, it was stressed that proprioception, joint position sense, and kinesthesia are critical to the neuromuscular control of body segments within the kinetic chain. To perform a motor skill, muscular forces, occurring at the correct moment and magnitude, interact to move body parts in a coordinated manner.[56] Coordinated movement is controlled by the central nervous system that integrates input from joint and muscle mechanoreceptors acting within the kinetic chain. Smooth coordinated movement requires constant integration of receptor, feedback, and control center information.[56]

In the lower extremity, a functional weightbearing activity requires muscles and joints to work in synchrony and in synergy with one another. For example, taking a single step requires concentric, eccentric, and isometric muscle contractions to produce supination and pronation in the foot; ankle dorsiflexion and plantarflexion; knee flexion, extension, and rotation; and hip flexion, extension, and rotation. Lack of normal motion secondary to injury in one joint will affect the way another joint or segment moves.[56]

To perform this single step in a coordinated manner, all of the joints and muscles must work together. Thus, exercises that act to integrate, rather than isolate, all of these functioning elements would seem to be the most appropriate. Closed-kinetic-chain exercises, which recruit foot, ankle, knee, and hip muscles in a manner that reproduces normal loading and movement forces in all of the joints within the kinetic chain, are similar to functional mechanics and would appear to be most useful.[56]

Quite often, open-kinetic-chain exercises are used primarily to develop muscular strength while little attention is given to the importance of including exercises that reestablish proprioception and joint position sense.[1] Closed-kinetic-chain activities facilitate the integration of proprioceptive feedback coming from Pacinian corpuscles, Ruffini endings, Golgi-Mazzoni corpuscles, Golgi-tendon organs, and Golgi-ligament endings through the functional use of multijoint and multiplanar movements.[13]

BIOMECHANICS OF OPEN- VERSUS CLOSED-KINETIC-CHAIN ACTIVITIES IN THE LOWER EXTREMITY

Open- and closed-kinetic-chain exercises have different biomechanical effects on the joints of the lower extremity.[18] Walking along with the ability to change direction require coordinated joint motion and a complex series of well-timed muscle activations. Biomechanically, shock absorption, foot flexibility, foot stabilization, acceleration and deceleration, multiplanar motion, and joint stabilization must occur in each of the joints in the lower extremity for normal function.[33,56] Some understanding of how these biomechanical events occur during both open- and closed-kinetic-chain activities is essential for the athletic trainer.

Foot and Ankle

The foot's function in the support phase of weight bearing during gait is twofold. At heel strike, the foot must act as a shock absorber to the impact or ground reaction forces and then adapt to the uneven surfaces. Subsequently, at push-off, the foot functions as a rigid lever to transmit the explosive force from the lower extremity to the ground.[77]

As the foot becomes weight bearing at heel strike, creating a closed kinetic chain, the subtalar joint moves into a pronated position in which the talus adducts and the plantar flexes while the calcaneous everts. Pronation of the foot

unlocks the midtarsal joint and allows the foot to assist in shock absorption. It is important during initial impact to reduce the ground reaction forces and distribute the load evenly on many different anatomical structures throughout the lower-extremity kinetic chain. As pronation occurs at the subtalar joint, there is obligatory internal rotation of the tibia and slight flexion at the knee. The dorsiflexors contract eccentrically to decelerate plantarflexion. In an open kinetic chain, when the foot pronates, the talus is stationary while the foot everts, abducts, and dorsiflexes. The muscles that evert the foot appear to be most active.[77]

The foot changes its function from being a shock absorber to being a rigid lever system as the foot begins to push off the ground. In weight bearing in a closed kinetic chain, supination consists of the talus abducting and dorsiflexing on the calcaneus while the calcaneus inverts on the talus. The tibia externally rotates and produces knee extension. During supination the plantarflexors stabilize the foot, decelerate the tibia, and flex the knee. In an open kinetic chain, supination consists of the calcaneus inverting as the talus adducts and plantarflexes. The foot moves into adduction. and plantarflexion, around the stabilized talus.[77] Changes in foot position (i.e., pronation or supination) appear to have little or no effect on the electromyogram (EMG) activity of the vastus medialis or the vastus lateralis.[37]

Knee Joint

It is essential for the athletic trainer to understand forces that occur around the knee joint. Palmitier et al. have proposed a biomechanical model of the lower extremity that quantifies two critical forces at the knee joint (Figure 12-2).[53] A *shear force* occurs in a posterior direction that would cause the tibia to translate anteriorly if not checked by soft tissue constraints—primarily the anterior cruciate ligament (ACL).[14] The second force is a *compressive force* directed along a longitudinal axis of the tibia. Weightbearing exercises increase joint compression, which enhances joint stability.

In an open-kinetic-chain seated knee-joint exercise, as a resistive force is applied to the distal tibia, the shear and compressive forces would be maximized (Figure 12-3A). When a resistive force is applied more proximally, shear force is significantly reduced, as is the compressive force[30] (Figure 12-3B). If the resistive force is applied in a more axial direction, the shear force is also smaller (Figure 12-3C). If a hamstring co-contraction occurs, the shear force is minimized (Figure 12-3D).

Closed-kinetic-chain exercises induce hamstring contraction by creating a flexion moment at both the hip and the knee, with the contracting hamstrings stabilizing the

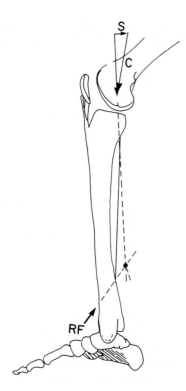

Figure 12-2   Mathematical model showing shear and compressive force vectors. S = shear, C = compressive.

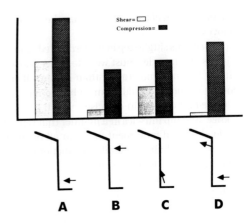

Figure 12-3   Resistive forces applied in different positions alter the magnitude of the shear and compressive forces. **A,** Resistive force applied distally. **B,** Resistive force applied proximally. **C,** Resistive force applied axially. **D,** Resistive force applied distally with hamstring co-contraction.

hip and the quadriceps stabilizing the knee.[74] A *moment* is the product of force and distance from the axis of rotation. Also referred to as torque, it describes the turning effect produced when a force is exerted on the body that is pivoted about some fixed point (Figure 12-4). Co-contraction of the hamstring muscles helps to counteract the tendency of the quadriceps to cause anterior tibial translation.[73] Co-contraction of the hamstrings is most efficient in reducing shear force when the resistive force is directed in an axial orientation relative to the tibia, as is the case in a weightbearing exercise.[53] Several studies have shown that co-contraction is useful in stabilizing the knee joint and decreasing shear forces.[36,41,54,68]

The tension in the hamstrings can be further enhanced with slight anterior flexion of the trunk.[50] Trunk flexion moves the center of gravity anteriorly, decreasing the knee flexion moment and thus reducing knee shear force and decreasing patellofemoral compression forces.[52] Closed-kinetic-chain exercises try to minimize the flexion moment at the knee while increasing the flexion moment at the hip.

A flexion moment is also created at the ankle when the resistive force is applied to the bottom of the foot. The soleus stabilizes ankle flexion and creates a knee extension moment, which again helps to neutralize anterior shear force (see Figure 12-4). Thus the entire lower-extremity kinetic chain is recruited by applying an axial force at the distal segment.

In an open-kinetic-chain exercise involving seated leg extensions, the resistive force is applied to the distal tibia, creating a flexion moment at the knee only.[70] This negates the effects of a hamstring co-contraction and thus produces maximal shear force at the knee joint. Shear forces created by isometric open-kinetic-chain knee flexion and extension at 30 degrees and 60 degrees of knee flexion are greater than those with closed-kinetic-chain exercises.[47] Decreased anterior tibial displacement during isometric closed-kinetic-chain knee flexion at 30 degrees when measured by knee arthrometry has also been demonstrated.[78]

Patellofemoral Joint

The effects of open- versus closed-kinetic-chain exercises on the patellofemoral joint must also be considered. In open-kinetic-chain knee extension exercise, the flexion moment increases as the knee extends from 90 degrees of flexion to full extension, increasing tension in the quadriceps and patellar tendon.[6] Thus the patellofemoral joint reaction forces are increased, with peak force occurring at 36 degrees of joint flexion.[25] As the knee moves toward full extension, the patellofemoral contact area decreases, causing increased contact stress per unit area.[7,38]

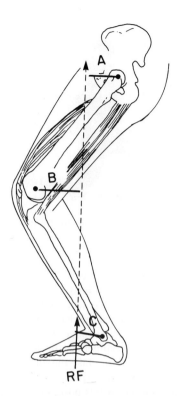

Figure 12-4   Closed-kinetic-chain exercises induce hamstring contraction by creating a flexion moment at **A**, Hip, **B**, Knee, **C**, Ankle.

In closed-kinetic-chain exercise, the flexion moment increases as the knee flexes, once again causing increased quadriceps and patellar tendon tension and thus an increase in patellofemoral joint reaction forces. However, the patella has a much larger surface contact area with the femur, and contact stress is minimized.[7,25,38] Closed-kinetic-chain exercises might be better tolerated in the patellofemoral joint because contact stress is minimized.[6]

CLOSED-KINETIC-CHAIN EXERCISES FOR REHABILITATION OF LOWER-EXTREMITY INJURIES

For many years, athletic trainers have made use of open-kinetic-chain exercises for lower-extremity strengthening. This practice has been partly due to design constraints of existing resistive exercise machines. However, the current popularity of closed-kinetic-chain exercises can be attributed primarily to a better understanding of the kinesiology and biomechanics, along with the neuromuscular

control factors, involved in rehabilitation of lower-extremity injuries.

For example, the course of rehabilitation after injury to the anterior ACL has changed drastically over the years. (Specific rehabilitation protocols will be discussed in detail in Chapter 21.) Technological advances have created significant improvement in surgical techniques, and this has allowed athletic trainers to change their philosophy of rehabilitation. The current literature provides a great deal of support for accelerated rehabilitation programs that recommend the extensive use of closed-kinetic-chain exercises.[9,15,20,25,48,62,75,82]

Because of the biomechanical and functional advantages of closed-kinetic-chain exercises described earlier, these activities are perhaps best suited to rehabilitation of the ACL.[35] The majority of these studies also indicate that closed-kinetic-chain exercises can be safely incorporated into the rehabilitation protocols very early. Some athletic trainers recommend beginning within the first few days after surgery.

Several different closed-kinetic-chain exercises have gained popularity and have been incorporated into rehabilitation protocols.[43] Among those exercises commonly used are the minisquat, wall slides, lunges, leg press, stair-climbing machines, lateral step-up, terminal knee extension using tubing, and stationary bicycling, slide boards, biomechanical ankle platform system (BAPS) boards, and the Fitter.

Minisquats, Wall Slides, and Lunges

The minisquat (Figure 12-5) or wall slide (Figure 12-6) involves simultaneous hip and knee extension and is performed in a 0- to 40-degree range.[82] As the hip extends, the

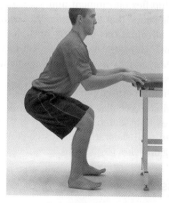

Figure 12-5   Minisquat performed in 0- to 40-degree range.

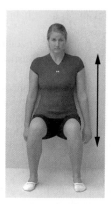

Figure 12-6   Standing wall slide.

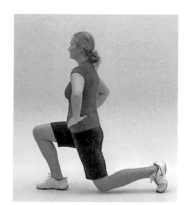

Figure 12-7   Lunges are done to strengthen quadriceps eccentrically.

rectus femoris contracts eccentrically while the hamstrings contract concentrically. Concurrently, as the knee extends, the hamstrings contract eccentrically while the rectus femoris contracts concentrically. Both concentric and eccentric contractions occur simultaneously at either end of both muscles, producing a concurrent shift contraction. This type of contraction is necessary during weightbearing activities. [63] It will be elicited with all closed-kinetic-chain exercises and is impossible with isolation exercises. [69]

These concurrent shift contractions minimize the flexion moment at the knee. The eccentric contraction of the hamstrings helps to neutralize the effects of a concentric quadriceps contraction in producing anterior translation of the tibia. [22] Henning et al. found that the half squat produced significantly less anterior shear at the knee than did an open-chain exercise in full extension. [31] A full squat markedly increases the flexion moment at the knee and thus increases anterior shear of the tibia. As mentioned previously, slightly flexing the trunk anteriorly will also increase the hip flexion moment and decrease the knee moment. It appears that increasing the width of the stance in a wall squat has no effect on EMG activity in the quadriceps. [2] However, moving the feet forward does seem to increase activity in the quadriceps as well as the plantarflexors. [11]

Lunges should be used later in a rehabilitation program to facilitate eccentric strengthening of the quadriceps to act as a decelerator (Figure 12-7). [24,81] Like the minisquat and wall slide, it facilitates co-contraction of the hamstring muscles. [23]

Leg Press

Theoretically, the leg press takes full advantage of the kinetic chain and at the same time provides stability, which

decreases strain on the lower back. [45] It also allows exercise with resistance lower than body weight and the capability of exercising each leg independently (Figure 12-8). [53] It has been recommended that leg-press exercises be performed in a 0- to 60-degree range of knee flexion. [82]

It has also been recommended that leg-press machines allow full hip extension to take maximum advantage of the kinetic chain. [5] Full hip extension can only be achieved in a supine position. In this position, full hip and knee flexion and extension can occur, thus reproducing the concurrent shift and ensuring appropriate hamstring recruitment. [53]

The foot plates should also be designed to move in an arc of motion rather than in a straight line. This movement would facilitate hamstring recruitment by increasing the hip flexion moment and decreasing the knee moment. Foot plates should be fixed perpendicular to the frontal plane of the hip to maximize the knee extension moment created by the soleus.

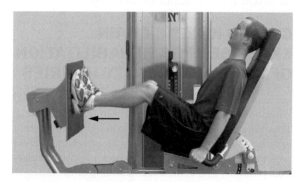

Figure 12-8   Leg-press.

Stair Climbing

Stair-climbing machines have gained a great deal of popularity, not only as a closed-kinetic-chain exercise device useful in rehabilitation, but also as a means of improving cardiorespiratory endurance (Figure 12-9). Stair-climbing machines have two basic designs. One involves a series of rotating steps similar to a department store escalator, while the other uses two foot plates that move up and down to simulate a stepping-type movement. With the latter type of stair climber, also sometimes referred to as a stepping machine, the foot never leaves the foot plate, making it a true closed-kinetic-chain exercise device.

Stair climbing involves many of the same biomechanical principles identified with the leg-press exercise.[51] When exercising on the stair climber, the body should be held erect with only slight trunk flexion, thus maximizing hamstring recruitment through concurrent shift contractions while increasing the hip flexion moment and decreasing the knee flexion moment.

Exercise on a stepping machine produces increased EMG activity in the gastrocnemius. Because the gastrocnemius attaches to the posterior aspect of the femoral condyles, increased activity of this muscle could produce a flexion moment of the femur on the tibia. This motion would cause posterior translation of the femur on the tibia, increasing strain on the ACL. Peak firing of the quadriceps might offset the effects of increased EMG activity in the gastronemius.[17]

Step-Ups

Lateral, forward, and backward step-ups are widely used closed-kinetic-chain exercises (Figure 12-10). Lateral

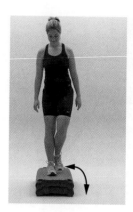

Figure 12-10   Lateral step-ups.

step-ups seem to be used more often clinically than forward step-ups. Step height can be adjusted to patient capabilities and generally progresses up to about 8 inches. Heights greater than 8 inches create a large flexion moment at the knee, increasing anterior shear force and making hamstring co-contraction more difficult.[12,17]

Step-ups elicit significantly greater mean hamstring EMG activity than a stepping machine, whereas the quadriceps are more active during stair climbing.[85] When performing a step-up, the entire body weight must be raised and lowered, whereas on the stepping machine the center of gravity is maintained at a relatively constant height. The lateral step-up can produce increased muscle and joint shear forces compared to stepping exercise.[17] Caution should be exercised by the athletic trainer in using the lateral step-up in cases where minimizing anterior shear forces is essential. Contraction of the hamstrings appears to be of insufficient magnitude to neutralize the shear force produced by the quadriceps.[12] In situations where strengthening of the quadriceps is the goal, the lateral step-up has been recommended as a beneficial exercise.[86] However, lateral stepping exercises have failed to increase isokinetic strength of the quadriceps muscle. It also appears that concentric quadricep contractions produce more EMG activity than eccentric contractions in a lateral step-up.[60]

Terminal Knee Extensions Using Surgical Tubing

It has been reported in numerous studies that the greatest amount of anterior tibial translation occurs between 0 degrees and 30 degrees of flexion during open-kinetic-chain exercise.[26,28,40,51,54,55,82] At one time, athletic trainers avoided open-kinetic-chain terminal knee extension after surgery.

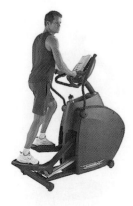

Figure 12-9   Stepping machine.
Source: Courtesy Diamandback Fitness.

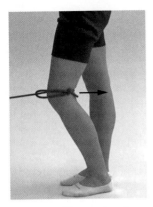

Figure 12-11 Terminal knee extensions using surgical tubing resistance.

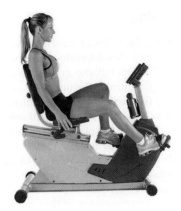

Figure 12-12 Stationary bicycle.

extension after surgery. Unfortunately, this practice led to quadriceps weakness, flexion contracture, and patellofemoral pain.[58]

Closed-kinetic-chain terminal knee extensions using surgical tubing resistance have created a means of safely strengthening terminal knee extension (Figure 12-11).[59] Application of resistance anteriorly at the femur produces anterior shear of the femur, which eliminates any anterior translation of the tibia. This type of exercise performed in the 0- to 30-degree range also minimizes the knee flexion moment, further reducing anterior shear of the tibia. The use of rubber tubing produces an eccentric contraction of the quadriceps when moving into knee flexion. Weightbearing terminal knee extensions with tubing increase the EMG activity in the quadriceps.[85]

Stationary Bicycling

The stationary bicycle can be of significant value as a closed-kinetic-chain exercise device (Figure 12-12).

The advantage of stationary bicycling over other closed-kinetic-chain exercises for rehabilitation is that the amount of the weightbearing force exerted by the injured lower extremity can be adapted within patient limitations. The seat height should be carefully adjusted to minimize the knee flexion moment on the downstroke. However, if the stationary bike is being used to regain range of motion in flexion, the seat height should be adjusted to a lowered position using passive motion of

the injured extremity. Toe clips will facilitate hamstring contractions on the upstroke.

BAPS Board and Minitramp

The BAPS board (Figure 12-13) and minitramp (Figure 12-14) both provide an unstable base of support that helps to facilitate reestablishing proprioception and joint position sense in addition to strengthening. Working on the BAPS board allows the athletic trainer to provide stress to the lower extremity in a progressive and controlled manner.[13] It allows the patient to work simultaneously on strengthening and range of motion, while trying to regain neuromuscular control and balance. The minitramp may

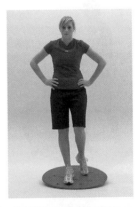

Figure 12-13 BAPS board exercise.

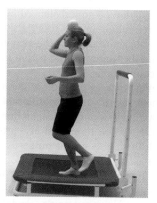

Figure 12-14   Minitramp provides an unstable base of support to which other functional plyometric activities may be added.

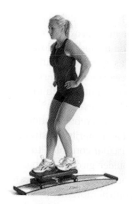

Figure 12-16   The Fitter is useful for weight shifting. Source: Courtesy Fitter First

be used to accomplish the same goals, but it can also be used for more advanced plyometric training.

Slide Boards and Fitter

Shifting the body weight from side to side during a more functional activity on either a slide board (Figure 12-15) or a Fitter (Figure 12-16) helps to reestablish dynamic control as well as improving cardiorespiratory fitness.[13] These motions produce valgus and varus stresses and strains to the joint that are somewhat unique to these two pieces of equipment. Lateral slide exercises have been shown to improve knee extension strength following ACL reconstruction.[10]

CLINICAL DECISION MAKING	Exercise 12–2

Why would the BAPS board and minitramp be good tools in a rehabilitation program for a dancer recovering from an Achilles tendon repair?

CLINICAL DECISION MAKING	Exercise 12–3

Why would a slide board not be an appropriate choice for someone beginning a rehabilitation program for an MCL sprain?

BIOMECHANICS OF OPEN- VERSUS CLOSED-KINETIC-CHAIN ACTIVITIES IN THE UPPER EXTREMITY

Although it is true that closed-kinetic-chain exercises are most often used in rehabilitation of lower-extremity injuries, there are many injury situations where closed-kinetic-chain exercises should be incorporated into upper-extremity rehabilitation protocols.[64] Unlike the lower extremity, the upper extremity is most functional as an open-kinetic-chain system. Most activities involve movement of the upper extremity in which the hand moves freely. These activities are generally dynamic movements. In these movements, the proximal segments of the kinetic chain are used for stabilization, while the distal segments have a high degree of mobility. Push-ups, chinning exercises, and handstands in gymnastics are all examples of closed-kinetic-chain activities in the upper extremity. In

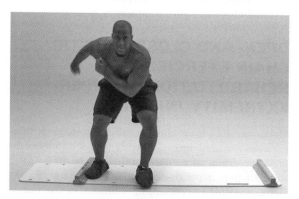

Figure 12-15   Slide board training.

these cases, the hand is stabilized, and muscular contractions around the more proximal segments, the elbow and shoulder, function to raise and lower the body. Still other activities such as swimming and cross-country skiing involve rapid successions of alternating open-and closed-kinetic-chain movements, much in the same way as running does in the lower extremity.[83]

For the most part in rehabilitation, closed-kinetic-chain exercises are used primarily for strengthening and establishing neuromuscular control of those muscles that act to stabilize the shoulder girdle.[76] In particular, the scapular stabilizers and the rotator cuff muscles function at one time or another to control movements about the shoulder. It is essential to develop both strength and neuromuscular control in these muscle groups, thus allowing them to provide a stable base for more mobile and dynamic movements that occur in the distal segments.[76]

It must also be emphasized that although traditional upper-extremity rehabilitation programs have concentrated on treating and identifying the involved structures, the body does not operate in isolated segments but instead works as a dynamic unit.[49] More recently rehabilitation programs have integrated closed-kinetic-chain exercises with core stabilization exercises and more functional movement programs.[65] Athletic trainers should recognize the need to address the importance of the legs and trunk as contributors to upper-extremity function and routinely incorporate therapeutic exercises that address the entire kinetic chain.[49]

CLINICAL DECISION MAKING   Exercise 12–4

A football player suffers from chronic shoulder dislocations. What type of exercises can be used to increase stability of the shoulder?

Shoulder Complex Joint

Closed-kinetic-chain weightbearing activities can be used to both promote and enhance dynamic joint stability. Most often closed-kinetic-chain exercises are used with the hand fixed and thus with no motion occurring. The resistance is then applied either axially or rotationally. These exercises produce both joint compression and approximation, which act to enhance muscular co-contraction about the joint producing dynamic stability.[83]

Two essential force couples must be reestablished around the glenohumeral joint: the anterior deltoid along with the infraspinatus and teres minor in the frontal plane,

and the subscapularis counterbalanced by the infraspinatus and teres minor in the transverse plane. These opposing muscles act to stabilize the glenohumeral joint by compressing the humeral head within the glenoid via muscular co-contraction.

The scapular muscles function to dynamically position the glenoid relative to the position of the moving humerus, resulting in a normal scapulohumeral rhythm of movement. However, they must also provide a stable base on which the highly mobile humerus can function. If the scapula is hypermobile, the function of the entire upper extremity will be impaired. Thus force couples between the inferior trapezius counterbalanced by the upper trapezius and levator scapula—and the rhomboids and middle trapezius counterbalanced by the serratus anterior—are critical in maintaining scapular stability. Again, closed-kinetic-chain activities done with the hand fixed should be used to enhance scapular stability.[44]

Elbow

The elbow is a hinged joint that is capable of 145 degrees of flexion from a fully extended position. In some cases of joint hyperelasticity, the joint can hyperextend a few degrees beyond neutral. The elbow consists of the humeroulnar, humeroradial, and radioulnar articulations. The concave radial head articulates with the convex surface of the capitellum of the distal humerus and is connected to the proximal ulna via the annular ligament. The proximal radioulnar joint constitutes the forearm that permits approximately 90 degrees of pronation and 80 degrees of supination when working in conjunction with the elbow joint.

In some activities, the elbow functions in an open kinetic chain. In other activities, the elbow must possess static stability and adequate dynamic strength to be able to transfer force to a hitting implement.[42]

OPEN- AND CLOSED-KINETIC-CHAIN EXERCISES FOR REHABILITATION OF UPPER-EXTREMITY INJURIES

Most typically, closed-kinetic-chain glenohumeral joint exercises are used during the early phases of a rehabilitation program, particularly in the case of an unstable shoulder to promote co-contraction and muscle recruitment, in addition to preventing shutdown of the rotator cuff secondary to pain and/or inflammation.[3,66] Likewise, closed-kinetic-chain exercise should be used during the late phases of a rehabilitation program to promote muscular endurance of muscles surrounding the glenohumeral and scapulothoracic joints. They may also be used during the later stages of rehabilitation in conjunction with open-kinetic-chain activities to enhance some degree of stability, on which highly dynamic and ballistic motions may be superimposed. At some point during the middle stages of the rehabilitation program, traditional open-kinetic-chain strengthening exercises for the rotator cuff, deltoid, and other glenohumeral and scapular muscles must be incorporated.[34,83]

In the elbow, exercises should also be designed to enhance muscular balance and neuromuscular control of the surrounding agonists and antagonists. Closed-kinetic-chain exercise should be used to improve dynamic stability of the more proximal muscles surrounding the elbow in those activities where the elbow must provide some degree of proximal stability. Open-kinetic-chain exercises for strengthening flexion, extension, pronation, and supination are essential to regain high-velocity dynamic movements of the elbow that are necessary in throwing-type activities.

> **CLINICAL DECISION MAKING**   Exercise 12–5
>
> A female basketball player has been experiencing some hip pain and general lower-extremity fatigue that you think is due to gluteus medius weakness. You want to improve her awareness of this muscle as well as improve her neuromuscular control. How can closed-and open-chain exercises both help you achieve your goals?

Weight Shifting

A variety of weight-shifting exercises can be done to assist in facilitating glenohumeral and scapulothoracic dynamic stability through the use of axial compression.[16] Weight shifting can be done in standing, quadruped, tripod, or biped (opposite leg and arm), with weight supported on a stable surface such as the wall or a treatment table (Figure 12-17A–D), or on a movable, unstable surface such as a BAPS board, a wobble board, stability ball, or a plyoball (Figure 12-18A–D). Shifting may be done side

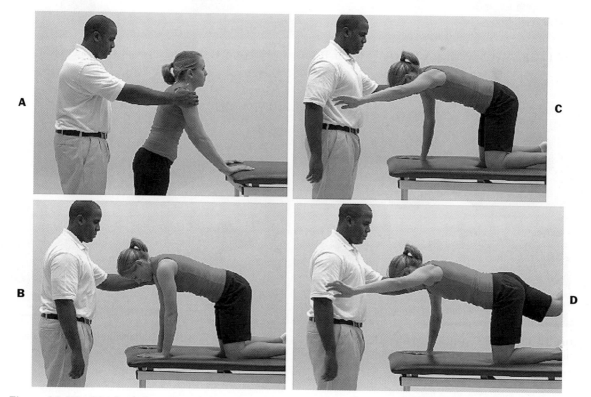

Figure 12-17   Weight shifting. **A**, Standing. **B**, Quadruped. **C**, Tripod. **D**, Opposite knee and arm.

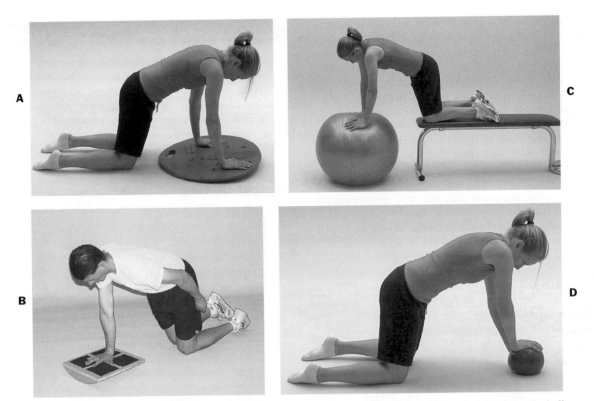

Figure 12-18 Weight shifting. **A,** On a BAPS board. **B,** On a wobble board. **C,** On a stability ball. **D,** On a Plyoball.

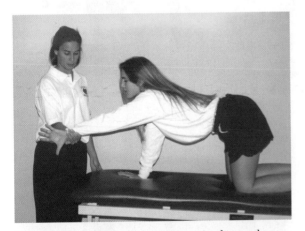

Figure 12-19 D2 PNF pattern in a tripod to produce stabilization in the contralateral support limb.

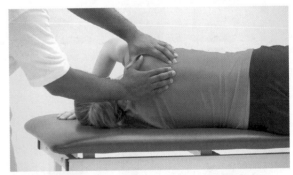

Figure 12-20 Rhythmic stabilization for the scapular muscles.

to side, forward and backward, or on a diagonal. Hand position may be adjusted from a wide base of support to one hand placed on top of the other to increase difficulty. The patient can adjust the amount of weight being supported as tolerated. The athletic trainer can provide manual force of resistance in a random manner to which the patient must rhythmically stabilize and adapt. A diagonal 2 (D2) proprioceptive neuromuscular facilitation pattern may be used in a tripod to force the contralateral support limb to produce a co-contraction and thus stabilization (Figure 12-19).[83] Rhythmic stabilization can also be used regain neuromuscular control of the scapular muscles with the hand in a closed kinetic chain and random pressure applied to the scapular borders (Figure 12-20).

Push-Ups, Push-Ups with a Plus, Press-Ups, Step-Ups

Push-ups and/or press-ups are also done to reestablish neuromuscular control. Push-ups done on an unstable surface such as on a Plyoball require a good deal of strength in addition to providing an axial load that requires co-contraction of agonist and antagonist force couples around the glenohumeral and scapulothoracic joints, while the distal part of the extremity has some limited movement (Figure 12-21). A variation of a standard push-up would be to have the patient use reciprocating contractions on a stair climber (Figure 12-22) or doing single-arm lateral step-ups onto a step (Figure 12-23). Also, the patient may perform push-ups in a variety of positions, including overhead position on the Shuttle 2000 (Figure 12-24).[72] Push-ups with a plus are done to strengthen the serratus anterior, which is critical for scapular dynamic stability in overhead activities

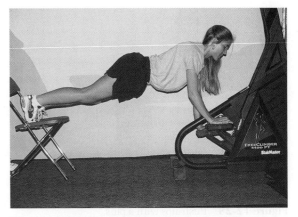

Figure 12-22   Push-ups done on a stair climber.

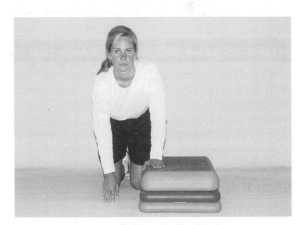

Figure 12-23   Single-arm lateral step-ups.

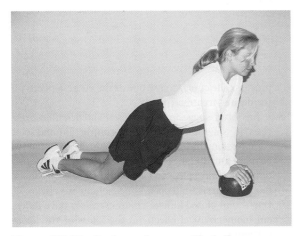

Figure 12-21   Push-ups done on a Plyoball.

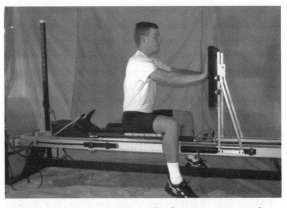

Figure 12-24   Push-ups can be done in a variety of positions on a Shuttle 2000.

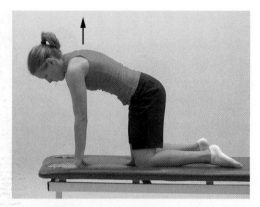

Figure 12-25 Push-ups with a plus.

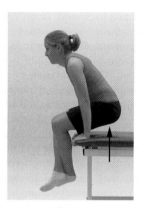

Figure 12-26 Press-ups

(Figure 12-25). Press-ups involve an isometric contraction of the glenohumeral stabilizers (Figure 12-26).

CLINICAL DECISION MAKING **Exercise 12–6**

An athlete has general back weakness. You think that this could be the cause for some anterior shoulder pain. He appears to have winging scapula, and he is having symptoms consistent with impingement. What type of exercises would you introduce to help him with this problem?

Slide Board

Upper-extremity closed-kinetic-chain exercises performed on a slide board are useful not only for promoting strength and stability but also for improving muscular endurance.[72,83] In a kneeling position, the patient uses a recip-

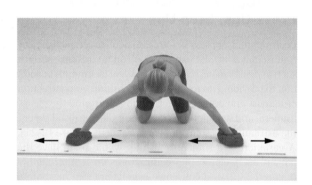

Figure 12-27 Slide board strengthening exercise.

rocating motion, sliding the hands forward and backward, side to side, in a "wax on-wax off" circular pattern, or both hands laterally (Figure 12-27). It is also possible to do wall slides in a standing position.

Summary

1. A closed-kinetic-chain exercise is one in which the distal segment of the extremity is fixed or stabilized. In an open kinetic chain, the distal segment is mobile and not fixed.
2. Both open- and closed-kinetic-chain exercises have their place in the rehabilitative process.
3. The concepts of the reversibility of muscle actions and the concurrent shift are hallmarks of closed-kinetic-chain exercises.
4. Open- and closed-kinetic-chain exercises offer distinct advantages and disadvantages in the rehabilitation

process. The choice to use one or the other depends on the desired treatment goal.
5. It has been suggested that closed-kinetic-chain exercises are safer due to muscle co-contraction and joint compression; that closed-kinetic-chain exercises tend to be more functional; and that they facilitate the integration of proprioceptive and joint position sense feedback more effectively than open-kinetic-chain exercises.
6. Open- and closed-kinetic-chain exercises have different biomechanical effects on the joints of the lower extremity.

7. Closed-kinetic-chain exercises in the lower extremity decrease the shear forces, reducing anterior tibial translation, and increase the compressive forces that increase stability around the knee joint.

8. Minisquat, wall slides, lunges, leg press, stair-climbing machines, lateral step-up, terminal knee extension using tubing, stationary bicycling, slide boards, BAPS boards, and the Fitter are all examples of closed-kinetic-chain activities for the lower extremity.

9. Although it is true that closed-kinetic-chain exercises are most often used in rehabilitation of lower-

extremity injuries, there are many injury situations where closed-kinetic-chain exercises should be incorporated into upper-extremity rehabilitation protocols.

10. Closed-kinetic-chain exercises in the upper extremity are used primarily for strengthening and establishing neuromuscular control of those muscles that act to stabilize the shoulder girdle.

11. Closed-kinetic-chain activities, such as push-ups, press-ups, weight shifting, and slide board exercises, are strengthening exercises used primarily for improving shoulder stabilization in the upper extremity.

......

References

1. Andersen, S., D. Terwilliger, and C. Denegar. 1995. Comparison of open- versus closed-kinetic-chain test positions for measuring joint position sense. *J Sport Rehab* 4(3):165–171.

2. Anderson, R., C. Courtney, and E. Carmeli. 1998. EMG analysis of the vastus medialis/vastus lateralis muscles utilizing the unloading narrow and wide-stance squats. *J Sport Rehab* 7(4):236.

3. Andrews, J., J. Dennison, and K. Wilk. 1995. The significance of closed-chain kinetics in upper extremity injuries from a physician's perspective. *J Sport Rehab* 5(1):64–70.

4. Augustsson, J., A. Esko, R. Thornee, and J. Karlsson. 1998. Weight training of the thigh muscles using closed vs. open kinetic chain exercises: A comparison of performance enhancement. *J Orthop Sports Phys Ther* 27(1):3.

5. Azegami, M., and R. Yanagihashi. 2007. Effects of multi-joint angle changes on EMG activity and force of lower extremity muscles during maximum isometric leg press exercises. *Journal of Physical Therapy Science* 19(1):65.

6. Bakhtiary, A., and E. Fatemi. 2008. Open versus closed kinetic chain exercises for patellar chondromalacia. *British Journal of Sports Medicine* 42(2):99.

7. Baratta, R., M. Solomonow, and B. Zhou. 1988. Muscular coactivation: The role of the antagonist musculature in maintaining knee stability. *Am J Sports Med* 16(2):113–122.

8. Blackburn, J.R., and M.C. Morrissey. 1988. The relationship between open and closed kinetic chain strength of the lower limb and jumping performance. *J Orthop Sports Phys Ther* 27(6):431.

9. Blair, D., and R. Willis. 1991. Rapid rehabilitation following anterior cruciate ligament reconstruction. *Athlet Train* 26(1):32–43.

10. Blanpied, P., R. Carroll, T. Douglas, and M. Lyons. 2000. Effectiveness of lateral slide exercise in an anterior cruciate ligament reconstruction rehabilitation home exercise program. *J Orthop Sports Physl Ther* 30(10):602.

11. Blanpied, P. 1999. Changes in muscle activation during wall slides and squat-machine exercise. *J Sport Rehab* 8(2):123.

12. Brask, B., R. Lueke, and G. Soderberg. 1984. Electromyographic analysis of selected muscles during the lateral step-up. *Phys Ther* 64(3):324–329.

13. Bunton, E., W. Pitney, and A. Kane. 1993. The role of limb torque, muscle action and proprioception during closed-kinetic-chain rehabilitation of the lower extremity. *J Athlet Train* 28(1):10–20.

14. Butler, D., F. Noyes, and E. Grood. 1980. Ligamentous restraints to anterior-posterior drawer in the human knee: A biomechanical study. *J Bone Joint Surg* 62(A):259–270.

15. Case, J., B. DePalma, and R. Zelko. 1991. Knee rehabilitation following anterior cruciate ligament repair/reconstruction: An update. *Athlet Train* 26(1):22–31.

16. Cipriani, D. 1994. Open- and closed-chain rehabilitation for the shoulder complex. In *The athlete's shoulder*, Andrews J., and K. Wilk, eds. New York: Churchill Livingston.

17. Cook, T., C. Zimmerman, and K. Lux, et al. 1992. EMG comparison of lateral step-up and stepping machine exercise. *J Orthop Sports Phys Ther* 16(3):108–113.

18. Cordova, M.L. 2001. Considerations in lower extremity closed kinetic chain exercise: A clinical perspective. *Athlet Ther Today* 6(2):46–50.

19. Davies, G. 1995. The need for critical thinking in rehabilitation. *J Sport Rehab* 4(1):1–22.

20. DeCarlo, M., D. Shelbourne, and J. McCarroll, et al. A traditional versus accelerated rehabilitation following ACL reconstruction: A one-year follow-up. *J Orthop Sports Phys Ther* 15(6):309–316.

21. Ellenbecker, T.S., and G.J. Davies. 2001. *Closed kinetic chain exercise: A comprehensive guide to multiple-joint exercise.* Champaign, IL: Human Kinetics.

22. Escamilla, R.F. 2001. Knee biomechanics of the dynamic squat exercise. *Med Sci Sports Exerc* 33(1):127–141.

23. Escamilla, R., and N. Zheng. 2008. Patellofemoral compressive force and stress during the forward and side lunges with and without a stride. *Clinical Biomechanics* 23(8):1026.

24. Farrokhi, S., and C. Pollard. 2008. Trunk position influences the kinematics, kinetics, and muscle activity of the lead lower

extremity during the forward lunge exercise. *Journal of Orthopaedic & Sports Physical Therapy* 38(7):403.

25. Fu, F., S. Woo, and J. Irrgang. 1992. Current concepts for rehabilitation following anterior cruciate ligament reconstruction. *J Orthop Sports Phys Ther* 15(6):270–278.

26. Fukubayashi, T., P. Torzilli, and M. Sherman. 1982. An in-vitro biomechanical evaluation of anterior/posterior motion of the knee: Tibial displacement, rotation, and torque. *J Bone Joint Surg* 64[B]:258–264.

27. Grahm, V., G. Gehlsen, and J. Edwards. 1993. Electromyographic evaluation of closed- and open-kinetic-chain knee rehabilitation exercises. *J Athlet Train* 28(1):23–33.

28. Grood, E., W. Suntag, and F. Noyes, et al. 1984. Biomechanics of knee extension exercise. *J Bone Joint Surg* 66[A]:725–733.

29. Harter, R. 1995. Clinical rationale for closed-kinetic-chain activities in functional testing and rehabilitation of ankle pathologies. *J Sport Rehab* 5(1):13–24.

30. Heijne, A., and B. Fleming. 2004. Strain on the anterior cruciate ligament during closed kinetic chain exercises. *Medicine & Science in Sports & Exercise* 36(6):935–941.

31. Henning, S., M. Lench, and K. Glick. 1985. An in-vivo strain gauge study of elongation of the anterior cruciate ligament. *Am J Sports Med* 13:22–26.

32. Herrington, L., and A. Al-Sherhi. 2007. Comparison of single and multiple joint quadriceps exercise in anterior knee pain rehabilitation. *Journal of Orthopaedic & Sports Physical Therapy* 37(4):155.

33. Herrington, L. 2005. Knee-joint position sense: The relationship between open and closed kinetic chain tests. *Journal of Sport Rehabilitation* 14(4):356.

34. Hillman, S. 1994. Principles and techniques of open-kinetic-chain rehabilitation: The upper extremity. *Journal of Sport Rehabilitation* 3(4): 319–30.

35. Hooper, D.M., M.C. Morrissey, and W. Drechsler. 2001. Open and closed kinetic chain exercises in the early period after anterior cruciate ligament reconstruction: Improvements in level walking, stair ascent, and stair descent. *Am J Sports Med* 29(2):167–174.

36. Hopkins, J.T., C.D. Ingersoll, and M.A. Sandrey 1999. An electromyographic comparison of 4 closed chain exercises. *J Athlet Train* 34(4):353.

37. Hung, Y.J., and M.T. Gross. 1999. Effect of foot position on electromyographic activity of the vastus medialis oblique and vastus lateralis during lower-extremity weight bearing activities. *Journal of Orthopaedic and Sports Physical Therapy* 29(2): 93–105.

38. Hungerford, D., and M. Barry. 1979. Biomechanics of the patellofemoral joint. *Clin Orthop* 144:9–15.

39. Irrgang, J., M. Safran, and F. Fu. 1995. The knee: Ligamentous and meniscal injuries. In *Athletic injuries and rehabilitation*, Zachazewski, J., D. McGee, and W. Quillen. Philadelphia: WB Saunders.

40. Jurist, K., and V. Otis. 1985. Anteroposterior tibiofemoral displacements during isometric extension efforts. The roles of external load and knee flexion angle. *Am J Sports Med* 13: 254–258.

41. Kaland, S., T. Sinkjaer, and L. Arendt-Neilsen, et al. 1990. Altered timing of hamstring muscle action in anterior cruciate ligament deficient patients. *Am J Sports Med* 18(3):245–248.

42. Kibler, W., and A. Sciascia. Kinetic chain contributions to elbow function and dysfunction in sports. *Clinics in Sports Medicine* 23(4):545–552.

43. Kleiner, D., T. Drudge, and M. Ricard. 1994. An electromyographic comparison of popular open- and closed-kinetic-chain knee rehabilitation exercises. *J Athlet Train* 29(2):156–157.

44. Kovaleski, J.E., R. Heitman, L. Gurchiek, and T. Tyundle. 1990. Reliability and effects of arm dominance on upper extremity isokinetic force, work, and power using the closed chain rider system. *J Athlet Train* 34(4):358.

45. LaFree, J., A. Mozingo, and T. Worrell. 1995. Comparison of open-kinetic-chain knee and hip extension to closed-kinetic-chain leg press performance. *J Sport Rehab* 3(2):99–107.

46. Lepart, S., and T. Henry. 1995. The physiological basis for open- and closed-kinetic-chain rehabilitation for the upper extremity. *J Sport Rehab* 5(1):71–87.

47. Lutz, G., M. Stuart, and H. Franklin. 1990. Rehabilitative techniques for athletes after reconstruction of the anterior cruciate ligament. *Mayo Clin Proc* 65:1322–1329.

48. Malone, T., and W. Garrett. 1992. Commentary and historical perspective of anterior cruciate ligament rehabilitation. *J Orthop Sports Phys Ther* 15(6):265–269.

49. McMullen, J., and T.L. Uhl. A kinetic chain approach for shoulder rehabilitation. *J Ath Train* 35(3): 329.

50. Mesfar, W., and A. Shirazi-Adl. 2008. Knee joint biomechanics in open-kinetic-chain flexion exercises. *Clinical Biomechanics* 23(4):477.

51. Nisell, R., M. Ericson, and G. Nemeth, et al. 1989. Tibiofemoral joint forces during isokinetic knee extension. *Am J Sports Med* 17:49–54.

52. Ohkoshi, Y., K. Yasuda, and K. Kaneda, et al. 1991. Biomechanical analysis of rehabilitation in the standing position. *Am J Sports Med* 19(6):605–611.

53. Palmitier, R., A. Kai-Nan, and S. Scott, et al. 1991. Kinetic-chain exercise in knee rehabilitation. *Sports Med* 11(6):402–413.

54. Renstrom, P., S. Arms, and T. Stanwyck, et al. 1986. Strain within the anterior cruciate ligament during hamstring and quadriceps activity. *Am J Sports Med* 14:83–87.

55. Reynolds, N., T. Worrell, and D. Perrin. 1992. Effect of lateral step-up exercise protocol on quadriceps isokinetic peak torque values and thigh girth. *J Orthop Sports Phys Ther* 15(3):151–56.

56. Rivera, J. 1994. Open- versus closed-kinetic-chain rehabilitation of the lower extremity: A functional and biomechanical analysis. *J Sport Rehab* 3(2):154–167.

57. Ross, M.D., C.R. Denegar, and J.A. Winzenried. 2001. Implementation of open and closed kinetic chain quadriceps strengthening exercises after anterior cruciate ligament reconstruction. *J Strength Cond Res* 15(4):466–473.

58. Sachs, R., D. Daniel, and M. Stone, et al. 1989. Patellofemoral problems after anterior cruciate ligament reconstruction. *Am J Sports Med* 17:760–765.

59. Schulthies, S.S., M.D. Ricard, K.J. Alexander, and J.W. Myrer. 1998. An electromyographic investigation of 4 elastic-tubing closed kinetic chain exercises after anterior cruciate ligament reconstruction. *J Athlet Train* 33(4):328–335.

60. Selseth, A., M. Dayton, M. Cardova, C. Ingersoll, and M. Merrick. 2000. Quadriceps concentric EMG activity is greater than eccentric EMG activity during the lateral step-up exercise. *J Sport Rehab* 9(2):124.

61. Sheehy, P., R.C. Burdett, J.J. Irrgang, and J. VanSwearingen. 1998. An electromyographic study of vastus medialis oblique and vastus lateralis activity while ascending and descending stairs. *J Orthop Sports Phys Ther* 27(6):423–429.

62. Shellbourne, D., and P. Nitz. 1990. Accelerated rehabilitation after anterior cruciate ligament reconstruction. *Am J Sports Med* 18:292–299.

63. Shields, and S. Madhavan. 2005. Neuromuscular control of the knee during a resisted single-limb squat exercise. *American Journal of Sports Medicine* 33(10):1520–1526.

64. Smith, D. 2006. Incorporating kinetic-chain integration, Part 1: Concepts of functional shoulder movement. *Athletic Therapy Today* 11(4):63.

65. Smith, D. 2006. Incorporating kinetic-chain integration, Part 2: Functional shoulder rehabilitation. *Athletic Therapy Today* 11(5):63.

66. Smith, J., D. Dahm, and B. Kotajarvi. 2007. Electromyographic activity in the immobilized shoulder girdle musculature during ipsilateral kinetic chain exercises. *Archives of Physical Medicine & Rehabilitation* 88(11):1377–1383.

67. Snyder-Mackler, L. 1995. Scientific rationale and physiological basis for the use of closed-kinetic-chain exercise in the lower extremity. *J Sport Rehab* 5(1): 2–12.

68. Solomonow, M., R. Barata, and B. Zhou, et al. 1987. The synergistic action of the anterior cruciate ligament and thigh muscles in maintaining joint stability. *Am J Sports Med* 15:207–213.

69. Steindler, A. 1977. *Kinesiology of the human body under normal and pathological conditions.* Springfield, IL: Charles C. Thomas.

70. Stensdotter, A., P. Hodges, and R. Mellor. 2003. Quadriceps activation in closed and in open kinetic chain exercise. *Medicine & Science in Sports & Exercise* 35(12):2043–2047.

71. Stiene, H., T. Brosky, and M. Reinking. 1996. A comparison of closed-kinetic-chain and isokinetic joint isolation exercise in patients with patellofemoral dysfunction. *J Orthop Phys Ther* 24(3):136–141.

72. Stone, J., J. Lueken, and N. Partin. 1993. Closed-kinetic-chain rehabilitation of the glenohumeral joint. *J Athlet Train* 28(1):34–37.

73. Tagesson, S., B. Öberg, and L. Good. 2008. A comprehensive rehabilitation program with quadriceps strengthening in closed versus open kinetic chain exercise in patients with anterior cruciate ligament deficiency. *American Journal of Sports Medicine* 36(2):298.

74. Tang, S.F.T., C.K. Chen, R. Hsu, S.W. Chou, W.H. Hong, and H.L. Lew. 2001. Vastus medialis obliquus and vastus lateralis activity in open and closed kinetic chain exercises in patients with patellofemoral pain syndrome: An electromyographic study. *Arch Phys Med Rehab* 82(10):1441–1445.

75. Tovin, B., T. Tovin, and M. Tovin. 1992. Surgical and biomechanical considerations in rehabilitation of patients with intra-articular ACL reconstructions. *J Orthop Sports Phys Ther* 15(6):317–322.

76. Ubinger, M.E., W.E. Prentice, and K.M. Guskiewicz. 1999. Effect of closed kinetic chain training on neuromuscular control in the upper extremity. *J Sport Rehab* 8(3):184–194.

77. Valmassey, R. 1996. *Clinical biomechanics of the lower extremities.* St. Louis: Mosby.

78. Voight, M., S. Bell, and D. Rhodes. 1992. Instrumented testing of tibial translation during a positive Lachman's test and selected closed-chain activities in anterior cruciate deficient knees. *J Orthop Sports Phys Ther* 15:49.

79. Voight, M., and G. Cook. 1995. Clinical application of closed-chain exercise. *J Sport Rehab* 5(1):25–44.

80. Voight, M., and S. Tippett. 1990. *Closed kinetic chain.* Paper presented at 41st Annual Clinical Symposium of the National Athletic Trainers Association, Indianapolis, June 12.

81. Wawrzyniak, J., J. Tracy, and P. Catizone. 1996. Effect of closed-chain exercise on quadriceps femoris peak torque and functional performance. *J Athlet Train* 31(4):335–345.

82. Wilk, K., and J. Andrew. 1992. Current concepts in the treatment of anterior cruciate ligament disruption. *J Orthop Sports Phys Ther* 15(6):279–293.

83. Wilk, K., C. Arrigo, and J. Andrews. 1995. Closed- and open-kinetic-chain exercise for the upper extremity. *J Sport Rehab* 5(1): 88–102.

84. Willett, G., G. Karst, E. Canney, D. Gallant, and J. Wees. 1998. Lower limb EMG activity during selected stepping exercises. *J Sport Rehab* 7(2):102.

85. Willett, G., J. Paladino, K. Barr, J. Korta, and G. Karst. 1998. Medial and lateral quadriceps muscle activity during weight-bearing knee extension exercise. *J Sport Rehab* 7(4):248.

86. Worrell, T.W., E. Crisp, and C. LaRosa. 1998. Electromyographic reliability and analysis of selected lower extremity muscles during lateral step-up conditions. *J Athlet Train* 33(2):156.

SOLUTIONS TO CLINICAL DECISION MAKING EXERCISES

12-1 An exercise bike is a good tool when rehabilitating lower-extremity injuries. The patient can work through a full ROM without bearing weight. The seat height can be adjusted to target a specific ROM. And most muscles of the leg are utilized. Most bikes have an option of upper-body activity as well. A stair-climber or elliptical machine provides weightbearing exercise that is nonimpact. Later in closed-chain progression, lateral step-ups can be used for neuromuscular control and increased quadriceps firing.

12-2 Neuromuscular control and balance are crucial to the performance of a dancer. The BAPS board and minitramp provide unstable surfaces on which the patient is required to stand. Such controlled systems are ideal because they challenge proprioception more than the stable ground. The patient who has mastered balance on an apparatus such as the minitramp can be progressed to functional activity such as catching a ball while balancing on an unstable surface.

12-3 Unique to the slide board are the valgus and varus strains elicited by the movement. Too much valgus stress while the ligament and musculature are still weak could exacerbate the injury.

12-4 Closed-chain exercises in which the arm is fixed and the shoulder joint is perturbed cause contraction of the scapular stabilizers and the rotator cuff. This encourages overall stability of the joint.

12-5 Open-chain exercises will allow you to apply significant resistance and isolate the muscle. With side-lying exercises it is easy to teach the patient to isolate the muscle. Once that is accomplished, more functional closed-chain exercises can be implemented. Closed-chain exercises will encourage neuromuscular control, as the patient is expected to balance in addition to targeting the particular muscle.

12-6 He needs to strengthen his scapular stabilizers so that his shoulder will not rest anteriorly. Any exercise that perturbs the shoulder complex will cause the scapular stabilizers to fue. Push-ups with a plus are done to strengthen the serratus anterior. Push-ups performed on a BAPS board or on a Plyoball also promote stability and neuromuscular control of the shoulder complex.

CHAPTER 13

Joint Mobilization and Traction Techniques in Rehabilitation

William E. Prentice

After completing this chapter, the athletic training student should be able to do the following:

- Differentiate between physiologic movements and accessory motions.

- Discuss joint arthrokinematics.

- Discuss how specific joint positions can enhance the effectiveness of the treatment technique.

- Discuss the basic techniques of joint mobilization.

- Identify Maitland's five oscillation grades.

- Discuss indications and contraindications for mobilization.

- Discuss the use of various traction grades in treating pain and joint hypomobility.

- Explain why traction and mobilization techniques should be used simultaneously.

- Demonstrate specific techniques of mobilization and traction for various joints.

Following injury to a joint, there will almost always be some associated loss of motion. That loss of movement may be attributed to a number of pathological factors including contracture of inert connective tissue (for example, ligaments and joint capsule), resistance of the contractile tissue or the musculotendinous unit (for example, muscle, tendon, and fascia) to stretch, or some combination of the two.[7,8] If left untreated, the joint will become hypomobile and will eventually begin to show signs of degeneration.[30]

Joint mobilization and traction are manual therapy techniques that are slow, passive movements of articulating surfaces.[33] They are used to regain normal active joint range of motion, restore normal passive motions that occur about a joint, reposition or realign a joint, regain a normal distribution of forces and stresses about a joint, or reduce pain—all of which will collectively improve joint function.[25] Joint mobilization and traction are two extremely effective and widely used techniques in injury rehabilitation.[3]

RELATIONSHIP BETWEEN PHYSIOLOGICAL AND ACCESSORY MOTIONS

For the athletic trainer supervising a rehabilitation program, some understanding of the biomechanics of joint movement is essential. There are basically two types of movements that govern motion about a joint. Perhaps the better known of the two types of movements are the *physiological movements* that result from either concentric or eccentric active muscle contractions that move a bone or a joint. This type of motion is referred to as *osteokinematic motion.* A bone can move about an axis of rotation, or

267

a joint into flexion, extension, abduction, adduction, and rotation. The second type of motion is *accessory motion.* Accessory motions refer to the manner in which one articulating joint surface moves relative to another. Physiological movement is voluntary, while accessory movements normally accompany physiological movement.[2] The two occur simultaneously. Although accessory movements cannot occur independently, they may be produced by some external force. Normal accessory component motions must occur for full-range physiological movement to take place. If any of the accessory component motions are restricted, normal physiological cardinal plane movements will not occur.[23,24] A muscle cannot be fully rehabilitated if the joint is not free to move and vice versa.[30]

Traditionally in rehabilitation programs, we have tended to concentrate more on passive physiological movements without paying much attention to accessory motions. The question is always being asked, "How much flexion or extension is this patient lacking?" Rarely will anyone ask "How much is rolling or gliding restricted?"

It is critical for the athletic trainer to closely evaluate the injured joint to determine whether motion is limited by physiological movement constraints involving musculotendinous units or by limitation in accessory motion involving the joint capsule and ligaments.[15] If physiological movement is restricted, the patient should engage in stretching activities designed to improve flexibility. Stretching exercises should be used whenever there is resistance of the contractile or musculotendinous elements to stretch. Stretching techniques are most effective at the end of physiological range of movement; they are limited to one direction, and they require some element of discomfort if additional range of motion is to be achieved. Stretching techniques make use of long-lever arms to apply stretch to a given muscle.[14] Stretching techniques are discussed in Chapters 8 and 14.

If accessory motion is limited by some restriction of the joint capsule or the ligaments, the athletic trainer should incorporate mobilization techniques into the treatment program. Mobilization techniques should be used whenever there are tight inert or noncontractile articular structures; they can be used effectively at any point in the range of motion, and they can be used in any direction in which movement is restricted. Mobilization techniques use a short-lever arm to stretch ligaments and joint capsules, placing less stress on these structures, and consequently are somewhat safer to use than stretching techniques.[5]

CLINICAL DECISION MAKING   **Exercise 13–1**

Following a grade 2 sprain of the lateral collateral ligament, a high jumper is having trouble regaining full knee extension. Describe a rehabilitation protocol that can help her regain full ROM.

JOINT ARTHROKINEMATICS

Accessory motions are also referred to as *joint arthrokinematics,* which include *spin, roll,* and *glide* (Figure 13-1).[1,17,19]

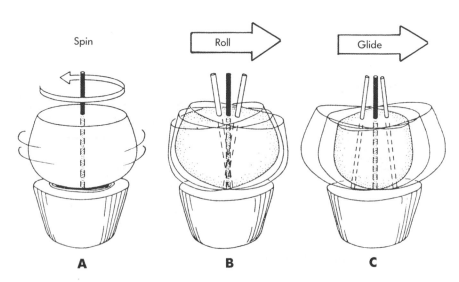

Figure 13-1 Joint arthrokinematics. **A,** Spin. **B,** Roll. **C,** Glide.

Spin occurs around some stationary longitudinal mechanical axis and may be in either a clockwise or counterclockwise direction. An example of spinning is motion of the radial head at the humeroradial joint as occurs in forearm pronation/supination (Figure 13-1A).

Rolling occurs when a series of points on one articulating surface come in contact with a series of points on another articulating surface. An analogy would be to picture a rocker of a rocking chair rolling on the flat surface of the floor. An anatomic example would be the rounded femoral condyles rolling over a stationary flat tibial plateau (Figure 13-1B).

Gliding occurs when a specific point on one articulating surface comes in contact with a series of points on another surface. Returning to the rocking chair analogy, the rocker slides across the flat surface of the floor without any rocking at all. Gliding is sometimes referred to as *translation*. Anatomically, gliding or translation would occur during an anterior drawer test at the knee when the flat tibial plateau slides anteriorly relative to the fixed rounded femoral condyles (Figure 13-1C).

Pure gliding can occur only if the two articulating surfaces are congruent, where either both are flat or both are curved. Since virtually all articulating joint surfaces are incongruent, meaning that one is usually flat while the other is more curved, it is more likely that gliding will occur simultaneously with a rolling motion. Rolling does not occur alone because this would result in compression or perhaps dislocation of the joint.

Although rolling and gliding usually occur together, they are not necessarily in similar proportion, nor are they always in the same direction. If the articulating surfaces are more congruent, more gliding will occur; whereas if they are less congruent, more rolling will occur. Rolling will always occur in the same direction as the physiological movement. For example, in the knee joint when the foot is fixed on the ground, the femur will always roll in an anterior direction when moving into knee extension and conversely will roll posteriorly when moving into flexion (Figure 13-2).

The direction of the gliding component of motion is determined by the shape of the articulating surface that is moving. If you consider the shape of two articulating surfaces, one joint surface can be determined to be convex in shape while the other may be considered to be concave in shape. In the knee, the femoral condyles would be considered the convex joint surface, while the tibial plateau would be the concave joint surface. In the glenohumeral joint, the humeral head would be the convex surface, while the glenoid fossa would be the concave surface.

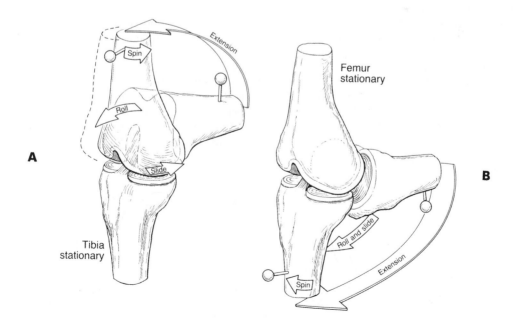

Figure 13-2   Convex-concave rule. **A,** Convex moving on concave. **B,** Concave moving on convex.

This relationship between the shape of articulating joint surfaces and the direction of gliding is defined by the *convex-concave rule*. If the concave joint surface is moving on a stationary convex surface, gliding will occur in the same direction as the rolling motion. Conversely, if the convex surface is moving on a stationary concave surface, gliding will occur in an opposite direction to rolling. Hypomobile joints are treated by using a gliding technique. Thus it is critical to know the appropriate direction to use for gliding.[9]

JOINT POSITIONS

Each joint in the body has a position in which the joint capsule and the ligaments are most relaxed, allowing for a maximum amount of *joint play.*[4,19] This position is called the *resting position*. It is essential to know specifically where the resting position is, because testing for joint play during an evaluation, and treatment of the hypomobile joint using either mobilization or traction, are usually performed in this position. Table 13-1 summarizes the appropriate resting positions for many of the major joints.

Placing the joint capsule in the resting position allows the joint to assume a *loose-packed position* in which the articulating joint surfaces are maximally separated. A *close-packed position* is one in which there is maximal contact of the articulating surfaces of bones with the capsule

and ligaments tight or tense. In a loose-packed position, the joint will exhibit the greatest amount of joint play, while the close-packed position allows for no joint play. Thus the loose-packed position is most appropriate for mobilization and traction (Figure 13-3).

Both mobilization and traction techniques use a translational movement of one joint surface relative to the other. This translation may be either perpendicular or parallel to the *treatment plane*. The treatment plane falls perpendicular to, or at a right angle to, a line running from the axis of rotation in the convex surface to the center of the concave articular surface (Figure 13-4).[17,19] Thus the treatment plane lies within the concave surface. If the convex segment moves, the treatment plane remains fixed. However, the treatment plane will move along with the concave segment. Mobilization techniques use glides that translate one articulating surface along a line parallel with the treatment plane. Traction techniques translate one of the articulating surfaces in a perpendicular direction to the treatment plane. Both techniques use a loose-packed joint position.[17]

JOINT MOBILIZATION TECHNIQUES

The techniques of joint mobilization are used to improve joint mobility or to decrease joint pain by restoring accessory movements to the joint and thus allowing full, nonrestricted, pain-free range of motion.[25,34]

Mobilization techniques may be used to attain a variety of either mechanical or neurophysiological treatment goals: reducing pain; decreasing muscle guarding; stretching or lengthening tissue surrounding a joint, in particular capsular and ligamentous tissue; reflexogenic effects that either inhibit or facilitate muscle tone or stretch reflex; and proprioceptive effects to improve postural and kinesthetic awareness.[1,12,18,24,28,30]

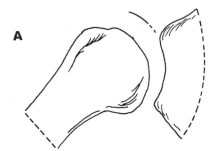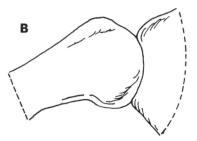

Figure 13-3 Joint capsule resting position. **A,** Loose-packed position. **B,** Close-packed position.

■ TABLE   13-1   Shape, Resting Position, and Treatment Planes of Various Joints

Joint	Convex Surface	Concave Surface	Resting Position (Loose-packed)	Close-packed Position	Treatment Plane
Sternoclavicular	Clavicle[a]	Sternum[a]	Anatomic position	Horizontal	In sternum
Acromioclavicular	Clavicle	Acromion	Anatomic position, in horizontal plane at 60 degrees to sagittal plane	Adduction	In acromion
Glenohumeral	Humerus	Glenoid	Shoulder abducted 55 degrees, horizontally adducted 30 degrees, rotated so that forearm is in horizontal plane	Abduction and lateral rotation	In glenoid fossa in scapular plane
Humeroradial	Humerus	Radius	Elbow extended, forearm supinated	Flexion and forearm production	In radial head perpendicular to long axis of radius
Humeroulnar	Humerus	Ulna	Elbow flexed 70 degrees, forearm supinated 10 degrees	Full extension and forearm supination	In olecranon fossa, 45 degrees to long axis of ulna
Radioulnar (proximal)	Radius	Ulna	Elbow flexed 70 degrees, forearm supinated 35 degrees	Full extension and forearm supination	In radial notch of ulna, parallel to long axis of ulna
Radioulnar (distal)	Ulna	Radius	Supinated 10 degrees	Extension	In radius, parallel to long axis of radius
Radiocarpal	Proximal carpal bones	Radius	Line through radius and third metacarpal	Extension	In radius, perpendicular to long axis of radius
Metacarpophalan-geal	Metacarpal	Proximal phalanx	Slight flexion	Full flexion	In proximal phalanx
Interphalangeal	Proximal phalanx	Distal phalanx	Slight flexion	Extension	In proximal phalanx
Hip	Femur	Acetabulum	Hip flexed 30 degrees, abducted 30 degrees, slight external rotation	Extension and medial rotation	In acetabulum
Tibiofemoral	Femur	Tibia	Flexed 25 degrees	Full extension	On surface of tibial plateau
Patellofemoral	Patella	Femur	Knee in full extension	Full flexion	Along femoral groove
Talocrural	Talus	Mortise	Plantarflexed 10 degrees	Dorsiflexion	In the mortise in anterior/posterior direction
Subtalar	Calcaneus	Talus	Subtalar neutral between inversion/eversion	Supination	In talus, parallel to foot surface
Intertarsal	Proximal articulating surface	Distal articulating surface	Foot relaxed	Supination	In distal segment
Metatarsophalan-geal	Tarsal bone	Proximal phalanx	Slight extension	Full flexion	In proximal phalanx
Interphalangeal	Proximal phalanx	Distal phalanx	Slight flexion	Extension	In distal phalanx

[a]In the sternoclavicular joint the clavicle surface is convex in a superior/inferior direction and concave in an anterior/posterior direction.

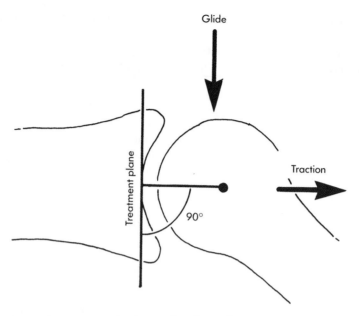

Figure 13-4 The treatment plane is perpendicular to a line drawn from the axis of rotation to the center of the articulating surface of the concave segment.

Movement throughout a range of motion can be quantified with various measurement techniques. Physiological movement is measured with a goniometer and composes the major portion of the range. Accessory motion is thought of in millimeters, although precise measurement is difficult.

Accessory movements may be hypomobile, normal, or hypermobile.[6] Each joint has a range-of-motion continuum with an anatomical limit (AL) to motion that is determined by both bony arrangement and surrounding soft tissue (Figure 13-5). In a hypomobile joint, motion stops at some point referred to as a pathological point of limitation (PL), short of the anatomical limit caused by pain, spasm, or tissue resistance. A hypermobile joint moves beyond its anatomical limit because of laxity of the surrounding structures. A hypomobile joint should respond well to techniques of mobilization and traction. A hypermobile joint should be treated with strengthening exercises, stability exercises, and if indicated, taping, splinting, or bracing.[29,30]

In a hypomobile joint, as mobilization techniques are used in the range-of-motion restriction, some deformation of soft-tissue capsular or ligamentous structures occurs. If a tissue is stretched only into its elastic range, no permanent structural changes will occur. However, if that tissue is stretched into its plastic range, permanent structural

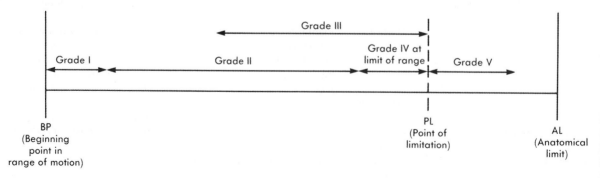

Figure 13-5 Maitland's five grades of motion. *PL* = point of limitation; *AL* = anatomical limit.

changes will occur. Thus, mobilization and traction can be used to stretch tissue and break adhesions. If used inappropriately, they can also damage tissue and cause sprains of the joint.[30]

Treatment techniques designed to improve accessory movement are generally slow, small-amplitude movements, the amplitude being the distance that the joint is moved passively within its total range. Mobilization techniques use these small-amplitude oscillating motions that glide or slide one of the articulating joint surfaces in an appropriate direction within a specific part of the range.[22]

CLINICAL DECISION MAKING   **Exercise 13–3**

Following shoulder surgery a swimmer is having trouble regaining full ROM. His stroke will be affected if he cannot regain full extension and lateral rotation. What type of joint mobilization protocol could you implement to help him?

Maitland has described various grades of oscillation for joint mobilization. The amplitude of each oscillation grade falls within the range-of-motion continuum between some beginning point (BP) and the AL.[23,24] Figure 13-5 shows the various grades of oscillation that are used in a joint with some limitation of motion. As the severity of the movement restriction increases, the PL will move to the left, away from the AL. However, the relationships that exist among the five grades in terms of their positions within the range of motion remain the same. The five mobilization grades are defined as follows:

Grade I. A small-amplitude movement at the beginning of the range of movement. Used when pain and spasm limit movement early in the range of motion.[37]

Grade II. A large-amplitude movement within the midrange of movement. Used when spasm limits movement sooner with a quick oscillation than with a slow one, or when slowly increasing pain restricts movement halfway into the range.

Grade III. A large-amplitude movement up to the PL in the range of movement. Used when pain and resistance from spasm, inert tissue tension, or tissue compression limit movement near the end of the range.

Grade IV. A small-amplitude movement at the very end of the range of movement. Used when resistance limits movement in the absence of pain and spasm.

Grade V. A small-amplitude, quick thrust delivered at the end of the range of movement, usually accompanied by a popping sound, called a manipulation. Used when minimal resistance limits the end of the range. Manipulation is most effectively accomplished by the velocity of the thrust rather than by the force of the thrust.[21] Most authorities agree that manipulation should be used only by individuals trained specifically in these techniques, because a great deal of skill and judgment is necessary for safe and effective treatment.[32]

CLINICAL DECISION MAKING   **Exercise 13–4**

How might a chiropractor apply the concepts of joint mobilization?

Joint mobilization uses these oscillating gliding motions of one articulating joint surface in whatever direction is appropriate for the existing restriction. The appropriate direction for these oscillating glides is determined by the convex-concave rule, described previously. When the concave surface is stationary and the convex surface is mobilized, a glide of the convex segment should be in the direction opposite to the restriction of joint movement (Figure 13-6A).[17,19,35] If the convex articular surface is stationary and the concave surface is mobilized, gliding of the concave segment should be in the same direction as the restriction of joint movement (Figure 13-6B). For example, the glenohumeral joint would be considered to be a convex joint with the convex humeral head moving on the concave glenoid. If shoulder abduction is restricted, the humerus should be glided in an inferior direction relative to the glenoid to alleviate the motion restriction. When mobilizing the knee joint, the concave tibia should be glided anteriorly in cases where knee extension is restricted. If mobilization in the appropriate direction exacerbates complaints of pain or stiffness, the athletic trainer should apply the technique in the opposite direction until the patient can tolerate the appropriate direction.[35]

Typical mobilization of a joint may involve a series of three to six sets of oscillations lasting between 20 and 60 seconds each, with one to three oscillations per second.[23,24]

CLINICAL DECISION MAKING   **Exercise 13–5**

Following an ankle sprain, accumulated scar tissue is preventing full plantar flexion. How can joint mobilization be used to help regain full ROM?

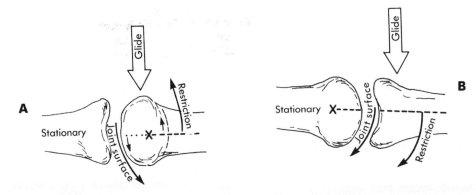

Figure 13-6   Gliding motions. **A,** Glides of the convex segment should be in the direction opposite to the restriction. **B,** Glides of the concave segment should be in the direction of the restriction.

Indications for Mobilization

In Maitland's system, grades I and II are used primarily for treatment of pain and grades III and IV are used for treating stiffness. Pain must be treated first and stiffness second.[24] Painful conditions should be treated on a daily basis. The purpose of the small-amplitude oscillations is to stimulate mechanoreceptors within the joint that can limit the transmission of pain perception at the spinal cord or brain stem levels.

Joints that are stiff or hypomobile and have restricted movement should be treated three to four times per week on alternating days with active motion exercise. The athletic trainer must continuously reevaluate the joint to determine appropriate progression from one oscillation grade to another.

Indications for specific mobilization grades are relatively straightforward. If the patient complains of pain before the athletic trainer can apply any resistance to movement, it is too early, and all mobilization techniques should be avoided. If pain is elicited when resistance to motion is applied, mobilization using grades I, II, and III is appropriate. If resistance can be applied before pain is elicited, mobilization can be progressed to grade IV. Mobilization should be done with both the patient and the athletic trainer positioned in a comfortable and relaxed manner. The athletic trainer should mobilize one joint at a time. The joint should be stabilized as near one articulating surface as possible, while moving the other segment with a firm, confident grasp.

Contraindications for Mobilization

Techniques of mobilization and manipulation should not be used haphazardly. These techniques should generally not be used in cases of inflammatory arthritis, malignancy, bone disease, neurological involvement, bone fracture, congenital bone deformities, and vascular disorders of the vertebral artery. Again, manipulation should be performed only by those athletic trainers specifically trained in the procedure, because some special knowledge and judgment are required for effective treatment.[24]

JOINT TRACTION TECHNIQUES

Traction refers to a technique involving pulling on one articulating segment to produce some separation of the two joint surfaces. While mobilization glides are done parallel to the treatment plane, traction is performed perpendicular to the treatment plane (see Figure 13-7). Like mobilization techniques, traction may be used either to decrease pain or to reduce joint hypomobility.[38]

Kaltenborn has proposed a system using traction combined with mobilization as a means of reducing pain or mobilizing hypomobile joints.[14] As discussed earlier, all joints have a certain amount of joint play or looseness. Kaltenborn referred to this looseness as *slack*. Some degree of slack is necessary for normal joint motion. Kaltenborn's three traction grades are defined as follows.[17] (Figure 13-8):

Grade I traction (loosen). Traction that neutralizes pressure in the joint without actual separation of the joint surfaces. The purpose is to produce pain relief by reducing the compressive forces of articular surfaces during mobilization and is used with all mobilization grades.

Grade II traction (tighten or "take up the slack"). Traction that effectively separates the articulating surfaces and takes up the slack or eliminates play in

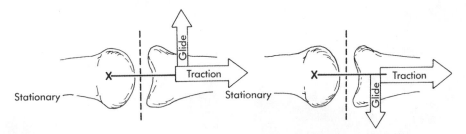

Figure 13-7   Traction vs. glides. Traction should be perpendicular to the treatment plane, while glides are parallel to the treatment plane.

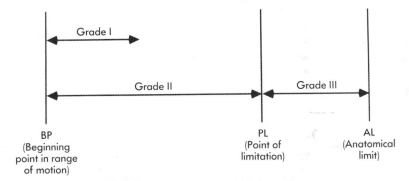

Figure 13-8   Kaltenborn's grades of traction. *PL* = point of limitation; *AL* = anatomical limit.

the joint capsule. Grade II is used in initial treatment to determine joint sensitivity.

Grade III traction (stretch). Traction that involves actual stretching of the soft tissue surrounding the joint to increase mobility in a hypomobile joint.

Grade I traction should be used in the initial treatment to reduce the chance of a painful reaction. It is recommended that 10-second intermittent grades I and II traction be used, distracting the joint surfaces up to a grade III traction and then releasing distraction until the joint returns to its resting position.[16]

Kaltenborn emphasizes that grade III traction should be used in conjunction with mobilization glides to treat joint hypomobility (Figure 13-7).[17] Grade III traction stretches the joint capsule and increases the space between the articulating surfaces, placing the joint in a loose-packed position. Applying grades III and IV oscillations within the patient's pain limitations should maximally improve joint mobility (Figure 13-9).[16]

CLINICAL DECISION MAKING   **Exercise 13–6**

A physician has diagnosed disc pathology in a field hockey player with low back pain. The disc is protruding and impinging on the spinal cord. How could traction help relieve pain for this athlete?

MOBILIZATION AND TRACTION TECHNIQUES

Figures 13-10 to 13-73 provide descriptions and illustrations of various mobilization and traction techniques. These figures should be used to determine appropriate hand positioning, stabilization (S), and the correct direction for gliding (G), traction (T), and/or rotation (R). The information presented in this chapter should be used as a reference base for appropriately incorporating joint mobilization and traction techniques into the rehabilitation program.

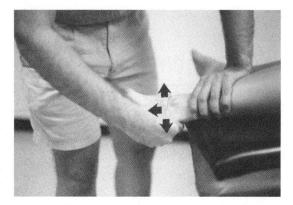

Figure 13-9 Traction and mobilization should be used together.

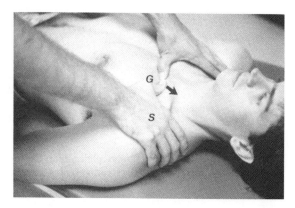

Figure 13-10 Posterior and superior clavicular glides. When posterior or superior clavicular glides are done at the sternoclavicular joint, use the thumbs to glide the clavicle. Posterior glides are used to increase clavicular retraction, and superior glides increase clavicular retraction and clavicular depression.

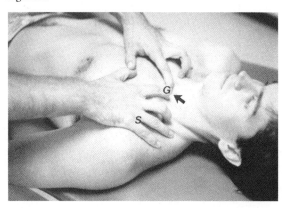

Figure 13-11 Inferior clavicular glides. Inferior clavicular glides at the sternoclavicular joint use the index fingers to mobilize the clavicle, which increases clavicular elevation.

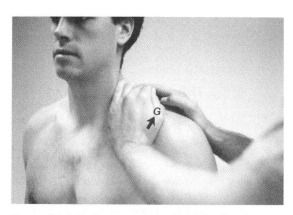

Figure 13-12 Posterior clavicular glides. Posterior clavicular glides done at the acromioclavicular (AC) joint apply posterior pressure on the clavicle while stabilizing the scapula with the opposite hand. They increase mobility of the AC joint.

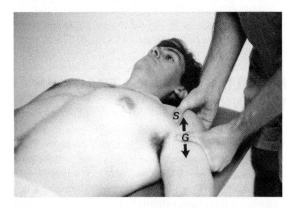

Figure 13-13 Anterior/posterior glenohumeral glides. Anterior/posterior glenohumeral glides are done with one hand stabilizing the scapula, and the other gliding the humeral head. They initiate motion in the painful shoulder.

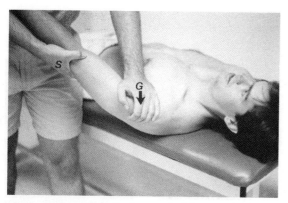

Figure 13-14   Posterior humeral glides. Posterior humeral glides use one hand to stabilize the humerus at the elbow and the other to glide the humeral head. They increase flexion and medial rotation.

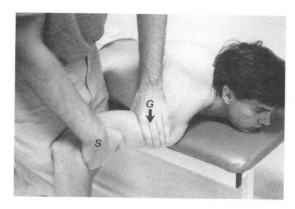

Figure 13-15   Anterior humeral glides. In anterior humeral glides the patient is prone. One hand stabilizes the humerus at the elbow, and the other glides the humeral head. They increase extension and lateral rotation.

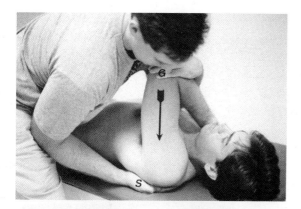

Figure 13-16   Posterior humeral glides. Posterior humeral glides may also be done with the shoulder at 90 degrees. With the patient in supine position, one hand stabilizes the scapula underneath while the patient's elbow is secured at the athletic trainer's shoulder. Glides are directed downward through the humerus. They increase horizontal adduction.

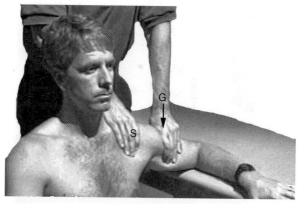

Figure 13-17   Inferior humeral glides. For inferior humeral glides the patient is in the sitting position with the elbow resting on the treatment table. One hand stabilizes the scapula, and the other glides the humeral head inferiorly. These glides increase shoulder abduction.

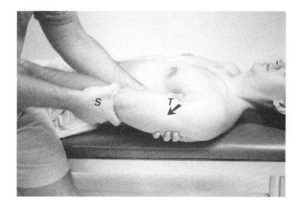

Figure 13-18 Lateral glenohumeral joint traction. Lateral glenohumeral joint traction is used for initial testing of joint mobility and for decreasing pain. One hand stabilizes the elbow while the other applies lateral traction at the upper humerus.

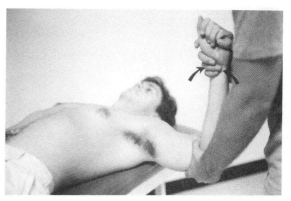

Figure 13-19 Medial and lateral rotation oscillations. Medial and lateral rotation oscillations with the shoulder abducted at 90 degrees can increase medial and lateral rotation in a progressive manner according to patient tolerance.

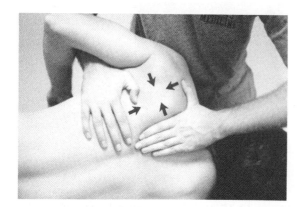

Figure 13-20 General scapular glides. General scapular glides may be done in all directions, applying pressure at either the medial, inferior, lateral, or superior border of the scapula. Scapular glides increase general scapulothoracic mobility.

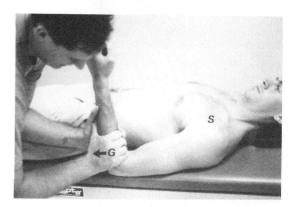

Figure 13-21 Inferior humeroulnar glides. Inferior humeroulnar glides increase elbow flexion and extension. They are performed using the body weight to stabilize proximally with the hand grasping the ulna and gliding inferiorly.

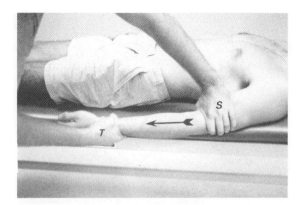

Figure 13-22   Humeroradial inferior glides. Humeroradial inferior glides increase the joint space and improve flexion and extension. One hand stabilizes the humerus above the elbow; the other grasps the distal forearm and glides the radius inferiorly.

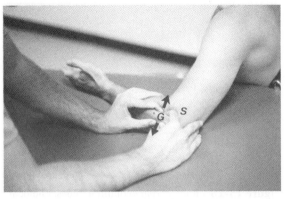

Figure 13-23   Proximal anterior/posterior radial glides. Proximal anterior/posterior radial glides use the thumbs and index fingers to glide the radial head. Anterior glides increase flexion, while posterior glides increase extension.

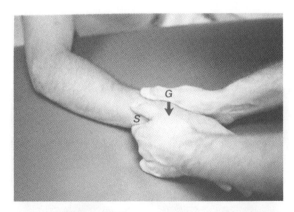

Figure 13-24   Distal anterior/posterior radial glides. Distal anterior/posterior radial glides are done with one hand stabilizing the ulna and the other gliding the radius. These glides increase pronation.

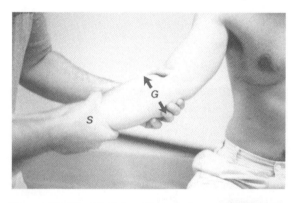

Figure 13-25   Medial and lateral ulnar oscillations. Medial and lateral ulnar oscillations increase flexion and extension. Valgus and varus forces are used with a short lever arm.

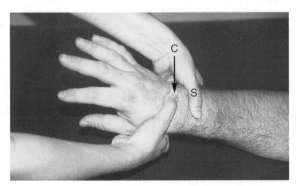

Figure 13-26   Radiocarpal joint anterior glides. Radiocarpal joint anterior glides increase wrist extension.

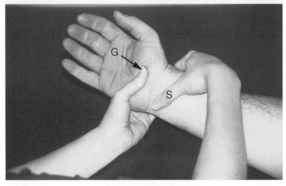

Figure 13-27   Radiocarpal joint posterior glides. Radiocarpal joint posterior glides increase wrist flexion.

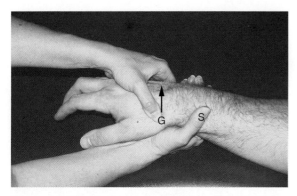

Figure 13-28 Radiocarpal joint ulnar glides. Radiocarpal joint ulnar glides increase radial deviation.

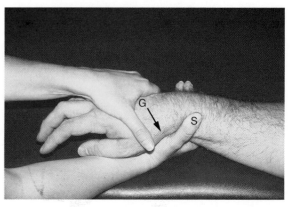

Figure 13-29 Radiocarpal joint radial glides. Radiocarpal joint radial glides increase ulnar deviation.

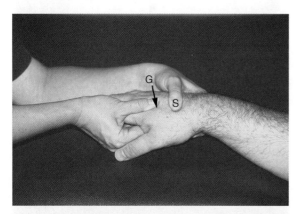

Figure 13-30 Carpometacarpal joint anterior/posterior glides. Carpometacarpal joint anterior/posterior glides increase mobility of the hand.

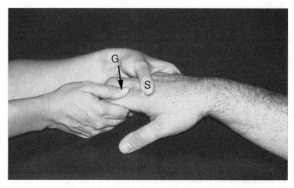

Figure 13-31 Metacarpophalangeal joint anterior/posterior glides. In metacarpophalangeal joint anterior or posterior glides, the proximal segment, in this case the metacarpal, is stabilized and the distal segment is mobilized. Anterior glides increase flexion of the MP joint. Posterior glides increase extension.

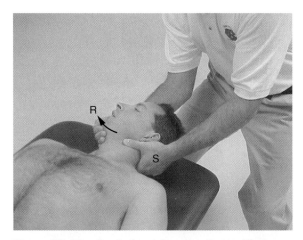

Figure 13-32   Cervical vertebrae rotation oscillations. Cervical vertebrae rotation oscillations are done with one hand supporting the weight of the head and the other rotating the head in the direction of the restriction. These oscillations treat pain or stiffness when there is some resistance in the same direction as the rotation.

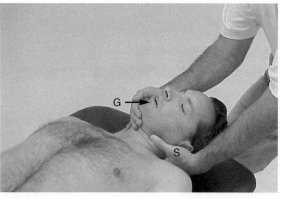

Figure 13-33   Cervical vertebrae sidebending. Cervical vertebrae sidebending may be used to treat paint or stiffness with resistance when sidebending the neck.

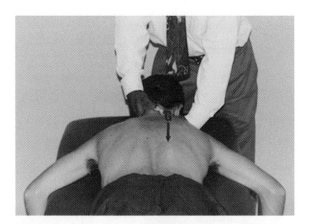

Figure 13-34   Unilateral cervical facet anterior/posterior glides. Unilateral cervical facet anterior/posterior glides are done using pressure from the thumbs over individual facets. They increase rotation or flexion of the neck toward the side where the technique is used.

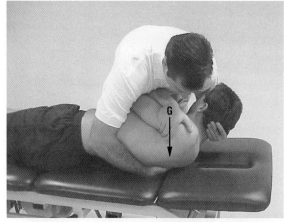

Figure 13-35   Thoracic vertebral facet rotations. Thoracic vertebral facet rotations are accomplished with one hand underneath the patient providing stabilization and the weight of the body pressing downward through the rib cage to rotate an individual thoracic vertebrae. Rotation of the thoracic vertebrae is minimal, and most of the movement with this mobilization involves the rib facet joint.

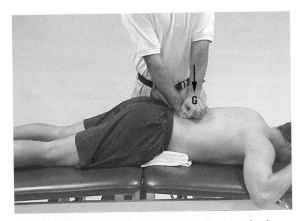

Figure 13-36 Anterior/posterior lumbar vertebral glides. In the lumbar region, anterior/posterior lumbar vertebral glides may be accomplished at individual segments using pressure on the spinous process through the pisiform in the hand. These decrease pain or increase mobility of individual lumbar vertebrae.

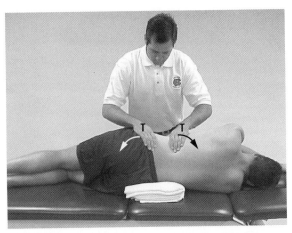

Figure 13-37 Lumbar lateral distraction. Lumbar lateral distraction increases the space between transverse processes and increases the opening of the intervertebral foramen. This position is achieved by lying over a support, flexing the athlete's upper knee to a point where there is gapping in the appropriate spinal segment, then rotating the upper trunk to place the segment in a close-packed position. Then finger and forearm pressure are used to separate individual spaces. This pressure is used for reducing pain in the lumber vertebrae associated with some compression of a spinal segment.

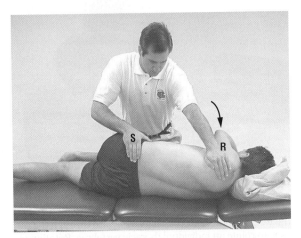

Figure 13-38 Lumbar vertebral rotations. Lumbar vertebral rotations decrease pain and increase mobility in lumbar vertebrae. These rotations should be done in a sidelying position.

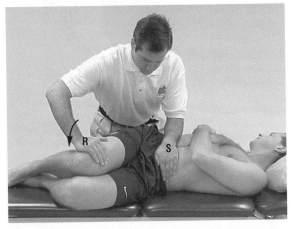

Figure 13-39 Lateral lumbar rotations. Lateral lumbar rotations may be done with the patient in supine position. In this position, one hand must stabilize the upper trunk, while the other produces rotation.

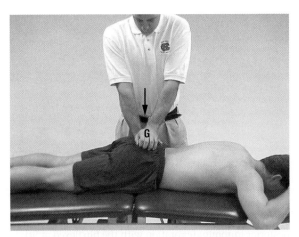

Figure 13-40   Anterior sacral glides. Anterior sacral glides decrease pain and reduce muscle guarding around the sacroiliac joint.

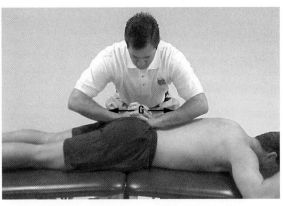

Figure 13-41   Superior/inferior sacral glides. Superior/inferior sacral glides decrease pain and reduce muscle guarding around the sacroiliac joint.

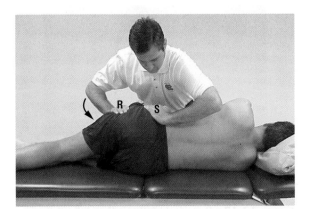

Figure 13-42   Anterior innominate rotation. An anterior innominate rotation in a sidelying position is accomplished by extending the leg on the affected side then stabilizing with one hand on the front of the thigh while the other applies pressure anteriorly over the posterosuperior iliac spine to produce an anterior rotation. This technique will correct a unilateral posterior rotation.

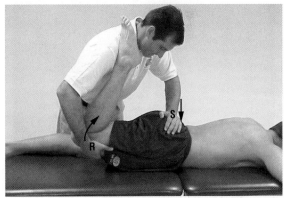

Figure 13-43   Anterior innominate rotation. An anterior innominate rotation may also be accomplished by extending the hip, applying upward force on the upper thigh, and stabilizing over the posterosuperior iliac spine. This technique is once again used to correct a posterior unilateral innominate rotation.

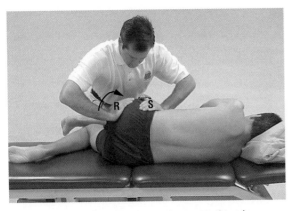

Figure 13-44 Posterior innominate rotation. A posterior innominate rotation with the patient in sidelying position is done by flexing the hip, stabilizing the antero-superior iliac spine, and applying pressure to the ischium in an anterior direction.

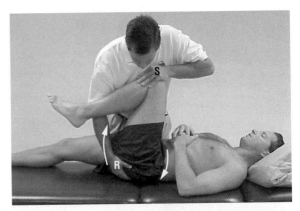

Figure 13-45 Posterior innominate rotation. Another posterior innominate rotation with the hip flexed at 90 degrees stabilizes the knee and rotates the innominate anteriorly through upward pressure on the ischium.

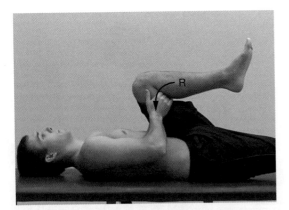

Figure 13-46 Posterior innominate rotation self-mobilization (supine). Posterior innominate rotation may be easily accomplished using self-mobilization. In a supine position the patient grasps behind the flexed knee and gently rocks the innominate in a posterior direction.

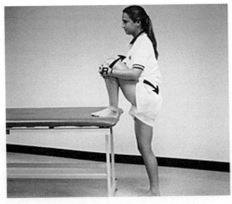

Figure 13-47 Posterior rotation self-mobilization (standing). In a standing position the patient can perform a posterior rotation self-mobilization by pulling on the knee and rocking forward.

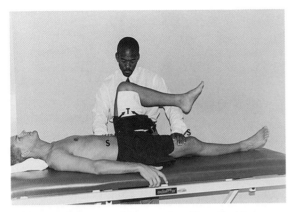

Figure 13-48   Lateral hip traction. Since the hip is a very strong, stable joint, it may be necessary to use body weight to produce effective joint mobilization or traction. An example of this would be in lateral hip traction. One strap should be used to secure the patient to the treatment table. A second strap is secured around the patient's thigh and around the therapist's hips. Lateral traction is applied to the femur by leaning back away from the patient. This technique is used to reduce pain and increase hip mobility.

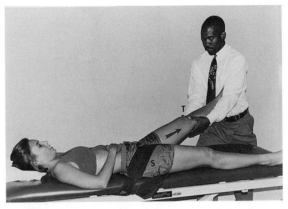

Figure 13-49   Femoral traction. Femoral traction with the hip at 0 degrees reduces pain and increases hip mobility. Inferior femoral glides in this position should be used to increase flexion and abduction.

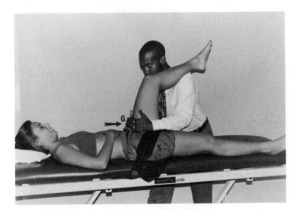

Figure 13-50   Inferior femoral glides. Inferior femoral glides at 90 degrees of hip flexion may also be used to increase abduction and flexion.

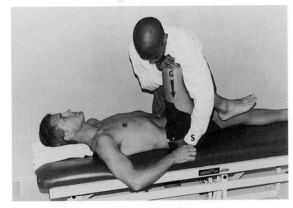

Figure 13-51   Posterior femoral glides. With the patient supine, a posterior femoral glide can be done by stabilizing underneath the pelvis and using the body weight applied through the femur to glide posteriorly. Posterior glides are used to increase hip flexion.

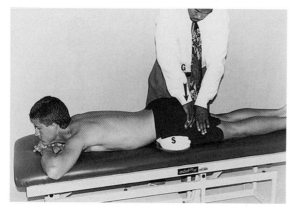

Figure 13-52 Anterior femoral glides. Anterior femoral glides increase extension and are accomplished by using some support to stabilize under the pelvis and applying an anterior glide posteriorly on the femur.

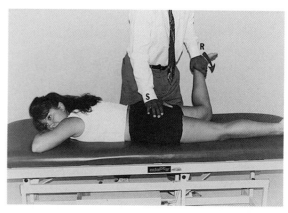

Figure 13-53 Medial femoral rotations. Medial femoral rotations may be used for increasing medial rotation and are done by stabilizing the opposite innominate while internally rotating the hip through the flexed knee.

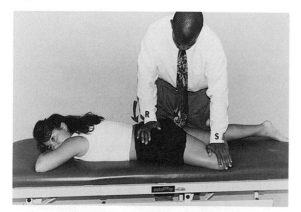

Figure 13-54 Lateral femoral rotation. Lateral femoral rotation is done by stabilizing a bent knee in the figure 4 position and applying rotational force to the ischium. This technique increases lateral femoral rotation.

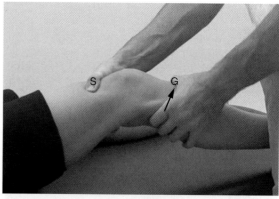

Figure 13-55 Anterior tibial glides. Anterior tibial glides are appropriate for the patient lacking full extension. Anterior glides should be done in prone position with the femur stabilized. Pressure is applied to the posterior tibia to glide anteriorly.

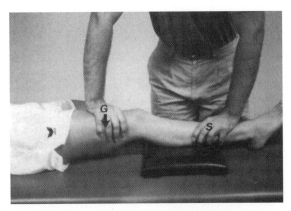

Figure 13-56 Posterior femoral glides. Posterior femoral glides are appropriate for the patient lacking full extension. Posterior femoral glides should be done in supine position with the tibia stabilized. Pressure is applied to the anterior femur to glide posteriorly.

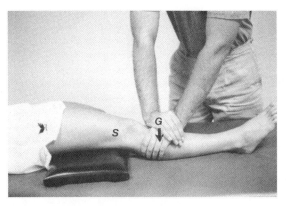

Figure 13-57 Posterior tibial glides. Posterior tibial glides increase flexion. With the patient in supine position, stabilize the femur, and glide the tibia posteriorly.

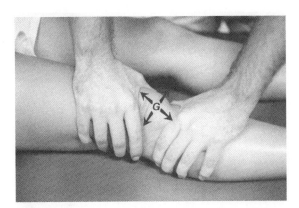

Figure 13-58 Patellar glides. Superior patellar glides increase knee extension. Inferior glides increase knee flexion. Medial glides stretch the lateral retinaculum. Lateral glides stretch tight medial structures.

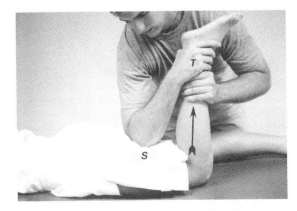

Figure 13-59 Tibiofemoral joint traction. Tibiofemoral joint traction reduces pain and hypomobility. It may be done with the patient prone and the knee flexed at 90 degrees. The elbow should stabilize the thigh while traction is applied through the tibia.

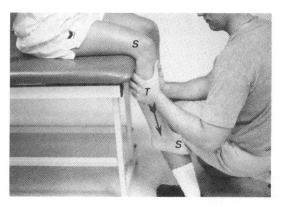

Figure 13-60 Alternative techniques for tibiofemoral joint traction. In very large individuals an alternative technique for tibiofemoral joint traction uses body weight of the athletic trainer to distract the joint once again for reducing pain and hypomobility.

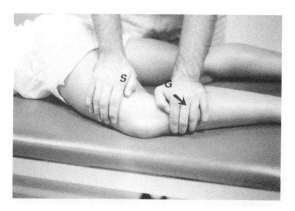

Figure 13-61 Proximal anterior and posterior glides of the fibula. Anterior and posterior glides of the fibula may be done proximally. They increase mobility of the fibular head and reduce pain. The femur should be stabilized. With the knee slightly flexed, grasp the head of the femur, and glide it anteriorly and posteriorly.

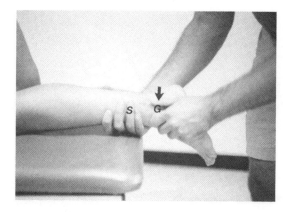

Figure 13-62 Distal anterior and posterior fibular glides. Anterior and posterior glides of the fibula may be done distally. The tibia should be stabilized, and the fibular malleolus is mobilized in an anterior or posterior direction.

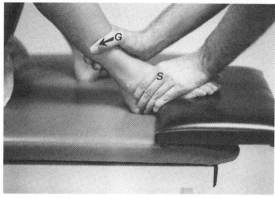

Figure 13-63 Posterior tibial glides. Posterior tibial glides increase plantarflexion. The foot should be stabilized, and pressure on the anterior tibia produces a posterior glide.

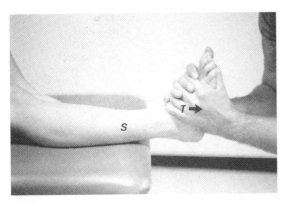

Figure 13-64 Talocrural joint traction. Talocrural joint traction is performed using the patient's body weight to stabilize the lower leg and applying traction to the midtarsal portion of the foot. Traction reduces pain and increases dorsiflexion and plantarflexion.

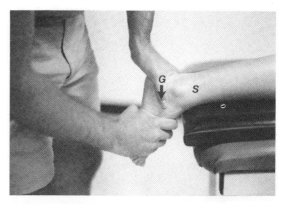

Figure 13-65 Anterior talar glides. Plantarflexion may also be increased by using an anterior talar glide. With the patient prone the tibia is stabilized on the table, and pressure is applied to the posterior aspect of the talus to glide it anteriorly.

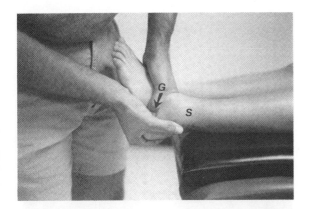

Figure 13-66 Posterior talar glides. Posterior talar glides may be used for increasing dorsiflexion. With the patient supine the tibia is stabilized on the table, and pressure is applied to the anterior aspect of the talus to glide it posteriorly.

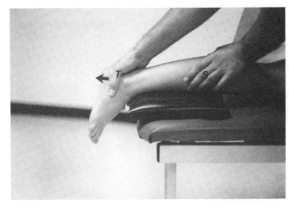

Figure 13-67 Subtalar joint traction. Subtalar joint traction reduces pain and increases inversion and eversion. The lower leg is stabilized on the table, and traction is applied by grasping the posterior aspect of the calcaneus.

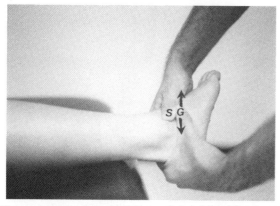

Figure 13-68 Subtalar joint medial and lateral glides. Subtalar joint medial and lateral glides increase eversion and inversion. The talus must be stabilized while the calcaneus is mobilized medially to increase inversion and laterally to increase eversion.

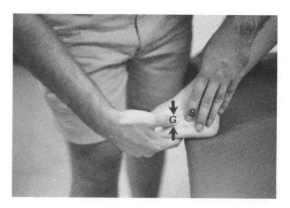

Figure 13-69 Anterior/posterior calcaneocuboid glides. Anterior/posterior calcaneocuboid glides may be used for increasing adduction and abduction. The calcaneus should be stabilized while the cuboid is mobilized.

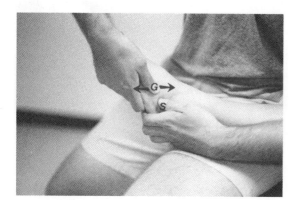

Figure 13-70 Anterior/posterior cuboidmetatarsal glides. Anterior/posterior cuboidmetatarsal glides are done with one hand stabilizing the cuboid and the other gliding the base of the fifth metatarsal. They are used for increasing mobility of the fifth metatarsal.

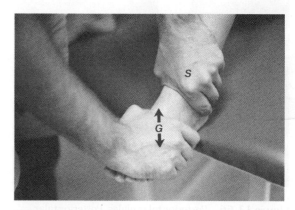

Figure 13-71 Anterior/posterior carpometacarpal glides. Anterior/posterior carpometacarpal glides decrease hypomobility of the metacarpals.

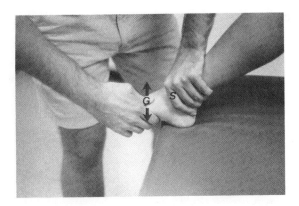

Figure 13-72   Anterior/posterior talonavicular glides. Anterior/posterior talonavicular glides also increase adduction and abduction. One hand stabilizes the talus while the other mobilizes the navicular bone.

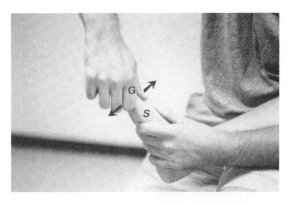

Figure 13-73   Anterior/posterior metacarpophalangeal glides. With anterior/posterior metacarpophalangeal glides, the anterior glides increase extension, and posterior glides increase flexion. Mobilizations are accomplished by isolating individual segments.

MULLIGAN JOINT MOBILIZATION TECHNIQUE

Brian Mulligan, an Australian physioathletic trainer proposed a concept of mobilizations based on Kaltenborn's principles. While Kaltenborn's technique relies on passive accessory mobilization, the Mulligan technique combines passive accessory joint mobilization applied by a athletic trainer with active physiological movement by the patient for the purpose of correcting positional faults and returning the patient to normal pain-free function.[27] It is a noninvasive and comfortable intervention, and has applications for the spine and the extremities. Mulligan's concept uses what are referred to as either *mobilizations with movement* (MWMs) for treating the extremities, or *sustained natural apophyseal glides* (SNAGs) for treating problems in the spine.[36] Instead of the athletic trainer using oscillations or thrusting techniques, the patient moves in a specific direction as the athletic trainer guides the restricted body part. MWMs and SNAGs have the potential to quickly restore functional movements in joints, even after many years of restriction.[27]

Principles of Treatment

A basic premise of the Mulligan technique for an athletic trainer choosing to make use of MWMs in the extremities or SNAGs in the spine is to never cause pain to the patient.[10] During assessment the athletic trainer should look for specific signs, which may include a loss of joint movement, pain associated with movement, or pain associated with

specific functional activities.[13] A passive accessory joint mobilization is applied following the principles of Kaltenborn discussed earlier in this chapter (i.e., parallel or perpendicular to the joint plane). The athletic trainer must continuously monitor the patient's reaction to ensure that no pain is recreated during this mobilization. The athletic trainer experiments with various combinations of parallel or perpendicular glides until the appropriate treatment plane and grade of movement are discovered, which together significantly improve range of motion, and/or significantly decrease or, better yet, eliminate altogether the original pain. Failure to improve range of motion or decrease pain indicates that the athletic trainer has not found the correct contact point, treatment plane, grade, or direction of mobilization. The patient then actively repeats the restricted and/or painful motion or activity while the athletic trainer continues to maintain the appropriate accessory glide. Further increases in range of motion or decreases in pain may be expected during a treatment session that typically involves three sets of 10 repetitions. Additional gains may be realized through the application of pain-free, passive overpressure at the end of available range.[20]

An example of MWM might be in a patient with restricted ankle dorsiflexion (Figure 13-74A). The patient is standing on a treatment table with the athletic trainer manually stabilizing the foot. A nonelastic belt passes around both the distal leg of the patient and the waist of the athletic trainer who applies a sustained anterior glide of the tibia by leaning backward away from the patient. The patient then performs a slow dorsiflexion movement

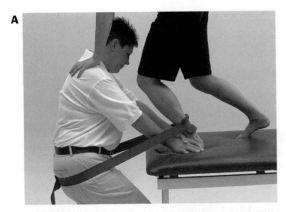

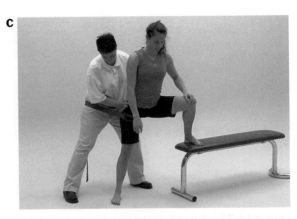

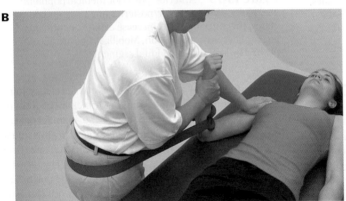

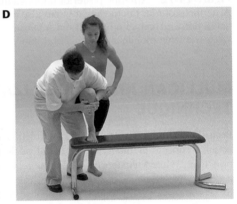

Figure 13-74   Mulligan Techniques **A,** Technique for increasing dorsiflexion. **B,** Treating elbow lateral epicondylitis. **C,** Technique for restricted hip abduction. **D,** Treating painful knee flexion.

until the first onset of pain or end of range. Once this end point is reached, the position is sustained for 10 seconds. The patient then relaxes and returns to the standing position followed by release of the anteroposterior glide, and then followed by a 20-second rest period. [27] Figure 13-74B, C, and D show several additional Mulligan techniques.

Summary

1. Mobilization and traction techniques increase joint mobility or decrease pain by restoring accessory movements to the joint.
2. Physiological movements result from an active muscle contraction that moves an extremity through traditional cardinal planes.
3. Accessory motions refer to the manner in which one articulating joint surface moves relative to another.
4. Normal accessory component motions must occur for full-range physiological movement to take place.
5. Accessory motions are also referred to as joint arthrokinematics, and include spin, roll, and glide.
6. The convex-concave rule states that if the concave joint surface is moving on the stationary convex surface, gliding will occur in the same direction as the rolling motion. Conversely, if the convex surface is

moving on a stationary concave surface, gliding will occur in an opposite direction to rolling.

7. The resting position is one in which the joint capsule and the ligaments are most relaxed, allowing for a maximum amount of joint play.

8. The treatment plane falls perpendicular to a line running from the axis of rotation in the convex surface to the center of the concave articular surface.

9. Maitland has proposed a series of five graded movements or oscillations in the range of motion to treat pain and stiffness.

10. Kaltenborn uses three grades of traction to reduce pain and stiffness.

11. Kaltenborn emphasizes that traction should be used in conjunction with mobilization glides to treat joint hypomobility.

12. Mulligan's technique combines passive accessory movement with active physiological movement to improve range of motion or to minimize pain.

References

1. Barak, T., E. Rosen, and R. Sofer. 1990. Mobility: Passive orthopedic manual therapy. In *Orthopedic and Sports Physical Therapy*, Gould, J. and G. Davies, eds. St. Louis, MO: Mosby.

2. Basmajian, J., and S. Banerjee. 1996. *Clinical decision making in rehabilitation: Efficacy and outcomes*. Philadelphia: Churchill-Livingstone.

3. Boissonnault, W., J. Bryan, and K.S. Fox. 2004. Joint manipulation curricula in physical therapist professional degree programs. *J Orthop Sports Phys Ther* 34(4):171–181.

4. Conroy, D.E., and K.W. Hayes. 1998. The effect of joint mobilization as a component of comprehensive treatment for primary shoulder impingement syndrome. *J Orthop Sports Phys Ther* 28(1):3–14.

5. Cookson, J. 1979. Orthopedic manual therapy: An overview, II. The spine. *J Am Phys Ther Assoc* 59:259.

6. Cookson, J., and B. Kent. 1979. Orthopedic manual therapy: An overview, I. The extremities. *J Am Phys Ther Assoc* 59:136.

7. Cyriax, J. 1996. *Cyriax's illustrated manual of orthopaedic medicine*. London: Butterworth.

8. Donatelli, R., and H. Owens-Burkhart. 1981. Effects of immobilization on the extensibility of periarticular connective tissue. *J Orthop Sports Phys Ther* 3:67.

9. Edmond, S. 2006. *Joint mobilization and manipulation: Extremity and spinal techniques*. Philadelphia: Elsevier Health Sciences.

10. Exelby, L. 2002. The Mulligan concept: Its application in the management of spinal conditions. *Man Ther* 7(2):64–70.

11. Green, T., K. Refshauge, J. Crosbie, and R. Adams. 2001. A randomized controlled trial of a passive accessory joint mobilization on acute ankle inversion sprains. *Phys Ther* 81(4):984–994.

12. Grimsby, O. 1981. *Fundamentals of manual therapy: A course workbook*. Vagsbygd, Norway: Sorlandets Fysikalske Institutt.

13. Hall, T. 2001. Effects of the Mulligan traction straight leg raise technique on range of movement. *J Man Manipulative Ther* 9(3):128–133.

14. Hollis, M. 1999. *Practical exercise*. Oxford: Blackwell Scientific.

15. Hsu, A.T., L. Ho, J.H. Chang, G.L. Chang, and T. Hedman. 2002. Characterization of tissue resistance during a dorsally directed translational mobilization of the glenohumeral joint. *Arch Phys Med Rehabil* 83(3):360–366.

16. Kaltenborn, F. 2003. *Manual mobilization of the joints, Vol. II: The spine*. Minneapolis, MN: Orthopedic Physical Therapy Products.

17. Kaltenborn, F., D. Morgan, and O. Evjenth. 2002. *Manual mobilization of the joints, Vol. I: The extremities*. Minneapolis, MN: Orthopedic Physical Therapy Products.

18. Kaminski, T., L. Kahanov, and M. Kato. 2007. Therapeutic effect of joint mobilization: Joint mechanoreceptors and nociceptors. *Athletic Therapy Today* 12(4):28.

19. Kisner, C., and L. Colby. 2007. *Therapeutic exercise: Foundations and techniques*. Philadelphia: FA Davis.

20. MacConaill, M., and J. Basmajian. 1977. *Muscles and movements: A basis for kinesiology*. Baltimore: Williams & Wilkins.

21. Maigne, R. 1976. *Orthopedic medicine*. Springfield, IL: Charles C Thomas.

22. Macintyre, J. 2002. Passive joint mobilization for acute ankle inversion sprains. *Clin J Sport Med* 12(1):54.

23. Maitland, G. 1991. *Extremity manipulation*. London, Butterworth.

24. Maitland, G. 2005. *Vertebral manipulation*. Philadelphia: Elsevier Health Science.

25. Mangus, B., L. Hoffman, and M. Hoffman. 2002. Basic principles of extremity joint mobilization using a Kaltenborn approach. *J Sport Rehabil* 11(4):235–250.

26. Mennell, J. 1991. *The musculoskeletal system: Differential diagnosis from symptoms and physical signs*. New York: Aspen.

27. Mulligan's Concept available at: http://www.bmulligan.com/about/concept.htm.

28. Paris, S. 1979. *The spine: Course notebook*. Atlanta: Institute Press.

29. Paris, S. 1979. Mobilization of the spine. *Phys Ther* 59:988.

30. Saunders, D. 2004. *Evaluation, treatment and prevention of musculoskeletal disorders*. Saunder Group Inc.

31. Schiotz, E., and J. Cyriax. 1978. *Manipulation past and present*. London: Heinemann.

32. Stevenson, J., and D. Vaughn. 2003. Four cardinal principles of joint mobilization and joint play assessment. *Journal of Manual & Manipulative Therapy* 11(3):146.

33. Stone, J.A. 1998. Joint mobilization. *Athlet Ther Today* 4(6):59–60.

34. Teys, P. 2008. The initial effects of a Mulligan's mobilization with movement technique on range of movement and pressure pain threshold in pain-limited shoulders. *Manual Therapy* 13(1):37.

35. Wadsworth, C. 1998. *Manual examination and treatment of the spine and extremities.* Baltimore: William & Wilkins.

36. Wilson, E. 2001. The Mulligan concept: NAGS, SNAGS and mobilizations with movement. *J Bodywork Mov Ther* 5(2):81–89.

37. Zohn, D., and J. Mennell. 1987. *Musculoskeletal pain: Diagnosis and physical treatment.* Boston: Little, Brown and Company.

38. Zusman, M. 1985. Reappraisal of a proposed neurophysiological mechanism for the relief of joint pain with passive joint movements. *Physiother Pract* 1:61–70.

Clinical Studies In The Literature

Bukowski, E. 1991. Assessing joint mobility. *Clin Manage* 11:48–56.

Cibulka, M., S. Rose, and A. Delitto. 1986. Hamstring muscle strain treated by mobilizing the sacroiliac joint. *Phys Ther* 66:1220–1223.

Cleland, J. 2006. Immediate effects of thoracic manipulation in patients with neck pain: a randomized clinical trial. *Manual Therapy* 10(2):127–135.

Cochrane, C. 1987. Joint mobilization principles: Considerations for use in the child with central nervous system dysfunction. *Phys Ther* 67:1105–1109.

Collins, N. 2004. The initial effects of a Mulligan's mobilization with movement technique on dorsiflexion and pain in subacute ankle sprains. *Manual Therapy* 9(2):77–82.

Don Tigny, R. 1990. Measuring PSIS movement. *Clin Manage* 10:43–44.

Eiff, M., A. Smith, and G. Smith. 1994. Early mobilization versus immobilization in the treatment of lateral ankle sprains. *Am J Sports Med* 22:83–88.

Gibson, H., J. Ross, and J. Allen. 1993. The effect of mobilization on forward bending range. *J Man Manipulative Ther* 1:142–147.

Gratton, P. 1993. Early active mobilization after flexor tendon repairs. *J Hand Ther* 6:285–289.

Hall, T. 2006. Mulligan bent leg raise technique—preliminary randomized trial of immediate effects after a single intervention. *Manual Therapy* 11(2):130–135.

Hall, T. 2006. Mulligan traction straight leg raise: A pilot study to investigate effects on range of motion in patients with low back pain. *Journal of Manual & Manipulative Therapy* 14(2):95.

Hanrahan, S., B. Van Lunen, and M. Tamburello. 2005. The short-term effects of joint mobilizations on acute mechanical low back dysfunction in collegiate athletes. *Journal of Athletic Training* 40(2):88.

Harding, L., M. Barbe, and K. Shepard. 2003. Posterior-anterior glide of the femoral head in the acetabulum: A cadaver study. *Journal of Orthopaedic & Sports Physical Therapy* 33(3):118–125.

Harris S., and B. Lundgren. 1991. Joint mobilization for children with central nervous system disorders: Indications and precautions. *Phys Ther* 71:890–896.

Johnson, A., J. Godges, and G. Zimmerman. 2007. The effect of anterior versus posterior glide joint mobilization on external rotation range of motion in patients with shoulder adhesive capsulitis. *Journal of Orthopaedic & Sports Physical Therapy* 37(3):88.

Konin, J. 2006. Joint mobilization to decrease glenohumeral-joint impingement. *Athletic Therapy Today* 11(3):50.

Landrum, E., B. Kelly, and W. Parente. 2008. Immediate effects of anterior-to-posterior talocrural joint mobilization after prolonged ankle immobilization: A preliminary study. *Journal of Manual & Manipulative Therapy* 16(2):100.

Lee, M., J. Latimer, and C. Maher. 1993. Manipulation: Investigation of a proposed mechanism. *Clin Biomech* 8:302–306.

Lee, R., and J. Evans. 1994. Towards a better understanding of spinal posteroanterior mobilisation. *Physiotherapy* 80:68–73.

Levin, S. 1993. Early mobilization speeds recovery. *Phys Sports Med* 21:70–74.

Macintyre, J. 2002. Passive joint mobilization for acute ankle inversion sprains. *Clinical Journal of Sport Medicine* 12(1):54.

Maitland, G. 1983. Treatment of the glenohumeral joint by passive movement. *Physiotherapy* 69:3–7.

Makofsky, H., and J. Abbruzzese. 2007. Immediate effect of grade IV inferior hip joint mobilization on hip abductor torque: A pilot study. *Journal of Manual & Manipulative Therapy* 15(2):103.

May, E. 1994. Controlled mobilization after flexor tendon repair in the hand: Techniques, methods and results. *Aust Occup Ther J* 41:143.

McCollam, R., and C. Benson. 1993. Effects of postero-anterior mobilization on lumbar extension and flexion. *J Man Manipulative Ther* 1:134–141.

McNair, P., and P. Portero. 2007. Acute neck pain: Cervical spine range of motion and position sense prior to and after joint mobilization. *Manual Therapy* 12(4):390.

Moss, P., and K. Sluka. 2007. The initial effects of knee joint mobilization on osteoarthritic hyperalgesia. *Manual Therapy* 12(2):109.

Moulson, A. 2006. A preliminary investigation into the relationship between cervical snags and sympathetic nervous system activity in the upper limbs of an asymptomatic population. *Manual Therapy* 11(3):214–224.

Mulligan, B. 1992. Extremity joint mobilisations combined with movements. *NZJPhysiother* 20:28–29.

Mulligan, B. 1993. Mobilisations with movement (MWM's). *J Man Manipulative Ther* 1:154–156.

Muraki, T. 2007. Strain on the repaired supraspinatus tendon during manual traction and translational glide mobilization on the glenohumeral joint: A cadaveric biomechanics study. *Manual Therapy* 12(3):231.

Nield, S., K. Davis, and J. Latimer. 1993. The effect of manipulation on the range of movement at the ankle joint. *Scand J Rehabil Med* 25:161–166.

Oates, D., and D. Draper. 2006. Restoring wrist range of motion using ultrasound and mobilization: A case study. *Athletic Therapy Today* 11(1):45.

Ottenbacher, K., and R. Difabio. 1985. Efficacy of spinal manipulation/mobilization therapy: A meta-analysis. *Spine* 10:833–837.

Petersen, P., S. Sites, and I. Grossman. 1992. Clinical evidence for the utilisation and efficacy of upper extremity mobilisation. *Br J Occup Ther* 55:112–116.

Prentice, W. 1992. Techniques of manual therapy for the knee. *J Sport Rehabil* 1:249–257.

Quillen, W., J. Halle, and L. Rouillier. 1992. Manual therapy: Mobilization of the motion-restricted shoulder. *J Sport Rehabil* 1:237–248.

Randall, T., L. Portney, and B. Harris. 1992. Effects of joint mobilization on joint stiffness and active motion of the metacarpalphalangeal joint. *J Orthop Sports Phys Ther* 16:30–36.

Schoensee, S., G. Jensen, and G. Nicholson. 1995. The effect of mobilization on cervical headaches. *J Orthop Sports Phys Ther* 21:184–196.

Smith, R., B. Sebastian, and R. Gajdosik. 1988. Effect of sacroiliac joint mobilization on the standing position of the pelvis in healthy men. *J Orthop Sports Phys Ther* 10:77–84.

Stuberg, W. 1993. Manual therapy in pediatrics: Some considerations. *PT—Mag Phys Ther* 1:54–56.

Taylor, N., and K. Bennell. 1994. The effectiveness of passive joint mobilisation on the return of active wrist extension following Colles' fracture: A clinical trial. *NZJ Physiother* 22:24–28.

Vicenzino, B. 2007. Mulligan's mobilization-with-movement, positional faults and pain relief: Current concepts from a critical review of literature. *Manual Therapy* 12(2):98.

Wilson, F. 1991. Manual therapy versus traditional exercises in mobilisation of the ankle post-ankle fracture: A pilot study. *NZJ Physiother* 19:11–16.

Wise, P. 1994. Mobilisation technique improves neural mobility. *Aust J Physiother* 40:51–54.

Yerys, S. 2002. Effect of mobilization of the anterior hip capsule on gluteus maximus strength. *Journal of Manual & Manipulative Therapy* 10(4):218.

Zito, M. 1996. Joint mobilization: Stretch specificity using a distraction. *J Orthop Sports Phys Ther* 23:65.

SOLUTIONS TO CLINICAL DECISION MAKING EXERCISES

13-1 Once the patient has progressed through the acute stage, exercises and active and passive stretching can be accompanied by joint mobilizations. Mobilization of the knee joint involves gliding the concave tibia anteriorly on the femur.

13-2 In addition to exercises and possibly friction massage, she would benefit from joint mobilization to break down the scar tissue. If plantar flexion is limited, the talus should be glided anteriorly to stretch the anterior capsule. To address her ankle instability she can be provided with a brace, taping, and exercises to increase stability. Exercises should also target the muscles responsible for ankle inversion and eversion.

13-3 If the patient is restricted in extension, and lateral rotation due to tightness in the anterior capsule is causing the restriction, then the humeral head should be glided anteriorly on the glenoid to stretch the restriction.

13-4 Most manipulations performed by a chiropractor are grade V. They take the joint to the end range of motion and then apply a quick, small-amplitude thrust that forces the joint just beyond the point of limitation. Grade V manipulations should be performed only by those specifically trained in this technique. Laws and practice acts relative to the use of manipulations vary considerably from state to state.

13-5 Grade IV mobilization can be used. The talus should be forced anteriorly until movement is restricted. Small-amplitude movements are then made at this end range causing structural changes in the scar tissue.

13-6 Traction applied to the spine increases space in between the vertebrae. The increased space reduces the pressure and compressive forces on the disc.

CHAPTER 14

Proprioceptive Neuromuscular Facilitation Techniques in Rehabilitation

William E. Prentice

After completing this chapter, the athletic training student should be able to do the following:

- Explain the neurophysiologic basis of proprioceptive neuromuscular facilitation (PNF) techniques.

- Discuss the rationale for use of PNF techniques.

- Identify the basic principles of using PNF in rehabilitation.

- Demonstrate the various PNF strengthening and stretching techniques.

- Describe PNF patterns for the upper and lower extremity, for the upper and lower trunk, and for the neck.

- Discuss the concept of muscle energy technique and explain how it is similar to PNF.

Proprioceptive neuromuscular facilitation (PNF) is an approach to therapeutic exercise based on the principles of functional human anatomy and neurophysiology.[10] It uses proprioceptive, cutaneous, and auditory input to produce functional improvement in motor output and can be a vital element in the rehabilitation process of many conditions and injuries.

The therapeutic techniques of PNF were first used in the treatment of patients with paralysis and various neuromuscular disorders in the 1950s. Originally the PNF techniques were used for strengthening and enhancing neuromuscular control. Since the early 1970s, the PNF techniques have also been used extensively as a technique for increasing flexibility and range of motion.[8,9,16,17,18,30,34,36,45,54,67,71]

This discussion should guide the athletic trainer using the principles and techniques of PNF as a component of a rehabilitation program.

PNF AS A TECHNIQUE FOR IMPROVING STRENGTH AND ENHANCING NEUROMUSCULAR CONTROL

Original Concepts of Facilitation and Inhibition

Most of the principles underlying modern therapeutic exercise techniques can be attributed to the work of Sherrington,[63] who first defined the concepts of facilitation and inhibition.

According to Sherrington, an impulse traveling down the corticospinal tract or an afferent impulse traveling up from peripheral receptors in the muscle causes an impulse volley, that results in the discharge of a limited number of specific motor neurons, as well as the discharge of additional surrounding (anatomically close) motor neurons in the subliminal fringe area. An impulse causing the recruitment and discharge of additional motor neurons within the subliminal fringe is said to be facilitatory. Any stimulus that causes motor neurons to drop out of the discharge zone and away from the subliminal fringe is said to be inhibitory.[40] Facilitation results in increased excitability, and inhibition results in decreased excitability of motor neurons.[75] Thus the function of weak muscles would be aided by facilitation, and muscle spasticity would be decreased by inhibition.[26]

Sherrington attributed the impulses transmitted from the peripheral stretch receptors via the afferent system as being the strongest influence on the alpha motor neurons.[63] Therefore, the athletic trainer should be able to modify the input from the peripheral receptors and thus influence the excitability of the alpha motor neurons. The discharge of motor neurons can be facilitated by peripheral stimulation, which causes afferent impulses to make contact with excitatory neurons and results in increased muscle tone or strength of voluntary contraction. Motor neurons can also be inhibited by peripheral stimulation, which causes afferent impulses to make contact with inhibitory neurons, resulting in muscle relaxation and allowing for stretching of the muscle.[63] To indicate any technique in which input from peripheral receptors is used to facilitate or inhibit, PNF should be used.[26]

Several different approaches to therapeutic exercise based on the principles of facilitation and inhibition have been proposed. Among these are the Bobath method,[5] Brunnstrom method,[60] Rood method,[58] and the Knott and Voss method,[37] which they called PNF. Although each of these techniques is important and useful, the PNF approach of Knott and Voss probably makes the most explicit use of proprioceptive stimulation.[37]

Rationale for Use

As a positive approach to injury rehabilitation, PNF is aimed at what the patient can do physically within the limitations of the injury. It is perhaps best used to decrease deficiencies in strength, flexibility, and neuromuscular coordination in response to demands that are placed on the neuromuscular system.[39] The emphasis is on selective reeducation of individual motor elements through development of neuromuscular control, joint stability, and coordinated mobility. Each movement is learned and then

reinforced through repetition in an appropriately demanding and intense rehabilitative program.[59]

The body tends to respond to the demands placed on it. The principles of PNF attempt to provide a maximal response for increasing strength and neuromuscular control. These principles should be applied with consideration of their appropriateness in achieving a particular goal. It is well accepted that the continued activity during a rehabilitation program is essential for maintaining or improving strength. Therefore an intense program should offer the greatest potential for recovery.[53]

The PNF approach is holistic, integrating sensory, motor, and psychological aspects of a rehabilitation program. It incorporates reflex activities from the spinal levels and upward, either inhibiting or facilitating them as appropriate.

The brain recognizes only gross joint movement and not individual muscle action. Moreover, the strength of a muscle contraction is directly proportional to the activated motor units. Therefore, to increase the strength of a muscle, the maximum number of motor units must be stimulated to strengthen the remaining muscle fibers.[30,37] This "irradiation," or overflow effect, can occur when the stronger muscle groups help the weaker groups in completing a particular movement. This cooperation leads to the rehabilitation goal of return to optimal function.[4,37] The principles of PNF, as discussed in the next section, should be applied to reach that ultimate goal.

CLINICAL DECISION MAKING	Exercise 14–1

A breaststroker is having trouble regaining strength after recovering from a hamstring strain. What can the athletic trainer do to help her?

BASIC PRINCIPLES OF PNF

Margret Knott, in her text on PNF,[37] emphasized the importance of the principles rather than specific techniques in a rehabilitation program. These principles are the basis of PNF that must be superimposed on any specific technique. The principles of PNF are based on sound neurophysiological and kinesiologic principles and clinical experience.[59] Application of the following principles can help promote a desired response in the patient being treated.

1. The patient must be taught the PNF patterns regarding the sequential movements from starting position to terminal position. The athletic trainer has to keep instructions brief and simple. It is sometimes helpful

for the athletic trainer to passively move the patient through the desired movement pattern to demonstrate precisely what is to be done. The patterns should be used along with the techniques to increase the effects of the treatment.

2. When learning the patterns, the patient is often helped by looking at the moving limb. This visual stimulus offers the patient feedback for directional and positional control.

3. Verbal cues are used to coordinate voluntary effort with reflex responses. Commands should be firm and simple. Commands most commonly used with PNF techniques are "Push" and "Pull," which ask for an isotonic contraction; "Hold," which asks for an isometric or stabilizing contraction; and "Relax."

4. Manual contact with appropriate pressure is essential for influencing direction of motion and facilitating a maximal response, because reflex responses are greatly affected by pressure receptors. Manual contact should be firm and confident to give the patient a feeling of security. The manner in which the athletic trainer touches the patient influences their confidence as well as the appropriateness of the motor response or relaxation.[59] A movement response may be facilitated by the hand over the muscle being contracted to facilitate a movement or a stabilizing contraction.

5. Proper mechanics and body positioning of the athletic trainer are essential in applying pressure and resistance. The athletic trainer should stand in a position that is in line with the direction of movement in the diagonal movement pattern. The knees should be bent and close to the patient such that the direction of resistance can easily be applied or altered appropriately throughout the range.

6. The amount of resistance given should facilitate a maximal response that allows smooth, coordinated motion. The appropriate resistance depends to a large extent on the capabilities of the patient. It may also change at different points throughout the range of motion. Maximal resistance may be applied with techniques that use isometric contractions to restrict motion to a specific point; it may also be used in isotonic contractions throughout a full range of movement.

7. Rotational movement is a critical component in all of the PNF patterns because maximal contraction is impossible without it.

8. Normal timing is the sequence of muscle contraction that occurs in any normal motor activity resulting in coordinated movement.[37] The distal movements of the patterns should occur first. The distal movement

components should be completed no later than halfway through the total PNF pattern. To accomplish this, appropriate verbal commands should be timed with manual commands. Normal timing may be used with maximal resistance or without resistance from the athletic trainer.

9. Timing for emphasis is used primarily with isotonic contractions. This principle superimposes maximal resistance, at specific points in the range, upon the patterns of facilitation, allowing overflow or irradiation to the weaker components of a movement pattern. The stronger components are emphasized to facilitate the weaker components of a movement pattern.

10. Specific joints may be facilitated by using traction or approximation. Traction spreads apart the joint articulations, and approximation presses them together. Both techniques stimulate the joint proprioceptors. Traction increases the muscular response, promotes movement, assists isotonic contractions, and is used with most flexion antigravity movements. Traction must be maintained throughout the pattern. Approximation increases the muscular response, promotes stability, assists isometric contractions, and is used most with extension (gravity-assisted) movements. Approximation may be quick or gradual and repeated during a pattern.

11. Giving a quick stretch to the muscle before muscle contraction facilitates a muscle to respond with greater force through the mechanisms of the stretch reflex. It is most effective if all the components of a movement are stretched simultaneously. However, this quick stretch can be contraindicated in many orthopedic conditions because the extensibility limits of a damaged musculotendinous unit or joint structure might be exceeded, exacerbating the injury.

CLINICAL DECISION MAKING　　　　Exercise 14–2

A baseball player has had shoulder surgery to correct an anterior instability. He is having difficulty regaining strength throughout a full range of movement following the surgery. How can PNF strengthening be beneficial to someone who has a loss of ROM due to pain?

BASIC STRENGTHENING TECHNIQUES

Each of the principles described in the previous section should be applied to the specific techniques of PNF. These techniques may be used in a rehabilitation program to strengthen or facilitate a particular agonistic muscle group.[29,43,44] The choice of a specific technique depends on the deficits of a particular patient.[56] Specific techniques or combinations of techniques should be selected on the basis of the patient's problem.[3]

CLINICAL DECISION MAKING Exercise 14–3

Weakness following immobilization because of a radial fracture leaves a fencer with weak wrist musculature. She is having trouble initiating wrist extension. What PNF technique might the athletic trainer employ to increase strength?

The following techniques are most appropriately used for the development of muscular strength and endurance, as well as for reestablishing neuromuscular control.

Rhythmic initiation. The rhythmic initiation technique involves a progression of initial passive, then active-assistive, followed by active movement against resistance through the agonist pattern. Movement is slow, goes through the available range of motion, and avoids activation of a quick stretch. It is used for patients who are unable to initiate movement and who have a limited range of motion because of increased tone. It may also be used to teach the patient a movement pattern.

Repeated contraction. Repeated contraction is useful when a patient has weakness either at a specific point or throughout the entire range. It is used to correct imbalances that occur within the range by repeating the weakest portion of the total range. The patient moves isotonically against maximal resistance repeatedly until fatigue is evidenced in the weaker components of the motion. When fatigue of the weak components becomes apparent, a stretch at that point in the range should facilitate the weaker muscles and result in a smoother, more coordinated motion. Again, quick stretch may be contraindicated with some musculoskeletal injuries. The amount of resistance to motion given by the athletic trainer should be modified to accommodate the strength of the muscle group. The patient is commanded to push by using the agonist concentrically and eccentrically throughout the range.

Slow reversal. Slow reversal involves an isotonic contraction of the agonist followed immediately by an isotonic contraction of the antagonist. The initial contraction of the agonist muscle group facilitates the succeeding contraction of the antagonist muscles. The slow-reversal technique can be used for developing active range of motion of the agonists and normal reciprocal timing between the antagonists and agonists, which is critical for normal coordinated motion.[55] The patient should be commanded to push against maximal resistance by using the antagonist and then to pull by using the agonist. The initial agonistic push facilitates the succeeding antagonist contraction.

Slow-reversal-hold. Slow-reversal-hold is an isotonic contraction of the agonist followed immediately by an isometric contraction, with a hold command given at the end of each active movement. The direction of the pattern is reversed by using the same sequence of contraction with no relaxation before shifting to the antagonistic pattern. This technique can be especially useful in developing strength at a specific point in the range of motion.

Rhythmic stabilization. Rhythmic stabilization uses an isometric contraction of the agonist, followed by an isometric contraction of the antagonist to produce co-contraction and stability of the two opposing muscle groups. The command given is always "Hold," and movement is resisted in each direction. Rhythmic stabilization results in an increase in the holding power to a point where the position cannot be broken. Holding should emphasize cocontraction of agonists and antagonists.

CLINICAL DECISION MAKING Exercise 14–4

A tennis player is complaining that when he serves, it feels like his shoulder "pops out" just after he hits the ball on the follow-through. How can PNF techniques be used to help this tennis player increase stability in his shoulder?

CLINICAL DECISION MAKING Exercise 14–5

A wrestler is recovering from a shoulder dislocation. He wants to know why the athletic trainer is using a manual PNF strengthening program instead of just letting him go to the weight room and work out on an exercise machine. What possible rationale might the athletic trainer give to the wrestler as to why PNF may be a more useful technique?

Treating Specific Problems with PNF Techniques

PNF-strengthening techniques can be useful in a variety of different conditions. To some extent the choice of the most effective technique for a given situation will be dictated by the state of the existing condition and the capabilities and limitations of the individual patient.[72] There are some advantages to using PNF techniques in general.

Relative to strengthening, the PNF techniques are not encumbered by the design constraints of commercial exercise machines, although some of the newer exercise machines have been designed to accommodate triplanar motion and thus will allow for PNF patterned motion.[9] With the PNF patterns, movement can occur in three planes simultaneously thus more closely resembling a functional movement pattern. The amount of resistance applied by the athletic trainer can be easily adjusted and altered at different points through the range of motion to meet patient capabilities. The athletic trainer can choose to concentrate on the strengthening through the entire range of motion or through a very specific range. Combinations of several strengthening techniques can be used concurrently within the same PNF pattern.[51] Rhythmic initiation is useful in the early stages of rehabilitation when the patient is having difficulty moving actively through a pain-free arc. Passive movement can allow the patient to maintain a full range while using an active contraction to move through the available pain-free range. Slow reversal should be used to help improve muscular endurance. Slow-reversal-hold is used to correct existing weakness at specific points in the range of motion through isometric strengthening.

Rhythmic stabilization is used to achieve stability and neuromuscular control about a joint.[11] This technique requires co-contraction of opposing muscle groups and is useful in creating a balance in the existing force couples.

CLINICAL DECISION MAKING   **Exercise 14–6**

A small female athletic trainer is attempting to do a D2 lower-extremity PNF strengthening pattern on a 300-pound offensive tackle. How can the athletic trainer ensure that proper resistance is applied when performing PNF strengthening even when the athlete is quite strong?

PNF PATTERNS

The PNF patterns are concerned with gross movement as opposed to specific muscle actions. The techniques identified previously can be superimposed on any of the PNF patterns. The techniques of PNF are composed of both rotational and

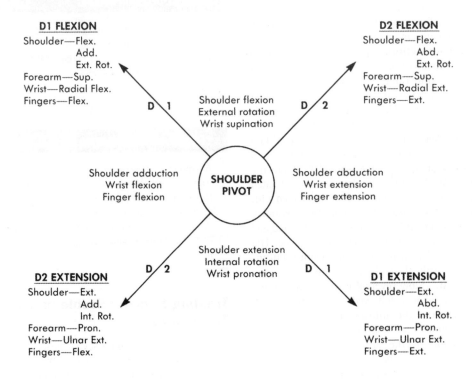

Figure 14-1 PNF patterns of the upper extremity.

diagonal exercise patterns that are similar to the motions required in most sports and normal daily activities.

The exercise patterns have three component movements: flexion-extension, abduction-adduction, and internal-external rotation. Human movement is patterned and rarely involves straight motion because all muscles are spiral in nature and lie in diagonal directions.

The PNF patterns described by Knott and Voss[37] involve distinct diagonal and rotational movements of the upper extremity, lower extremity, upper trunk, lower trunk, and neck. The exercise pattern is initiated with the muscle groups in the lengthened or stretched position. The muscle group is then contracted, moving the body part through the range of motion to a shortened position.

The upper and lower extremities all have two separate patterns of diagonal movement for each part of the body, which are referred to as the diagonal 1 (D1) and diagonal 2 (D2) patterns. These diagonal patterns are subdivided into D1 moving into flexion, D1 moving into extension, D2 moving into flexion, and D2 moving into extension. Figures 14-1 and 14-2 illustrate the PNF patterns for the upper and lower extremities, respectively. The patterns are named according to the proximal pivots at either the

shoulder or the hip (for example, the glenohumeral joint or femoralacetabular joint).

Tables 14-1 and 14-2 describe specific movements in the D1 and D2 patterns for the upper extremities. Figures 14-3 through 14-10 show starting and terminal positions for each of the diagonal patterns in the upper extremity.

Tables 14-3 and 14-4 describe specific movements in the D1 and D2 patterns for the lower extremities. Figures 14-11 through 14-18 show the starting and terminal positions for each of the diagonal patterns in the lower extremity.

Table 14-5 describes the rotational movement of the upper trunk moving into extension (also called chopping) and moving into flexion (also called lifting). Figures 14-19 and 14-20 show the starting and terminal positions of the upper-extremity chopping pattern moving into flexion to the right. Figures 14-21 and 14-22 show the starting and terminal positions for the upper-extremity lifting pattern moving into extension to the right.

Table 14-6 describes rotational movement of the lower extremities moving into positions of flexion and extension. Figures 14-23 and 14-24 show the lower-extremity pattern moving into flexion to the left. Figures 14-25 and 14-26

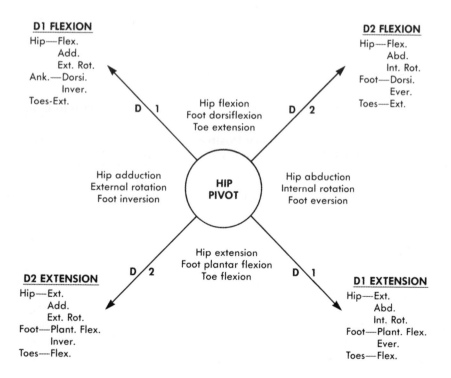

Figure 14-2 PNF patterns of the lower extremity.

■ **TABLE 14-1** D1 Upper-Extremity Movement Patterns

Body Part	Moving Into Flexion		Moving Into Extension	
	Starting Position (Figure 14-3)	Terminal Position (Figure 14-4)	Starting Position (Figure 14-5)	Terminal Position (Figure 14-6)
Shoulder	Extended Abducted Internally rotated	Flexed Adducted Externally rotated	Flexed Adducted Externally rotated	Extended Adducted Internally rotated
Scapula	Depressed Retracted Downwardly rotated	Flexed Protracted Upwardly rotated	Elevated Protracted Upwardly rotated	Depressed Retracted Downwardly rotated
Forearm	Pronated	Supinated	Supinated	Pronated
Wrist	Ulnar extended	Radially flexed	Radially flexed	Ulnar extended
Finger and thumb	Extended Abducted	Flexed Adducted	Flexed Adducted	Extended Abducted
Hand position for athletic trainer[*]	Left and inside of volar surface of hand. Right hand underneath arm in cubital fossa of elbow		Left hand on back of elbow on humerus. Right hand on dorsum of hand	
Verbal command	Pull		Push	

[*] For patient's right arm.

■ **TABLE 14-2** D2 Upper-Extremity Movement Patterns

Body Part	Moving Into Flexion		Moving Into Extension	
	Starting Position (Figure 14-7)	Terminal Position (Figure 14-8)	Starting Position (Figure 14-9)	Terminal Position (Figure 14-10)
Shoulder	Extended Abducted Internally rotated	Flexed Adducted Externally rotated	Flexed Adducted Externally rotated	Extended Adducted Internally rotated
Scapula	Depressed Retracted Downwardly rotated	Flexed Protracted Upwardly rotated	Elevated Protracted Upwardly rotated	Depressed Retracted Downwardly rotated
Forearm	Pronated	Supinated	Supinated	Pronated
Wrist	Ulnar extended	Radially flexed	Radially flexed	Ulnar extended
Finger and thumb	Flexed Abducted	Extended Adducted	Extended Adducted	Flexed Abducted
Hand position for athletic trainer[*]	Left and on back of humerus. Right hand on dorsum of hand		Left hand on volar surface of humerus. Right hand on cubital fossa of elbow	
Verbal command	Push		Pull	

[*] For patient's right arm.

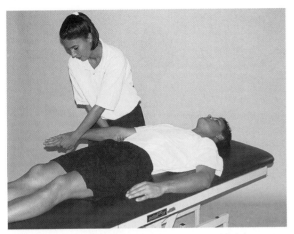

Figure 14-3   D1 upper-extremity movement pattern moving into flexion. Starting position.

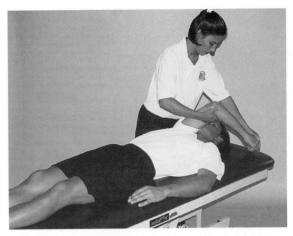

Figure 14-4   D1 upper-extremity movement pattern moving into flexion. Terminal position.

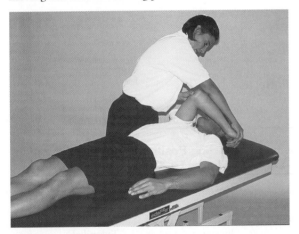

Figure 14-5   D1 upper-extremity movement pattern moving into extension. Starting position.

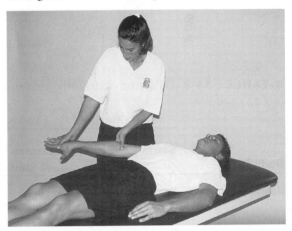

Figure 14-6   D1 upper-extremity movement pattern moving into extension. Terminal position.

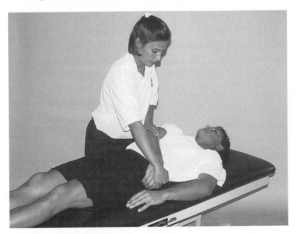

Figure 14-7   D2 upper-extremity movement pattern moving into flexion. Starting position.

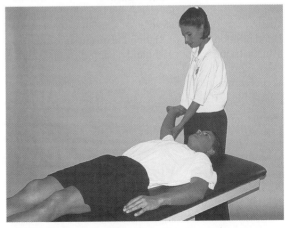

Figure 14-8   D2 upper-extremity movement pattern moving into flexion. Terminal position.

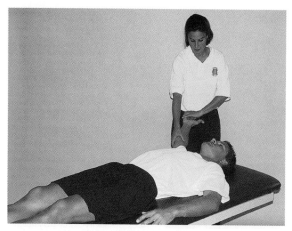

Figure 14-9 D2 upper-extremity movement pattern moving into extension. Starting position.

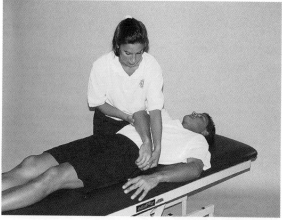

Figure 14-10 D2 upper-extremity movement pattern moving into extension. Terminal position.

■ **TABLE** **14-3** D1 Lower-Extremity Movement Patterns

	Moving Into Flexion		**Moving Into Extension**	
Body Part	**Starting Position (Figure 14-11)**	**Terminal Position (Figure 14-12)**	**Starting Position (Figure 14-13)**	**Terminal Position (Figure 14-14)**
Hip	Extended	Flexed	Flexed	Extended
	Abducted	Adducted	Adducted	Abducted
	Internally rotated	Externally rotated	Externally rotated	Internally rotated
Knee	Extended	Flexed	Flexed	Extended
Position of tibia	Externally rotated	Internally rotated	Internally rotated	Externally rotated
Ankle and foot	Plantarflexed	Dorsiflexed	Dorsiflexed	Plantarflexed
	Everted	Inverted	Inverted	Everted
Toes	Flexed	Extended	Extended	Flexed
Hand position for athletic trainer[*]	Right hand on dorsimedial surface of foot. Left hand on anteromedial thigh near patella		Right hand on lateralplantar surface of foot. Left hand on posteriolateral thigh near popliteal crease	
Verbal command	Pull		Push	

[*] For patient's right leg.

■ TABLE 14-4 D2 Lower-Extremity Movement Patterns

Body Part	Moving Into Flexion		Moving Into Extension	
	Starting Position (Figure 14-15)	Terminal Position (Figure 14-16)	Starting Position (Figure 14-17)	Terminal Position (Figure 14-18)
Hip	Extended	Flexed	Flexed	Extended
	Adducted	Abducted	Abducted	Adducted
	Externally rotated	Internally rotated	Internally rotated	Externally rotated
Knee	Extended	Flexed	Flexed	Extended
Position of tibia	Externally rotated	Internally rotated	Internally rotated	Externally rotated
Ankle and foot	Plantarflexed	Dorsiflexed	Dorsiflexed	Plantarflexed
	Inverted	Everted	Everted	Inverted
Toes	Flexed	Extended	Extended	Flexed
Hand position for athletic trainer*	Right hand on dorsilateral surface of foot. Left hand on anterolateral thigh near patella		Right hand on medialplantar surface of foot. Left hand on posteriomedial thigh near popliteal crease	
Verbal command	Pull		Push	

* For patient's right leg.

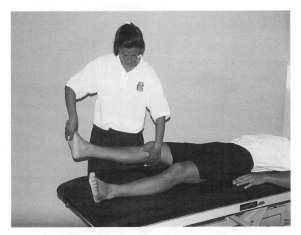

Figure 14-11 D1 lower-extremity movement pattern moving into flexion. Starting position.

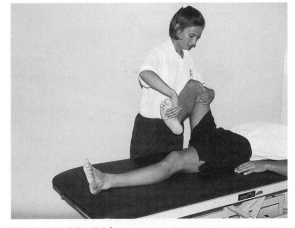

Figure 14-12 D1 lower-extremity movement pattern moving into flexion. Terminal position.

show the lower-extremity pattern moving into extension to the left.

The neck patterns involve simply flexion and rotation to one side (Figures 14-27 and 14-28) with extension and rotation to the opposite side (Figures 14-29 and 14-30). The patient should follow the direction of the movement with their eyes.

The principles and techniques of PNF, when used appropriately with specific patterns, can be an extremely effective tool for rehabilitation of injuries.[65] They can be used to strengthen weak muscles or muscle groups and to improve the neuromuscular control about an injured joint. Specific techniques selected for use should depend on individual patient needs and may be modified accordingly.[14,15]

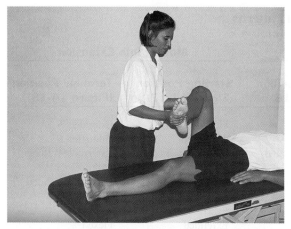

Figure 14-13 D1 lower-extremity movement pattern moving into extension. Starting position.

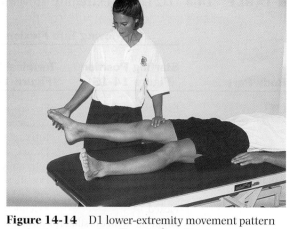

Figure 14-14 D1 lower-extremity movement pattern moving into extension. Terminal position.

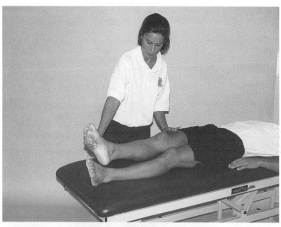

Figure 14-15 D1 lower-extremity movement pattern moving into flexion. Starting position.

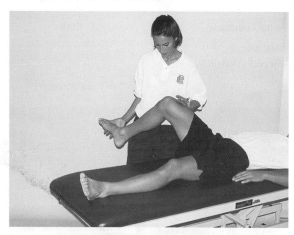

Figure 14-16 D2 lower-extremity movement pattern moving into flexion. Terminal position.

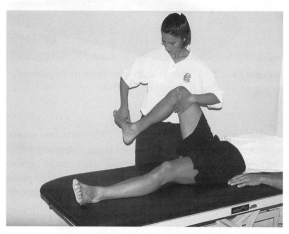

Figure 14-17 D2 lower-extremity movement pattern moving into extension. Starting position.

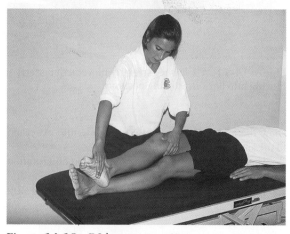

Figure 14-18 D2 lower-extremity movement pattern moving into extension. Terminal position.

■ **TABLE   14-5** Upper-Trunk Movement Patterns

| Body Part | Moving Into Flexion (Chopping)* | | Moving Into Extension (Lifting)* | |
	Starting Position (Figure 14-19)	Terminal Position (Figure 14-20)	Starting Position (Figure 14-21)	Terminal Position (Figure 14-22)
Right upper extremity	Flexed	Extended	Extended	Flexed
	Adducted	Abducted	Adducted	Abducted
	Internally rotated	Externally rotated	Internally rotated	Externally rotated
Left upper extremity (left hand grasps right forearm)	Flexed	Extended	Extended	Flexed
	Abducted	Adducted	Abducted	Adducted
	Externally rotated	Internally rotated	Externally rotated	Internally rotated
Trunk	Rotated and extended to left	Rotated and flexed to right	Rotated and flexed to left	Rotated and extended to right
Head	Rotated and extended to left	Rotated and flexed to right	Rotated and flexed to left	Rotated and extended to right
Hand position of athletic trainer	Left hand on right anterolateral surface of forehead. Right hand on dorsum of right hand		Right hand on dorsum of right hand. Left hand on posteriolateral surface of head.	
Verbal command	Pull down		Push up	

* Patient's rotation is to the right.

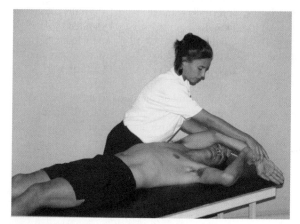

Figure 14-19   Upper-trunk pattern moving into flexion or chopping. Starting position.

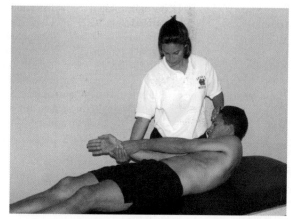

Figure 14-20   Upper-trunk pattern moving into flexion or chopping. Terminal position.

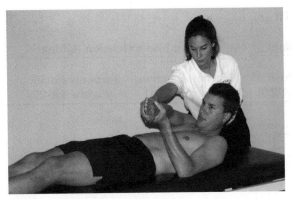

Figure 14-21 Upper-trunk pattern moving into flexion or lifting. Starting position.

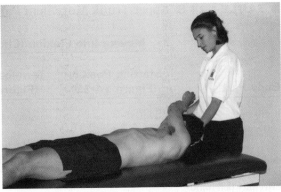

Figure 14-22 Upper-trunk pattern moving into flexion or lifting. Terminal position.

■ **TABLE 14-6** Lower Trunk Movement Patterns

Body Part	Moving Into Flexion*		Moving Into Extension†	
	Starting Position (Figure 14-23)	**Terminal Position (Figure 14-24)**	**Starting Position (Figure 14-25)**	**Terminal Position (Figure 14-26)**
Right hip	Extended	Flexed	Flexed	Extended
	Abducted	Adducted	Adducted	Abducted
	Externally rotated	Internally rotated	Internally rotated	Externally rotated
Left hip	Extended	Flexed	Flexed	Extended
	Adducted	Abducted	Abducted	Adducted
	Internally rotated	Externally rotated	Externally rotated	Internally rotated
Ankles	Plantarflexed	Dorsiflexed	Dorsiflexed	Plantarflexed
Toes	Flexed	Extended	Extended	Flexed
Hand position of athletic trainer	Right hand on dorsum of feet. Left hand on anterolateral surface of left knee		Right hand on plantar surface of foot. Left hand on posteriolateral surface of right knee	
Verbal command	Pull up and in		Push down and out	

* Patient's rotation is to the right.
† Patient's rotation is to the right in extension.

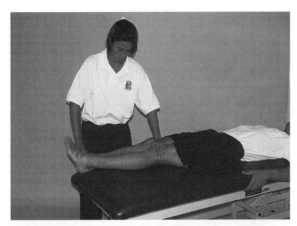

Figure 14-23   Lower-trunk pattern moving into flexion to the left. Starting position.

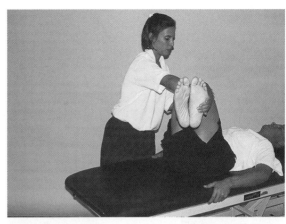

Figure 14-24   Lower-trunk pattern moving into flexion to the left. Terminal position.

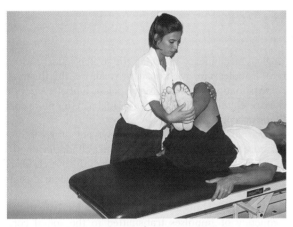

Figure 14-25   Lower-trunk pattern moving into extension to the left. Starting position.

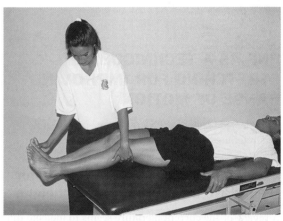

Figure 14-26   Lower-trunk pattern moving into extension to the left. Terminal position.

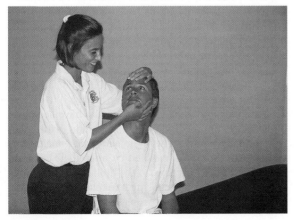

Figure 14-27   Neck flexion and rotation to the left. Starting position.

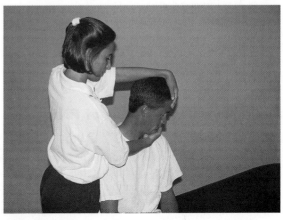

Figure 14-28   Neck flexion and rotation to the left. Terminal position.

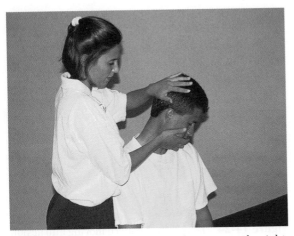

Figure 14-29 Neck extension and rotation to the right. Starting position.

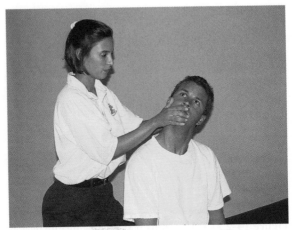

Figure 14-30 Neck extension and rotation to the right. Terminal position.

PNF AS A TECHNIQUE OF STRETCHING FOR IMPROVING RANGE OF MOTION

As indicated previously, PNF techniques can also be used for stretching to increase range of motion.

Evolution of the Theoretical Basis for Using PNF as a Stretching Technique

A review of the current literature seems to indicate that many clinicians feel that the PNF-stretching techniques can be an effective treatment modality for improving flexibility and thus use them regularly in clinical practice.[4,18,26,35,49,52,61,62] Over the years, various theories have been proposed to explain the neurological and physical mechanisms through which the PNF techniques improve flexibility.[13] However, to date no consensus agreement exists that embraces a single theoretical explanation.

Neurophysiological Basis of PNF Stretching

PNF gained popularity as a stretching technique in the 1970s.[45,54,71] The PNF research that has traditionally appeared in the literature since that time has attributed increases in range of motion primarily to neurophysi-

ological mechanisms involving the stretch reflex.[13] More recent studies have questioned the validity of this theoretical explanation.[1,13,32,33,68] Nevertheless, a brief review of the stretch reflex will serve as a springboard for more currently accepted theories.

The stretch reflex involves two types of receptors: (1) muscle spindles that are sensitive to a change in length, as well as the rate of change in length of the muscle fiber; and (2) Golgi tendon organs that detect changes in tension (Figure 14-31).

Stretching a given muscle causes an increase in the frequency of impulses transmitted to the spinal cord from the muscle spindle along Ia fibers, which in turn produces an increase in the frequency of motor nerve impulses returning to that same muscle, along alphamotor neurons, thus reflexively resisting the stretch. However, the development of excessive tension within the muscle activates the Golgi tendon organs, whose sensory impulses are carried back to the spinal cord along Ib fibers. These impulses have an inhibitory effect on the motor impulses returning to the muscles and cause that muscle to relax.[12]

Two neurophysiological phenomena have been proposed to explain facilitation and inhibition of the neuromuscular systems. The first, *autogenic inhibition*, is defined as inhibition mediated by afferent fibers from a stretched muscle acting on the alpha motor neurons supplying that muscle, causing it to relax. When a muscle is stretched, motor neurons supplying that muscle

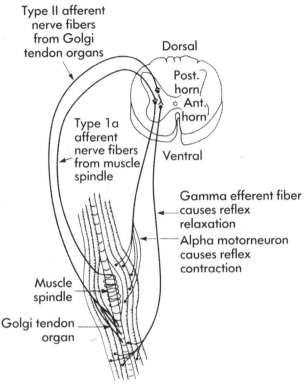

Figure 14-31   Diagrammatic representation of the stretch reflex.

A second mechanism, *reciprocal inhibition,* deals with the relationships of the agonist and antagonist muscles (Figure 14-32.) The muscles that contract to produce joint motion are referred to as agonists, and the resulting movement is called an agonistic pattern. The muscles that stretch to allow the agonist pattern to occur are referred to as antagonists. Movement that occurs directly opposite to the agonist pattern is called the antagonist pattern.

When motor neurons of the agonist muscle receive excitatory impulses from afferent nerves, the motor neurons that supply the antagonist muscles are inhibited by afferent impulses.[4] Thus contraction or extended stretch of the agonist muscle has been said to elicit relaxation or inhibit the antagonist. Likewise, a quick stretch of the antagonist muscle facilitates a contraction of the agonist.

The PNF literature has traditionally asserted that isometric or isotonic submaximal contraction of a target muscle (muscle to be stretched) prior to a passive stretch of that same muscle, or contraction of opposing muscles (agonists) during muscle stretch, produces relaxation of

receive both excitatory and inhibitory impulses from the receptors. If the stretch is continued for a slightly extended period of time, the inhibitory signals from the Golgi tendon organs eventually override the excitatory impulses and therefore cause relaxation. Because inhibitory motor neurons receive impulses from the Golgi tendon organs while the muscle spindle creates an initial reflex excitation leading to contraction, the Golgi tendon organs apparently send inhibitory impulses that last for the duration of increased tension (resulting from either passive stretch or active contraction) and eventually dominate the weaker impulses from the muscle spindle. This inhibition seems to protect the muscle against injury from reflex contractions resulting from excessive stretch.

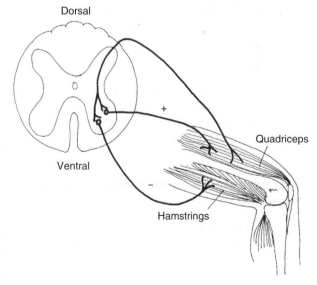

Figure 14-32   Diagrammatic representation of reciprocal inhibition.

the stretched muscle through activation of the mechanisms of the stretch reflex that include autogenic inhibition and reciprocal inhibition.[13]

However, a number of studies done since the early 1990s have suggested that relaxation following a contraction of a stretched muscle is not due to the inhibition of muscle spindle activity or to subsequent activation of Golgi tendon organs.[1,2,12,13,23,24,29,46,51]

Conclusions are based on the fact that when slowly stretching a muscle to a long length, as in the PNF-stretching techniques, the reflex-generated muscle electrical activation from the muscle spindles (as indicated by electromyogram) is very small and clinically insignificant, and not likely to effectively resist an applied muscle lengthening force.[13,28,31,35,41] Furthermore, when a muscle relaxes following an isometric contraction, Golgi tendon organ firing is decreased or even becomes silent.[20,73] Thus, Golgi tendon organs would not be able to inhibit the target muscle in the seconds following contraction when the slow therapeutic stretch would be applied.[13] It is apparent that, in general, there is a lack of research-based evidence to support the theory that Golgi tendon organ and muscle spindle reflexes are able to relax target muscles during any of the PNF-stretching techniques.[13] Thus, other mechanisms have been proposed that may explain increases in range of motion with PNF-stretching exercises.

Presynaptic Inhibition

In the PNF-stretching techniques, the contraction and subsequent relaxation of the target muscle is followed by a slow passive stretch of that muscle to a longer length. It has been suggested that lengthening is associated with an increase in presynaptic inhibition of the sensory signal from the muscle spindle.[13,22,25] This occurs with inhibition of the release of a neurotransmitter from the synaptic terminals of the muscle spindle Ia sensory fibers that limits activation in that muscle.

Viscoelastic Changes in Response to Stretching

It has been proposed that viscoelastic changes that occur in a muscle, and not a decrease in muscle activation mediated by Gogi tendon organs, is the mechanism that may explain increases in range of motion associated with the PNF techniques.[8] The viscoelastic properties of collagen in muscle were discussed briefly in Chapter 8. The force that is required to produce a change in length of a muscle is determined by its *elastic stiffness*.[72] Because of the viscous

properties of muscle, less force is needed to elongate a muscle if that force is applied slowly rather than rapidly.[72] Also, the force that resists elongation is reduced if the muscle is held at a stretched length over a period of time thus producing *stress relaxation*.[64] As stress relaxation occurs, the muscle will elongate further producing *creep*. These properties have been demonstrated in muscles with no significant electrical activity.[41,42,47]

As the viscoelastic properties within a muscle are changed during a PNF-stretching procedure, there is an altered perception of stretch and a greater range of motion and greater torque can be achieved before the onset of pain is perceived.[42] This is thought to occur because lengthening interrupts the actin-myosin bonds within the intrafusal fibers of the muscle spindle thus reducing their sensitivity to stretch.[22,27,73]

Stretching Techniques

The following techniques should be used to increase range of motion, relaxation, and inhibition.

Contract-relax. Contract-relax is a stretching technique that moves the body part passively into the agonist pattern. The patient is instructed to push by contracting the antagonist (muscle that will be stretched) isotonically against the resistance of the athletic trainer. The patient then relaxes the antagonist while the athletic trainer moves the part passively through as much range as possible to the point where limitation is again felt. This contract-relax technique is beneficial when range of motion is limited by muscle tightness.

Hold-relax. Hold-relax is very similar to the contract-relax technique. It begins with an isometric contraction of the antagonist (muscle that will be stretched) against resistance, followed by a concentric contraction of the agonist muscle combined with light pressure from the athletic trainer to produce maximal stretch of the antagonist. This technique is appropriate when there is muscle tension on one side of a joint and may be used with either the agonist or antagonist.

Slow-reversal-hold-relax. Slow-reversal-hold-relax technique begins with an isotonic contraction of the agonist, which often limits range of motion in the agonist pattern, followed by an isometric contraction of the antagonist (muscle that will be stretched) during the push phase. During the relax phase, the antagonists are relaxed while the agonists are contracting, causing movement in the direction of the agonist pattern and thus stretching the antagonist. The technique, like the contract-relax and hold-relax, is useful for increasing range of motion

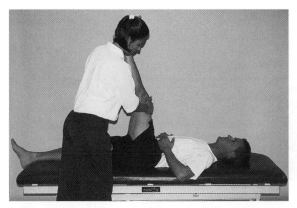

figure 14-33   PNF–stretching technique.

when the primary limiting factor is the antagonistic muscle group.

Because a goal of rehabilitation with most injuries is restoration of strength through a full, nonrestricted range of motion, several of these techniques are sometimes combined in sequence to accomplish this goal.[50] Figure 14-33 shows a PNF–stretching technique in which the athletic trainer is stretching an injured patient.

MUSCLE ENERGY TECHNIQUES

Muscle energy is a manual therapy technique, which is a variation of the PNF contract-relax and hold-relax techniques. Like the PNF techniques, the muscle energy techniques are based on the same neurophysiological mechanisms involving the stretch reflex discussed earlier in this chapter. Muscle energy techniques involve a voluntary contraction of a muscle in a specifically controlled direction at varied levels of intensity against a distinctly executed counterforce applied by the athletic trainer.[30,48] The patient provides the corrective *intrinsic* forces and controls the intensity of the muscular contractions while the athletic trainer controls the precision and localization of the procedure.[48] The amount of patient effort can vary from a minimal muscle twitch to a maximal muscle contraction.[30]

Five components are necessary for muscle energy techniques to be effective[30]:

1. Active muscle contraction by the patient
2. A muscle contraction oriented in a specific direction
3. Some patient control of contraction intensity
4. Athletic trainer control of joint position
5. Athletic trainer application of appropriate counterforce

Clinical Applications

It has been proposed that muscles function not only as flexors, extenders, rotators, and side-benders of joints but also as restrictors of joint motion. In situations where the muscle is restricting joint motion, muscle energy techniques use a specific muscle contraction to restore physiological movement to a joint.[48] Any articulation, whether in the spine or extremities, that can be moved by active muscle contraction can be treated using muscle energy techniques.[48,57]

Muscle energy techniques can be used to accomplish a number of treatment goals[30]:

1. Lengthening of a shortened, contracted, or spastic muscle
2. Strengthening of a weak muscle or muscle group
3. Reduction of localized edema through muscle pumping
4. Mobilization of an articulation with restricted mobility
5. Stretching of fascia

Treatment Techniques

Muscle energy techniques can involve four types of muscle contraction: isometric, concentric isotonic, eccentric isotonic, and *isolytic*. An isolytic contraction involves a concentric contraction by the patient while the athletic trainer applies an external force in the opposite direction, overpowering the contraction and lengthening that muscle.[48]

Isometric and concentric isotonic contractions are most frequently used in treatment.[66] Isometric contractions are most often used in treating hypertonic muscles in the spinal vertebral column, while isotonic contractions are most often used in the extremities. With both types of contraction, the idea is to inhibit antagonistic muscles producing more symmetrical muscle tone and balance.

A concentric contraction can also be used to mobilize a joint against its *motion barrier* if there is motion restriction.

For example, if a strength imbalance exists between the quadriceps and hamstrings, with weak quadriceps limiting knee extension, the following concentric isotonic muscle energy technique may be used (Figure 14-34A):

1. The patient should lie prone on the treatment table.
2. The athletic trainer stabilizes the patient with one hand and grasps the ankle with the other.
3. The athletic trainer fully flexes the knee.
4. The patient is instructed to actively extend the knee, using as much force as possible.

A

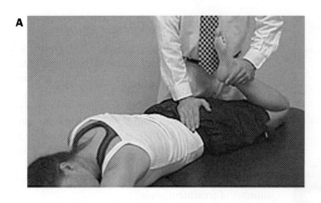

B

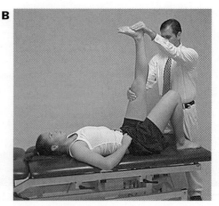

Figure 14-34 Positions for muscle energy techniques for improving **A,** Weak quadriceps that limit knee extension and/or hip flexion; and **B,** Weak hamstrings that limit knee flexion and or hip extension.

5. The athletic trainer provides a resistant counterforce that allows slow knee extension throughout the available range.
6. Once the patient has completely relaxed, the athletic trainer moves the knee back to full flexion and the patient repeats the contraction with additional resistance applied through the full range of extension. This is repeated three to five times with increasing resistance on each repetition.

If a knee has a restriction due to tightness in the hamstrings that is limiting full extension, the following isometric muscle energy technique should be used (Figure 14-34B):

1. The patient should lie supine on the treatment table.
2. The athletic trainer stabilizes the knee with one hand and grasps the ankle with the other.
3. The athletic trainer fully extends the knee until an extension barrier is felt.
4. The patient is instructed to actively flex the knee using a minimal sustained force.
5. The athletic trainer provides an equal resistant counterforce for 3 to 7 seconds, after which the patient completely relaxes.
6. The athletic trainer once again extends the knee until a new extension barrier is felt.
7. This is repeated three to five times.

Summary

1. The PNF techniques may be used to increase both strength and range of motion and are based on the neurophysiology of the stretch reflex.
2. The motor neurons of the spinal cord always receive a combination of inhibitory and excitatory impulses from the afferent nerves. Whether these motor neurons will be excited or inhibited depends on the ratio of the two types of incoming impulses.
3. The PNF techniques emphasize specific principles that may be superimposed on any of the specific techniques.

4. The PNF–strengthening techniques include repeated contraction, slow-reversal, slow-reversal-hold, rhythmic stabilization, and rhythmic initiation.
5. The PNF–stretching techniques include contract-relax, hold-relax, and slow-reversal-hold-relax.
6. The techniques of PNF are rotational and diagonal movements in the upper extremity, lower extremity, upper trunk, and the head and neck.
7. Muscle energy techniques involve a voluntary contraction of a muscle in a specifically controlled direction at varied levels of intensity against a distinctly executed counterforce applied by the athletic trainer.

References

1. Alter, M. 2004. *Science of flexibility,* 3rd ed. Champaign, IL: Human Kinetics.
2. Anderson, B., and E.R. Burke. 1991. Scientific, medical, and practical aspects of stretching. *Clin Sports Med* 10:63–86.
3. Barak, T., E. Rosen, and R. Sofer. 1990. Mobility: Passive orthopedic manual therapy. In *Orthop Sports Phys Ther,* Gould, J., and G. Davies, eds. St. Louis: Mosby.
4. Barry, D. 2005. Proprioceptive neuromuscular facilitation for the scapula, Part 1: Diagonal 1. *Athletic Therapy Today* 10(2):54.
5. Basmajian, J. 1990. *Therapeutic exercise.* Baltimore, MD: Lippincott, Williams & Wilkins.
6. Bobath, B. 1955. The treatment of motor disorders of pyramidal and extrapyramidal tracts by reflex inhibition and by facilitation of movement. *Physiotherapy* 41:146.
7. Bonnar, B., R. Deivert, and T. Gould. 2004. The relationship between isometric contraction durations during hold-relax stretching and improvement of hamstring flexibility. *J Sports Med Phys Fitness* 44(3):258–261.
8. Bradley, P., P. Olsen, and M. Portas. 2007. The effect of static ballistic and PNF stretching on vertical jump performance. *Journal of Strength & Conditioning Research* 21(1):223.
9. Burke, D.G., C.J. Culligan, and L.E. Holt. 2000. Equipment designed to stimulate proprioceptive neuromuscular facilitation flexibility training. *Journal of Strength and Conditioning Research* 14(2):135–39.
10. Burke, D.G., C.J. Culligan, and L.E. Holt. 2000. The theoretical basis of proprioceptive neuromuscular facilitation. *J Strength Cond Res* 14(4):496–500.
11. Burke, D.G., L.E. Holt, and R. Rasmussen. 2001. Effects of hot or cold water immersion and modified proprioceptive neuromuscular facilitation flexibility exercise on hamstring length. *J Athlet Train* 36(1):16–19.
12. Carter, A.M., S.J. Kinzey, L.E. Chitwood, and J.L. Cole. 2000. Proprioceptive neuromuscular facilitation decreases muscle activity during the stretch reflex in selected posterior thigh muscles. *Journal of Sport Rehabilitation* 9(4):269–78.
13. Chalmers, G. 2004. Re-examination of the possible role of Golgi tendon organ and muscle spindle reflexes in proprioceptive neuromuscular facilitation muscle stretching. *Sports Biomech* 3(1):159–183.
14. Cookson, J., and B. Kent. 1979. Orthopedic manual therapy: An overview, I. The extremities. *J Am Phys Ther Assoc* 59:136.
15. Cookson, J. 1979. Orthopedic manual therapy: An overview, II. The spine. *J Am Phys Ther Assoc* 59:259.
16. Cornelius, W., and A. Jackson. 1984. The effects of cryotherapy and PNF on hip extension flexibility. *Athlet Train* 19(3):184.
17. Davis, D., M. Hagerman-Hose, and M. Midkiff. 2004. The effectiveness of 3 proprioceptive neuromuscular facilitation stretching techniques on the flexibility of the hamstring muscle group (Abstract). *Journal of Orthopaedic & Sports Physical Therapy* 34(1):A33–A34.
18. Decicco, P.V., and M.M. Fisher. 2005. The effects of proprioceptive neuromuscular facilitation stretching on shoulder range of motion in overhand athletes. *J Sports Med Phys Fitness* 45(2):183–187.
19. Decicco, P., and M. Fisher. 2005. The effects of proprioceptive neuromuscular facilitation stretching on shoulder range of motion in overhand athletes. *Journal of Sports Medicine & Physical Fitness* 45(2):183-187.
20. Edin, B.B., and A.B. Vallbo. 1990. Muscle afferent responses to isometric contractions and relaxations in humans. *J Neurophys* 63:1307–1313.
21. Engle, R., and G. Canner. 1989. Proprioceptive neuromuscular facilitation (PNF) and modified procedures for anterior cruciate ligament (ACL) instability. *J Orthop Sports Phys Ther* 11(6):230–236.
22. Enoka, R. 2008. *Neuromechanics of Human Movement,* 4th ed. Champaign, IL: Human Kinetics.
23. Enoka, R.M., R.S. Hutton, and E. Eldred. 1980. Changes in excitability of tendon tap and Hoffmann reflexes following voluntary contractions. *Electroencephalogr Clin Neurophysiol* 48:664–672.
24. Ferber, R., L. Osternig, and D. Gravelle. 2002. Effect of PNF stretch techniques on knee flexor muscle EMG activity in older adults. *J Electromyogr Kinesiol* 12:391–397.
25. Gollhofer, A., A. Schopp, W. Rapp, and V. Stroinik. 1998. Changes in reflex excitability following isometric contraction in humans. *Eur J Appl Physiol Occup Physiol* 77:89–97.
26. Greenman, P. 2003. *Principles of manual medicine.* Baltimore, MD: Lippincott, Williams & Wilkins.
27. Gregory, J.E., R.F. Mark, D.L. Morgan, A. Patak, B. Polus, and U. Proske. 1990. Effects of muscle history on the stretch reflex in cat and man. *J Physiol* 424:93–107.
28. Halbertsma, J.P., I. Mulder, L.N. Goeken, and W.H. Eisma. 1999. Repeated passive stretching: Acute effect on the passive muscle moment and extensibility of short hamstrings. *Arch Phys Med Rehab* 80:407–414.
29. Holcomb, W.R. 2000. Improved stretching with proprioceptive neuromuscular facilitation. *Strength Cond J* 22(1):59–61.
30. Hollis, M. 1981. *Practical exercise.* Oxford: Blackwell Scientific.
31. Houk, J.C., W.Z. Rymer, and P.E. Crago. 1981. Dependence of dynamic response of spindle receptors on muscle length and velocity. *J Neurophysiol* 46:143–166.
32. Hultborn, H. 2001. State-dependent modulation of sensory feedback. *J Physiol* 533(Pt 1):5–13.
33. Jankowska, E. 1992. Interneuronal relay in spinal pathways from proprioceptors. *Prog Neurobiol* 38:335–378.
34. Johnson, G.S. 2000. PNF and knee rehabilitation. *J Orthop Sports Phys Ther* 30(7):430–431.
35. Kitani, I. 2004. The effectiveness of proprioceptive neuromuscular facilitation (PNF) exercises on shoulder joint position sense in baseball players (Abstract). *Journal of Athletic Training* 39(2):S-62.

36. Knappstein, A., S. Stanley, and C. Whatman. 2004. Range of motion immediately post and seven minutes post, PNF stretching hip joint range of motion and PNF stretching. *New Zealand Journal of Sports Medicine* 32(2):42–46.

37. Knott, M., and D. Voss. 1985. *Proprioceptive neuromuscular facilitation: Patterns and techniques.* Baltimore: Lippincott, Williams and Wilkins.

38. Kofotolis, N., and E. Kellis. 2007. Cross-training effects of a proprioceptive neuromuscular facilitation exercise program on knee musculature. *Physical Therapy in Sport* 8(3):109.

39. Kofotolis, N., and E. Kellis. 2006. Effects of two 4-week proprioceptive neuromuscular facilitation programs on muscle endurance, flexibility, and functional performance in women with chronic low back pain. *Physical Therapy* 86(7):1001.

40. Lloyd, D. 1946. Facilitation and inhibition of spinal motorneurons. *J Neurophysiol* 9:421

41. Magnusson, S.P., E.B. Simonsen, P. Aagaard, P. Dyhre-Poulsen, M.P. McHugh, and M. Kjaer. 1996. Mechanical and physiological responses to stretching with and without preisometric contraction in human skeletal muscle. *Arc Phys Med Rehab* 77:373–378.

42. Magnusson, S.P., E.B. Simonsen, P. Dyhre-Poulsen, P. Aagaard, T. Mohr, and M. Kjaer. 1996. Viscoelastic stress relaxation during static stretch in human skeletal muscle in the absence of EMG activity. *Scand J Med Sci Sports* 6:323–328.

43. Manoel, M., M. Harris-Love, and J. Danoff. 2008. Acute effects of static, dynamic and proprioceptive neuromuscular facilitation stretching on muscle power in women. *Journal of Strength & Conditioning Research* 22(5):1528.

44. Marek, S., J. Cramer, and L. Fincher. 2005. Acute effects of static and proprioceptive neuromuscular facilitation stretching on muscle strength and power output. *Journal of Athletic Training* 40(2):94.

45. Markos, P. 1979. Ipsilateral and contralateral effects of proprioceptive neuromuscular facilitation techniques on hip motion and electromyographic activity. *Phys Ther* 59(11) P:66–73.

46. McAtee, R., and J. Charland. 2007. *Facilitated stretching,* 3rd ed. Champaign, IL: Human Kinetics.

47. McHugh, M.P., S.P. Magnusson, G.W. Gleim, and J.A. Nicholas. 1992. Viscoelastic stress relaxation in human skeletal muscle. *Med Sci Sports Exerc* 24:1375–1382.

48. Mitchell, F. 1993. Elements of muscle energy technique. In *Rational manual therapies*, Basmajian, J., and R. Nyberg, eds. Baltimore, MD: Lippincott, Williams & Wilkins.

49. Mitchell, U., J. Myrer, and T. Hopkins. 2007. Acute stretch perception alteration contributes to the success of the PNF "contract-relax" stretch. *Journal of Sport Rehabilitation* 16(2):85.

50. Osternig, L., R. Robertson, and R. Troxel, et al. 1990. Differential responses to proprioceptive neuromuscular facilitation stretch techniques. *Med Sci Sports Exerc* 22:106–111.

51. Osternig, L., R. Robertson, R. Troxel, and P. Hansen. 1987. Muscle activation during proprioceptive neuromuscular facilitation (PNF) stretching techniques … stretch-relax (SR), contract-relax (CR) and agonist contract-relax (ACR). *Am J Phys Med* 66(5):298–307.

52. Padua, D., K. Guskiewicz, and W. Prentice. 2004. The effect of select shoulder exercises on strength, active angle reproduction, single-arm balance, and functional performance. *J Sport Rehab* 13(1):75–95.

53. Prentice, W., and E. Kooima. 1986. The use of proprioceptive neuromuscular facilitation techniques in the rehabilitation of sport-related injuries. *Athlet Train* 21:26–31.

54. Prentice, W. 1983. A comparison of static stretching and PNF stretching for improving hip joint flexibility. *Athlet Train* 18(1):56–59.

55. Prentice, W. 1988. A manual resistance technique for strengthening tibial rotation. *Athlet Train* 23(3):230–233.

56. Prentice, W. 1993. Proprioceptive neuromuscular facilitation [Videotape]. St. Louis: Mosby.

57. Roberts, B.L. 1997. Soft tissue manipulation: Neuromuscular and muscle energy techniques. *J Neurosci Nurs* 29(2):123–127.

58. Rood, M. 1954. Neurophysiologic reactions as a basis of physical therapy. *Phys Ther Rev* 34:444.

59. Saliba, V., G. Johnson, and C. Wardlaw. 1993. Proprioceptive neuromuscular facilitation. In *Rational manual therapies.* Basmajian, J., and R. Nyberg, eds. Baltimore, MD: Lippincott Williams & Wilkins.

60. Sawner, K., and J. LaVigne. 1992. Brunstrom's movement therapy in hemiplegia. Baltimore: Lippincott, Williams and Wilkins.

61. Schuback, B., J. Hooper, and L. Salisbury. 2004. A comparison of a self-stretch incorporating proprioceptive neuromuscular facilitation components and a therapist-applied PNF-technique on hamstring flexibility. *Physiotherapy* 90(3):151.

62. Sharman, M., Cresswell, T and G. Andrew. 2006. Proprioceptive neuromuscular facilitation stretching: Mechanisms and clinical implications. *Sports Medicine* 36(11):929.

63. Sherrington, C. 1947. *The integrative action of the nervous system.* New Haven: Yale University Press.

64. Shrier, I. 2002. Does stretching help prevent injuries? In *Evidence based sports medicine.* MacAuley, D., and T. Best, eds. London: BMJ Books.

65. Spernoga, S.G., T.L. Uhl, B.L. Arnold, and B.M. Gansneder. 2001. Duration of maintained hamstring flexibility after a one-time, modified hold-relax stretching protocol. *J Athlet Train* 36(1):44–48.

66. Stone, J. 2000. Muscle energy technique. *Athlet Ther Today* 5(5):25.

67. Stone, J.A. 2000. Prevention and rehabilitation: Proprioceptive neuromuscular facilitation. *Athlet Ther Today* 5(1):38–39.

68. Stuart, D.G. 2002. Reflections of spinal reflexes. *Adv Exp Med Biol* 508:249–257.

69. Surberg, P. 1954. Neuromuscular facilitation techniques in sports medicine. *Phys Ther Rev* 34:444.

70. Surburg, P., and J. Schrader. 1997. Proprioceptive neuromuscular facilitation techniques in sports medicine: A reassessment. *J Athlet Train* 32(1):34–39.

71. Taniqawa, M. 1972. Comparison of the hold-relax procedure and passive mobilization on increasing muscle length. *Phys Ther* 52(7):725–735.

72. Taylor, D.C., J.D. Dalton, and A. Seaber. 1990. Viscoelastic properties of muscle-tendon units: The biomechanical effects of stretching. *Am J Sports Med* 18:300–309.

73. Wilson L.R., S.C. Gandevia, and D. Burke. 1995. Increased resting discharge of human spindle afferents following voluntary contractions. *J Physiol* 488(Pt 3):833–840.

74. Worrell, T., T. Smith, and J. Winegardner. 1994. Effect of hamstring stretching on hamstring muscle performance. *J Orthop Sports Phys Ther* 20(3):154–159.

75. Zohn, D., and J. Mennell. 1987. *Musculoskeletal pain: Diagnosis and physical treatment.* Boston: Little, Brown.

SOLUTIONS TO CLINICAL DECISION MAKING EXERCISES

14-1 A breaststroke kick involves multiplanar movements. Because PNF is used to strengthen gross motor patterns instead of specific muscle actions, it may help her regain strength and control in her kick.

14-2 The athletic trainer can apply resistance and encourage movement within the pain-free ROM. This strengthening technique will help prevent loss of coordination due to inactivity.

14-3 The rhythmic initiation technique promotes strength by first introducing the movement pattern passively. The patient will slowly progress to active assistive and then resistive exercises through the movement pattern.

14-4 Rhythmic stabilization can be used to facilitate strength and stability at a joint by stimulating co-contraction of the opposing muscles that support the joint. PNF strengthening using the D1 and D2 patterns will encourage control in the player's overhead serve.

14-5 The movements required for sport are not single-plane movements. PNF strengthening is more functional and is not limited by the design constraints of an exercise machine. Also, PNF technique allows the athletic trainer to adjust the amount of manual resistance throughout the range of motion according to the patient's capabilities.

14-6 Proper body and hand positioning will maximize the athletic trainer's ability to provide sufficient resistance. The athletic trainer should stand in a position that is in line with the direction of movement in the diagonal movement pattern. The knees should be bent and the stance close to the patient, so that the direction and amount of resistance can easily be applied or altered appropriately throughout the range of movement.

CHAPTER 15

Aquatic Therapy in Rehabilitation

Barbara J. Hoogenboom
Nancy E. Lomax

After completing this chapter, the athletic training student should be able to do the following:

- Explain the principles of buoyancy and specific gravity and the role they have in the aquatic environment.

- Identify and describe the three major resistive forces at work in the aquatic environment.

- Apply the principles of buoyancy and resistive forces to exercise prescription and progression.

- Contrast the advantages and disadvantages of aquatic therapy in relation to traditional land-based exercise.

- Identify and describe techniques of aquatic therapy for the upper extremity, lower extremity, and trunk.

- Select and utilize various types of equipment for aquatic therapy.

- Incorporate functional, work- and sport-specific movements and exercises performed in the aquatic environment into rehabilitation.

- Understand and describe the necessity for transition from the aquatic environment to the land environment.

In recent years, widespread interest has developed in the area of aquatic therapy. It has rapidly become a popular rehabilitation technique for treatment of a variety of patient populations.[27,38] This newfound interest has sparked numerous research efforts to evaluate the effectiveness of aquatic therapy as a therapeutic intervention. Current research shows aquatic therapy to be beneficial in the treatment of everything from orthopedic injuries to spinal cord damage, chronic pain, cerebral palsy, multiple sclerosis, and many other conditions, making it useful in a variety of settings.[24,32] It is also gaining acceptance as a preventative maintenance tool to facilitate overall fitness, cross-training, and sport-specific skills for healthy athletes (Figure 15-1).[28,29] General conditioning, strength, and a wide variety of movement skills can all be enhanced by aquatic therapy.[14,44,49]

Water healing techniques have been traced back through history as early as 2400 b.c. but it was not until the late nineteenth century that more traditional types of aquatic therapy came into existence.[7] The development of the Hubbard tank in 1920 sparked the initiation of present-day therapeutic use of water by allowing aquatic therapy to be conducted in a highly controlled clinical setting.[6] Loeman and Roen took this a step farther in 1924 and stimulated interest in actual pool therapy or what we

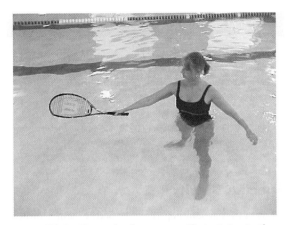

Figure 15-1 Example of sport-specific training in the aquatic environment.

now call aquatic therapy. Only recently, however, has water come into its own as a therapeutic exercise medium.[7]

Aquatic therapy is believed to be beneficial because it decreases joint compression forces. The perception of weightlessness experienced in the water assists in decreasing pain and eliminating or drastically reducing the body's protective muscular spasm and pain that can carry over into the patient's daily functional activities.[49,51] The primary goal of aquatic therapy is to teach the patient how to use water as a modality for improving movement, strength, and fitness.[2,49] Then, along with other therapeutic modalities and treatments, aquatic therapy can become one link in the patient recovery chain.[1]

PHYSICAL PROPERTIES AND RESISTIVE FORCES

The athletic trainer must understand several physical properties of the water before designing an aquatic therapy program. Land exercise cannot always be converted to aquatic exercise, because buoyancy rather than gravity is the major force governing movement. A thorough understanding of buoyancy, specific gravity, the resistive forces of the water, and their relationships must be the groundwork of any therapeutic aquatic program. The program must be individualized to the patient's particular injury or condition and activity level if it is to be successful.

Buoyancy

Buoyancy is one of the primary forces involved in aquatic therapy. All objects, on land or in the water, are subjected to the downward pull of the earth's gravity. In the water, however, this force is counteracted to some degree by the upward buoyant force. According to Archimedes' Principle, any object submerged or floating in water is buoyed upward by a counterforce that helps support the submerged object against the downward pull of gravity. In other words, the buoyant force assists motion toward the water's surface and resists motions away from the surface.[20,49] Because of this buoyant force, a person entering the water experiences an apparent loss of weight.[12] The weight loss experienced is nearly equal to the weight of the liquid that is displaced when the object enters the water (Figure 15-2).

For example, a 100-pound individual, when almost completely submerged, displaces a volume of water that weighs nearly 95 pounds; therefore, that person feels as though she/he weighs less than 5 pounds. This sensation occurs because, when partially submerged, the individual only bears the weight of the part of the body that is above the water. With immersion to the level of the seventh cervical vertebra, both males and females only bear approximately 6 to 10 percent of their total body weight (TBW). The percentages increase to 25 to 31 percent TBW for females and 30 to 37 percent TBW for males at the xiphisternal level, and 40 to 51 percent TBW for females and 50 to 56 percent TBW for males at the anterosuperior iliac spine (ASIS) level (Table 15-1).[21] The percentages differ slightly for males and females due to the differences in their centers of gravity. Males carry a higher percentage of their weight in the upper body, whereas females carry a higher percentage of their weight in the lower body. The center of gravity on land corresponds with a center of buoyancy in the water.[39,40] Variations of build and body type only minimally affect weightbearing values. Due to the decreased percentage of weight bearing offered by the buoyant force, each joint that is below the water is decompressed or unweighted. This allows ambulation and vigorous exercise

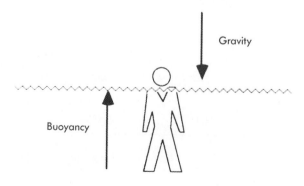

Figure 15-2 The buoyant force.

■ **TABLE 15-1** Weightbearing Percentages

Body Level	Percentage of Weight Bearing	
	Male	**Female**
C7	8	8
Xiphisternal	28	35
ASIS	47	54

to be performed with little impact and drastically reduced friction between joint articular surfaces.

Through careful use of Archimedes' Principle, a gradual increase in the percentage of weight bearing can be undertaken. Initially, the patient would begin nonweightbearing in the deep end of the pool. A flotation vest, kickboard, or other buoyancy device might be used to help the patient remain afloat for the desired exercises (Figure 15-3). Other commercial equipment available for use in the aquatic environment will be discussed later in the section "Facilities and Equipment."

Specific Gravity

Buoyancy is partially dependent on body weight. However, the weight of different parts of the body is not constant. Therefore, the buoyant values of different body parts will vary. Buoyant values can be determined by several factors. The ratio of bone weight to muscle weight, the amount and distribution of fat, and the depth and expansion of the chest all play a role. Together, these factors determine the specific gravity of the individual body part. On the average, humans have a specific gravity slightly less than

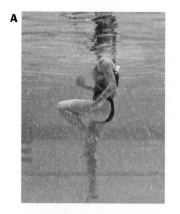
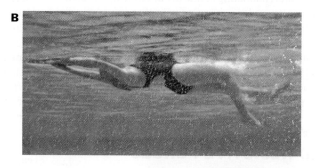
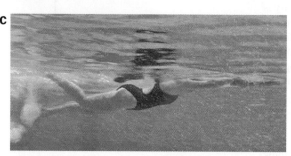
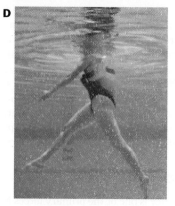

Figure 15-3   Underwater exercise using either a floatation vest or a Kickboard **A,** Running, **B,** Supine Kicking, **C,** Prone Kicking, **D,** Scissors.

that of water. Any object with a specific gravity less than that of water will float. An object with a specific gravity greater than that of water will sink. However, as with buoyant values, the specific gravity of all body parts is not uniform. Therefore, even with a total-body specific gravity of less than the specific gravity of water, the individual might not float horizontally in the water. Additionally, the lungs, when filled with air, can further decrease the specific gravity of the chest area. This allows the head and chest to float higher in the water than the heavier, denser extremities. Many athletes tend to have a low percentage of body fat (specific gravity greater than water) and are "sinkers." Therefore, compensation with flotation devices at the extremities and trunk might be necessary for some athletes.[3,49]

Resistive Forces

Water has 12 times the resistance of air.[46] Therefore, when an object moves in the water, several resistive forces are at work that must be considered. Forces must be considered for both their potential benefits and precautions. These forces include the cohesive force, the bow force, and the drag force.

Cohesive Force.   There is a slight but easily overcome cohesive force that runs in a parallel direction to the water surface. This resistance is formed by the water molecules loosely binding together, creating a surface tension. Surface tension can be seen in still water, because the water remains motionless with the cohesive force intact unless disturbed.

Bow Force.   A second force is the bow force, or the force that is generated at the front of the object during movement. When the object moves, the bow force causes an increase in the water pressure at the front of the object and a decrease in the water pressure at the rear

of the object. This pressure change causes a movement of water from the high-pressure area at the front to the low-pressure area behind the object. As the water enters the low-pressure area, it swirls in to the low-pressure zone and forms eddies, or small whirlpool turbulences.[7] These eddies impede flow by creating a backward force, or drag force (Figure 15-4).

Drag Force   This third force, the fluid drag force, is very important in aquatic therapy. The bow force, and therefore also the drag force, on an object can be controlled by changing the shape of the object or the speed of its movement (Figure 15-5).

Frictional resistance can be decreased by making the object more streamlined. This change minimizes the surface area at the front of the object. Less surface area causes less bow force and less of a change in pressure between the front and rear of the object, resulting in less drag force. In a streamlined flow, the resistance is proportional to the velocity of the object. When working with a patient with generalized weakness, consideration of the aquatic environment is necessary. Increased activity occurring around the patient and turbulence of the water will make walking a challenging activity (Figure 15-6).

On the other hand, if the object is not streamlined, a turbulent situation (also referred to as pressure or form drag) exists. In a turbulent situation, drag is a function of the velocity squared. Therefore by increasing the speed of movement two times, the resistance the object must overcome is increased four times.[12] This provides a method to increase resistance progressively during aquatic rehabilitation. Considerable turbulence can be generated when the speed of movement is increased, causing muscles to work harder to keep the movement going. Another method to increase resistance is to change directions of movement, creating increased drag. Finally, by simply changing the shape of a limb through the addition of

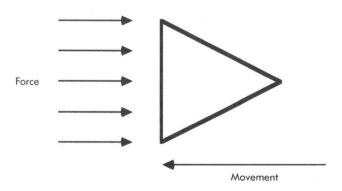

Figure 15-4   The bow force.

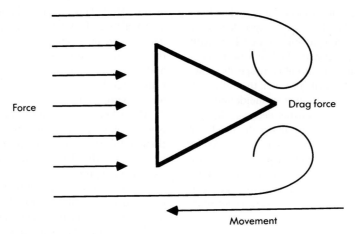

Figure 15-5   Drag force.

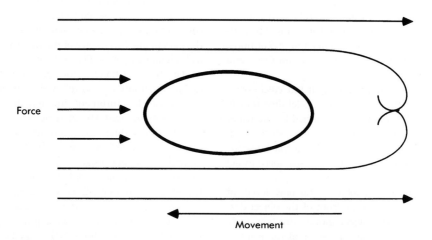

Figure 15-6   Streamlined movement. This creates less drag force and less turbulence.

rehabilitation equipment that increases surface area, the athletic trainer can modify the patient's workout intensity to match strength increases (Figure 15-7).

Drag force must also be considered when portions of a limb or joint must be protected after injury or surgery. For example, when working with a patient with an acutely injured medial collateral ligament, or anterior crucial ligament of the knee, resistance must not be placed distal to the knee, due to the increased torque that occurs due to drag forces.

Quantification of resistive forces that occur during aquatic exercise has been a challenge. Pöyhönen et al. examined knee flexion and extension in the aquatic environment using an anatomic model in barefoot and hydroboot-wearing conditions. They found that the highest drag forces and drag coefficients occurred during early extension from a flexed position (150 degrees to 140 degrees of flexion) while wearing the hydroboot (making the foot less streamlined), and that faster velocity was associated with higher drag forces.[41]

Once therapy has progressed, the patient could be moved to neck-deep water to begin light weight bearing. Gradual increases in the percentage of weight bearing are accomplished by systematically moving the patient to shallower water. Even when in waist-deep water, both male and female patients are only bearing

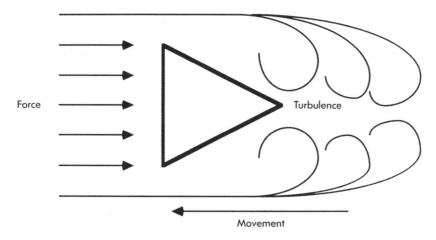

Figure 15-7   Turbulent flow.

approximately 50 percent of their TBW. By placing a sinkable bench or chair in the shallow water, step-ups can be initiated under partial-weightbearing conditions long before the patient is capable of performing the same exercise in full-weightbearing on land. Thus the advantages of low-weightbearing are coupled with the proprioceptive benefits of closed-kinetic-chain exercise, making aquatic therapy an excellent functional rehabilitation activity.

ADVANTAGES AND BENEFITS OF AQUATIC REHABILITATION

The addition of an aquatic therapy program can offer many advantages to a patient's therapy (Table 15-2).[16,49] The buoyancy of the water allows active exercise while providing a sense of security and causing little discomfort.[47] Utilizing a combination of the water's buoyancy, resistance, and warmth, the patient can typically achieve more in the aquatic environment than is possible on land.[29] Early in the rehabilitation process, aquatic therapy is useful in restoring range of motion and flexibility. As normal function is restored, resistance training and sport-specific activities can be added.

Following an injury, the aquatic experience provides a medium where early motions can be performed in a supportive environment.[18] The slow motion effect of moving through water provides extra time to control movement, which allows the patient to experience multiple movement errors without severe consequences.[45] This is especially helpful in lower-extremity injuries where balance and proprioception are impaired.[39,40] Geigle et al. demonstrated

a positive relationship between use of a supplemental aquatic therapy program and unilateral tests of balance when treating athletes with inversion ankle sprains.[16] The increased amount of time to react to and correct movement errors, combined with a medium in which the fear of falling is removed, assists the patient's ability to regain proprioception.

Turbulence functions as a destabilizer and as a tactile sensory stimulus. The stimulation from the turbulence generated during movement provides feedback and perturbation challenge that aids in the return of proprioception and balance. There is also an often overlooked benefit of edema reduction due to hydrostatic pressure. This would benefit pain reduction and increase range of motion.

By understanding buoyancy and utilizing its principles, the aquatic environment can provide a gradual transition from non-weightbearing to full-weightbearing land exercises. This gradual increase in percentage of weight bearing helps provide a return to smooth coordinated movements that are pain-free. By utilizing the buoyancy force to decrease apparent weight and joint compressive forces, locomotor activities can begin much earlier following an injury to the lower extremity.[23] This provides an enormous advantage to the athletic population. The ability to work out hard without fear of reinjury provides a psychological boost to the athlete. This helps keep motivation high and can help speed the athlete's return to normal function.[29] Psychologically, aquatic therapy increases confidence, because the patient experiences increased success at locomotor, stretching, or strengthening activities while in the water. Tension and anxiety are decreased, and the patient's morale increases, as does post-exercise vigor.[7,12]

■ **TABLE   15-2** Indications and Benefits of Aquatic Therapy

Indications for Use of Aquatic Therapy	Illustration of Benefits
Swelling/peripheral edema	Assist in edema control, decrease pain, increase mobility as edema decreases
Decreased range of motion	Earlier initiation of rehabilitation, controlled active movements
Decreased strength	Strength progression from assisted to resisted to functional; gradual increase in exercise intensity
Decreased balance, proprioception, coordination	Earlier return to function in supported, forgiving environment, slower movements
Weightbearing restrictions	Can partially or completely unweight the lower extremities; regulate weightbearing progressions
Cardiovascular deconditioning or potential deconditioning due to inability to train	Gradual increase of exercise intensity, alternative training environment for lower weight bearing
Gait deviations	Slower movements, easier assessment, and modification of gait
Difficulty or pain with land interventions	Increased support, decreased weight bearing, assistance due to buoyancy, more relaxed environment

Source: Reproduced from Irion, J. M. 2001. Aquatic therapy. In *Therapeutic exercise: Techniques for intervention*, Bandy, W. D., and B. Sanders, eds. Baltimore; Lippincott; Williams & Wilkins; Sova, R. 1993. *Aquatic activities handbook*. Boston; Jones & Bartlett; and Thein, J. M., and Thein. L. Brody 1998. Aquatic-based rehabilitation and training for the elite athlete. *Orthop Sports Phys Ther* 27(1):32–41.

CLINICAL DECISION MAKING   Exercise 15-2

A collegiate football player sustained a severe ACL/MCL and medial meniscus injury to the right knee. The injury to the medial meniscus was so severe that it was deemed nonrepairable, and the surgeon determined that a staged surgery (ACL reconstruction first, later a meniscal allograft) would best serve the athlete. The MCL is allowed to heal without surgical intervention. Despite well-designed and well-executed rehabilitation after the ACL reconstruction, it is likely that after the meniscal transplant a clinical "regression" in strength, ROM, and function will occur due to postoperative restrictions. What rehabilitation techniques can the athletic trainer utilize to maximize the rehabilitation after the meniscal allograft during the requisite non-weightbearing and partial weightbearing phases?

Muscular strengthening and reeducation can also be accomplished through aquatic therapy.[36,49] Progressive resistance exercises can be increased in extremely small increments by using combinations of different resistive forces. The intensity of exercise can be controlled by manipulating the flow of the water (turbulence), the body's position, or through the addition of exercise equipment. This allows individuals with minimal muscle contraction capabilities to do work and see improvement. The aquatic environment can also provide a challenging resistive workout to an athlete nearing full recovery.[49] Additionally, water serves as an accommodating resistance medium. This allows the muscles to be maximally stressed through the full range of motion available. One drawback to this, however, is that strength gains depend largely on the effort exerted by the patient, which is not easily quantified.

In another study, Pöyhönen et al.[41] studied the biomechanical and hydrodynamic characteristics of the therapeutic exercise of knee flexion and extension using kinematic and electromyographic analyses in flowing and still water. They found that the flowing properties of water modified the agonist/antagonist neuromuscular function of the quadriceps and hamstrings in terms of early reduction of quadriceps activity and concurrent increased activation of the hamstrings. They also found that flowing water (turbulence) causes additional resistance when moving the limb opposite the flow. They concluded that when prescribing aquatic exercise, the turbulence of the water must be considered in terms of both resistance and alterations of neuromuscular recruitment of muscles.

Strength gains through aquatic exercise are also brought about by the increased energy needs of the body working in an aquatic environment. Studies have shown that aquatic exercise requires higher energy expenditure than the same exercise performed on land.[7,9,12,49] The patient not only has to perform the activity but must also maintain a level of buoyancy and overcome the resistive forces of the water. For example, the energy cost for water running is four times greater than the energy cost for running the same distance on land.[7,12,26]

A simulated run in either shallow or deep water assisted by a tether or flotation devices can be an effective means of alternate fitness training (cross-training) for the injured athlete. It should be noted that a study of shallow-water running (xiphoid level) and deep-water running (using an aqua jogger), at the same rate of perceived exertion, found a significant difference of 10 beats per minute in heart rate, with shallow-water running demonstrating a greater heart rate. The authors of this study point out that aquatic rehabilitation professionals should not prescribe shallow-water working heart rates from heart rates values obtained during deep-water exercise.[44] All patients should be instructed how to accurately monitor their heart rate while exercising in water, whether deep or shallow.[9]

Not only does the patient benefit from early intervention, but aquatic exercise also helps prevent cardiorespiratory deconditioning through alterations in cardiovascular dynamics as a result of hydrostatic forces.[5,22,48] The heart actually functions more efficiently in the water than on land. Hydrostatic pressure enhances venous return, leading to a greater stroke volume and a reduction in the heart rate needed to maintain cardiac output.[50] There is also a decrease in ventilations and an increase in central blood volume. This means that the injured athlete can maintain a near-normal maximal aerobic capacity with aquatic exercise.[13,33] Due to the hydrostatic effects on heart efficiency, it has been suggested that an environment-specific exercise prescription is necessary.[28,48,52] Some research suggests the use of perceived exertion as an acceptable method for controlling exercise intensity. Other research suggests the use of target heart rate values as with land exercise, but compensates for the hydrostatic changes by setting the target range 10 percent lower than what would be expected for land exercise.[46,49] (Figure 15-8). Regardless of the method used, the keys to successful use of aquatic therapy are supervision and monitoring of the patient or patient during activity, and good communication between patient and athletic trainer.

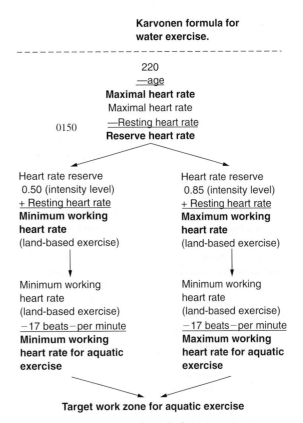

Figure 15-8 Karvonen formula for water exercise. Source: Adapted from R. Sova. 1993. *Aquatic activities handbook*. Boston: Jones & Bartlett, p. 55.

CLINICAL DECISION MAKING   **Exercise 15-3**

A high school cross-country runner sustained a small second-metatarsal stress reaction/fracture during the short 3-month season in response to increased volume and intensity of training. She has been cleared by her physician to finish out the remaining 3 weeks of the competitive season but is only allowed to run in meets. What might the athletic trainer suggest for alternate training to allow her to maintain aerobic function and enable her to compete?

DISADVANTAGES OF AQUATIC REHABILITATION

Disadvantages

As with any therapeutic intervention, aquatic therapy has its disadvantages. The cost of building and maintaining a rehabilitation pool, if there is no access to an existing facility, can be very high. Also, qualified pool attendants must be present, and the athletic trainer involved in the treatment must be trained in aquatic safety and therapy procedures.[10,26]

An athlete who requires high levels of stabilization will be more challenging to work with, because stabilization in water is considerably more difficult than on land. Thermo-regulation issues exist for the patient who exercises in an aquatic environment. Because the patient cannot always choose the temperature of the pool, the effects of water temperature must be noted for both cool and warm or hot pool temperatures. Water temperatures greater than body temperature cause increase in core body temperature greater than that in a land environment, due to differences in thermoregulation. Water temperatures less than body temperature will decrease core temperature and cause shivering in athletes faster and to a greater degree than in the general population, due to athletes' low body fat.[9] Another disadvantage of aquatic exercise utilized for cross-training is that training in water does not allow the athletes to improve or maintain their tolerance to heat while on land.

Contraindications and Precautions

The presence of any open wounds or sores on the patient is a contraindication to aquatic therapy, as are contagious

■ TABLE 15-3 Contraindications for Aquatic Therapy

Untreated infectious disease (patient has a fever/temperature)
Open wounds or unhealed surgical incisions
Contagious skin diseases
Serious cardiac conditions
Seizure disorders (uncontrolled)
Excessive fear of water
Allergy to pool chemicals
Vital capacity of 1 liter
Uncontrolled high- or low blood pressure
Uncontrolled bowel or bladder incontinence
Menstruation without internal protection

Source: Reproduced from Irion, J.M. 2001. Aquatic therapy. In *Therapeutic exercise: Techniques for Intervention,* Bandy, W.D. and B. Sanders, eds. Baltimore: Lippincott, Williams & Wilkins; Sova, R. 1993. *Aquatic activities handbook.* Boston; Jones & Bartlett; Giesecke, C. 1997. In *Aquatic rehabilitation,* Ruoti, R.G., D.M. Morris and A.J. Cole, eds. Philadelphia; Lippincott-Raven; and Thein, J.M., and Thein, L. Brody. 1998. Aquatic-based rehabilitation and training for the elite athlete. *J Orthop Sports Phys Ther* 27(1):32–41.

■ TABLE 15-4 Precautions for the Use of Aquatic Therapy

Recently healed wound or incision, incisions covered by moisture-proof barrier
Altered peripheral sensation
Respiratory dysfunction (asthma)
Seizure disorders controlled with medications
Fear of water

Source: Reproduced from Irion, J.M. 2001. Aquatic therapy. In *Therapeutic exercise techniques for intervention,* Bandy, W.D. and B. Sanders B, eds. Baltimore; Lippincott, Williams & Wilkins; Sova, R. 1993. *Aquatic activities handbook.* Boston: Jones & Bartlett; and Thein, J.M., and Thein L. Brody. 1998. Aquatic-based rehabilitation and training for the elite athlete. *J Orthop Sports Phys Ther* 27(1):32–41.

skin diseases. This restriction is obvious for health reasons to reduce the chance of infection of the patient or others who use the pool.[24,25,32,46] Because of this risk, all surgical wounds must be completely healed or adequately protected using a waterproof barrier before the patient enters the pool. An excessive fear of the water would also be a reason to keep a patient out of an aquatic exercise program. Fever, urinary tract infections, allergies to the pool chemicals, cardiac problems, and uncontrolled seizures are also contraindications (Tables 15-3 and 15-4). Use caution (or waterproof barrier) with medical equipment access sites such as an insulin pump, osteomies, suprapubic appliances, and G tubes. Patients with a tracheotomy need special consideration; they need to remain in waist to chest depth of water to exercise safely in an aquatic environment.

FACILITIES AND EQUIPMENT

When considering an existing facility or when planning to build one, certain characteristics of the pool should be taken into consideration. The pool should not be smaller than 10 feet by 12 feet. It can be in-ground or above-ground as long as access for the patient is well planned. Both a shallow area (2.5 feet) and a deep area (5+feet) should be present to allow standing exercise and swimming or non-standing exercise.[7] The pool bottom should be flat and the depth gradations clearly marked. Water temperature will vary depending on the clientele that is served. For the athlete, recommended pool temperature should be 26 to 28 degrees Celsius (79 to 82 degrees Fahrenheit) but may depend on the available facility.[49] The water temperature suggested by the Arthritis Foundation for their programs is 29 to 31 degrees Celsius (85 to 89 degrees Fahrenheit).

Depending on the type of condition, the patient's perception of the water temperature may differ.

Some prefabricated pools come with an in-water treadmill, exercise bike, or current-producing device (Figures 15-9 to 15-11). These devices can be beneficial but are not essential to treatment. An aquatic program will benefit from variety of types of equipment to allow increasing levels of resistance and assistance, and also to motivate the patient.[37] Catalog companies and sporting goods stores are good resources for obtaining equipment. There are many styles and variations available

in regard to equipment: the athletic trainer will need to select equipment depending on the needs of the program. Creative use 1 of floation support or even the use of actual sport equipment (baseball bats, tennis racquets, golf clubs, etc.) (see Figures 15-1 and 15-12) is helpful to incorporate sport-specific activities that challenge the athlete. Use of mask and snorkel will allow options for prone activities/swimming (see Figures 15-13 and 15-14). Instruction in the proper use of the mask and snorkel is essential for the patient's comfort and safety. Equipment aids for aquatic therapy or so-called pool toys

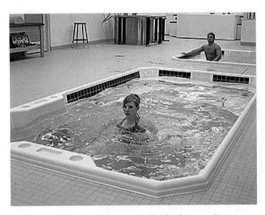

Figure 15-9   The Hydroworx Pool. This pool's even, controllable water flow allows for the application of individualized prescriptive exercise and therapeutic programs. As many as three patients can be treated simultaneously.

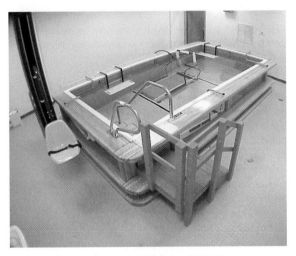

Figure 15-10   Custom pool with treadmill.

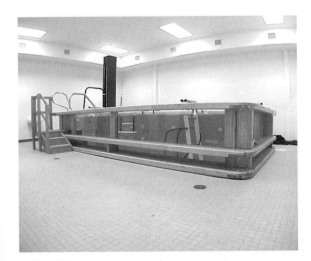

Figure 15-11   Custom pool environment.

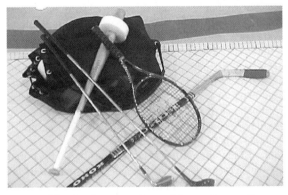

Figure 15-12   Sports equipment for use in aquatic environment.

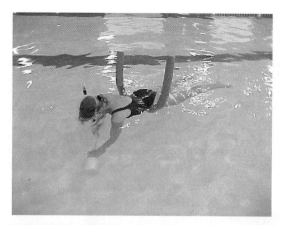

Figure 15-13   Prone kayak movement using mask and snorkel. Challenges the upper extremities and promotes stabilization of the trunk.

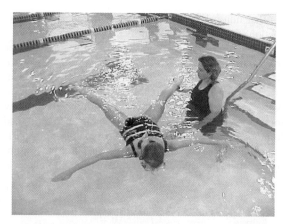

Figure 15-14   Prone hip abduction/adduction with manual resistance by athletic trainer. Note use of mask and snorkel, allowing the patient to maintain proper trunk and head/neck position.

are limited in their utilization only by the imagination of the athletic trainer. What is important is to stimulate the patient's interest in therapy and to keep in mind what goals are to be accomplished.

The clothing of the athletic trainer is an important consideration. Secondary to the close proximity of the athletic trainer to the patient with some treatments, wearing swimwear that covers portions of the lower extremities and upper trunk/upper extremities is an important aspect of professionalism in the aquatic environment. Footwear is another important consideration for the athletic trainer as well as the patient. Proper aquatic footwear provides stability and traction, prevents injuries, and maintains good foot position.

WATER SAFETY

There are a number of patients referred for aquatic therapy that are uncomfortable in the water due to minimal experience in an aquatic environment. Swimming ability is not necessary to participate in an aquatic exercise program, but instruction of water safety skills will allow for a satisfying experience for the patient. Initially, patients may need an exercise bar or flotation noodle to assist with balance during ambulation in water. When adding supine or prone activities into the patient's program, it is important to instruct the individual how to assume that position and return to upright position. This initial act will decrease fear and stress for the patient and also decrease stress to the injured area.

AQUATIC TECHNIQUES

Aquatic techniques and activities can be designed to begin as active assistive movements and progress to strengthening and eccentric control. Activities are selected based on several factors:

Type of injury/surgery/condition
Treatment protocols, if appropriate
Results/muscle imbalances found in evaluation
Goals/expected return to activities as stated by the patient
Aquatic programs are designed similar to land-based
    programs, with the following components:
Warm-up
Mobility activities
Strengthening activities
Balance or neuromuscular-response type of activities
Endurance/cardiovascular activities
Cool down/stretching

With these general considerations in mind, the following sections provide examples of aquatic exercises for the upper extremity, trunk, and lower extremity in a three-phase rehabilitation progression. What has been omitted in the current discussion, from the four-phase rehabilitation scheme used throughout this textbook, is the initial pain-control phase. It is assumed that by the time the patient arrives for aquatic therapy, he or she has undergone previous treatment to manage acute injuries and painful conditions. Subsequently, the patient is ready to begin phases two through four of the four-phase approach.

Upper Extremity

The goal of rehabilitation is to restore function by restoring motion and rhythm of movement of all joints of the upper extremity. Aquatic therapy may be used for treatment of the shoulder complex, elbow, wrist, and hand as one of the interventions to accomplish goals along with a land-based program. The following sections describe a rehabilitation progression for shoulder complex dysfunction.

Initial Level.   The patient can be started at chest-deep water to allow for support of the scapular/thoracic area. Walking forward, backward, and sideways will allow for warm-up, working on natural arm swing, and restoration of normal scapulothoracic motions, rotation, and rhythm. Initiation of activities to work on glenohumeral motions can be started at the wall (patient with back against the wall); having the patient in neck- or shoulder-deep water gives the patient physical cues as to posture and quality of movement. The primary goal during the early phase is for the athletic trainer and patient to be aware of the amount of movement available without compensatory shoulder elevation. The other options for positions during early treatment are supine and prone. The patient will need flotation equipment for cervical, lumbar, and lower-extremity support in order to have good positioning when supine (Fig. 15-15).

Supine activities include stretching, mobilization, and range of motion. Stabilizing the scapula with one hand, the athletic trainer can work on glenohumeral motion with the patient (Figure 15-16). The patient can initiate active movement in shoulder abduction and extension.

Prone activity can be done depending on the patient's comfort in water and use of mask and snorkel. Flotation support around the pelvis allows the patient to concentrate on movement. The patient is able to perform pendulum-type movements, proprioceptive neuromuscular facilitation (PNF) diagonals, and straight-plane movement patterns (flexion/extension and horizontal abduction/adduction) in pain-free range. For the patient not comfortable with the prone position, an alternative position is the pendulum position or the standing position.

Deep-water activity can also be integrated for conditioning/endurance building in early stages of rehabilitation. It is important for the patient to perform in the pain-free range when performing endurance type activities.

Intermediate Level.   The program can be progressed to challenge strength by using equipment to resist motion through the pain-free range. Increasing the surface area of the extremity or increasing the length of the lever arm will increase the difficulty of the activity. As the patient progresses into this phase, the limitations of the standing position become apparent. The athlete can work to the 90 degree angle but not overhead without exiting the water. It is important for the patient to maintain a neutral position of the spine and pelvic area to avoid injury and substitution patterns when performing strengthening activities while standing.

The patient will be able to progress with scapular stabilization from standing to supine and prone positions. Supine and prone positioning can allow for more functional movement patterns and core stabilization of the scapular muscles. Flotation assistance from equipment (Fig. 15-17) as well as use of mask and snorkel will allow

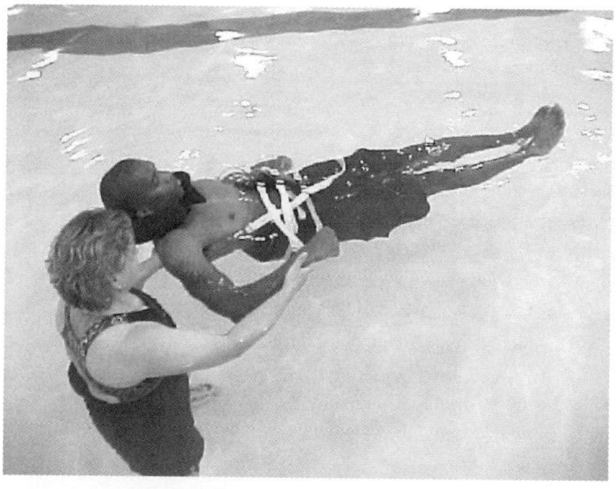

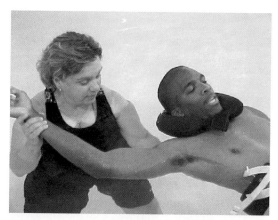

Figure 15-15   Internal and external rotation in supine position. Note appropriate floatation support for the patient.

Figure 15-16   Range of motion with scapular stabilization.

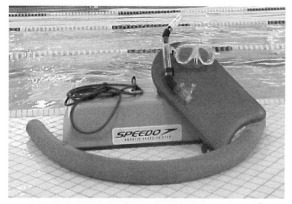

Figure 15-17 Other pool equipment: underwater step, mask and snorkel, kickboard, and tubing.

for proper cervical and spine positioning during prone activities (Refer to Figures 15-13, and 15-14). Activities such as PNF diagonal patterns can be performed with resistance in the pain-free range. Alternate shoulder flexion, "kayaking" type motion (Figure 15-13), and horizontal shoulder abduction/adduction can all be performed using various types of equipment or manual resistance provided by the athletic trainer. Supine positioning allows for work on shoulder extension as well as activities to work on internal and external rotation, at varying degrees of abduction (Figure 15-18). The land-based program and aquatic program should be coordinated to ensure continued improvement of strength, endurance, and function. The goal of treatment in the intermediate-level activities is development of strength and eccentric control throughout increasing ranges of motion.

Final Level. The goal of this level of treatment is high-level functional strengthening and training. Equally important is the transition from the aquatic environment to the land environment. Utilizing sport equipment in treatment, if applicable, will keep an athlete motivated and working toward the goal of returning to sport. Increasing the resistance by using elastic or flotation attachments will keep it challenging (Figures 15-19 and 15-20). As in the intermediate level, the patient needs to be involved in a strengthening and training program on land.

CLINICAL DECISION MAKING	Exercise 15–4

A 17-year-old high school baseball pitcher has undergone an ulnar collateral ligament repair of his dominant (right) elbow that used an autogenous graft. According to the post-operative protocol, resistive exercises at the elbow must be avoided for the next 4 weeks and a motion-limiting elbow brace must be worn during all activities for 5 weeks after surgery. How might aquatic exercises be used for this patient after the fifth week? Are there any precautions that must be observed?

Spine Dysfunction

The unloading capability of water allows the patient ease of movement and some potential relief of symptoms. Patients will need to be shown how to obtain and maintain the neutral spine position in the water even if they have been instructed on land. The neutral spine position is the basis of treatment in land and water and will be progressed in level of difficulty. Activities of the trunk, upper

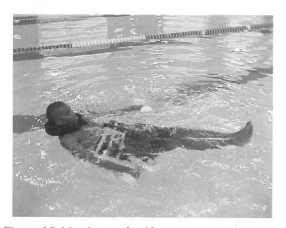

Figure 15-18 Supine shoulder extension can be done at multiple angles.

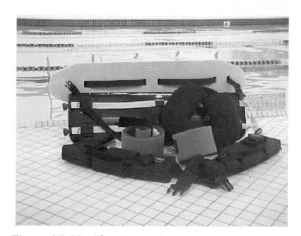

Figure 15-19 Flotation equipment.

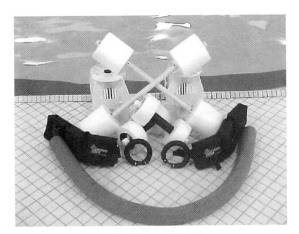

Figure 15-20   Equipment used for resistance or floatation.

extremities, and lower extremities all challenge trunk stability, strength, total body balance, and neuromuscular control. Directional movement preferences for relief of symptoms, such as extension- or flexion-based exercises, can be integrated into the program. Pregnant patients and patients who experience back pain would benefit from exercising in an aquatic environment.

Initial Level.   The patient in neutral spine position is instructed to take a partial squat position with back against the wall. Use of the pool wall provides the patient with a mechanism to monitor his or her ability to maintain the neutral position during activities. Upper- and lower-extremity activities can be progressed to incorporate the patient's ability to stabilize without increasing symptoms.

Use of deep-water activities can be initiated early in rehabilitation. The patient should maintain a vertical

position while performing small controlled movements of the upper and lower extremities. The Burdenko approach to aquatic activities utilizes deep-water activities before activities in shallow water. If dealing with radicular (sciatica) type symptoms, a trial of deep-water traction can be done. Flotation support of the upper body and trunk and placement of light weights on the ankles allows for gentle distraction of the lumbar spine. The patient can hang while performing small pedaling motions as if bicycling/walking.[30]

Working on normalizing the gait pattern and developing the ability to bear weight equally on the lower extremities in any depth of water comfortable to the patient is important early in the therapeutic progression. Incorporation of activities to help centralize the symptoms are important, as well as encouraging the patient to perform only activities that maintain or diminish symptoms during the session. Gentle stretching and rotation movements can be performed in the pain-free range to increase pelvic and lumbar spine mobility.

Intermediate Level.   At this level the patient is progressed away from the wall, and equipment is used to challenge the patient's ability to stabilize. Kickboards can be used to mimic pushing, pulling, and lifting motions (Figures 15-21 and 15-22). Equipment that resists upper-extremity or lower-extremity movements in a single-leg stance or lunge positions challenges the patient's balance and stabilization of abdominal and pelvic muscles (Figure 15-23).

The patient's ability to stabilize can be further challenged using deep-water activities that require maintaining a vertical position while bringing knees to chest and progressing to tucking and rolling type movement (Figures 15-24 to 15-26). Activities can be created to

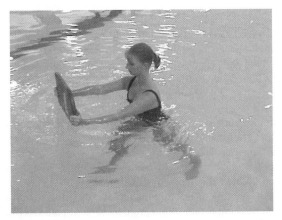

Figure 15-21   Trunk stabilization against anterior/posterior forces.

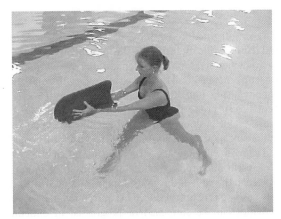

Figure 15-22   Trunk stabilization against oblique/diagonal forces.

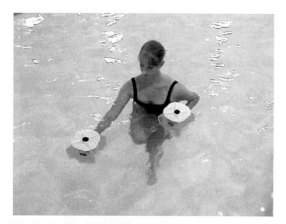

Figure 15-23 Challenging lower-extremity neuro-muscular control and balance as well as trunk control in single-limb stance, utilizing upper-extremity resistance.

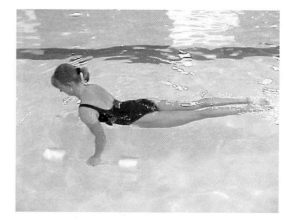

Figure 15-24 Tuck-and-roll exercise, extended position.

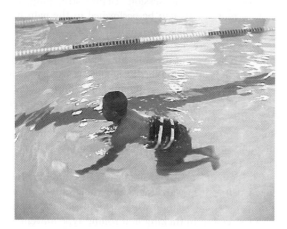

Figure 15-25 Tuck-and-roll exercise, tuck position.

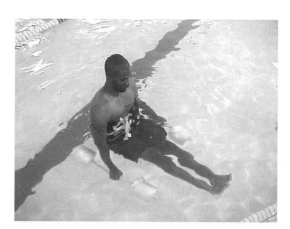

Figure 15-26 Tuck-and-roll exercise, pike position.

work on diagonal and rotational motions of the spine and trunk, while maintaining the neutral position.

Activities in a supine position are effective for increasing trunk mobility and then progressing to work on trunk stability using Bad Ragaz techniques (Figure 15-27).[15] Activities in prone position allow for challenges to the neutral spine position, and the patient may need flotation equipment to accomplish that goal. The use of the mask and snorkel will allow for proper positioning of the spine while performing the activities. It is important to monitor and teach the patient the neutral spine position with each new position that is introduced in the treatment program. Activities can be simplified or progressed in difficulty according to patient's level of function or their ability to maintain the neutral spine position.

Final Level. Depending on the patient's needs and functional goals related to return to a desired level of activity, the program can be modified and progressed. For the patient returning to a demanding occupation, development of a program of lifting/pushing/pulling or other needs described by the patient can complement a work-conditioning program. For the patient returning to a sport, the athletic trainer and athlete can work together to develop specific challenging activities. The athletic trainer needs to be creative with the use of aquatic equipment and should use equipment specific to the athlete's sport to challenge him or her to a higher level of trunk stabilization. It is important to integrate movement patterns that are opposites of the ones the athlete normally performs in his or her sport. (For example, if a gymnast or ice skater

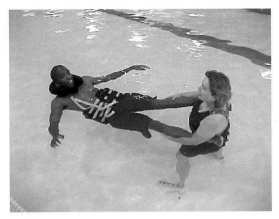

Figure 15-27 Bad Ragaz technique for oblique trunk stabilization.

predominantly turns or rotates in one direction, have them practice turns in the opposite direction.) The aquatic environment provides the athlete an alternate environment in which to train, which should be encouraged for the serious athlete to avoid overuse-type of conditions that can occur. Especially important in this phase is the reintegration of the patient into treatment and training on land, as the water environment does not allow for normal speeds and forces experienced on land.

Lower-Extremity Injuries

Aquatic therapy is a common modality for rehabilitation of many injuries of the lower extremity because of the properties of unloading and hydrostatic pressure. At an early phase of healing, the patient may need to use a flotation belt, vest, exercise bars, noodles, and various other buoyancy devices to provide support (Figure 15-20), depending on pain and how long they have been non-weightbearing. The aquatic environment allows for limited weight bearing and restoration of gait by calculating the percentage of weight bearing allowed and weight of the patient and then placing the patient in an appropriate depth of water.

Initial Level. The expected goals at this phase of rehabilitation are the return of normal motion and early strengthening of affected and unaffected muscles. The restoration of normal and functional gait pattern is also desired. Performing backward- and sideways walking adds a functional dimension to the program in addition to traditional forward walking. Range-of-motion activities may involve active motions of the hip, knee, and ankle. Utilizing cuffs, noodles, or kickboards under the foot will assist with increasing motion. Exercises for strengthening

noninvolved joints such as hips or ankles can be done with the patient who has had a knee injury. However, it is important to remember that resistance may need to be placed above the injured knee to decrease torque forces on the knee. It is important to integrate conditioning and balance activities within this initial level. Standing activities are to be performed with attention to maintaining the spine in a neutral position as well as to challenging balance and neuromuscular control in the lower extremity (Figure 15-23).

Deep-water activities will allow for conditioning and cross-training opportunities (Figures 15-3 and 15-28). The patient may need more assistance initially with flotation devices, but can progress to decreasing the amount of flotation when able. For the patient who must be non-weightbearing secondary to an injury or surgery, the deep water allows for a workout along with maintaining strength in uninvolved joints. Activities can involve running, bicycling, cross-country skiing, and incorporating sport-specific activities (Figure 15-29).

The athletic trainer can also incorporate activities performed in the supine position. The patient will need to be supported with flotation equipment that will allow him or her to float evenly. The athletic trainer can stabilize at the feet and have the patient work on active hip and knee flexion and extension to work on increasing range of motion at the affected joint (Figure 15-30). Resistance of hip abduction and adduction can also be performed in a supine position. Again, attention must be paid to the location of applied force. Resistance of the uninvolved leg movement will also allow for strengthening of the injured extremity.

Intermediate Level. Depending on the injury, surgery, or condition, the patient can be progressed to the

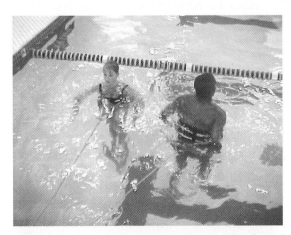

Figure 15-28 Patients running forward and backward against tubing resistance.

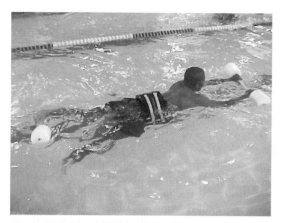

Figure 15-29 Supported single-lower-extremity running movement. Note the appropriate support of the patient with buoyancy belts and upper-extremity bell and lower-extremity bell under the stationary LE. Also challenges trunk stabilization.

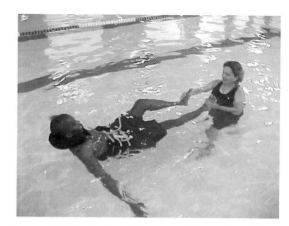

Figure 15-30 Supine alternating hip and knee flexion and extension, using Bad Ragaz technique. Hand contact by athletic trainer gives the athlete cues for movement.

intermediate level when appropriate. The activities can be progressed by use of weights or flotation cuffs to increase difficulty. As in the initial level, resistance may need to be placed more proximally with anterior crucial ligament injuries/surgeries and other ligament injuries. Performing circuits of straight-plane and diagonal patterns with both lower extremities can be progressed by performing with upper-extremity support on the wall and progressing to no support. The patient can stand on an uneven surface, such as a noodle or cuff, to challenge balance and stabilization. Eccentric, closed-chain activities can be performed in the shallow water with the patient standing on a noodle or kickboard for single-leg reverse squats, and utilizing a noodle, kickboard, or bar for bilateral reverse-squat motions in

deep water (Figure 15-31) and progressing to a single-leg reverse squat.

Performing deep-water tether running or sprinting forward and backward for increasing periods of time will allow for overall conditioning. The patient can progress to running in shallower water depending upon the condition of injury or surgery (Fig. 15-32).

Supine activities can be continued with emphasis on strengthening and stabilization of the trunk, pelvis, and lower extremities. Placement of the athletic trainer's resistance will depend on the patient's strength, ability to stabilize, and how much time has elapsed since surgery or injury. Increasing the number of repetitions and/or speed of movement will provide more resistance and work on fatiguing muscle groups of the lower extremity. The prone

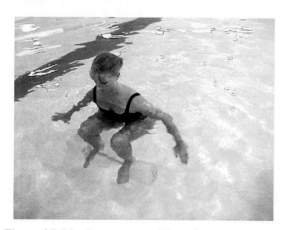

Figure 15-31 Reverse squat, bilateral.

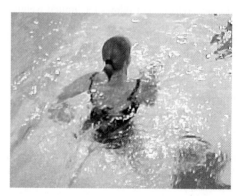

Figure 15-32 Patient running against tether.

position provides increased challenges to the patient to perform hip abduction and adduction along with hip and knee flexion and extension. The patient can use mask and snorkel or flotation equipment to help with positioning while in the prone position.

Sport-specific activities can be integrated into the program for the athlete. While practicing movement patterns needed for sport, the patient can start at chest depth and progress to shallow water. As with spine rehabilitation, there is benefit from practicing opposite movement patterns such as turns and jumps. The aquatic environment will allow for early initiation of a structured jumping and landing program. Some adaptations and proper instruction to the patient will provide positive effects similar to those seen in land-based programs.[34] Progression to the land-based jump and land program is recommended when appropriate.

Final Level. In the final level, the patient is involved with a high-level strengthening and training program. The aquatic program can and should be used to complement the land program. The patient can continue to practice sport-specific activities in varying levels of water. Decreasing the use of flotation equipment can increase the difficulty with deep-water activities. Using buoyancy cuffs on the ankles without using a flotation belt will challenge the athlete's ability to stabilize and perform running in deep water. Endurance training in an aquatic environment is a good alternative for the healthy athlete's conditioning programs and may help prevent further injuries. As with the upper extremity, this phase also requires integration of aquatic- and land-based exercises to successfully transition the athlete to full participation in sport on land.

CLINICAL DECISION MAKING   **Exercise 15–5**

A 20-year-old female collegiate basketball player was injured and sustained a left ACL tear. She had a surgical repair utilizing the hamstring graft. How soon can she begin with activities in the aquatic environment, and what would be the goals of early intervention?

SPECIAL TECHNIQUES

Bad Ragaz Ring Method

Bad Ragaz technique originated in the thermal pools of Bad Ragaz, Switzerland in the 1930s, but continues to evolve through the years. As a method, it focuses on muscle reeducation, strengthening, spinal traction/elongation, relaxation, and tone inhibition.[15] The properties of water—including buoyancy, turbulence, hydrostatic pressure, and surface tension—provide dynamic environmental forces during activities. The PNF patterns (see Chapter 14) add a three-dimensional aspect to this method. Movement of the patient's body through the water provides the resistance.[40] The turbulent drag produced from movement is in direct relation to the patient's speed of movement. The athletic trainer provides the movement when the patient works on isometric (stabilization) patterns, but the athletic trainer is in the stable/fixed position when the patient is performing isokinetic or isotonic activities (Figures 15-27 and 15-30).[15] Stretching and lengthening responses can be obtained with passive or relaxed response from patient; the athletic trainer needs to support and stabilize body segments to obtain desired response.

Awareness of body mechanics and prevention of injury are important to the athletic trainer when performing resistive Bad Ragaz type activities. The athletic trainer should stand in waist-deep water, not deeper than T8-10[15] and wear aqua shoes for traction and stability. The athletic trainer should stand with one foot in front of the other, with knees slightly bent and legs shoulder-width apart, to compensate for the long-lever arm force of the patient.

Burdenko Method

The Burdenko method utilizes motion as the principle healing intervention. According to Burdenko,[5,43] the components of dynamic healing include patterns of movement, injury assessment, and rehabilitation exercises that occur with the patient in a standing position; the psychology of the injured patient benefiting from pain-free movement, and blood flow and neural stimulation being enhanced by activity.[5] Six essential qualities are necessary for perfecting and maintaining the art of movement: balance, coordination, flexibility, endurance, speed, and strength. Burdenko advocates the presentation of these qualities in exercise activities in the previously stated order. The activities are designed to challenge the center of buoyancy and center of gravity. Treatments/activities are initiated in deep water and incorporate shallow-water activities as the patient succeeds by demonstrating control of movement while maintaining neutral vertical position. Integration of land exercise along with the aquatic activity addresses functional movement patterns. For further information on this technique, see the suggested readings at the end of the chapter.

Halliwick Method

The Halliwick method is commonly used to teach individuals with physical disabilities to swim and to learn balance control in water.[19] Developed by James McMillan, the Halliwick method or concept is based on a "Ten Point Programme."[8] This method is frequently utilized with the pediatric population but portions of the technique can be utilized to improve and restore a patient's balance. Use of turbulence forces can assist in developing strategies for maintaining balance, or challenge the patient to maintain a stable posture during a change in the direction of force. For example, the patient maintains a single-leg stance while the athletic trainer or another person runs around the patient (Figure 15-33). More information on the Halliwick technique is also available in the suggested readings at the end of the chapter.

CLINICAL DECISION MAKING　　　　　**Exercise 15–6**

A 12-year-old female involved in high-level gymnastics has complaints of low back pain with 5- to 6-hour training sessions 5 to 6 days per week. She is diagnosed with grade 1 spondylolisthesis at L4-5. What is a key principle or position that she needs to be taught, and how can aquatic activities complement your land program?

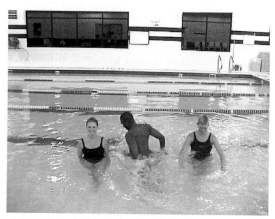

Figure 15-33 Balance and neuromuscular control restoration technique for trunk and single lower extremity. This exercise demonstrates the use of the principle of turbulence, generated in the Halliwick technique to challenge the stability of the patient.

CONCLUSIONS

Aquatic rehabilitation is usually not the exclusive intervention option for most patients. The aquatic environment offers many positive psychological and physiological effects during the early rehabilitation phase of injury.[31,40] However, in subsequent phases of rehabilitation, it is typical to use combinations of land- and water-based interventions to achieve rehabilitation goals. Because humans function in a "gravity environment," the transition from water to land is necessary for full rehabilitation for most patients. Some patients utilize the aquatic environment for continued strengthening and conditioning programs secondary to a painful response to land-based activities. Examples of this include those patients with pain that occurs with compressive forces at joints (such as cases of disc dysfunction, spinal stenosis, and osteoarthritis), as well as chronic neuromuscular dysfunction such as multiple sclerosis.

This chapter provides information regarding indications and benefits as well as contraindications and precautions of the aquatic environment for rehabilitation. Suggestions and exercises are offered to help the athletic trainer to incorporate aquatic exercise into a rehabilitation program. Utilizing the principles provided and the examples of activities, the athletic trainers can use their judgment, skill, and especially their creativity to develop an exercise program to meet their patient's goals. The old English proverb says "We never know the worth of water 'til the well is dry.'" The worth and value of aquatic therapy as an intervention cannot be fully understood and appreciated until experienced and additional research is completed.

Summary

1. The buoyant force counteracts the force of gravity as it assists motion toward the water's surface and resists motion away from the surface.
2. Because of differences in the specific gravity of the body, the head and chest tend to float higher in the water than the heavier, denser extremities, making compensation with floatation devices necessary.

3. The three forces that oppose movement in the water are the cohesive force, the bow force, and the drag force.
4. Aquatic therapy allows for fine gradations of exercise, increased control over the percentage of weight bearing, increased range of motion and strength in weak patients, and decreased pain and increased confidence in functional movements.

5. Pool size and depth, water temperature, and specific pool equipment will vary depending on the patients being treated and resources available to the athletic trainer.

6. Application of the principle of buoyancy allows for progression of exercises.

7. Upper- and lower-extremity activities both require and provide a challenge to trunk and core stability.

8. The special techniques exclusive to the aquatic environment can be used to complement traditional land-based therapeutic interventions.

9. Aquatic therapy can help stimulate interest, motivation, and exercise compliance in pediatric, geriatric, neurological, and athletic patients.

10. The aquatic environment is an excellent medium to facilitate speedy functional return to work, activities of daily living, and sport.

11. It is typical to use a combination of land- and water-based therapeutic exercise protocols to achieve rehabilitation goals.

References

1. Arrigo, C., ed. 1992. Aquatic rehabilitation. *Sports Med Update* 7(2).

2. Arrigo, C. C. S. Fuller and K. E., Wilk 1992. Aquatic rehabilitation following ACL-PTG reconstruction. *Sports Med Update* 7(2):22–27.

3. Broach, E.D., Groff R., Yaffe J., Dattilo and D., Gast. 1995. Effects of aquatics therapy on physical behavior of adult with multiple sclerosis. Paper presented at the 1995 Leisure Research Symposium, San Antonio, TX. Available at www.indiana.edu/?lrs/lrs95/ebroach95.html. Accessed on October 5, 2005.

4. Burdenko, I.N. 2002. Sport-specific exercises after injuries—the Burdenko method. Paper presented at the Aquatic Therapy Symposium 2002, August 22–25, Orlando, FL.

5. Butts, N.K., M. Tucker, and C. Greening. 1991. Physiologic responses to maximal treadmill and deep water running in men and women. *Am J Sports Med* 19(6):612–614.

6. Campion, M.R. 1997. *Hydrotherapy: Principles and practice.* New York: Butterworth-Heinemann.

7. Cole, A., and B. Becker. 2004. *Comprehensive aquatic therapy,* 2nd ed. Philadelphia: Butterworth-Heinemann.

8. Cunningham, J. 1997. Halliwick method. In *Aquatic rehabilitation,* Ruoti, R., and D. Morris, eds. Philadelphia: Lippincott-Raven.

9. Cureton, K.J. 1997. Physiologic responses to water exercise. In *Aquatic rehabilitation,* Ruoti, R., and D. Morris, eds. Philadelphia: Lippincott-Raven.

10. Dioffenbach, L. 1991. Aquatic therapy services. *Clin Manage* 11(1):14–19.

11. Dougherty, N.J. 1990. Risk management in aquatics. *J Health Phys Educ Recreation Dance* (May/June):46–48.

12. Edlich, R.F., M.A. Towler, and R.J. Goitz, et al. 1987. Bioengineering principles of hydrotherapy. *J Burn Care Rehabil* 8(6):580–584.

13. Eyestone, E.D., G. Fellingham, J. George, and G. Fisher. 1993. Effect of water running and cycling on maximum oxygen consumption and 2 mile run performance. *Am J Sports Med* 21(1):41–44.

14. Fawcett, C.W. 1992. Principles of aquatic rehab: A new look at hydrotherapy. *Sports Med Update* 7(2):6–9.

15. Garrett, G. 1997. Bad Ragaz ring method. In *Aquatic rehabilitation,* Ruoti, R.G., and D.M. Morris, and A.J., Cole, eds. Philadelphia: Lippincott-Raven.

16. Geigle, P., K. Daddona, and K. Finken, et al. 2001. The effects of a supplemental aquatic physical therapy program on balance and girth for NCAA division III athletes with a grade I or II lateral ankle sprain. *J Aquatic Phys Ther* 9(1):13–20.

17. Genuario, S.E., and J.J. Vegso. 1990. The use of a swimming pool in the rehabilitation and reconditioning of athletic injuries. *Contemp Orthop* 20(4):381–387.

18. Grosse, G. 2004. Safety standards for aquatic therapy and rehabilitation practitioners. *Aquatic Therapy Journal* 6(2):24–26.

19. Grosse, S., and J. Lambeck. 2004. The Halliwick method: A comparison of applications to swim instruction and aquatic therapy. *Journal of the International Council for Health, Physical Education, Recreation, Sport & Dance* 40(4):31.

20. Haralson, K.M. 1985. Therapeutic pool programs. *Clin Manage* 5(2):10–13.

21. Harrison, R., and S. Bulstrode. 1987. Percentage weight bearing during partial immersion in the hydrotherapy pool. *Physiother Pract* 3:60–63.

22. Hertler, L., M. Provost-Craig, D. Sestili, A. Hove, and M. Fees. 1992. Water running and the maintenance of maximal oxygen consumption and leg strength in runners. *Med Sci Sports Exerc* 24(5):S23.

23. Hinesly, D. 2008. Water-based work rehab. *Rehab Management: The Interdisciplinary Journal of Rehabilitation* 21(5):20.

24. Hurley, R., and C. Turner. 1991. Neurology and aquatic therapy. *Clin Manage* 11(1):26–27.

25. Irion, J.M. Aquatic therapy. In *Therapeutic exercise: Techniques for intervention,* Bandy, W.D., and B. Sanders, eds. Baltimore: Lippincott, Williams & Wilkins.

26. Kersey, R., and S. West. 2005. Aquatic therapy. *Athletic Therapy Today* 10(5):48–49.

27. Kittell, S. 2006. In the swim: Aquatic therapy has recently grown in popularity as a favored course of rehabilitation. *Rehab Management: The Interdisciplinary Journal of Rehabilitation* 19(10):28–30.

28. Koszuta, L.E. 1989. From sweats to swimsuits: Is water exercise the wave of the future? *Physician Sports Med* 17(4):203–206.

29. Levin, S. 1991. Aquatic therapy. *Physician Sports Med* 19(10):119–126.

30. McNamara, C., and L. Thein. 1997. Aquatic rehabilitation of musculoskeletal conditions of the spine. In *Aquatic rehabilitation*, Ruoti, R.G., D.M. Morris, and A.J. Cole, eds. Philadelphia: Lippincott-Raven.

31. McWaters, J.G. 1992. For faster recovery just add water. *Sports Med Update* 7(2):4–5.

32. Meyer, R.I. 1990. Practice settings for kinesiotherapy-aquatics. *Clin Kinesiol* 44(1):12–13.

33. Michaud, T.L., D.K. Brennan, R.P. Wilder, and N.W. Sherman. 1992. Aquarun training and changes in treadmill running maximal oxygen consumption. *Med Sci Sports Exerc* 24(5):S23.

34. Miller, M.G., D.C. Berry, R. Gilders, and S. Bullard. 2001. Recommendations for implementing an aquatic plyometric program. *Strength Cond J* 23(6):28–35.

35. Morris, D.M. 2004. Aquatic rehabilitation for the treatment of neurologic disorders. In *Comprehensive aquatic therapy*, Cole, A.J., and B.E. Becker, eds. Philadelphia: Butterworth-Heinemann.

36. Nolte-Heuritsch, I. 1990. *Aqua rhythmics: Exercises for the swimming pool*. New York: Sterling.

37. Paterson, C. 2006. Using an underwater exercise bike: therapeutics and fitness combined. *Aquatic Therapy Journal* 9(2):11–14.

38. Petersen, T.M. 2004. Pediatric aquatic therapy. In *Comprehensive aquatic therapy*, Cole, A.J., and B.E. Becker, eds. Philadelphia: Butterworth-Heinemann.

39. Pigliapoco, P. and P. Benelli. 2005. Aquatic rehabilitation for orthopedic trauma: Part one. *Aquatic Therapy Journal* 7(2):21–24.

40. Pigliapoca, P. and P. Benelli. 2006. Aquatic rehabilitation for orthopedic trauma: Part two. *Aquatic Therapy Journal* 8(2):17–19.

41. Pöyhönen, T., H. Kyröläinen, K.L. Keskinen, A. Hautala, J. Savolainen, and E. Mälkiä. 2001. Electromyographic and kinematic analysis of therapeutic knee exercises under water. *Clin Biomech* 16:496–504.

42. Pöyhönen, T.K., L. Keskinen A., Hautala, and E. Mälkiä. 2000. Determination of hydrodynamic drag forces and drag coefficients on human leg/foot model during knee exercise. *Clin Biomech* 19:256–260.

43. Ray, P., and T. Galloway. 2006. Implementing the Burdenko Method with children. *Aquatic Therapy* 9(2):16–20.

44. Robertson, J.M., E.A. Brewster, and K.I. Factora 2001. Comparison of heart rates during water running in deep and shallow water at the same rating of perceived exertion. *J Aquatic Phys Ther* 9(1):21–26.

45. Simmons, V. and P.D. Hansen. 1996. Effectiveness of water exercise on postural mobility in the well elderly: An experimental study on balance enhancement. *J Gerontol* 51A(5): M233–M238.

46. Sova, R. 1993. *Aquatic activities handbook*. Boston: Jones & Bartlett.

47. Speer, K., J.T. Cavanaugh, R.F. Warren, L. Day, and T.L. Wickiewicz. 1993. A role for hydrotherapy in shoulder rehabilitation. *Am J Sports Med* 21(6):850–853.

48. Svendenhag, J., and J. Seger. 1992. Running on land and in water: Comparative exercise physiology. *Med Sci Sports Exerc* 24(10):1195–1160.

49. Thein, J.M., L. Thein Brody. 1998. Aquatic-based rehabilitation and training for the elite athlete. *J Orthop Sports Phys Ther* 27(1):32–41.

50. Town, G.P., and S.S. Bradley. 1991. Maximal metabolic responses of deep and shallow water running in trained runners. *Med Sci Sports Exerc* 23(2):238–241.

51. Triggs, M. 1991. Orthopedic aquatic therapy. *Clin Manage* 11(1):30–31.

52. Wilder, R.P., D. Brennan, and D. Schotte. 1993. A standard measure for exercise prescription and aqua running. *Am J Sports Med* 21(1):45–48.

Suggested Readings

Berger, M.A., G. deGroot, and A.P. Hollander. 1995. Hydrodynamic drag and lift forces on human hand/arm models. *J Biomech* 28(2):125–133.

Burdenko, J., and E. Connors. 1990. *Ultimate power of resistance*. Igor Publishing. [available only through mail order].

Burdenko, J., and J. Miller. 2001. *Defying gravity*. Igor Publishing. [available only through mail order].

Campion, M.R. 1990. *Adult hydrotherapy: A practical approach*. Oxford: Heinemann Medical.

Cassady, S.L., and D.H. Nielsen. 1992. Cardiorespiratory responses of healthy subjects to calisthenics performed on land versus in water. *Phys Ther* 72(7):532–538.

Christie, J.L., L.M. Sheldahl, and F.E. Tristani. 1990. Cardiovascular regulation during head-out water immersion exercise. *J Appl Physiol* 69(2):657–664.

Frangolias, D.D., and E.C. Rhodes. 1995. Maximal and ventilatory threshold responses to treadmill and water immersion running. *Med Sci Sports Exerc* 27(7):1007–1013.

Green, J.H., N.T. Cable, and N. Elms. 1990. Heart rate and oxygen consumption during walking on land and in deep water. *J Sports Med Phys Fitness* 30(1):49–52.

Martin, J. 1981. The Halliwick method. *Physiotherapy* 67:288–291.

Sova, R. 1993. *Aquatic activities handbook*. Boston: Jones & Bartlett.

SOLUTIONS TO CLINICAL DECISION MAKING EXERCISES

16-1 This individual can begin initial activities when active assistive motion is allowed. Activities in this phase might include shoulder elevation (flexion and abduction) while standing in shoulder-deep water utilizing the assistance of buoyancy. He will be able to benefit from strengthening and stabilization activities when he progresses to being able to do resistive activities.

16-2 It is important in this example to honor the prescribed weightbearing restrictions imposed after surgery. The aquatic environment is an excellent choice for implementation of early rehabilitation after sufficient incisional healing or adequate coverage with a moisture-proof dressing. This environment is ideal for maintaining or improving range of motion and strength without full weight bearing. Also, the aquatic environment offers the possibility of gradual weightbearing progression and restoration of balance, neuromuscular control, and function.

16-3 The athletic trainer should recommend an alternate environment for maintenance of aerobic function. The aquatic environment is ideal for cross-training applications that decrease or eliminate weight bearing in the lower extremities. Excellent choices might include deep-water running and sport-specific lower-extremity strengthening in a diminished weightbearing application (chest-deep water).

16-4 Initially the aquatic environment is ideal for developing range of motion for elbow flexion and extension.

It can also be used for light resistance training for elbow and shoulder musculature, being very cautious about valgus forces that might occur at the elbow due to drag forces that could occur during upper-extremity adduction and internal rotation motions against water resistance. Exercises could be progressed appropriately to include exercise directed at development of endurance, power, and sport-specific movements (pitching).

16-5 She could begin as soon as incisions are healed, or sooner if a moisture-barrier dressing is used. Goals would be these:
- To control and decrease swelling because of the property of hydrostatic pressure
- To restore gait pattern in an unloaded environment
- To normalize motion in the left knee
- To normalize neuromuscular control
- To initiate and maintain her conditioning level with deep-water activities

Awareness of graft vulnerability occurring at 4 to 8 weeks after surgery must be integrated into the program.

16-6 She needs to be taught neutral position and core strengthening. Activities that are specific to gymnastics and the events she participates in can be practiced and challenged in the aquatic environment. Integrating activities utilizing opposite movement patterns can assist in developing core stabilization.

CHAPTER 16

Functional Progressions and Functional Testing in Rehabilitation

Michael McGee

After completion of this chapter, the athletic training student should be able to do the following:

- Develop the concept of a functional progression.

- Identify the goals of a functional progression.

- Recognize how and when functional progressions should be used in the rehabilitation process.

- Describe the physical benefits associated with a functional progression.

- Identify and describe the psychological benefits associated with a functional progression.

- Generalize the disadvantages associated with a functional progression.

- Incorporate the components of a functional progression.

- Develop a functional progression for a patient.

- Analyze various functional tests.

- Design a functional test for a patient.

In the athletic community, injuries and subsequent disability frequently occur. Disabilities can be described as restrictive influences that "disease and injury exert upon neuromotor performances."[15] Thus, in an effort to reduce the lasting effects of injury, the athletic trainer should direct rehabilitation toward improving neuromuscular coordination and agility, and not simply toward increasing strength and endurance. If rehabilitation is directed toward regaining range of motion, flexibility, strength, and endurance, and perhaps primarily toward increasing neuromuscular coordination and agility, a full return to activity is possible. However, if the program simply provides a means for reducing signs and symptoms associated with the injury, the patient will not return to a safe and effective level of activity.[3] As a result, rehabilitation of athletic injuries needs to focus on return to preinjury activity levels.[26]

Function refers to patterns of motion that use multiple joints acting with various axes and in multiple planes.[19] Traditional rehabilitation techniques, although vital to the return of function, often stress single joints in single planes of motion. To complement traditional rehabilitation, the athletic trainer can use functional rehabilitation techniques. Functional rehabilitation, along with traditional methods, will ready the patient for activity and competition more successfully than if either method is employed alone.

THE ROLE OF FUNCTIONAL PROGRESSIONS IN REHABILITATION

Athletic trainers must adapt rehabilitation to the sports-specific demands of each individual sport and playing position. But rehabilitation programs in a clinical setting cannot predict the ability of the injured part to endure the demands of full competition on the playing field. For example, the complex factors surrounding a solid tackle in competition play cannot be produced in the clinical setting.

The role of the functional progression is to improve and complete the clinical rehabilitation process.[32] A **functional progression** is a succession of activities that simulate actual motor and sport skills, enabling the patient to acquire or reacquire the skills needed to perform athletic endeavors safely and effectively. The athletic trainer takes the activities involved in a given sport and breaks them down into individual components. In this way the patient concentrates on individual parts of the game or activity in a controlled environment before combining them together in an uncontrolled environment as would exist during full competition. The functional progression places stresses and forces on each body system in a well-planned, positive, and progressive fashion, ultimately improving the patient's overall ability to meet the demands of daily activities as well as sport competition. The functional progression is essential in the rehabilitation process, because tissues not placed under performance-level stresses do not adapt to the sudden return of such stresses with the resumption of full activity. Thus, the functional progression is integrated into the normal rehabilitation scheme, as one component of exercise therapy, rather than replacing traditional rehabilitation altogether.[16]

BENEFITS OF USING FUNCTIONAL PROGRESSIONS

Using a functional progression in a rehabilitation program will help the patient and the athletic trainer reach the goals of the entire program. The goals of the functional progression generally include a restoration of (1) joint range of motion, (2) strength, (3) proprioception, (4) agility, and (5) confidence. Achieving these goals allows the patient to reach the desired level of activity safely and effectively.[24] Functional progressions provide both physical and psychological benefits to the injured patient. The physical benefits include improvements in muscular strength and endurance, mobility and flexibility, cardiorespiratory endurance, and neuromuscular coordination, along with an increase in the functional stability of an injured joint. Psychologically, the progression can reduce the feelings of anxiety, apprehension, and deprivation commonly observed in the injured patient.

Improving Functional Stability

Functional stability is provided by (1) passive restraints on the ligaments, (2) joint geometry, (3) active restraints

generated by muscles, and (4) joint compressive forces that occur with activity and force the joint together.[29] Stability is maintained by the neuromuscular control mechanisms involved in proprioception and kinesthesia (as discussed in Chapter 5). Functional stability cannot always be determined by examining the patient in the clinic. Therefore, the functional progression can be used to evaluate functional stability both objectively and subjectively. Can the patient complete all tasks with no adverse affects? Does the patient appear to perform at the same level, or close to the same level, as prior to injury? Performance during a functional task can be evaluated for improvement, and functional testing can be incorporated to provide an objective measure of ability.[16] The patient can also give important feedback regarding function, pain, and stability while performing the functional tasks.

Muscular Strength

Increased strength is a physical benefit of the functional progression. Strength is the ability of the muscle to produce tension or apply force maximally against resistance. This occurs statically or dynamically, in relation to the imposed demands. Strength increases are possible if the load imposed on a muscle exceeds that muscle's anatomic capabilities during exercise. This is commonly referred to as the overload principle and is possible due to increased efficiency in motor unit recruitment and muscle fiber hypertrophy.[20] To see these improvements, the muscle must be worked to the point of fatigue with either high or low resistance. The functional progression will develop strength using the SAID (Specific Adaptation to Imposed Demands) principle. The muscles involved will be strengthened dynamically, under stresses similar to those encountered in competition.

Endurance

Muscular and cardiorespiratory endurance can both be enhanced with a functional progression. Endurance is necessary for long-duration activity, whether in daily living or in the repeated motor functions found with sport participation. The functional progression will enhance muscular endurance through the repetition of the individual activities and their combination into one general activity. The progression provides an environment for improving muscular strength and endurance without using more than one program. Cardiorespiratory endurance can be improved through the repetition of movements involved in the progression in the same way as regular fitness levels improve with continuous exercise.

Flexibility

With injury, tissues will shorten or tighten in response to immobilization. This can inhibit proper function. With a functional progression, the injured area is stressed within a controlled range. This stress should be significant enough to allow the tissue to elongate and return to proper length. This improved mobility and flexibility is crucial to the patient. Strength and endurance do not mean much if the injured body part cannot move through a full range of motion. Tissues also become stronger with consistent stresses, so tissues other than muscle can also be improved with the functional progression.[20]

Muscle Relaxation

Relaxation involves the concerted effort to reduce muscle tension. The functional progression can teach an individual to recognize this tension and eventually control or remove it by consciously relaxing the muscles after exercise. The total body relaxation that can ensue relaxes the injured area, helping to relieve the muscle guarding that can inhibit the joint's full range of motion.[20]

Motor Skills

Coordination, agility, and motor skills are complex aspects of normal function defined as appropriate contractions at the most opportune time and with the appropriate intensity.[20] A patient needs coordination, agility, and motor skills to transform strength, flexibility, and endurance into full-speed performance. This is especially important for an injured patient. If the patient does not regain or improve their coordination and agility, their performance is hampered and can in itself lead to further injury. Repetition and practice are important to learning motor skills. Regular motions that are consciously controlled develop into automatic reactions via motor learning. This is possible due to the constant repetition and reinforcement of a particular skill.[15] To acquire these "automatic reactions," one needs an intact and functional neuromuscular system. Because this system is disturbed by injury, decreases in performance will occur, increasing the potential for injury. The functional progression can be used to minimize the loss of normal neuromuscular control by providing exercises that stress proprioception, motor-skill integration, and proper timing. The functional progression is indicated for improvement in agility and skill because of the constant repetition of sport-specific motor skills, use of sensory cues, and progressive increases in activity levels. Proprioception can be enhanced by stimulating the intra-articular and intramuscular mechanoreceptors. These are all components of, or general principles for, enhancing neuromuscular coordination.[15] The practice variations used with functional progressions allow the patient to relearn the various aspects of their sport that they might encounter in competition.

Rehabilitative exercise programs must stress neuromuscular coordination and agility. Increases in strength, endurance, and flexibility are unquestionably necessary for a safe and effective return to play, but without the neuromuscular coordination to integrate these aspects into proper function, little performance enhancement can occur. For this reason, functional progressions should become an integral part of the long-term rehabilitation stage so that injured patients can maximize their ability to return to competition at their pre-injury level.

PSYCHOLOGICAL AND SOCIAL CONSIDERATIONS

Functional progressions can also provide psychological benefits to the patient. Anxiety, apprehension, and feelings of deprivation are all common emotions found with injuries. The functional progression can aid the rehabilitation process and facilitate the return to play by diminishing these emotions. Chapter 4 discusses the psychological aspects of the rehabilitative process in more detail. This chapter will focus on the specific contributions of the functional progression.

Anxiety

Uncertainty about the future is a reason many patients give for their feelings of anxiety. Patients experience this insecurity because they have only a vague understanding of the severity of their injury and the length of time it will take for them to fully recover.[17] The progression can lessen anxiety because the patient is gradually placed into more demanding situations that allow the patient to experience success and not be concerned as much with failure in the future.

Deprivation

The patient might experience feelings of deprivation after losing direct contact with his team and coaches for an extended period of time. The functional progression can limit such feelings of deprivation, because the patient can exercise during regular team practice times at the practice site. By engaging in an activity that can be completed during practice, the patient remains close in proximity and socially feels little loss in team cohesion.[17]

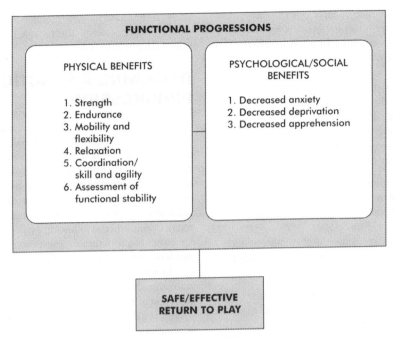

Figure 16-1   Physical and psychological benefits of using functional progressions.

Apprehension

Apprehension is often listed as an obstacle to performance and many times serves as a precursor to reinjury.[17] Functional progressions enable patients to adapt to the imposed demands of their sports in a controlled environment, helping to restore confidence, thus decreasing apprehension. Each success builds on past success, allowing the patient to feel in control as they return to full activity. Figure 16-1 provides a list of the physical and psychological benefits of functional progressions.

COMPONENTS OF A FUNCTIONAL PROGRESSION

Functional progressions can begin early post-injury. In general, the early focus of phase 1 in the progression is on restoration of joint range of motion, muscular strength, and muscle endurance. The next phase of the progression focuses on incorporating proprioception and agility exercises into the program. These two phases can be two separate phases or, as is often the case, they may overlap. By including proprioception and agility exercises into the program, the injured area is positively stressed to improve the neurovascular, neurosensory, and kinetic functions.[24]

The functional progression should allow for planned sequential activities that challenge the patient while allowing for success. The success will give the patient confidence in his or her ability to complete tasks and motivate the patient to attain the next goal. Neglecting to plan and use a simple progression can lead to reinjury, pain, effusion, tendinitis, or a plateau in performance. To plan appropriately, each decision for a patient should be based on individual results and performance rather than solely on time factors.[24]

Several factors must be addressed to provide a safe and effective return to play with the use of functional progressions. First, what are the physician's expectations for the patient's return to activity? Second, what are the patient's expectations for his or her return to activity? Third, what is the total disability of the patient? And fourth, what are the parameters of physical fitness for this patient? Keeping the total well-being of the injured patient in perspective is a significant factor.[34]

Activity Considerations

Exercise can be viewed from two perspectives. From one perspective, exercise is a single activity involving simple motor skills. From the second perspective, exercise involves the training and conditioning effect of repetitive activity.[15] It is well accepted that preinjury status can be regained only if appropriate activities of sufficient intensity are used to train and condition the patient. To provide the patient with these activities, four principles must be observed. First, the individuality of the patient, the sport, and the injury must be addressed. Second, the activities should be positive, not negative; no increased signs and symptoms should occur. Third, an orderly progressive program should be utilized. And fourth, the program should be varied to avoid monotony.[20] Steps to minimize monotony include these:

1. Vary exercise techniques used
2. Alter the program at regular intervals
3. Maintain fitness base to avoid reinjury with return to play
4. Set achievable goals, reevaluate, and modify regularly
5. Use clinical, home, and on-field programs to vary the activity[15]

Patients are continually exposed to situations that make reinjury likely, so every effort should be made to understand and incorporate the inherent demands of the sport into the rehabilitation program. The athletic trainer can emphasize the importance of sport-specific activities to enhance the patient's return to activity rather than simply concentrating on traditional rehabilitation methods involving only weight machines and analgesics.

The components of fitness are listed in Figure 16-2. There are two distinct components in this model. The physical fitness items used in more traditional rehabilitation programs should be merged with the athletic fitness items of functional progressions to maximize the patient's chance to regain preinjury fitness levels.

The components of a functional progression should aim to incorporate all the factors listed in Figure 16-2 under athletic fitness items.

DESIGNING A FUNCTIONAL PROGRESSION

Athletic trainers should consider all aspects of a patient's situation when designing a functional progression. There is no "cookbook" method that meets the needs of all patients. Athletic trainers should use their creativity when it comes to developing progressions for the patient. As previously mentioned, functional progressions may start early in the rehabilitation process and then culminate in a full return to participation. The following guidelines are suggestions for designing functional progressions that can meet the needs of various injury situations.

As with any rehabilitation program, the patient's current state should be evaluated first. This step may include a review of the patient's medical history, physician notes and/or rehabilitation protocols, a physical exam or injury evaluation, diagnostic testing, and functional testing. Once the status of the patient is established, planning for proper progression may occur. The planning will involve reviewing the expectations of the patient and the physician. What are the rehabilitation goals and parameters? At this point the athletic trainer must determine whether the injury situation, the patient's goals, and the physician's expectations will work together. If not, the athletic trainer must work to bring the three together. The athletic trainer will also need to understand the demands of the sport and the position played by the patient. The patient, coaches,

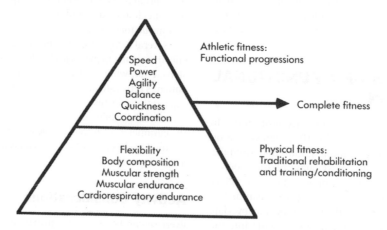

Figure 16-2   Combining components of physical fitness with components of athletic fitness in functional progressions.

and other athletic trainers may serve as valuable resources for successful completion of this step.

A complete analysis of the demands that will be placed on the patient and the injured body part once return to play is achieved must be completed. All of the tasks involved in the activity should be ranked on a continuum from simple to difficult. Simple tasks may involve isolated joints, assisted techniques, or low-impact activities, whereas difficult tasks often group simple tasks together into one activity and involve higher-impact activity-related skills. Primary concerns should include the intention of the activity, what activities should be included, and the order in which the activities should occur.[10] For example, if throwing a baseball is the purpose, the progression can be broken into an ordered sequence like this:

1. Grip the ball
2. Stance
3. Backswing of the upper limb
4. Forward swing of the upper limb
5. Release of the ball
6. Follow-through[10]

It is imperative that the athletic trainer assesses the patient periodically throughout the progression prior to moving to the next level in the progression. Assessment of present functional status of the injury should serve as a guide to a safe progression.[20] The assessment should be based on traditional assessment methods, such as goniometry, along with knowledge of the healing process and the patient's response to activity, functional testing, and subjective evaluation. Aggressive activities that lead to pain, effusion, or patient anxiety can be replaced with less-aggressive activities. Achieving a certain skill level in a functional progression occurs when the skill can be completed at functional speed with high repetitions and no associated increase in pain or effusion or decrease in range of motion. The athletic trainer and the patient should realize, however, that setbacks will occur and are common. Sometimes it takes two steps forward and one step back to achieve the needed level of improvement.

Full Return to Play

Deciding whether a patient is ready to return to play at full participation is a difficult task. The decision requires a complete evaluation of the patient's condition, including objective observations and subjective evaluation. The athletic trainer should feel that the patient is ready both physically and mentally before allowing a return to play.[8] Return to activity should not be attempted too soon, in order to avoid added stress to the injury, which can slow healing and result in a long, painful recovery or reinjury.[7] The following are criteria for allowing a full return to activity:

1. Physician's release
2. Free of pain
3. No swelling
4. Normal ROM
5. Normal strength (in reference to contralateral limb)
6. Appropriate functional testing completed with no adverse reactions

FUNCTIONAL TESTING

Functional testing involves having the patient perform certain tasks appropriate to his or her stage in the rehabilitation process in order to isolate and address specific deficits. As a result the athletic trainer is able to determine the patient's current functional level and set functional goals.[27] According to Harter, functional testing is an indirect measure of muscular strength and power. Function is "quantified" using maximal performance of an activity.[14] Harter describes three purposes of functional testing as follows:

1. Determine risk of injury due to limb asymmetry
2. Provide objective measure of progress during a treatment or rehabilitation program
3. Measure the ability of the individual to tolerate forces[14]

Functional testing can provide the athletic trainer with objective data for review. Traditional rehabilitation programs and improvements in strength and range of motion do not always correlate with functional ability.[18] Functional testing should have a better correlation with functional ability.

When contemplating the use of a functional test or battery of tests, the athletic trainer must evaluate the test(s) chosen. Validity and reliability must be considered. A test should measure what it intends to measure (validity) and should consistently provide similar results (reliability) regardless of the evaluator. Other factors must be considered before releasing a patient to full activity. These include a subjective evaluation of the injury, performance on functional tests, presence or absence of signs and symptoms, other recognized clinical tests (isokinetic testing, special tests, etc.), and the physician's approval. Functional testing should attempt to look at unilateral function and bilateral function in an attempt to determine whether the patient is compensating with the uninjured limb. Other considerations should include the stage of healing for the patient, appropriate rest time, and self-evaluation.[27]

Functional testing might be limited if the athletic trainer does not have normative values or preinjury baseline values for comparison. Obviously, a patient who cannot complete the test(s) is not ready for a return to play. However, what happens to the patient who can complete the test(s) but has no preinjury data available for comparison? The athletic trainer has to make a subjective decision based on the test results. If the normative data or preinjury data are available, the athletic trainer can make an objective decision. If a soccer player is able to complete a sprint test with a mean of 20 seconds but her preinjury time was 16 seconds, then she is only 85-percent functional. Without the preinjury data, the athletic trainer might be unable to determine the patient's functional level. Of course, the athletic trainer can always compare to the mean functional level of the uninjured team members to aid in the decision making. Other methods that will aid in objective decision making include limb symmetry and error scores. Limb symmetry can include strength, ROM, and other traditional measurements; however, in this case, limb symmetry refers to the functional ability of the limbs. For example, a single-leg hop that compares the ipsilateral limb with the contralateral limb using the following formula

$$(\text{ipsilateral limb}/\text{contralateral limb})(100) = \text{limb symmetry percentage}$$

An 85-percent or better goal is the recognized standard for limb symmetry scores.[9,11,27] Error scores typically calculate the number of times an error is made during the testing time frame. Bernier describes an error test with the Stork Stand for the ankle. Over the 20-second time frame, the number of errors is recorded and compared to the score for the contralateral limb.[5]

Functional testing should be an easy task for athletic trainers and should be equally simple for patients to understand. Cost efficiency, time demands, and space demands are important concepts when considering the tests to use.

CLINICAL DECISION MAKING   **Exercise 16–1**

A soccer midfielder is recovering from a grade 2 MCL sprain and has been cleared for sport-specific training. What types of activities could you use for this patient?

EXAMPLES OF FUNCTIONAL PROGRESSIONS AND TESTING

The Upper Extremity

Functional activities that will enhance the healing and performance of the upper extremity might include PNF patterns, swimming motions, closed-kinetic-chain activities,

and using pulley machines or rubber tubing to simulate sport activity.[8] Functional rehabilitation for the shoulder joint needs to focus on proprioception and neuromuscular control. Myers and Lephart report that four "facets of functional rehabilitation must be addressed: awareness of proprioception, dynamic stabilization restoration, preparatory and reactive muscle facilitation, and replication of functional activities."[28] Activities that promote awareness of proprioception are described as activities that promote restoration of interrupted afferent pathways while facilitating compensatory afferent pathways. This improvement in afferent pathways will result in a return of kinesthesia and joint position sense at an early stage in the rehabilitation process. Dynamic stabilization involves training the muscular and tendinous structures to work together as "force-couples." The muscles of the glenohumeral joint along with the scapular stabilizers work together using co-contraction as a way of providing stability to the upper extremity. Preparatory and reactive muscle facilitation involves stressing the upper extremity with unexpected forces. These activities will allow the patient to improve both muscle stiffness and muscle reflex action. Finally, functional activities that mimic actual sport or activity participation should be included.[28]

Numerous activities can promote joint position sense. Isokinetic exercise, proprioception testing devices, goniometry, and electromagnetic motion analysis are all reported by Myers and Lephart[28] as potential means for achieving this goal. Patients can practice reproducing joint positions with visual cues and progress to using no external cues. Activities can be passive, where the patient attempts to recognize certain joint positions when passively moved by the athletic trainer, or active in nature, where the patient attempts to actively reproduce a specific position. The patient can also attempt to reproduce specific motion paths in an attempt to increase the functional component of the activity. All activities need to stress the joint at both the end range of motion and midrange of motion. The end-range motion will stress the capsuloligamentous afferents; the midrange motion will stress the musculotendinous mechanoreceptors. Attention to full range of motion will maximize the functional training for complete joint position sense.[28]

Kinesthesia training can use activities similar to those for joint position sense. To stress kinesthetic awareness, the athletic trainer needs to remove external visual and auditory cues. During motion, the patient is instructed to signal when they first notice joint motion. The athletic trainer notes what degree of error occurs before the patient senses the motion.[28]

Dynamic stability stresses the training of the force couples provided by the scapular stabilizers and the muscles of the glenohumeral joint. Closed-kinetic chain activities are believed to enhance coactivation of these force couples. Common examples of activities would include push-ups and variations on the push-up, slide board activities, weight-shifting activities, and press-ups.[28]

The athletic trainer can improve the patient's muscle preparation and reaction skills by incorporating rhythmic stabilization activities into the program along with the closed-kinetic-chain activities previously discussed. Rhythmic stabilization helps the patient prepare for motion, thus improving muscle stiffness, while also training for muscle reaction. Simple rhythmic stabilization activities are discussed in Chapter 14. Plyometric training is an excellent alternative activity to include for training the muscle for reaction and preparation. Finally, functional activities that stress sport-specific skills should be included in the progression. PNF patterns can be used as an early alternative to sport-specific activity to simulate the sport motions with less stress.[28]

King advocates that upper-extremity rehabilitation should focus on the glenohumeral joint, the scapulothoracic articulation, and the core. An effort should be made to coordinate the rehabilitation process and incorporate activities that stress glenohumeral improvements along with scapular and core stability. The quadruped position allows the patient to work the muscles that connect the trunk and scapula in both a concentric and an eccentric manner.[19] This idea is consistent with Myers and Lephart's plan for improving dynamic stability and muscle readiness. King suggests using activities that use a quadruped position with stable and unstable surfaces along with movement patterns.[19]

Although many sport-specific skills for the upper extremity are completed in the open kinetic chain, closed-kinetic-chain activities are important factors for proper function. Athletic trainers should work to incorporate these activities into the rehabilitation process as a part of the functional progression. Open-kinetic-chain sport-specific activities are important as well. A functional progression for the throwing shoulder should include the following steps. First, the patient must be instructed in and complete a proper warm-up. During the warm-up, the patient should practice the throwing motion at a slow velocity and with low stress. The activity can then progress through increasingly difficult stages as indicated in Table 16-1 and in more detail in Chapter 17. Table 16-2 provides an example of a functional progression for hitting a golf ball, and Table 16-3 provides a program for return to hitting a tennis ball. Any upper-extremity injury can benefit from one of these programs or can be exercised in similar fashion using any sport equipment needed for that sport.[3]

| **CLINICAL DECISION MAKING** | **Exercise 16–2** |

A volleyball player has chronic impingement syndrome due to poor scapular stabilization. What types of functional activities would help this patient?

The shoulder joint serves as a template for upper-extremity rehabilitation and functional progressions. Many of the activities for the shoulder are equally effective for rehabilitation of the elbow, wrist, and hand. Other activities that can be used for upper-extremity rehabilitation may focus more on the elbow or wrist/hand. An excellent example of functional elbow rehabilitation can be found with Uhl, Gould, and Geick's work with a football lineman. The progression started with simulated lineman drills for the upper extremity in the pool. The patient then progressed to proprioception and endurance work using a basketball bounced against a wall and progressed to a medicine ball thrown against a plyoback.[35] There are many ways to functionally test a patient. The most common and often the simplest ways include timed performance. For the upper extremity, a throwing velocity test is often used. This can be accomplished two ways, depending on the athletic trainer's budget and the availability of complex testing tools.

1. Test velocity in a controlled environment, preferably indoors to decrease effects of the weather.
2. Set up a standard pitching distance (60 feet 6 inches).
3. Have the patient use a windup motion.
4. Measure a maximum of five throws—measured in miles per hour with a calibrated Magnum X ban radar gun (CMI Corporation, Owensburg, KY) placed 36 inches high and to the right of the catcher.
5. Compute the mean of the five throws and compare to the pretest value.

Many athletic trainers do not have access to such equipment. A second way to test the upper extremity using velocity would be to use a similar setup but minus the radar gun. In this situation the athletic trainer needs a stopwatch to time the flight of the ball. The athletic trainer begins timing as the patient releases the ball and stops when the catcher receives the ball. Again, a mean of five throws should be computed to help decrease testing error. The first method will be the most accurate, but the second method can be used as an effective testing tool.

Other upper-extremity tests are possible. The closed-kinetic-chain upper-extremity stability test (CKC UE ST) can be used for an objective measure of upper extremity readiness for sport. In the CKC UE ST the athletic trainer

■ **TABLE 16-1** Upper-Extremity Progression for Throwing

1. Functional activity can begin early with assisted PNF techniques
2. Rubber tubing exercises simulating PNF patterns and/or sport motions
3. Swimming
4. Push-ups
5. Sport drills:
   Interval throwing program
   45 ft phase

Step 1:
1. Warm-up throwing
2. 25 throws
3. Rest 10 minutes
4. Warm-up throwing
5. 25 throws

Step 2:
1. Warm-up throwing
2. 25 throws
3. 15 minute rest
4. Warm-up throwing
5. 25 throws
6. Rest 10 minutes
7. Warm-up throwing
8. 25 throws

Repeat steps 1 and 2 for 60, 90, 120, 150, and 180 feet, until full throwing from the mound or respective position is achieved. See Chapter 19 for a more detailed program.

■ **TABLE 16-2** Interval Golf Rehabilitation Program

	Day 1	Day 2	Day 3
Week 1	5 min chipping/putting 5 min rest 5 min chipping	5 min chipping/putting 5 min rest 5 min chipping 5 min rest 5 min chipping	5 min chipping/putting 5 min rest 5 min chipping 5 min rest 5 min chipping
Week 2	10 min chipping 10 min rest 10 min short iron	10 min chipping 10 min rest 10 min short iron 10 min rest 10 min short iron	10 min short iron 10 min rest 10 min short iron 10 min rest 10 min short iron
Week 3	10 min short iron 10 min rest 10 min long iron 10 min rest 10 min long iron	10 min short iron 10 min rest 10 min long iron 10 min rest 10 min long iron	10 min short iron 10 min rest 10 min long iron 10 min rest 10 min long iron
Week 4	Repeat week 3, day 2	Play 9 holes	Play 18 holes

■ **TABLE   16-3** Interval Tennis Program

	Day 1	Day 2	Day 3
Week 1			
	12 FH	15 FH	15 FH
	8 BH	8 BH	10 BH
	10 min rest	10 min rest	10 min rest
	13 FH	15 FH	15 FH
	7 BH	7 BH	10 BH
Week 2			
	25 FH	30 FH	30 FH
	15 BH	20 BH	25 BH
	10 min rest	10 min rest	10 min rest
	25 FH	30 FH	30 FH
	15 BH	20 BH	15 BH
			10 Overheads (OH)
Week 3			
	30 FH	30 FH	30 FH
	25 BH	25 BH	30 BH
	10 OH	15 OH	15 OH
	10 min rest	10 min rest	10 min rest
	30 FH	30 FH	30 FH
	25 BH	25 BH	15 OH
	10 OH	15 OH	10 min rest
			30 FH
			30 BH
			15 OH
Week 4			
	30 FH	30 FH	30 FH
	30 BH	30 BH	30 BH
	10 OH	10 OH	10 OH
	10 min rest	10 min rest	10 min rest
	Play 3 games	Play set	Play 1.5 sets
	10 FH	10 FH	10 FH
	10 BH	10 BH	10 BH
	5 OH	5 OH	3 OH

FH = Forehand
BH = Backhand
OH = Overhead

sets up a course using two strips of athletic tape placed on the ground parallel to each other 36 inches apart. The patient assumes a push-up position with hands on the appropriate tape strips. The patient then has 15 seconds to alternately reach across and touch the opposite tape strip. The patient should complete 3 trials with a maximal effort. The mean value is calculated as the patient's score. A standard 1:3 work : rest ratio is used allowing the patient to rest for 45 seconds in between each trial. Assessment of the score can be the total number of touches, the number of touches divided by body weight to normalize the data, or determining a power score by multiplying the mean score by 68 percent of the patient's body weight (weight of arms, head, and trunk) then dividing by 15 seconds. Goldbeck and Davies found that the CKC UE ST has a test–retest reliability of 0.922 and a coefficient of stability of 0.859, indicating that the test is a reliable evaluation tool.[12]

Uhl et al. used sport-specific testing to determine the readiness for return of the football lineman. The patient completed up–down drills, drive-blocking on a dummy (5 × 4 yards), blocking drill with a butt roll to both the right and the left, and finally a snap-pass protection drill against an opponent. Both athletic trainer and patient satisfaction and no report of pain indicated successful completion.[35] This is a great example of how the athletic training staff used sport-specific tasks to determine the functional level of the patient.

To functionally test the upper extremity, the key concept is to focus on the sport demand for the patient. Careful attention should focus on the skill involved with the sport. Does the patient perform a primarily open-kinetic-chain skill, or is the skill performed in a closed kinetic chain? A gymnast might need more closed-kinetic-chain testing than a tennis player. Similarly, the athletic trainer will not test a volleyball player using a pitching test. The athletic trainer will have to consult with the coach and determine what the patient needs to do, and from this devise a test battery. For the volleyball player, a serving test would obviously be better than the pitching test.

CLINICAL DECISION MAKING   **Exercise 16–3**

A gymnast has a recurrent anterior dislocation of the glenohumeral joint. She has excellent muscular strength in both the glenohumeral muscles and the scapular muscles. She has had no problem regaining full range of motion. She is extremely worried that the shoulder will dislocate again. Because strength and range of motion are normal for this patient, what type of rehabilitation activities should the patient concentrate on to help improve her dynamic stability?

The Lower Extremity

The lower extremity follows the same basic pattern, with different exercises. The activities used should provide functional stress to the injured limb. An example of a functional progression for the lower extremity is found in Table 16-4. The lower extremity can be tested in many ways; sprint times, agility run times, jumping or hopping heights/distances, co-contraction tests, carioca runs, and shuttle runs. The following are brief introductions to a variety of these tests.

Sprint Tests. The sprint test is exactly what the name implies:

1. A set distance is measured.
2. The patient then runs the distance with a time-per-run recorded.
3. Three to five sprints should be completed and the mean computed.
4. Pretest and posttest means are compared.

Agility Tests. Agility runs involve the same premise. The run is timed, and a mean is taken for five runs. The difference is the course. Rather than concentrating on straight-ahead motion, the agility run incorporates changes of direction, acceleration/deceleration, and quick starts and stops. For example, a simple figure eight can be set up with cones and the patient is instructed to travel the cones as fast as possible while being timed for performance. Gross et al. described a figure-eight course that was 5 by 10 meters. Each subject in their study was instructed to complete three trips around the figure eight while being timed. Two trials were conducted, and the best time was recorded.[13] Anderson and Foreman point out that no standard in the literature dictates testing procedures for the figure eight.[2] A standard procedure should be developed

A 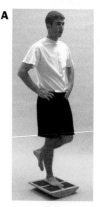   B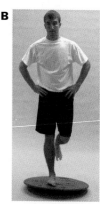

Figure 16-3 Board exercises. **A,** Wobble board exercise. **B,** BAPS board exercise.

■ TABLE   16-4 Lower-Extremity Functional Progression

1. Functional activity can begin early in the rehabilitation process with:
   - Assisted proprioceptive neuromuscular facilitation (PNF) techniques
   - Cycling
   - Non-weightbearing (NWB) BAPS board or tilt board exercises
   - Partial-weightbearing (PWB) BAPS board or tilt board exercises
   - Full-weightbearing (FWB) BAPS board or tilt board exercise (Figure 16-3)
   - Walking
        Normal
        Heel
        Toe
        Sidestep/shuffle slides (Figure 16-4)
2. Lunges:
   - 90° Pivot (Figure 16-5)
   - 180° Pivot (Figure 16-6)
3. Step-ups:
   - Forward step-up, 50–75% max speed (Figure 16-7A)
   - Lateral step-up, 50–75% max speed (Figure 16-7B)
4. Jogging:
   - Straight-aways on track; jog in turns (goal = 2miles)
   - Complete oval of track (goal =2–4 miles)
   - 100 yd–"S" course 75–100% max speed with gradual increase in number of curves (Figure 16-8)
   - 100 yd–"8" course 75–100% max speed with gradual decrease in size of "8" to fit 5–10 yd (Figure 16-9)
   - 100 yd–"Z" course 75–100% max speed with gradual increase in number of "Zs"(Figure 16-10)
   - Sidestep/shuffle slides
5. Lunges:
   - 90° Pivot with weight or increased speed
   - 180° Pivot with weight or increased speed
6. Sprints:
   - 10 yd × 10
   - 20 yd × 10
   - 40 yd × 10
   - Acceleration/deceleration; 50 yd × 10 (Figure 16-11)
   - "W" sprints × 10 (Figure 16-12)
7. Box runs: (Figure 16-13)
   - 5 yd clockwise/counterclockwise × 10
8. Carioca: (Figure 16-14)
   - 30 yd × 5 right lead-off; 30 yd × 5 left lead-off
9. Jumping: (Figure 16-15)
   - Rope
   - Lines
   - Boxes, balls, etc.
10. Hopping: (Figure 16-18)
    - Two feet
    - One foot
    - Alternate
11. Cutting, jumping, hopping on command
12. Sport drills used for preseason or in-season practice

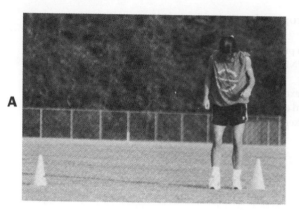
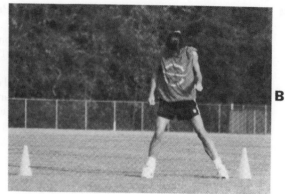

Figure 16-4   Shuffle slides. **A,** Starting position. **B,** Finish position.

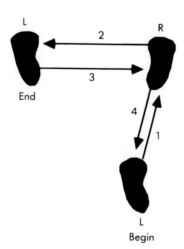

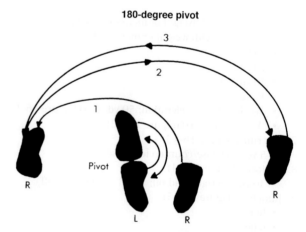

Figure 16-5   90-degree pivot. The patient pushes off with the left foot, landing on the right foot directly in front, then steps immediately laterally landing on the left foot, then back laterally in the opposite direction landing on the right foot, then backward onto the left foot.

Figure 16-6   180-degree pivot. The patient pushes off the right foot, pivoting on the left, thus rotating the body 180 degrees, landing on the right foot. Then pushing off the right foot, the body pivots on the left foot 180 degrees in the other direction, landing on the right foot.

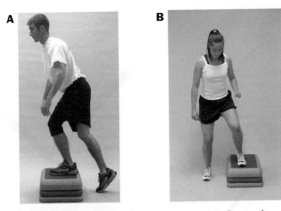

Figure 16-7   Step-ups. The patient steps **A,** forward, or **B,** laterally onto a step.

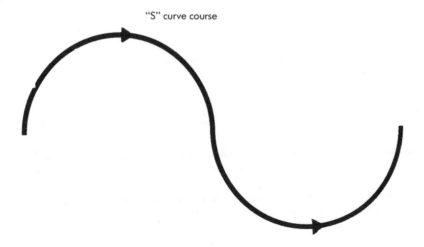

Figure 16-8   S Curve. The patient runs a set distance in a curving S pattern rather than straight ahead.

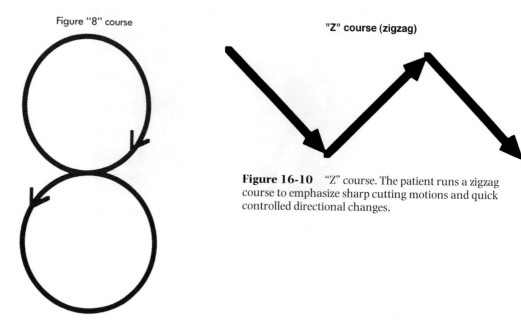

Figure 16-9 Figure 8. The patient walks, jogs, or runs a figure 8 pattern around cones or markers.

Figure 16-10 "Z" course. The patient runs a zigzag course to emphasize sharp cutting motions and quick controlled directional changes.

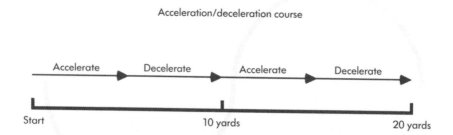

Figure 16-11 Acceleration/deceleration. The patient accelerates to a maximum, then decelerates almost to a stop, then repeats this within a relatively short distance.

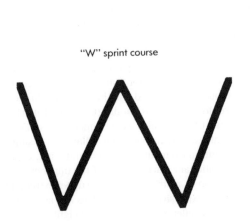

Figure 16-12   "W" sprints. The patient sprints forward to the first marker, then backpedals to the second, then sprints forward to the third, and so on.

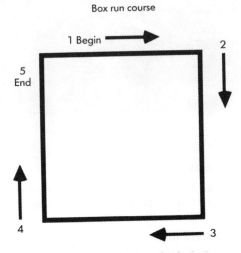

Figure 16-13   Box runs. Running both clockwise and counterclockwise, the patient runs around four markers set in a box shape, concentrating on abrupt directional changes at each corner.

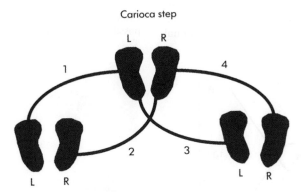

Figure 16-14   Carioca. The patient sidesteps onto the right foot, then steps across with the left foot in front of the right, then steps back onto the right foot, then the left foot steps across in back of the right, then back onto the right, and so on.

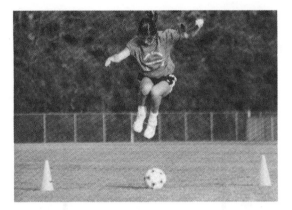

Figure 16-15 Timed exercise. The patient jumps side to side over a ball or other obstacle in a timed exercise.

by each athletic trainer or each institution to ensure the validity and reliability of the test.

Box runs are also beneficial as agility runs, because they emphasize pivoting and change of direction. The patient is instructed to travel around four cones arranged in a box formation. The time to complete the box is recorded. Again, variations are prominent, with single laps versus multiple laps and the use of multiple movements (run, carioca, backpedal, etc.). The Barrow zigzag run is a variation of the box run using five cones. The four cones of the box are set as usual, and the fifth cone is set in the center of the box. The box course is 16 feet by 10 feet. The patient travels around the cones as shown in Figure 16-16.

Nussbaum reports that the use of sprinting, cutting maneuvers, figure-eight runs, and backpedaling drills are all excellent means for assessing the functional performance of the lower extremity.[30] It is beneficial to use agility runs because the level of difficulty can be changed. Early in the rehabilitation process, large figure eights that are more circular in shape can be used to provide functional data with low stress to the injury. As the injury heals, the figure eight can be tighter to provide greater stress to the injured body part.

Vertical Jump. The vertical jump test can also be used to evaluate the lower extremity.[4] In this test, the patient has chalked fingertips and jumps to touch a piece of paper (of a different color than the chalk). Three to five jumps should be attempted and the mean height recorded (measured from fingertips standing to the chalk mark).[2,6,33] Variations in the test also exist. Anderson and Foreman mention alterations that include "bilateral vs. single leg jump, countermovement vs. static squat start, approach steps vs. stationary start, and use of the upper extremities for propulsion vs. restricted use of the upper extremities."[2] Many, more expensive, testing devices are available that measure time differentials, force, and height.

Co-contraction Semicircular Test. The co-contraction semicircular test involves securing the patient in a 48-inch resistance strap (TheraBand) that is attached to the wall 60 inches above the floor (see Figure 16-17). The strap is then stretched to twice its recoil length and the patient completes five 180-degree semicircles, with a radius of 96 inches, around a tape line. The patient is instructed to use a forward-facing lateral shuffle step. If the patient starts on the left, she or he will travel around the semicircle until reaching the right boundary. This semicircle counts as one repetition. The patient must complete five repetitions in the shortest amount of time possible. Three trials can be used, and the mean time is

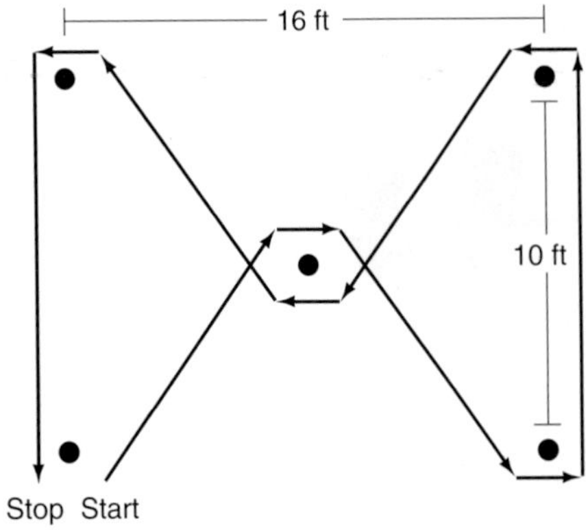

Figure 16-16 Barrow Zigzag Run test. The patient essentially runs a figure 8 with sharp turns at the corners.

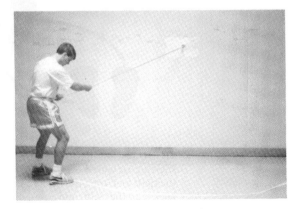

Figure 16-17 Co-contraction test. The patient moves in a sidestep or shuffle fashion around the periphery of a semicircle, using surgical tubing for resistance.

calculated. This test is designed to provide a dynamic pivot shift for the ACL-insufficient knee.[5,21,22,23,26]

Hopping Tests.   Hopping tests are also found in the literature (Figure 16-18). Booher et al. and Worrell et al. report that hopping tests might not be sensitive enough to evaluate the functional abilities of patients.[6,37] However, hopping tests are noted in the literature and are used for clinical determination of function. Noyes et al. used a variety of hop tests to determine lower-extremity limb symmetry.[2,26,29] The more common hopping tests are the single-leg hop for distance, the timed hop test, the triple hop for distance, and the crossover hop for distance. The single-leg hop for distance requires the patient to attempt to hop as far as possible while landing on the same limb.[4] The timed hopping test measures the amount time it takes the patient to hop a distance of 6 meters. The triple hop for distance measures the distance traveled by the patient with three consecutive hops. And finally the crossover hop for distance measures the distance traveled using three consecutive hops while crossing over a strip 15 centimeters wide.[2,5,6,9,18,26,29,37]

Carioca Test.   Carioca runs can be timed to measure improvement in function (see Figure 16-14). The carioca run involves a lateral grapevine or crossover step over a total distance of 80 feet. First, choose which direction to face and maintain the stance. The patient will then carioca 40 feet, change direction without turning around, and return to the starting position. The time to complete the 80-foot course is recorded. Three trials should be used and the mean time calculated.[21,22,23,26]

Shuttle Runs.   Shuttle runs can involve many different drills. The most common requires the patient to complete four 20-foot spints, for a total of 80 feet, incorporating three direction changes. It is common to take three trials, and the mean should be calculated.[21,22,23,26] Another common shuttle run is the line drill, sometimes called "suicide sprints" or "death warmed over." The course is set with markers at various distances from the starting line. The patient is instructed to sprint and touch the first marker and then return to the starting position. The patient then continues the course, touching each marker and returning to the starting position. A total time is recorded.[2] This test is very flexible and can be used on basketball, volleyball, or tennis courts, as well as football, soccer, or other playing fields.

Balance Tests.   Balance is an important component of any motor skill activity. Following injury, many patients exhibit deficits in proprioception, which translate into a loss of balance. A simple single-leg balance test is a valid test. The patient is instructed to stand on one leg, and timing begins. Timing stops when the patient alters his or her position in order to maintain balance. This test can be modified to include eyes open or closed to eliminate visual

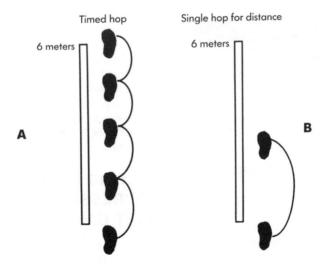

Figure 16-18   Hop tests. **A,** In the timed hop test, time required to cover a 6-meter distance is measured in seconds. **B,** The single hop for distance test measures the distance covered in a single hop. Both tests use a percentage of the injured leg compared to the uninjured leg.

cues. Also, changes in surface can be made that require greater balance. Instead of testing on a floor surface, the athletic trainer might choose to use a foam surface or a minitrampoline.[2,5,16] The athletic trainer can also incorporate sport skills into a balance test (see Chapter 7).

Subjective Evaluation. Subjective evaluations of performance have been correlated with functional performance testing to determine predictive capabilities. Wilk et al. found strong correlations between subjective scores and knee extension peak torques, knee extension acceleration, and functional testing; however, no significant relationship was noted with hamstring function.[36] This is in contrast to Shelbourne's research, which showed a poor relationship between subjective evaluation, functional tests, and knee strength. Shelbourne concluded that knee strength was a good measure of ability.[31] Subjective questionnaires or numeric scales might or might not be beneficial in the functional assessment of patients, based on the correlations. A low subjective score might indicate that the patient is apprehensive, which should serve as a warning sign of psychological unreadiness to return to play. The athletic trainer should determine whether subjective evaluation is useful with respect to the given patient.

Obviously, budget considerations and availability of equipment will determine the types of tests the athletic trainer can use, but simple timed sprints can indicate improved performance just as well as the more complicated tests that involve expensive equipment.[1,21,22,23]

CLINICAL DECISION MAKING **Exercise 16–4**

What type of functional testing could you use for a football receiver who has sustained a second-degree acromioclavicular sprain? What criteria for a return to play would you use?

CAROLINA FUNCTIONAL PERFORMANCE INDEX (CFPI)

The CFPI has been developed to help the athletic trainer evaluate lower-extremity functional performance. The CFPI evaluates the patient's existing functional performance capability. McGee and Futtrell evaluated 200 collegiate athletes and nonathletes using a battery of tests that included the co-contraction test, carioca test, shuttle run test, and one-legged timed hopping test. Table 16-5 shows the mean and standard deviation for each of these tests for males and for females. From this series of tests, a normative CFPI index was determined for males and females

■ **TABLE 16-5** CFPI Mean Index and Performance Test Means

	Males Means/standard deviation	Females Means/standard deviation
CFPI	31.551/2.867	36.402/3.489
Carioca	7.812/1.188	8.899/1.124
Co-contraction test	11.188/1.391	13.218/1.736
One-legged hop test	4.953/0.53	5.746/0.63
Shuttle run	7.596/0.654	8.539/0.69

that can be used in accurately assessing functional performance based on the results of only two of the tests—the carioca test and the co-contraction test.[26]

Using stepwise regression techniques, the following prediction equations were established:

$$\text{Males: } 1.09(x_1) + 1.415(x_2) + 8.305 = \text{CFPI}$$
$$\text{Females: } 1.26(x_1) + 1.303(x_2) + 8.158 = \text{CFPI}$$
$$\text{(Where } x_1 = \text{co-contraction score in seconds,}$$
$$\text{and } x_2 = \text{carioca score in seconds)}$$

The athletic trainer can test any individual using these two tests (co-contraction and carioca) and determine their individual CFPI. The CFPI value for that individual can be compared to the mean normative CFPI indices of 31.551 for males and 36.402 for females. If baseline preinjury testing was done, then the preinjury CFPI can be compared to the postinjury CFPI to determine how the patient is progressing in their rehabilitation program. The CFPI provides a reliable objective criteria for functional performance testing.

APPLYING FUNCTIONAL PROGRESSIONS TO A SPECIFIC SPORT CASE

The following is an example of how a functional progression may be applied to a specific sport-related injury:

Subject: 20-year-old female soccer player

History: Sustained anterior cruciate ligament (ACL) rupture of left knee while performing a cutting motion in practice. ACL reconstruction using an intra-articular patellar tendon graft was performed.

Rehabilitation for the first 2 months was conducted both at home and in a clinical setting. Emphasis of program concentrated on increasing range of motion (ROM) and decreasing pain and swelling, with some minor considerations to improving strength.

At 2 months postsurgery, the rehabilitation protocol consisted of emphasizing general physical fitness, strengthening via traditional rehabilitation means and strength testing, as well as improving ROM. At approximately 3 months postsurgery a functional progression was initiated. The progression included the following activities an average of three times per week:

- Walking
- Proprioceptive neuromuscular facilitation techniques—using lower extremity D1, D2 patterns
- Jogging on track with walking of curves
- Jogging full track
- Running on track with jogging of curves
- Running full track

This progression occupied the majority of the next 2 months, coupled with traditional rehabilitation techniques to increase strength and maintain ROM. At 4 months the progression intensified to a 5-day-a-week program including the following:

- Running for fitness—2 to 3 miles three times per week
- Lunges—90 degree, pivot, 180 degree
- Sprints—"W," triangle, 6 second, 20 yd, 40 yd, 120 yd
- Acceleration/deceleration runs (see Figure 16-11)
- Shuffle slides progressing to shuffle run
- Carioca
- Ball work—Turn/stop the pass; turn/mark opponent; mark/steal/shoot the ball; two-touch and shoot; one-touch and shoot; volley and shoot; passing; pass/knock/move; coerver drills; light drill work at practice; one-on-one; scrimmage (begin with short period, progress to full game); full active participation.

CLINICAL DECISION MAKING   **Exercise 16–5**

A patient had surgery 2 weeks ago for an ACL rupture. Acute inflammation is controlled, and he is clear to begin the next phase of rehabilitation. The physician prefers an accelerated protocol for the patient. What types of functional activities could you suggest for the patient?

CLINICAL DECISION MAKING   **Exercise 16–6**

A male patient has a CFPI of 42.00 following an ACL reconstruction. At what percentage of the norm is the patient? What decision would you make about his return to play? What type of activities may help this patient improve his score?

CONCLUSION

Once the patient can safely and effectively perform all specific tasks leading up to the motor skill, they can return to activity. For example, a patient might progress from cycling, to walking, to jogging, to running, before returning to sprinting activities and competition in a 4×400 relay.

The athletic trainer must note that these are only examples. No one program will benefit every patient and every condition. Athletic trainers should use these activities, along with others they develop, to help maximize the patient's recovery. By providing patients with every option available in rehabilitation, the athletic trainer can return the patient to participation at preinjury status. The preinjury status achieved with the functional progression not only can return the patient to competition, but also can ensure a safer, more effective return to play.

Summary

1. Complete rehabilitation should strive to improve neuromuscular coordination and agility, strength, endurance, and flexibility.
2. The role of the functional progressions is to improve and complete the traditional rehabilitation process by providing sport-specific exercise.
3. The functional progression is a sequence of activities that simulate sport activity. The progression will begin easy and progress to full sport participation.

4. Each sport activity can be divided into smaller components, allowing the patient to progress from easy to difficult.
5. Functional progressions are highly effective exercise therapy techniques that should be incorporated in the long-term rehabilitation stage.
6. Functional progressions allow for improvements in strength, endurance, mobility/flexibility, relaxation,

coordination/agility/skill, and assessment of functional stability.

7. Functional progression can benefit the patient psychologically and socially by decreasing the patient's feelings of anxiety, deprivation, and apprehension.

8. Components of a functional progression that should be addressed include development, choice of activity, implementation, and termination.

9. Many functional tests exist and should be administered when deciding whether to return a patient to competition.

References

1. Anderson, M. 1991. The relationships among isometric, isotonic, and isokinetic concentric and eccentric quadriceps and hamstring force and three components of athletic performance. *Journal of Orthopaedic and Sports Physical Therapy* 14:3.

2. Anderson, M. A., and T. L. Foreman. 1996. Return to competition: Functional rehabilitation. In *Athletic injuries and rehabilitation,* edited by J. E. Zachazewski, D. J. Magee, and W. S. Quillen. Philadelphia: W. B. Saunders.

3. Andrews, J. R. 1990. *Preventive and rehabilitative exercises for the shoulder and elbow.* Birmingham: American Sports Medicine Institute.

4. Augustsson, J., R. Thomeé, and R. Lindén. 2006. Single-leg hop testing following fatiguing exercise: Reliability and biomechanical analysis. *Scandinavian Journal of Medicine & Science in Sports* 16(2):111, 2006.

5. Bernier, J. N., K. Sieracki, and S. Levy. 2000. Functional rehabilitation of the ankle. *Athletic Therapy Today* 5(2): 38–44.

6. Booher, L. D., K. M. Hench, T. W. Worrell, and J. Stikeleather. 1993. Reliability of three single-leg hop tests. *Journal of Sport Rehabilitation* 2:165–70.

7. Davies, G, and J. Matheson. 2007. Functional testing as the basis for ankle rehabilitation progression. In *The unstable ankle,* Nyska, M., ed. Champaign, IL: Human Kinetics.

8. Drouin, J., and B. Riemann. 2004. Lower extremity functional performance testing, Part 2. *Athletic Therapy Today* 9(3):49.

9. Fitzgerald, G. K., S. M. Lephart, J. H. Hwang, R. Maj, and S. Wainner. 2001. Hop tests as predictors of dynamic knee stability. *Journal of Orthopaedic and Sports Physical Therapy* 31(10): 588–97.

10. Galley, J. 1991. *Human movement: An introductory text for physiotherapists.* London: UK Limited.

11. Goh, S., and J. Boyle. 1997. Self evaluation and functional testing two to four years post ACL reconstruction. *Australian Physiotherapy* 43(4): 255–62.

12. Goldbeck, T. G., and G. J. Davies. 2000. Test-retest reliability of the closed kinetic chain upper extremity stability test: A clinical field test. *Journal of Sport Rehabilitation* 9(1): 35–45.

13. Gross, M. T., J. R. Everts, and S. E. Roberson. 1994. Effect of DonJoy ankle ligament protector and Aircast Sport-Stirrup orthoses on functional performance. *Journal of Orthopaedic and Sports Physical Therapy* 19(3): 150–56.

14. Harter, R. 1996. Clinical rationale for closed kinetic chain activities in functional testing and rehabilitation of ankle pathologies. *Journal of Sport Rehabilitation* 5(1): 13–24.

15. Jokl, E. 1964. *The scope of exercise in rehabilitation.* Lexington, MA: Charles C. Thomas.

16. Kaikkonen, A., P. Kannus, and M. Jarvinen. 1994. A performance test protocol and scoring scale for the evaluation of ankle injuries. *American Journal of Sports Medicine* 22(4):462–69.

17. Kegerreis, S. 1983. The construction and implementation of functional progressions as a component of athletic rehabilitation. *Journal of Orthopaedic and Sports Physical Therapy* 63(4):14–19.

18. Keskula, D. R., J. B. Duncan, and V. L. Davis. 1996. Functional outcome measures for knee dysfunction assessment. *Journal of Athletic Training* 31(2): 105–10.

19. King, M. A. 2000. Functional stability for the upper quarter. *Athletic Therapy Today* 15(2):16–21.

20. Kisner, C., and L. Colby. 1985. *Therapeutic exercise foundations and techniques.* Philadelphia: F. A. Davis.

21. Lephart, S. 1992. Relationship between selected physical characteristics and functional capacity in the anterior cruciate ligament-insufficient patient. *Journal of Orthopaedic and Sports Physical Therapy* 16(4): 164–81.

22. Lephart, S. M., and T. Henry. 1995. Functional rehabilitation for the upper and lower extremity. *Orthopedic Clinics of North America* 26(3): 579–92.

23. Lephart, S., D. Perrin, and K. Minger, et al. 1991. Functional performance tests for the anterior cruciate ligament-insufficient patient. *Journal of Athletic Training* 26:44–50.

24. MacLean, C., and J. Taunton. 2001. Functional rehabilitation for the PCL-deficient knee. *Athletic Therapy Today* 6(6): 32–8.

25. Melliam, M. 1988. *Office management of sports injuries and athletic problems.* Philadelphia: Handy & Belfus.

26. McGee, M. R., and M. D. Futtrell. 1993. Functional testing of patients and non-patients using the Carolina Functional Performance Index. Unpublished master's thesis, University of North Carolina, Chapel Hill.

27. Mullin, M. J. 2000. Functional rehabilitation of the knee. *Athletic Therapy Today* 5(2): 28–35.

28. Myers, J. B., and S. M. Lephart. 2000. The role of the sensorimotor system in the athletic shoulder. *Journal of Athletic Training* 35(3): 35–63.

29. Noyes, F., S. Barber, and R. Mangine. 1991. Abnormal limb symmetry determined by function hop tests after anterior cruciate ligament rupture. *American Journal of Sports Medicine* 19(5): 513–18.

30. Nussbaum, E. D., T. M. Hosea, S. D. Sieler, B. R. Incremona, and D. E. Kessler. 2001. Prospective evaluation of syndesmotic ankle sprains without diastasis. *American Journal of Sports Medicine* 29(1): 31–35.

31. Shellbourne, D. 1987. Functional ability in athletes with anterior cruciate deficiency, *American Journal of Sports Medicine.* 15:628.

32. Tegner, Y., J. Lysholm, and M. Lysholm, et al. 1986. A performance test to monitor rehabilitation and evaluate anterior cruciate ligament injuries. *American Journal of Sports Medicine* 14:156–59.

33. Tibone, J. M., M. S. Antich, and G. S. Fanton, et al. 1986. Functional analysis of anterior cruciate ligament instability. *American Journal of Sports Medicine* 13:34–39.

34. Torg, J., J. Vegso, and E. Torg. 1987. *Rehabilitation of athletic injuries: An atlas of therapeutic exercise.* Chicago: Year Book.

35. Uhl, T. L., M. Gould, and J. H. Geick. 2000. Rehabilitation after posterolateral dislocation of the elbow in a collegiate football player: A case report. *Journal of Athletic Training* 35(1):108–110.

36. Wilk, K. E., W. T. Romaniello, S. M. Soscia, and C. A. Arrigo. 1994. The relationship between subjective knee scores, isokinetic testing, and functional testing in the ACL-reconstructed knee. *Journal of Orthopaedic and Sports Physical Therapy* 20(2): 60–71.

37. Worrell, T. W., L. D. Booher, and K. M. Hench. 1994. Closed kinetic chain assessment following inversion ankle sprain. *Journal of Sport Rehabilitation* 3(3): 197–203.

SOLUTIONS TO CLINICAL DECISION MAKING EXERCISES

16-1 Agility runs would be the most beneficial for this patient to allow for improvement in speed and direction change.

16-2 Closed-kinetic-chain (CKC) activities that stress coactivation of the core, scapular stabilizers, and rotator cuff muscles would help the patient correct the strength deficits with the scapular stabilizers. Once improvements are noted with the CKC activities, sport-specific open-kinetic-chain activities would be indicated.

16-3 The patient is probably deficient in her proprioception and kinesthetic awareness. Upper-extremity closed-kinetic-chain activities, rhythmic stabilization, and PNF diagonal patterns may benefit this patient.

16-4 Sport-specific and position-specific testing would be indicated. Open- and closed-kinetic-chain testing would be necessary in order to evaluate all aspects of the patient's position. Criteria for return: no pain, full ROM, bilaterally equal strength, successful completion of functional test, self-evaluation, and physician's release.

16-5 Although it is early in the rehabilitation process, functional activities could begin. Closed-kinetic-chain activities such as mini-squats could be initiated safely. Gait training and functional activities in the pool could also benefit the patient in this stage.

16-6 The patient is at approximately 75 percent of function. Based on this score, the patient would continue his rehabilitation program and not return to full participation. Agility training, along with continuation of his strengthening program, will help the patient reach his goals.